Th... ...
Training Manual

D1587016

Aung Myat • Sarah Clarke
Nick Curzen • Stephan Windecker
Paul A. Gurbel

Editors

The Interventional Cardiology Training Manual

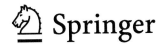

Editors
Aung Myat
Brighton and Sussex Medical School
and the Sussex Cardiac Centre
Brighton and Sussex University
Hospitals NHS Trust
Brighton
UK

Nick Curzen
Wessex Cardiothoracic Centre
University Hospital Southampton NHS
Foundation Trust
Southampton
UK

Paul A. Gurbel
Inova Center for Thrombosis Research
and Drug Development
Inova Heart and Vascular Institute
Falls Church, VA
USA

Sarah Clarke
Royal Papworth Hospital NHS
Foundation Trust
Papworth Everard
Cambridge
UK

Stephan Windecker
Department of Cardiology
Bern University Hospital
Bern
Switzerland

ISBN 978-3-319-71633-6   ISBN 978-3-319-71635-0   (eBook)
https://doi.org/10.1007/978-3-319-71635-0

Library of Congress Control Number: 2018945487

This Springer imprint is published by Springer Nature, under the registered company Springer International Publishing AG
The registered company address is: Gewerbestrasse 11, 6330 Cham, Switzerland

Foreword

It is with great pleasure that I introduce *The Interventional Cardiology Training Manual*, co-edited by Drs. Myat, Clarke, Curzen, Windecker, and Gurbel.

Tailored to the needs of the cardiology fellow and junior consultants, this is a welcome addition to the training literature. It combines a comprehensive coverage of the curriculum with a very practical and concise presentation of the individual topics.

Ever since the first coronary angioplasty with a balloon catheter in 1977, interventional cardiology has developed into a subspeciality that is defined by increasingly sophisticated technology, improved pharmacological options, and evidence-driven treatment strategies. Today's interventional cardiologist needs to have a good understanding of the underlying pathophysiology in acute and chronic conditions, manage the medical strategies for patients, master the different device technologies in the cath lab, and translate the ever growing trial evidence and guideline recommendations into their clinical practice. A compendium summarizing the most relevant information for training and accreditation has been missing.

The present *Interventional Cardiology Training Manual* comprises 33 chapters, all written by leading experts in the field. A unique touch is that we get to know about the professional background of the authors and the institutions they represent at the beginning of each chapter. The topics are brought to life by explaining the relevance for clinical practice, adding evidence and bullet point lists for easy learning. All supported by excellent graphical illustrations and clinical examples. This manual will serve equally as a learning platform and a reference tool for quick consultation. I am sure it will become a standard work, to be found on every interventional cardiology fellows' shelf or computer.

Andreas Baumbach
Queen Mary University of London
and the Barts Heart Centre
London, UK

Yale School of Medicine
New Haven, CT, USA

European Association of
Percutaneous Cardiovascular Interventions (EAPCI)
Sophia Antipolis, France

Preface

The evolution of interventional cardiology has been rapid and unrelenting. We owe a huge debt of gratitude to the founding fathers of our subspecialty: Werner Forssmann, André Cournand, Dickinson Richards, Mason Sones, Charles Dotter, Melvin Judkins, Andreas Gruentzig, Richard Schatz, Julio Palmaz, Jacques Puel, and Ulrich Sigwart, to name but a few. These pioneers, along with the many thousands of practising physicians and clinician scientists past and present from across the world, have allowed interventional cardiology to grow into the dynamic and evidence-rich field of medicine that it is today.

Interventional cardiology incorporates a requirement for both technical and decision-making skillsets. It demands consistently high personal and professional standards to provide optimal care and offers frequent opportunities to provide life-saving and life-modifying therapy. We have tried to encapsulate the very essence of this ethos into *The Interventional Cardiology Training Manual*.

Our aim has been to create a readily accessible educational tool for all fellows undertaking subspecialty training in interventional cardiology. The text will also serve as a refresher to early-career consultant (attendings in) interventional cardiologists. The key objective is to equip the reader with an expert-led guideline-mandated resource to be used as an aide-mémoire focused primarily on preprocedural planning of, periprocedural decision-making during, and the salient technical aspects of coronary intervention so that it is performed safely, appropriately, effectively, and with reference to the evidence base. The intention was not to produce a comprehensive reference text. The intention has been to produce a book that an interventional cardiologist can use to solidify their therapeutic thought process in the emergency room, the coronary care unit, or the catheterization laboratory so that the best possible care can be given to patients.

Each chapter covers a specific aspect of interventional cardiology, written by authors from leading cardiac centers across Europe, the United States, and Asia. Uniquely, each chapter has been written in a center-specific manner, affording the reader an opportunity to learn how each individual center performs a specific procedure, which algorithms and guidelines they follow, and what evidence they utilize to optimize patient outcome. To that end, we thank wholeheartedly all our contributors for their enthusiasm, wisdom, diligence, and attention to detail.

We very much hope you enjoy reading this book. We very much hope reading this book will help to improve and consolidate your clinical practice.

Brighton, UK   Aung Myat

Contents

Coronary Heart Disease

Diana Gorog

About Us The National Heart and Lung Institute of Imperial College, based in South Kensington, London, is recognized for its excellence in cardiovascular research both nationally and internationally, in both basic science and translational research.

Professor Diana Gorog is a Consultant Cardiologist with an interest in coronary intervention and research interest in coronary thrombosis. She has been Clinical Director of Cardiology for the last 8 years and currently Clinical Director of Research at East and North Hertfordshire NHS Trust, Professor of Cardiovascular Medicine at the University of Hertfordshire and Visiting Professor at Imperial College. Based just outside north London, the Trust comprises 4 hospitals, with a large catchment area of some 700,000 patients and 24/7 PPCI is provided at the 720-bedded Lister Hospital.

Introduction

- Globally, cardiovascular disease (CVD) remains the leading cause of mortality and morbidity, despite many preventative and therapeutic advances. CVD accounted for some 18 million deaths worldwide in 2015, and this number is expected to grow to >23.6 million by 2030.

D. Gorog
National Heart and Lung Institute, Imperial College London, London, UK
e-mail: d.gorog@imperial.ac.uk

- The predominant cause of cardiovascular death is ischemic heart disease, for both men and women. Advancing age is the strongest risk factor.
- Global CVD rates rose by 12.5% between 2005 and 2015, with deaths attributable to ischemic heart disease (IHD) increasing by 16.6% to 8.9 million deaths. Over the same time period, age-standardized mortality rates for IHD fell by 12.8%, reflecting improved survival of patients.
- Recent data from the Office for National Statistics in 2015 show that in England and Wales, more people now die from dementia than heart disease, with dementia being the leading cause of death in women, although IHD continues to be the leading cause of death in men.
- There is, therefore, an important ongoing need to further reduce mortality and morbidity from IHD, and an appreciation of the pathophysiology of IHD is essential to enable this.

Pathophysiology

Atherosclerosis

Risk Factors for Development of Coronary Artery Disease

- Both genetic and environmental factors contribute to the development of coronary atherosclerosis. Genome-wide association studies have revealed more than 55 loci related to

© Springer International Publishing AG, part of Springer Nature 2018
A. Myat et al. (eds.), *The Interventional Cardiology Training Manual*,
https://doi.org/10.1007/978-3-319-71635-0_1

coronary atherosclerosis, and it is mainly individuals with combinations of multiple variants who are at greatest risk.

- Several of the genes implicated encode proteins that relate to cardiovascular risk factors, such as lipids, lipoproteins, systemic inflammation, and hypertension. Some of the more recently identified loci encode genes with well-documented roles in vessel wall biology.
- ABO blood type impacts the risk of myocardial infarction. Individuals with blood type A or B are at greater risk of MI compared to individuals with blood type O.
- The demonstration of a genetic link between a mutation in the LDL-C receptor and development of premature coronary atherosclerosis culminated in the development of statins.
- The enzyme proprotein convertase subtilisin kexin 9 (PCSK9), located on chromosome 1p32.3, increases the degradation of LDL-C receptors. Mutations that increase the function of PCSK9 are associated with high levels of LDL-C and increase the incidence of coronary atherosclerosis. In contrast, mutations that result in loss of function of PCSK9 are associated with low levels of LDL-C and decrease the incidence of coronary atherosclerosis. These observations resulted in the development of monoclonal antibodies that inhibit the function of the PCSK9 enzyme and dramatically decrease LDL-C.
- Smoking impacts all phases of atherosclerosis from endothelial dysfunction to acute thrombotic cardiovascular events, particularly myocardial infarction. Both active and passive cigarette smoke, as well as air pollution, increases inflammation and thrombosis risk.
- Hypertension and diabetes mellitus (DM) are major risk factors contributing to the development of coronary atherosclerosis.
- Renal impairment, in particular end-stage renal disease, confers an excess cardiovascular risk, with a significant increase in the burden of coronary atherosclerosis and thrombosis risk, over and above that predicted by traditional risk factor models.

- A sedentary lifestyle may predispose to obesity and DM, which are associated with hyperlipidemia and an inflammatory process. Thus, moderate exercise and a balanced diet, particularly a Mediterranean diet, are recommended and have been shown to be associated with reduced cardiovascular risk.

Coronary Atherosclerosis

- Subclinical coronary atherosclerosis in the form of early intimal hyperplasia, usually near arterial branch points, may be apparent in infancy. Lesions can progress to pathological intimal thickening, which may be seen initially as "fatty streaks," namely subendothelial lipid deposits, even in adolescents.
- Atherosclerosis is considered to be the result of a complex, chronic inflammatory process. Coronary atheroma is classified in order of increasing severity in descriptive terminology as adaptive intimal thickening, intimal xanthoma (fatty streak), pathological intimal thickening, and fibroatheroma.
- Immune cell infiltration is most apparent in early atherosclerotic lesions, while uptake of monocytes and differentiation into macrophages, together with smooth muscle cell (SMC) infiltration and proliferation, accelerate atheroma progression (Fig. 1.1).
- Activation of inflammation can precipitate acute coronary syndromes (ACS) due to plaque rupture. The invasion of lipid pools by macrophages leads to foam cell formation and conversion of plaques into early and late fibroatheromas with large necrotic cores. Necrotic cores, arising from macrophage infiltration of lipid pools, further develop and expand, sometimes rapidly through intraplaque hemorrhage (IPH) from leaky vasa vasorum, principally from intimal microvessels originating within the adventitia, accompanied by free cholesterol derived from erythrocyte membranes and secondary macrophage response (Fig. 1.2).
- A fibrous cap separates the necrotic core from the vessel lumen and its structure and composition determine the potential for coronary thrombosis. Infiltrating macrophages and

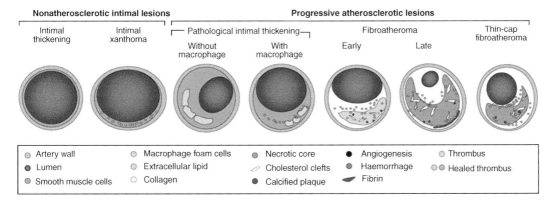

Fig. 1.1 Human coronary lesion morphologies categorized as nonatherosclerotic intimal lesions, progressive atherosclerotic lesions, lesions with acute thrombi, and complications of hemorrhage and/or thrombus with healing and stabilization. Yahagi, K. *et al.* (2015) Pathophysiology of native coronary, vein graft, and in-stent atherosclerosis. *Nat. Rev. Cardiol.* https://doi.org/10.1038/nrcardio.2015.164

release of active proteases can result in thinning of the fibrous cap, which may lead to plaque rupture, the most frequent cause of acute coronary thrombosis. Not all thin caps eventually go on to rupture; mechanical stress is probably critical to this process.

- When an atherosclerotic plaque initially develops, the artery undergoes remodeling in which the luminal area of the artery may not be diminished. The degree of luminal stenosis, therefore, may not be directly related to the atherosclerotic plaque burden. Coronary calcification, often used as a screening test for coronary artery disease, is directly related to total plaque burden, but not to percent stenosis.

- Many high-grade stenosis may have little calcium content, particularly in younger individuals. Significantly more calcification is seen in stable than in unstable plaque, and with advancing age.

Progression of Coronary Atherosclerosis

- Morphological features of plaque progression include infiltration with macrophage foam cells, IPH, and reduction in fibrous cap thickness. However, plaque progression is not linear and advances through episodic rupture and healing.

- Atherosclerotic plaques can be stable or unstable. Unstable atherosclerotic plaques are characterized by a large lipid core, abundant macrophages, small amount of collagen, and a thin fibrous cap. In contrast, stable atherosclerotic plaques contain a small lipid pool, large amounts of collagen, few macrophages, and a thick fibrous cap.

- In a dynamic process, stable plaques at any time may become unstable, while an unstable plaque may be stabilized. Unstable plaques are prone to rupture, and this leads to initiation of intraluminal thrombosis, manifesting in ACS (Fig. 1.3).

- Subtotal or short-lived vessel occlusion may result in unstable angina or a non-ST-elevation MI (NSTEMI), while sudden complete occlusion without a supportive collateral circulation results in a ST-elevation MI (STEMI).

- While plaque rupture may manifest in ACS, more often it will be clinically silent, giving rise to repetitive cycles of nonocclusive thrombosis and healing. Organization of such nonocclusive thrombi with granulation tissue, with SMC infiltration and deposition of proteoglycans and collagen, converts this into a fibrous plaque, with repetitive cycles leading to progressive luminal narrowing.

Thin-Cap Fibroatheroma

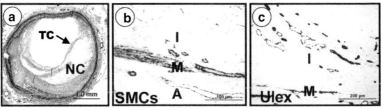

Plaque Rupture

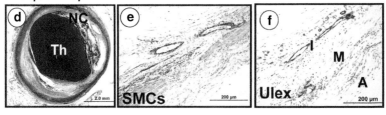

Stable Plaque

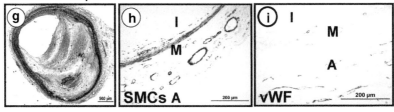

Fig. 1.2 Vasa vasorum in thin-cap fibroatheroma and plaque rupture compared with that in stable plaque in human.

Unstable atherosclerotic plaques thin-cap fibroatheroma (**a–c**) and rupture (**d–f**) are associated with marked neoangiogenesis. The microvessels close to the adventitial and medial layers (**b** and **e**) tend to be in contact with surrounding smooth muscle cells compared with intimal vessels closer to the lumen, which are characterized by a single lining of luminal endothelium (**c** and **f**). The main pathologic feature of the vulnerable plaque is an intact thin fibrous cap heavily infiltrated by macrophages (**a**). In plaque rupture (**d**), the fibrous cap is disrupted with a superimposed luminal thrombus. The adventitial vessels in unstable plaques often show perivascular smooth mus-

cle cells (**b** and **e**). In contrast, the vasa vasorum close to the necrotic core is abnormal, consisting mostly of endothelial cells overlying a disrupted "leaky" basement membrane. (**g–i**) Stable plaques contain mostly collagen, proteoglycans, and calcium, and show fewer vasa vasorum in the intima, media, and adventitia. Endothelial markers: *Ulex europaeus* (Ulex) and anti-von Willebrand factor (vWF) antibody immunohistochemical staining; smooth muscle cell (SMC) marker: -actin. (**a**, **d**, and **g**) Movat pentachrome staining. *A* adventitia, *I* intima, *M* media, *NC* necrotic core, *TC* thin cap, *Th* thrombus. Jain RK, et al. Antiangiogenic therapy for normalization of atherosclerotic plaque vasculature: a potential strategy for plaque stabilization. Nat Clin Pract Cardiovasc Med. 2007;4:491–502. https://doi.org/10.1038/ncpcardio0979

Coronary Thrombosis

Vulnerable Plaque/Thin-Cap Fibroatheroma

- ACS is generally precipitated by a sudden increase in atherosclerotic lesion size with accumulation of erythrocytes and fibrin within the necrotic core, predominantly due to IPH, luminal thrombus, or plaque fissure.

- Postmortem studies revealed a frequent association between acute MI and rupture or erosion of a coronary atherosclerotic plaque, most often a thin-cap fibroatheroma (TCFA). Thus, the TCFA, the lesion most frequently associated with plaque rupture and coronary thrombosis, has been termed the "vulnerable plaque."
- Such plaques consist of a thin fibrous cap (<65 µm thick) overlying a large necrotic core.

Fig. 1.3 Angiogram of left anterior descending coronary artery in a patient presenting with an acute coronary syndrome and anterior ST-segment depression, showing ulcerated plaque with rupture of the plaque shoulder in the proximal left anterior descending artery

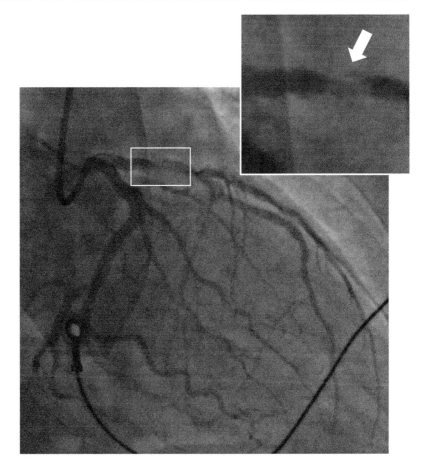

The fibrous cap is composed predominantly of type 1 collagen with variable contents of macrophages and T-lymphocytes, and notable for the paucity or absence of SMCs.

- TCFA are more common in patients with high cholesterol, smokers, women aged >50 years, and patients with inflammation as evidenced by elevated hs-CRP.

Plaque rupture is the main mechanism responsible for coronary thrombosis. Rupture, usually affecting TCFA, occurs at the weakest point of the fibrous cap involving the shoulder regions of the plaque (Fig. 1.4). The intraluminal thrombus at the site of rupture, which may or may not be occlusive, is predominantly composed of platelets ("white thrombus'") (Fig. 1.5). The majority of plaque ruptures occur in vessels with >75% luminal narrowing.

Plaque erosion is responsible for some 25–30% of cases of coronary thrombosis, and occur usually on an underlying fibroatheroma, or less frequently on a background of underlying pathological intimal thickening. The intimal surface becomes denuded and luminal thrombi come into direct contact with a denuded intimal surface consisting of SMCs and a proteoglycan matrix. In the majority of erosions, the medial wall is intact and less inflamed than in ruptures. Additionally, in contrast to ruptures, which generally show positive remodeling, erosions involve negative remodeling. Such lesions are seen most frequently in women aged <50 years.

Calcified nodule is the least frequent cause of coronary thrombosis (<5%). It is a noted complication of highly calcified coronary arteries and more common in older patients. Calcified nodules typically occur in eccentric lesions, in areas

Fig. 1.4 Acute plaque rupture in the left anterior descending coronary artery. Low magnification showing acute occlusive thrombus overlying atheroma with rupture on shoulder (arrow, main figure, and inset) and communication of the thrombus with atheroma core. Hematoxylin and eosin, original magnification 20×. Tavora F et al. Frequency of acute plaque ruptures and thin cap atheromas at sites of maximal stenosis. Arq Bras Cardiol. 2010;94:143–9

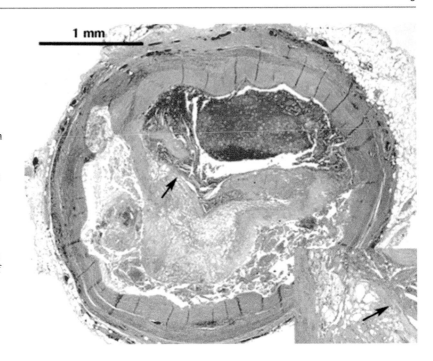

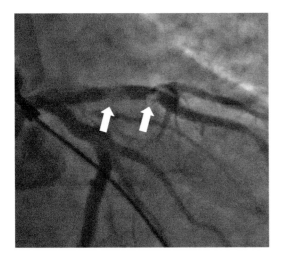

Fig. 1.5 Coronary angiogram showing filling defects representing thrombus in the left anterior descending coronary artery

of high torsion stress, where the protrusion causes disruption of the overlying luminal endothelium, which is likely to trigger platelet adherence.

Effect of Flow Dynamics
- At the pathologically high shear rates that exist in stenosed coronary arteries, thrombin and high shear stress play the most important roles in activation and aggregation of platelets leading to occlusive thrombus formation.
- The shear rates in severely stenosed arteries are determined by stenosis length, height, and plaque roughness. If shear rates exceed $10,000$ s^{-1}, changes occur in the glycoprotein Ibα (GPIbα) receptors on the platelet surface and plasma von Willebrand factor (vWF) undergoes conformational transformation allowing creation of vWF-GPIbα adhesive bonds. This leads to the formation of aggregates downstream, in the post-stenotic segment where there is low shear (shear deceleration zone) and turbulent flow.
- Above shear rates of $>10,000$ s^{-1}, microvesicles are formed on the platelet surface, which are responsible for abundant thrombin generation.

Current View of ACS Causation
- Many vulnerable plaque ruptures are silent, without clinical sequelae, and frequently transition to *thick*-cap fibroatheromas or fibrotic plaques, leading to progressive luminal narrowing through repeated rupture and healing.

- In ACS patients, recurrent major adverse cardiovascular events occurring during follow-up are equally attributable to recurrence at the site of culprit lesions and to non-culprit lesions. Plaque ruptures are frequently observed in non-culprit lesions, indicating not only widespread vulnerability/inflammation, but also a "vulnerable patient" rather than a vulnerable plaque. It is probably for this reason that identifying individual lesions prone to rupture has not translated into ACS reduction.
- Most non-culprit lesions associated with recurrent events are angiographically mild at baseline (mean [±SD] diameter stenosis, 32.3 ± 20.6%), characterized by a large plaque burden of ≥70% or a minimal luminal area of ≤4.0 mm^2 or classified as TCFA on intravascular ultrasonography.
- ACS typically occur when an atherosclerotic plaque, usually TCFA, undergoes rupture or erosion, but for this to cause an ACS it needs to occur in association with a prothrombotic milieu.
- Coronary thrombosis is the result of an imbalance between prothrombotic drivers, namely enhanced platelet reactivity and activation of coagulation, and the natural defense system to prevent lasting thrombosis, namely endogenous thrombolysis.
- While many studies have shown markers of enhanced platelet reactivity and coagulation to predict thrombotic events, altering antiplatelet medication for an individual based on the results of platelet function tests has thus far not translated into a clinical benefit.
- Both prevention and treatment of ACS are aimed at stabilizing vulnerable plaques, as well as promoting a less prothrombotic milieu.

Terminology and Definitions

Ischemia/Reperfusion Injury

- It is well recognized that the deleterious effects of hypoxia (ischemia) during STEMI are attenuated by prompt restoration of blood flow (reperfusion), leading to reduction in myocardial infarct size. However, reperfusion could paradoxically induce and exacerbate tissue injury and necrosis.
- Reperfusion injury, first described in 1960 in a canine model, is the term used to describe detrimental effects associated with reestablishing the blood supply over and above that sustained during the preceding ischemic period.
- The endothelial layer of distal microvasculature is particularly susceptible to the deleterious consequences of ischemia and reperfusion (ischemia/reperfusion, IR). The mechanisms underlying this phenomenon are complex and multifactorial, including calcium overload, generation of reactive oxygen species, endoplasmic reticulum and mitochondrial dysfunction, activation of protein kinases, inflammation, endothelial dysfunction, and appearance of a prothrombogenic phenotype.
- The presence of coexisting cardiovascular risk factors and events occurring during fetal life (fetal programming) markedly enhances the susceptibility to IR. The response to IR is bimodal, depending on the length of IR. While prolonged episodes of ischemia, conventionally taken as >20 min, cause persistent deleterious downstream effects despite reperfusion, brief periods of IR may be cardioprotective (see below).
- The RISK pathway refers to a group of protein kinases that, when activated, attenuate reperfusion injury. In animal models, activation of the RISK pathway by pharmacological or mechanical interventions such as ischemic preconditioning or postconditioning can reduce infarct size by up to 50%.
- While pharmacological modulation of IR through activation of the RISK pathway by administration of atrial natriuretic peptide, protein kinase C-delta inhibitor, glucagon-like peptide 1, darbepoetin alfa and atorvastatin, or pharmacological inhibition of mitochondrial permeability transition pore opening with cyclosporine has shown initially encouraging results in small studies, these manoeuvres have not translated into tangible benefits in patients with STEMI.

Preconditioning, Postconditioning, and Remote Conditioning

- Brief exposure of the heart to short bouts of ischemia and reperfusion (IR) prior to prolonged reductions in coronary blood flow (index ischemia) exerts powerful infarct-sparing effects (ischemic preconditioning, IP). This cardioprotective mechanism has been demonstrated in other organs as well.
- Preconditioning exerts a biphasic effect, with an acute cardioprotective effect becoming apparent within minutes and lasting up to 2 h after the brief preconditioning ischemia and a second window of *delayed preconditioning* that becomes apparent 24–72 h after the initial insult.
- While the exact mechanisms are likely multifaceted and not fully understood, adenosine release appears to play a role in the initiation of acute preconditioning which is protein synthesis independent, while nitric oxide appears to play a major role in delayed preconditioning, effects that require protein synthesis.
- IP diminishes the effects of prolonged ischemia in animal models by reducing microvascular endothelial dysfunction, capillary plugging, leukocyte adhesion and emigration, and protein leakage.
- Cardioprotection can also be achieved by inflicting brief repetitive episodes of IR to an organ or a tissue remote from the heart; this is known as remote ischemic conditioning. Repetitive cycles of IR can be applied before the major (index) ischemic event (preconditioning), during the event (perconditioning), or shortly after reperfusion (postconditioning).
- Studies on perconditioning have applied remote ischemia in patients with STEMI either pre- or during PPCI, with mixed results, and further studies are ongoing.

Warm-Up Angina

- Warm-up angina refers to the attenuation or abolition of angina on a second period of exercise, when separated from the first period of exercise by a brief rest. It is evidenced by reduced symptoms of chest pain, reduced ST-segment depression, and reduced ischemic ventricular arrhythmias on the second compared to the first exercise. It has been likened to ischemic preconditioning; however, warm-up ischemia does not seem to be mediated by adenosine or by cardiac adenosine triphosphate-sensitive potassium channels.

Myocardial Stunning

- The ventricular contractile dysfunction that temporarily persists following a period of ischemia and after restoration of normal, or near-normal coronary flow, despite the absence of irreversible damage, is termed myocardial stunning.
- Such contractile dysfunction is relatively short-lived and followed by full functional recovery. It has been proposed that myocardial stunning appears to result from reperfusion and may be an adaptive response that affords protection against the effects of prolonged IR.
- Interventionalists and intensivists should be aware of this phenomenon, since it explains why assessment of myocardial function may not be reliable for some time after PPCI for STEMI, and why supportive measures with inotropic or mechanical support may need to be continued for some time after successful reperfusion before maximal ventricular functional recovery can be expected.

Myocardial Viability/Hibernation

- Myocardial hibernation describes an adaptive phenomenon observed in patients with coronary artery disease, where repeated episodes of ischemia lead to cumulative stunning, culminating in significant downgrading of myocardial contractility to better withstand reductions in oxygen and nutrient delivery, and prevent cardiomyocyte death.
- This adaptation involves reduction in myocyte contractility as well as a metabolic switch to use of carbohydrates as an energy source, to reduce energy demand.
- At a cellular level, characteristic changes include the appearance of polymorphic mitochondria, increase in lysosomes and reduction in myofibrils, as well as observation of

apoptosis and autophagy, regulating destruction of nonviable cells to enhance survival of hibernating ones.

- Hibernating myocardium demonstrates significant improvement in response to revascularization manoeuvres with PCI or CABG, with restoration of normal metabolism and contractile function. Assessment of myocardial viability, using echocardiographic, CMR, or nuclear perfusion modalities, is used to guide revascularization decision in patients with LV impairment.
- In patients with a similar extent of ventricular dysfunction, significant differences may exist in the relative extent of hibernation or scarring, which will impact the response to revascularization.

Special Circumstances

Saphenous Vein Graft Disease

- While native coronary atherosclerosis develops over decades, saphenous vein grafts (SVG) demonstrate accelerated atherosclerosis within months to years of surgery.
- Cardiovascular risk factors, including hypertension and cholesterol, predispose to SVG disease. Other predictors of SVG failure include graft diameter, target vessel characteristics, and grafting onto the right coronary artery.
- Vein graft attrition rate is 2% per annum from the 1st to the 7th postoperative years, increasing to 5% per annum from the 7th to the 12th years; at 10 years, only 38–45% of SVGs remain patent.
- Typical SVG atherosclerosis is concentric and diffuse, low in calcium content, and heavily lipid laden, with a thin fibrous cap (Fig. 1.6).
- The extensive lipid core is attributable to macrophage foam cell infiltration, resulting in apoptosis and formation of necrotic cores within 2–5 years after surgery. Subsequently IPH contributes to expansion of the necrotic core. Plaque rupture is observed between 5 and 10 years after surgery.
- SVG plaque is highly "friable" and prone to distal embolization. This can manifest in no reflow phenomenon and periprocedural MI in up to 15% of cases during PCI, mandating distal embolic protection where technically feasible.
- Accelerated atherosclerosis also affects SVG stents.
- High-dose statin therapy significantly reduces SVG atherosclerosis, but whilst antiplatelet therapy has been shown to reduce thrombosis-induced graft failure, it has not improved long-term patency.

Saphenous vein graft

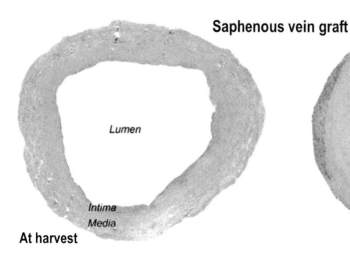

At harvest

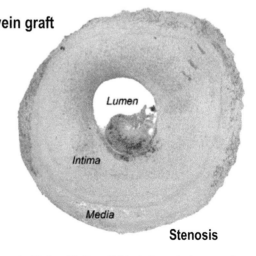

Stenosis

Fig. 1.6 Histology of saphenous vein graft cross section, showing concentric diffuse atherosclerosis with prominent neointima and remodeled media, causing significant stenosis. Garbey M, Berceli SA. A dynamical system that describes vein graft adaptation and failure. J Theor Biol. 2013;336:209–20

In-Stent Restenosis

- In-stent restenosis (ISR) is seen in 20–40% of bare metal stent (BMS) implantation. Early randomized controlled trials using drug-eluting stents (DES) showed ISR <6%, and subsequent real-world registries including longer and more complex lesions and patient subsets have shown this to occur in up to 20% of cases.
- ISR is the result of accelerated atherosclerosis, similar to that occurring in SVG. Whilst with BMS neointimal hyperplasia with smooth muscle cell hypertrophy characterizes ISR, with DES neoatherosclerosis is also very frequently seen.
- In-stent atherosclerosis or "neoatherosclerosis" is typified by macrophage foam cell infiltration. Such lipid-laden foam cells undergo apoptosis, resulting in the creation of necrotic cores. Necrotic cores of neoatherosclerosis do not communicate with the underlying native plaque.
- ISR is associated with neointimal calcification, with both BMS and DES, although it is more common with DES.
- Risk factors for ISR include procedural variables (including stent under-expansion, stent fracture, drug resistance, and hypersensitivity reactions), lesion characteristics (long lesions, bifurcations, small vessels, calcified or ostial lesions), as well as patient factors (age, diabetes, hyperlipidemia). The predominant pattern of angiographic restenosis with DES is focal (≤10 mm in length) in 70–80% of cases, whereas with BMS only <45% were focal and the rest diffuse.
- Whilst ISR occurs on average 5 months post-implant with BMS, it occurs later with DES up to 12 months.

Current Concepts and Future Directions

Despite significant advances in the understanding of complex atherosclerotic plaque morphology and alterations in plaque morphology associated with acute coronary thrombotic events, the recognition that plaque rupture occurs frequently without clinical sequelae has led to the realization that it is not an individual vulnerable plaque, but the co-occurrence of adverse alterations in plaque morphology in concert with a prothrombotic milieu that results in acute coronary thrombosis.

Thus future studies must look to both identify and favorably modulate not only local but also more widespread coronary and systemic atherosclerosis, as well as identify patients who are prothrombotic, with appropriate tailoring of antithrombotic and antiplatelet medications to those at risk.

References

Epidemiology

GBD 2015 Mortality and Causes of Death Collaborators. Global, regional, and national life expectancy, all-cause mortality, and cause-specific mortality for 249 causes of death, 1980–2015: a systematic analysis for the Global Burden of Disease Study 2015. Lancet. 2016;388:1459–544.

Atherosclerosis

Ambrose JA, Barua RS. The pathophysiology of cigarette smoking and cardiovascular disease: an update. J Am Coll Cardiol. 2004;43(10):1731–7.

Arbab-Zadeh A, Fuster V. The myth of "the vulnerable plaque": transitioning from a focus on individual lesions to atherosclerotic disease burden for coronary artery disease risk assessment. J Am Coll Cardiol. 2015;65(8):846–55.

Boudoulas KD, Triposciadis F, Geleris P, Boudoulas H. Coronary atherosclerosis: pathophysiologic basis for diagnosis and management. Prog Cardiovasc Dis. 2016;58(6):676–92.

GW Stone for PROSPECT Investigators. A prospective natural-history study of coronary atherosclerosis. N Engl J Med. 2011;364:226–35.

Hansson GK. Inflammation, atherosclerosis, and coronary artery disease. N Engl J Med. 2005;352:1685–95.

Michel J-B, Martin-Ventura JL, et al. Pathology of human plaque vulnerability: Mechanisms and consequences of intraplaque haemorrhages. Atherosclerosis. 2014;234:311e319.

Nikpay M, et al. A comprehensive 1000 Genomes–based genome-wide association meta-analysis of coronary artery disease. Nat Genet. 2015;47(10): 1121–30.

Yahagi K, et al. Pathophysiology of native coronary, vein graft, and in-stent atherosclerosis. Nat Rev Cardiol. 2016;13:79–98.

Ischemia Reperfusion, Preconditioning, Postconditioning

Carden DL, Granger DN. Pathophysiology of ischaemia-reperfusion injury. J Pathol. 2000;190(3): 255–66.

Kalogeris T, Baines CP, Krenz M, Korthuis RJ. Cell biology of ischemia/reperfusion injury. Int Rev Cell Mol Biol. 2012;298:229–317.

Vinten-Johansen J, Shi W. Perconditioning and postconditioning: current knowledge, knowledge gaps, barriers to adoption, and future directions. J Cardiovasc Pharmacol Ther. 2011;16(3-4):260–6.

Yellon DM, Hausenloy DJ. Myocardial reperfusion injury. N Engl J Med. 2007;357:1121–35.

Stunning, Hibernation

Bolli R, Marbán E. Molecular and cellular mechanisms of myocardial stunning. Physiol Rev. 1999;79:609–34.

Camici PG, Prasad SK, Rimoldi OE. Stunning, hibernation, and assessment of myocardial viability. Circulation. 2008;117:103–14.

Depre C, Vatner SF. Cardioprotection in stunned and hibernating myocardium. Heart Fail Rev. 2007;12(3–4):307–17.

Slezak J, Tribulova N, Okruhlicova L, Dhingra R, Bajaj A, Freed D, Singal P. Hibernating myocardium: pathophysiology, diagnosis, and treatment. Can J Physiol Pharmacol. 2009;87(4):252–65.

SVG Disease

Yahagi K, Kolodgi FD, Otsuka F, Finn AV, Davis HR, Joner M, Virmani R. Pathophysiology of native coronary, vein graft, and in-stent atherosclerosis. Nat Rev Cardiol. 2016;13(2):79–98.

ISR

Alfonso F, Byrne RA, Rivero F, Kastrati A. Current treatment of in-stent restenosis. J Am Coll Cardiol. 2014;63:2659–73.

Dangas GD, Claessen BE, Caixeta A, Sanidas EA, Mintz GS, Mehran R. In-stent restenosis in the drug-eluting stent era. J Am Coll Cardiol. 2010;56:1897–907.

Clinical Assessment of Coronary Heart Disease

Evangelos Giannitsis and Hugo A. Katus

About Us The cardiology department of the Heidelberg University Hospital is a tertiary referral center covering a population of 500,000 inhabitants with almost 12,000 hospitalized cases per year and more than annual 68,000 outpatient visits.

The Chest Pain Unit, part of the internal medicine Emergency Department, is visited by almost 9000 patients/year, with 1300 undergoing an evaluation for suspected acute coronary syndrome (ACS).

The department provides interventional and noninvasive services. The interventional spectrum includes more than 9000 coronary angiographies, >4000 PCI, >350 TAVI, 100 MitraClip, and >400 peripheral interventions of arteries and veins.

Noninvasive imaging includes cardiac MRI including stress MRI and contrast MR angiography, cardiac CT, and full spectrum of 2/3-D echocardiography and transoesophageal echocardiography.

Other services provided include implantations of pacemaker, ICD, CRT-P/D, complex EP studies, RF, and cryoablation procedures.

There are several active research groups with a focus on molecular genetics, epigenetics, and omics-based technologies, with a particular interest on genetic cardiomyopathies. Research activities are also on diagnosis and management of ACS, and cardiac imaging with MRI/CT.

Introduction

- The number of patients presenting with chest pain to emergency departments is increasing exponentially whereas numbers of patients with unstable angina or confirmed myocardial infarction (MI) remain stable or are even declining over the past two decades [1]. The rush to emergency departments of patients who present with chest pain leads to crowding and dissatisfaction of both medical staff and patients [2, 3].
- In order to provide an accurate diagnosis ensuring timely and appropriate treatment or discharge to avoid unnecessary hospitalization, clinical assessment to establish a working diagnosis is paramount.
- However, in patients presenting with suspected MI to the emergency department, the diagnostic performance of chest pain characteristics for MI is limited [4–7]. Atypical complaints are more often observed in the elderly, in women, and in patients with diabetes, chronic renal disease, or dementia. Atypical presentations include epigastric pain, indigestion-like symptoms, and isolated dyspnea.

E. Giannitsis (✉) · H. A. Katus
Department of Internal Medicine III, Cardiology,
University Hospital Heidelberg, Heidelberg, Germany
e-mail: evangelos.giannitsis@med.uni-heidelberg.de;
hugo.katus@med.uni-heidelberg.de

© Springer International Publishing AG, part of Springer Nature 2018
A. Myat et al. (eds.), *The Interventional Cardiology Training Manual*,
https://doi.org/10.1007/978-3-319-71635-0_2

- For this reason the 2015 European Society of Cardiology (ESC) guidelines [8] recommend that in patients with suspected non ST-elevation-acute coronary syndromes (NSTE-ACS), diagnosis of ACS should be based on a combination of clinical history, symptoms, physical findings, ECG, and biomarkers, preferentially cardiac troponin I or T.
- Although diagnostic algorithms are based on biomarker measurements, ECG, and clinical assessment, guidelines can vary widely across continents and even within Europe.

Chest Pain Assessment

- The dilemma starts with the limited ability of chest pain characteristics alone to predict the presence of obstructive coronary artery disease (CAD). Therefore, classical prediction rules or more refined rules, such as the modified Diamond Forrest rule [9] recommended by the ESC [8], include age, gender, and other risk factors for assessment of pretest probability.
- The classification of angina into typical angina, atypical angina, or non-anginal chest pain is old and standardized to an insensitive reference for MI (World Health Organization—WHO—definition). At that time, chest pain duration of 20 min or more at rest was found to be associated with NSTEMI [10].
- Typical angina was diagnosed in the presence of substernal chest pain, occurring during exercise and relieved following rest. If only two criteria are applied the chest pain was labeled as atypical, and in the presence of one or none of the three criteria symptoms were classified as non-anginal chest pain.
- Historically, unstable angina was further subclassified using the Braunwald classification scheme that had been prospectively validated for short-term outcomes [11]. In

the troponin era, atypical features do not exclude ACS [12].
- The relief of chest pain with nitroglycerin is not predictive of ACS [13]. Conversely the relief of chest pain by antacids, anticholinergic drugs, or lidocaine-containing agents does not predict the absence of ACS [14].
- Using cardiac troponins in the context of a Universal MI definition instead of the WHO definition of MI changed the spectrum of ACS with increasing numbers of NSTEMI while numbers of unstable angina declined [15].
- Using more sensitive and cardio-specific troponins improved detection of patients with atypical presentations.
- Women, elderly, younger patients, and patients with diabetes mellitus have been reported to present with atypical presentations. Chest pain is decreasing with increasing age and dyspnea becomes more prevalent in the elderly [16]. Dyspnea is associated with acute heart failure and indicates a higher mortality rate [17].
- More recent data suggest that at least five chest pain characteristics are very similar between men and women [18]. Rubini-Gimenez et al. [18] evaluated the predictive ability of 34 chest pain characteristics to predict the likelihood for an adjudicated diagnosis of MI in 2475 consecutive patients with suspected ACS. Interestingly, chest pain characteristics were not very helpful to predict final MI. In particular, there were only five chest pain characteristics that significantly decreased the likelihood of the diagnosis of AMI, with similar likelihood in women and men. These characteristics included stabbing pain; aggravation of the pain by breathing, movement, or palpation; pain located in the left side of the chest and infra-mammillary pain; pain without radiation; and pain duration of less than 2 min.
- An updated definition of angina and classification of chest pain established from findings of numerous trials is shown in Table 2.1.

Table 2.1 Definition of angina and classification of chest pain [4]

Finding	Definition
Typical angina	Substernal discomfort Precipitated by exertion Improved with rest or nitroglycerin (or both) in less than 10 min (many patients also report radiation to shoulders, jaw, or inner arm)
Atypical angina	Substernal discomfort with atypical features Nitroglycerin not always effective Inconsistent precipitating factors Relieved after 15–20 min of rest
Non-anginal chest pain	Pain unrelated to activity Unrelieved by nitroglycerin Otherwise not suggestive of angina

Differential Diagnoses of Chest Pain

- Assessment and interpretation of clinical symptoms require clinical expertise as some differential diagnoses of chest pain may be life threatening.
- The "Big Five" include:
  - Acute myocardial infarction (AMI)
  - Aortic dissection
  - Pulmonary embolism
  - Tension pneumothorax
  - Boerhaave syndrome (mediastinitis following esophageal rupture)
- A multitude of benign differential diagnoses have to be considered as well. These differential diagnoses include:
  - Cardiac
  - Vascular
  - Gastrointestinal
  - Orthopedic causes [8]
- In some cases the clinical picture may be straightforward but sometimes symptoms and clinical signs are equivocal or absent.

Therefore, cardiac imaging and testing for noncardiac acute conditions have been recommended for the workup and differential diagnoses of chest pain patients (see Table 2.2).

- These imaging modalities include:
  - Cardiac computed tomography (CT)
  - Echocardiography
  - X-ray
  - Cardiac magnetic resonance (CMR)
  - Various stress imaging tests
  - Laboratory testing [8, 19, 20]
- In order to differentiate an acute from a chronic troponin elevation, serial troponin measurements are mandatory, with few exceptions, to disclose a rise and/or fall of troponin.
- In addition, the diagnosis of MI according to the 3rd version of the Universal MI definition [21] requires the presence of myocardial ischemia as the reason of myocardial necrosis. Therefore, interpretation of troponin values cannot be made in isolations, and elevated troponin in the absence of a significant obstruction should not be labeled false positive but should be interpreted in the appropriate clinical context.
- Differential diagnoses with regard to elevated troponin include an almost endless list of cardiac, noncoronary but also extra-cardiac disorders [22].
- Reasons for acute troponin elevations should also include:
  - Acute myocarditis
  - Aortic dissection
  - Acute pulmonary embolism
  - Stress cardiomyopathy (Tako Tsubo)
  - Heart failure
  - Structural heart disease, e.g., aortic stenosis
  - Hypertensive emergencies and atrial tachyarrhythmias [22]

Table 2.2 Overview of selected guideline recommendations

Variable	NICE 2014 [19]	ACC/AHA 2014 [20]	ESC 2015 [8]
ECG	12-lead immediately	12-lead immediately	12-lead immediately
Preferred biomarker Baseline measurement	Cardiac troponin At presentation	Cardiac troponin At presentation	Cardiac troponin At presentation
Standard protocol for repeat measurement	10–12 h after onset of symptoms	3–6 h after symptom onset	3 h after admission if hsTn available
Serial change criteria	At least one value above the 99th percentile	If cTn below or close to 99th percentile: Change ≥3 standard deviations If cTn >99th percentile: increase or decrease ≥20%	If hsTn <99th percentile: increase by >50% of ULN (e.g., 7 ng/L for hsTnT) If cTn >99th percentile: increase or decrease ≥20%
Early rule-out protocols:	Recommended	Not recommended	Recommended (except in patients presenting very early, i.e., within 1 h from chest pain onset, then second cardiac troponin level should be obtained at 3 h
Option A	Presentation and 3 h if hsTnT or hsTnI (Abbott architect) available	hsTn not available	1-h rule-out if hsTnT or hsTnI (Abbott Architect) available
Option B	—	—	2 h ADP together with TIMI score and ECG
Option C	—	—	Instant if normal cTn (<99th percentile but >limit of detection) and copeptin <95% percentile
Specific recommendations with hsTn cutoff: hsTnT	99th percentile cutoff, i.e., 14 ng/L	99th percentile cutoff	99th percentile cutoff, for 1-h rule-out <12 ng/L and delta <3 ng/L
hsTnI (Abbott Architect)	99th percentile 26.2 ng/L Sex-specific cutoff: 34.2 ng/L for men and 15.6 ng/L for women		99th percentile, for 1-h rule-out <5 ng/L and delta 0–1 h <2 ng/L
Clinical risk score recommendation	*General:* Prediction of 6-month mortality such as GRACE score	*Undifferentiated chest pain (including discomfort, pressure, and squeezing):* TIMI risk score PURSUIT score GRACE score NCDR-ACTION *Chest pain:* Sanchis score Vancouver rule HEART score HEARTS₃ score Hess prediction rule	*General:* GRACE score, preferentially over TIMI risk score

Table 2.2 (continued)

Variable	NICE 2014 [19]	ACC/AHA 2014 [20]	ESC 2015 [8]
Management Invasive:	*General:* Offer coronary angiography (with follow-on PCI if indicated) within 96 h of first admission to hospital to patients who have an intermediate or higher risk of adverse cardiovascular events (predicted 6-month mortality above 3.0%)	*Stabilized high-risk patient:* Early invasive strategy within 24 h of admission (preferred) or delayed invasive strategy within 25–72 h Not high/intermediate risk: delayed invasive approach is reasonable	*General:* Immediate invasive strategy (<2 h): Paralleling the STEMI pathway, this strategy should be undertaken for patients with ongoing ischemia, characterized by at least one very-high-risk criterion Early invasive strategy (<24 h): patients qualify if they have at least one high-risk criterion Invasive strategy (<72 h): maximal delay for coronary angiography in patients without recurrence of symptoms but with at least one intermediate-risk criterion
Conservative:	Offer conservative management without early coronary angiography to patients with a low risk of adverse cardiovascular events (predicted 6-month mortality 3.0% or less)	Extensive comorbidities Acute chest pain and a low likelihood of ACS who are troponin negative, especially women	In low-risk patients, a noninvasive stress test (preferably with imaging) for inducible ischemia is recommended before deciding on an invasive strategy
Selective:	Offer coronary angiography (with follow-on PCI if indicated) to patients initially assessed to be at low risk of adverse cardiovascular events (predicted 6-month mortality 3.0% or less) if ischemia is subsequently experienced or is demonstrated by ischemia testing	Ischemia-guided strategy may be considered for patients with NSTE-ACS (without serious comorbidities or contraindications to this approach) who have an elevated risk for clinical events	Patients with no recurrence of chest pain, no signs of heart failure, no abnormalities in the initial or subsequent ECG, and no increase in (preferably high-sensitivity) cardiac troponin level are at low risk of subsequent CV events In this setting, a noninvasive stress test (preferably with imaging) for inducible ischemia is recommended before deciding on an invasive strategy
Discharge recommendations	*Non-high risk:* To detect and quantify inducible ischemia, consider ischemia testing before discharge for patients whose condition has been managed conservatively and who have not had coronary angiography	*Possible ACS who have normal serial ECGs and cardiac troponins:* Treadmill ECG, stress myocardial perfusion imaging, or stress echocardiography before discharge or within 72 h after discharge	*Unstable angina:* Regular ward or discharge, no rhythm monitoring

(continued)

Table 2.2 (continued)

Variable	NICE 2014 [19]	ACC/AHA 2014 [20]	ESC 2015 [8]
Cardiac imaging	Echocardiography and coronary CT	*Possible ACS and a normal ECG, normal cardiac troponins, and no history of CAD:* Coronary CT angiography to assess coronary artery anatomy, or rest myocardial perfusion imaging with technetium-99m to assess coronary artery anatomy, or to exclude myocardial ischemia	Echocardiography, X-ray, CT, CMR Stress imaging is preferred over exercise ECG due to its greater diagnostic accuracy

Key: *cTn* cardiac troponin, *hsTn* high-sensitivity troponin, *hsTnT* high-sensitivity troponin T, *hsTnI* high-sensitivity troponin I, *ULN* upper limit of normal, *ADP* adenosine diphosphate, *TIMI* thrombolysis in myocardial infarction, *ACS* acute coronary syndrome, *CT* computed tomography, *ECG* electrocardiogram, *NSTE* non-ST elevation, *CV* cardiovascular, *CMR* cardiac magnetic resonance, *CAD* coronary artery disease

Clinical Scores

Acute Coronary Syndrome

- A number of risk-scoring systems have been developed to predict short- and medium-term outcome in patients with acute coronary syndromes [23–25]. Many of these risk-scoring systems were derived from clinical trial populations, which generally excluded the highest risk patients.
- Other risk scores were derived from large patient databases in an attempt to model a more representative ACS population with a broader spectrum of risk.
- Most of the risk scores include ECG signs of myocardial ischemia and cardiac biomarkers of necrosis, as well as other clinical features at presentation.
- In NSTE-ACS, quantitative assessment of ischemic risk by means of scores is superior to the clinical assessment. There are numerous clinical scores that have been established in different populations. Endpoints and duration of follow-up as well as performance of the scores vary widely.
- The GRACE risk score [26] provides the most accurate stratification of risk both on admission and at discharge, and has been validated in prospective registries on patients with acute coronary syndrome [8, 27].

- The TIMI risk score is simple to use and has also been validated in several clinical trials [28, 29]. Its discriminative accuracy is inferior to that of the GRACE risk score and the GRACE 2.0 risk calculation [8].
- More recently the HEART score has been established and validated prospectively [30, 31]. An overview on the different multivariable clinical scores is given in Table 2.2.
- The usefulness of clinical scores is to estimate increased individual risk and accordingly guide need and timing of coronary angiography and coronary intervention [27], or as a tool to identify a low-risk patient who might be safely discharged after rule-out of MI [24].

Prediction of Cardiovascular Disease Risk in Individuals Without Known CVD

- In all individuals without known cardiovascular disease (CVD), several risk scores have been developed to estimate the risk of CVD including the Framingham score(s), the PROCAM score, and more recently the ESC-score [32–41].
- There are several review articles providing a critical overview of an incomplete number of available risk scores with advantages and limitations [32, 33].

- Briefly, the Framingham Risk Score is a gender-specific algorithm used to estimate the 10-year cardiovascular risk of an individual [34]. The Framingham Risk Score was first developed based on the data obtained from the Framingham Heart Study, to estimate the 10-year risk of developing coronary heart disease.
- The ESC-SCORE is a cardiovascular disease risk assessment and management tool developed by the European Society of Cardiology, using data from 12 European cohort studies (N = 205,178) covering a wide geographic spread of countries at different levels of cardiovascular risks [35]. The score includes gender, age, smoking, systolic blood pressure, and total cholesterol as risk factors, and estimates fatal cardiovascular disease events over a 10-year period.
- The SCORE data contains some three million person-years of observation and 7934 fatal cardiovascular events. Three different formats have been developed including:
  - A Web-based version, offering graphical display of absolute CVD risk, including relative risk for younger patients, patient data history, and progress monitoring
  - A downloadable PC version since 2008
  - A quick calculator
- In the USA, the American Heart Association (AHA) and the American College of Cardiology (ACC) introduced a new atherosclerotic cardiovascular disease (ASCVD) risk score in the year 2013 to guide ASCVD risk-reducing therapy [36].
- The ideal target populations to estimate the 10-year risk of ASCVD events are non-Hispanic African-American and non-Hispanic white men and women from 40 to 79 years of age.
- 10-year risk was defined as the risk of developing a first ASCVD event, defined as nonfatal myocardial infarction or coronary heart disease (CHD) death or fatal or nonfatal stroke. The recommendation to calculate 30-year or lifetime risk for ASCVD events is weak [36].
- The Joint British Societies rather recommend use of the JBS3 score as a risk calculator provided conveniently on an smartphone "app" that intends to help healthcare practitioners to better illustrate the risk of CVD and the gains that can be made from interventions such as reducing blood pressure, or stopping smoking [37].
- In contrast to other scores, the JBS3 score extends estimation of CVD risk over a lifetime and considers death from competing diseases such as cancer.
- This risk calculator is based on the concept that early lifestyle interventions and drug treatment can decrease or slow down CVD and thereby the risk of future CVD events. Therefore, it is recommended to estimate both 10-year risk and lifetime risk of CVD in all individuals, except for those with existing CVD or certain high-risk diseases, i.e., diabetes age >40 years, patients with chronic kidney disease (CKD) stages 3–5, or familial hypercholesterolemia.
- Although this score is still relatively new for the medical community, particularly outside the UK, it has been applied by the insurance industry for many years to determine appropriate levels of insurance premium risk over a lifetime to help inform prevention strategies with lifestyle changes (interventions) and, where necessary, drug therapy.
- JBS3 includes estimation of the widely used 10-year risk estimation, as previously recommended in JBS2, but now extends this to include CVD risk over a lifetime.
- Another risk score for estimation of CVD that is recommended in the UK by the National Institute for Health and Care Excellence (NICE) guidelines instead of the Framingham Risk Score [38] is the QRISK2 [39].
- The most recent version of QRISK is a prediction algorithm for cardiovascular disease (CVD) that—in analogy to the Framingham Risk Score—includes traditional risk factors (age, systolic blood pressure, smoking status, and ratio of total serum cholesterol to high-density lipoprotein cholesterol).
- However, the QRISK also includes body mass index, family history of cardiovascular disease, chronic kidney failure, rheumatoid

arthritis, atrial fibrillation, social deprivation (Townsend score), and use of antihypertensive treatment.

- QRISK excludes patients with a preexisting diagnosis of diabetes and does not include electrocardiogram assessment of left ventricular hypertrophy. The second version also accounts for statin use and a method to adjust for missing data. The algorithm has been validated using an external dataset [40, 41].

- QRISK has also been developed further to estimate individualized lifetime risk of cardiovascular disease [42].

High-Sensitivity Troponins

- Several years ago manufacturers started to develop novel high-sensitivity generations of cardiac troponin (cTn) assays in order to comply with the precision criteria of the 2000 ESC/ACC consensus document on the redefinition of myocardial infarction [43].

- It has been proposed that a cTn assay should be designated as a "high-sensitivity" assay if cTn can be measured in at least 50% of healthy individuals, in order to ensure a high clinical sensitivity [44].

- These high-sensitivity assays are characterized by a substantially higher analytical sensitivity than conventional sensitive assays, allowing the measurement of cTn in ng/L, rather than microgram/L [45].

- The more sensitive high-sensitivity troponin (hsTn) assays differ regarding their analytical characteristics. In direct comparison, 19 cTn assays were found to show very heterogenous analytical characteristics regarding the 99th percentile value and their analytical sensitivity, as reflected by the proportion of detectable cTn concentrations in a healthy reference population [46].

- Whether the clinical performance of the different hsTn assays is similar is unsettled as yet only a few studies have directly compared hscTn assays head to head for the detection of reversible ischemia, diagnosis, and prognosis.

- The key differentiating feature of hsTn assays, when compared to the conventional sensitive cTn assays, is not apparent at higher values but is restricted to the area around the 99th percentile cutoff.

- The clinical interpretation of hsTn concentrations in this range is challenging, but important, as most of the increased sensitivity for the detection of myocardial injury is at the low concentration level.

- In clinical routine, there is substantial evidence that the use of more sensitive cTn assays enables more accurate and earlier detection of myocardial infarction (MI) [47–50]. Numerous trials [49, 50] and a recent meta-analysis [51] now provide substantial evidence that high-sensitivity assays, using the 99th percentile as the threshold for positivity, can achieve sensitivity at presentation of 90% or more.

- A higher analytical sensitivity changes the spectrum of ACS, as hsTn assays used at lower thresholds increase the incidence of non-ST-segment elevation myocardial infarction (NSTEMI), particularly small MI, that would have been mislabeled as unstable angina (UA) [52, 53].

- Maximizing early sensitivity results in some loss of clinical specificity [22]. Thus, lowering the diagnostic cutoff increases the number of patients with analytically true cTn elevations that are related to myocardial injury, but not to MI.

- Compared to conventional sensitive assays, the prevalence of detectable and elevated cTn values increases with the use of hsTn assays in various study populations, including patients with acute [54] or chronic heart failure [55–57], and stable CAD [58], and in general populations of middle-aged individuals [59–61], and patients with structural heart disease are identified at earlier clinical stages [55, 62].

- Not uncommonly, patients with suspected ACS may present with symptoms other than typical chest pain. Therefore, the diagnosis may be uncertain in many patients who require strategies to overcome the loss of clinical specificity. Such strategies to increase the clinical specificity without a loss of sensitivity include a strict adherence to the Universal MI definition, use of recommended cutoffs, and relevant concentration change in serial testing.

- A working group of the ESC [45] recommends, by consensus, an increase of >50% of the 99th percentile value if the baseline value lies below the 99th percentile and the second value exceeds the 99th percentile.
- In cases where the initial cTn value is already above the 99th percentile value, an increase of only 20% on the second sample is necessary to diagnose NSTEMI [45].
- The most recent achievement with biomarker testing is the implementation of hsTn assays, instead of the conventional, less sensitive troponin assays, in patients with suspected ACS [8].
- The higher analytical sensitivity and precision of the more sensitive assays have facilitated an earlier and more accurate detection of NSTEMI [47–50]. Accordingly, recent ESC guidelines [8] recommend the use of hsTn assays with a second sample after 3 h, or optionally after 6 h, in order to rule out NSTEMI earlier than with standard cardiac troponin (cTn) assays.
- As an alternative, a 1-h diagnostic protocol can be used if validated hsTn assays are available, a 2-h accelerated diagnostic protocol with cTn, or an instant rule-out using a single hsTn with a cutoff at the limit of detection (LoD), or a combination of a normal cTn or hsTn together with a normal copeptin.
- An overview on differences regarding diagnosis, risk estimation, and management of ACS without ST-segment elevation across guidelines, i.e., NICE 2014 [19] versus ACC/AHA 2014 [20] versus ESC 2015 [8], is provided in Table 2.2.

References

1. Goodacre S, Cross E, Arnold J, Angelini K, Capewell S, Nicholl J. The health care burden of acute chest pain. Heart. 2005;91:229–30.
2. Guttmann A, Schull MJ, Vermeulen MJ, Stukel TA. Association between waiting times and short term mortality and hospital admission after departure from emergency department: population based cohort study from Ontario, Canada. BMJ. 2011;342:d2983.
3. Diercks DB, Roe MT, Chen AY, Peacock WF, Kirk JD, Pollack CV Jr, Gibler WB, Smith SC Jr, Ohman M, Peterson ED. Prolonged emergency department stays of non-ST-segment-elevation myocardial infarction patients are associated with worse adherence to the American College of Cardiology/American Heart Association guidelines for management and increased adverse events. Ann Emerg Med. 2007;50:489–96.
4. Chun AA, McGee SR. Bedside diagnosis of coronary artery disease: a systematic review. Am J Med. 2004;117:334–43.
5. Brieger D, Eagle KA, Goodman SG, Steg PG, Budaj A, White K, Montalescot G. Acute coronary syndromes without chest pain, an underdiagnosed and undertreated high-risk group: insights from the global registry of acute coronary events. Chest. 2004;126:461–9.
6. Canto JG, Shlipak MG, Rogers WJ, Malmgren JA, Frederick PD, Lambrew CT, Ornato JP, Barron HV, Kiefe CI. Prevalence, clinical characteristics, and mortality among patients with myocardial infarction presenting without chest pain. JAMA. 2000;283: 3223–9.
7. Body R, Carley S, Wibberley C, McDowell G, Ferguson J, Mackway-Jones K. The value of symptoms and signs in the emergent diagnosis of acute coronary syndromes. Resuscitation. 2010;81:281–6.
8. Roffi M, Patrono C, Collet JP, Mueller C, Valgimigli M, Andreotti F, Bax JJ, Borger MA, Brotons C, Chew DP, Gencer B, Hasenfuss G, Kjeldsen K, Lancellotti P, Landmesser U, Mehilli J, Mukherjee D, Storey RF, Windecker S, Baumgartner H, Gaemperli O, Achenbach S, Agewall S, Badimon L, Baigent C, Bueno H, Bugiardini R, Carerj S, Casselman F, Cuisset T, Erol Ç, Fitzsimons D, Halle M, Hamm C, Hildick-Smith D, Huber K, Iliodromitis E, James S, Lewis BS, Lip GY, Piepoli MF, Richter D, Rosemann T, Sechtem U, Steg PG, Vrints C, Luis Zamorano J. 2015 ESC guidelines for the management of acute coronary syndromes in patients presenting without persistent ST-segment elevation: Task Force for the Management of Acute Coronary Syndromes in Patients Presenting without Persistent ST-Segment Elevation of the European Society of Cardiology (ESC). Management of Acute Coronary Syndromes in Patients Presenting without Persistent ST-Segment Elevation of the European Society of Cardiology. Eur Heart J. 2016;37:267–315.
9. Diamond GA, Forrester JS. Analysis of probability as an aid in the clinical diagnosis of coronary-artery disease. N Engl J Med. 1979;300:1350–8.
10. Braunwald E. Unstable angina. A classification. Circulation. 1989;80:410–4.
11. Hamm CW, Braunwald E. A classification of unstable angina revisited. Circulation. 2000;102:118–22.
12. Lee TH, Cook EF, Weisberg M, Sargent RK, Wilson C, Goldman L. Acute chest pain in the emergency

room. Identification and examination of low-risk patients. Arch Intern Med. 1985;145:65–9.

13. Henrikson CA, Howell EE, Bush DE, Miles JS, Meininger GR, Friedlander T, Bushnell AC, Chandra-Strobos N. Chest pain relief by nitroglycerin does not predict active coronary artery disease. Ann Intern Med. 2003;139:979–86.

14. Swap CJ, Nagurney JT. Value and limitations of chest pain history in the evaluation of patients with suspected acute coronary syndromes. JAMA. 2005;294:2623–9.

15. Braunwald E, Morrow DA. Unstable angina: is it time for a requiem? Circulation. 2013;127:2452–7.

16. Alexander KP, Newby LK, Cannon CP, Armstrong PW, Gibler WB, Rich MW, Van de Werf F, White HD, Weaver WD, Naylor MD, Gore JM, Krumholz HM, Ohman EM, American Heart Association Council on Clinical Cardiology; Society of Geriatric Cardiology. Acute coronary care in the elderly, part I: Non-ST-segment-elevation acute coronary syndromes: a scientific statement for healthcare professionals from the American Heart Association Council on Clinical Cardiology: in collaboration with the Society of Geriatric Cardiology. Circulation. 2007;115:2549–69.

17. Mockel M, Searle J, Muller R, Slagman A, Storchmann H, Oestereich P, Wyrwich W, Ale-Abaei A, Vollert JO, Koch M, Somasundaram R. Chief complaints in medical emergencies: do they relate to underlying disease and outcome? The Charité Emergency Medicine Study (CHARITEM). Eur J Emerg Med. 2013;20:103–8.

18. Rubini Gimenez M, Reiter M, Twerenbold R, Reichlin T, Wildi K, Haaf P, Wicki K, Zellweger C, Hoeller R, Moehring B, Sou SM, Mueller M, Denhaerynck K, Meller B, Stallone F, Henseler S, Bassetti S, Geigy N, Osswald S, Mueller C. Sex-specific chest pain characteristics in the early diagnosis of acute myocardial infarction. JAMA Intern Med. 2014;174:241–9.

19. National Institute for Health and Clinical Excellence: Guidance. Unstable Angina and NSTEMI: The Early Management of Unstable Angina and Non-ST-Segment-Elevation Myocardial infarction. National Clinical Guideline Centre (UK). London: Royal College of Physicians (UK); 2010 niceorguk/guidance/cg94, last update November 2013, online access November 16 2016.

20. Amsterdam EA, Wenger NK, Brindis RG, Casey DE Jr, Ganiats TG, Holmes DR Jr, Jaffe AS, Jneid H, Kelly RF, Kontos MC, Levine GN, Liebson PR, Mukherjee D, Peterson ED, Sabatine MS, Smalling RW, Zieman SJ, Members AATF. 2014 aha/acc guideline for the management of patients with non-stelevation acute coronary syndromes: executive summary: a report of the American College of Cardiology/American Heart Association Task Force on Practice Guidelines. Circulation. 2014;130:2354–94.

21. Thygesen K, Alpert JS, Jaffe AS, Simoons ML, Chaitman BR, White HD, Joint ESC/ACCF/AHA/WHF Task Force for the Universal Definition of Myocardial Infarction, Katus HA, Lindahl B, Morrow DA, Clemmensen PM, Johanson P, Hod H, Underwood R, Bax JJ, Bonow RO, Pinto F, Gibbons RJ, Fox KA, Atar D, Newby LK, Galvani M, Hamm CW, Uretsky BF, Steg PG, Wijns W, Bassand JP, Menasché P, Ravkilde J, Ohman EM, Antman EM, Wallentin LC, Armstrong PW, Simoons ML, Januzzi JL, Nieminen MS, Gheorghiade M, Filippatos G, Luepker RV, Fortmann SP, Rosamond WD, Levy D, Wood D, Smith SC, Hu D, Lopez-Sendon JL, Robertson RM, Weaver D, Tendera M, Bove AA, Parkhomenko AN, Vasilieva EJ, Mendis S Collaborators: Bax JJ, Baumgartner H, Ceconi C, Dean V, Deaton C, Fagard R, Funck-Brentano C, Hasdai D, Hoes A, Kirchhof P, Knuuti J, Kolh P, McDonagh T, Moulin C, Popescu BA, Reiner Ž, Sechtem U, Sirnes PA, Tendera M, Torbicki A, Vahanian A, Windecker S. Third universal definition of myocardial infarction. Circulation. 2012;126:2020–35.

22. Giannitsis E, Katus HA. Cardiac troponin level elevations not related to acute coronary syndromes. Nat Rev Cardiol. 2013;10:623–34.

23. Backus BE, Six AJ, Kelder JH, Gibler WB, Moll FL, Doevendans PA. Risk scores for patients with chest pain: evaluation in the emergency department. Curr Cardiol Rev. 2011;7:2–8.

24. Carlton EW, Khattab A, Greaves K. Identifying patients suitable for discharge after a single-presentation high-sensitivity troponin result: a comparison of five established risk scores and two high-sensitivity assays. Ann Emerg Med. 2015;66:635–45.

25. D'Ascenzo F, Biondi-Zoccai G, Moretti C, Bollati M, Omedè P, Sciuto F, Presutti DG, Modena MG, Gasparini M, Reed MJ, Sheiban I, Gaita F. TIMI, GRACE and alternative risk scores in acute coronary syndromes: a meta-analysis of 40 derivation studies on 216,552 patients and of 42 validation studies on 31,625 patients. Contemp Clin Trials. 2012;33:507–14.

26. Granger CB, Goldberg RJ, Dabbous O, Pieper KS, Eagle KA, Cannon CP, Van De Werf F, Avezum A, Goodman SG, Flather MD, Fox KA, Global Registry of Acute Coronary Events Investigators. Predictors of hospital mortality in the global registry of acute coronary events. Arch Intern Med. 2003;163: 2345–53.

27. Fox KA, Dabbous OH, Goldberg RJ, et al. Prediction of risk of death and myocardial infarction in the 6 months after presentation with acute coronary syndrome: prospective multinational observational study (GRACE). BMJ. 2006;333:1091–4.

28. Antman EM, Cohen M, Bernink PJ, McCabe CH, Horacek T, Papuchis G, Mautner B, Corbalan R, Radley D, Braunwald E. The TIMI risk score for unstable angina/non-ST elevation MI: a method for prognostication and therapeutic decision making. JAMA. 2000;284:835–42.

29. Pollack CV Jr, Sites FD, Shofer FS, Sease KL, Hollander JE. Application of the TIMI risk score for unstable angina and non-ST elevation acute coronary syndrome to an unselected emergency depart-

ment chest pain population. Acad Emerg Med. 2006;13:13–8.

30. Six AJ, Backus BE, Kelder JC. Chest pain in the emergency room: value of the heart score. Neth Heart J. 2008;16:191–6.

31. Backus BE, Six AJ, Kelder JC, Bosschaert MA, Mast EG, Mosterd A, Veldkamp RF, Wardeh AJ, Tio R, Braam R, Monnink SH, van Tooren R, Mast TP, van den Akker F, Cramer MJ, Poldervaart JM, Hoes AW, Doevendans PA. A prospective validation of the heart score for chest pain patients at the emergency department. Int J Cardiol. 2013;168:2153–8.

32. Erbel R, Budoff M. Improvement of cardiovascular risk prediction using coronary imaging: subclinical atherosclerosis: the memory of lifetime risk factor exposure. Eur Heart J. 2012;33:1201–13.

33. Mureddu GF, Brandimarte F, Faggiano P, Rigo F, Nixdorff U. Between risk charts and imaging: how should we stratify cardiovascular risk in clinical practice? Eur Heart J Cardiovasc Imaging. 2013;14:401–16.

34. Wilson PW, D'Agostino RB, Levy D, Belanger AM, Silbershatz H, Kannel WB. Prediction of coronary heart disease using risk factor categories. Circulation. 1998;97(18):1837–47.

35. Conroy RM, Pyörälä K, Fitzgerald AE, Sans S, Menotti A, De Backer G, De Bacquer D, Ducimetiere P, Jousilahti P, Keil U, Njølstad I. Estimation of ten-year risk of fatal cardiovascular disease in Europe: the SCORE project. Eur Heart J. 2003;24: 987–1003.

36. Goff DC Jr, Lloyd-Jones DM, Bennett G, Coady S, D'Agostino RB, Gibbons R, Greenland P, Lackland DT, Levy D, O'Donnell CJ, Robinson JG, Schwartz JS, Shero ST, Smith SC Jr, Sorlie P, Stone NJ, Wilson PW, Jordan HS, Nevo L, Wnek J, Anderson JL, Halperin JL, Albert NM, Bozkurt B, Brindis RG, Curtis LH, DeMets D, Hochman JS, Kovacs RJ, Ohman EM, Pressler SJ, Sellke FW, Shen WK, Smith SC Jr, Tomaselli GF. 2013 ACC/AHA guideline on the assessment of cardiovascular risk: a report of the American College of Cardiology/American Heart Association Task Force on Practice Guidelines. Circulation. 2014;129(Suppl. 2):S49–73.

37. JBS3 Board. Joint British Societies' consensus recommendations for the prevention of cardiovascular disease (JBS3). Heart. 2014 Apr;100(Suppl 2):ii1–ii67. https://doi.org/10.1136/heartjnl-2014-305693.

38. Anderson KM, Odell PM, Wilson PWF, Kannel WB. Cardiovascular disease risk profiles. Am Heart J. 1991;121:293–8.

39. Hippisley-Cox J, Coupland C, Vinogradova Y, Robson J, Brindle P. Performance of the QRISK cardiovascular risk prediction algorithm in an independent UK sample of patients from general practice: a validation study. Heart. 2008;94:34–9.

40. Collins GS, Altman DG. An independent external validation and evaluation of QRISK cardiovascular risk prediction: a prospective open cohort study. BMJ. 2009;339:b2584.

41. Collins GS, Altman DG. An independent and external validation of QRISK2 cardiovascular disease risk score: a prospective open cohort study. BMJ. 2010;340:c2442.

42. Hippisley-Cox J, Coupland C, Robson J, Brindle P. Derivation, validation, and evaluation of a new QRISK model to estimate lifetime risk of cardiovascular disease: cohort study using QResearch database. BMJ. 2010;341:c6624.

43. Alpert JS, Thygesen K, Antman E, Bassand JP. Myocardial infarction redefined—a consensus document of the Joint European Society of Cardiology/American College of Cardiology Committee for the redefinition of myocardial infarction. J Am Coll Cardiol. 2000;36:959–69.

44. Apple FS, Ler R, Murakami MM. Determination of 19 cardiac troponin I and T assay 99th percentile values from a common presumably healthy population. Clin Chem. 2012;58:1574–81.

45. Thygesen K, Mair J, Giannitsis E, Mueller C, Lindahl B, Blankenberg S, Huber K, Plebani M, Biasucci LM, Tubaro M, Collinson P, Venge P, Hasin Y, Galvani M, Koenig W, Hamm C, Alpert JS, Katus H, Jaffe AS, Study Group on Biomarkers in Cardiology of ESC Working Group on Acute Cardiac Care. How to use high-sensitivity cardiac troponins in acute cardiac care. Eur Heart J. 2012;33:2252–7.

46. Apple FS. A new season for cardiac troponin assays: it's time to keep a scorecard. Clin Chem. 2009;55:1303–6.

47. Melanson SE, Morrow DA, Jarolim P. Earlier detection of myocardial injury in a preliminary evaluation using a new troponin I assay with improved sensitivity. Am J Clin Pathol. 2007;128:282–6.

48. Giannitsis E, Kurz K, Hallermayer K, Jarausch J, Jaffe AS, Katus HA. Analytical validation of a high sensitivity cardiac troponin T assay. Clin Chem. 2010;56:254–61.

49. Keller T, Zeller T, Peetz D, Tzikas S, Roth A, Czyz E, Bickel C, Baldus S, Warnholtz A, Fröhlich M, Sinning CR, Eleftheriadis MS, Wild PS, Schnabel RB, Lubos E, Jachmann N, Genth-Zotz S, Post F, Nicaud V, Tiret L, Lackner KJ, Münzel TF, Blankenberg S. Sensitive troponin I assay in early diagnosis of acute myocardial infarction. N Engl J Med. 2009;361: 868–77.

50. Reichlin T, Hochholzer W, Bassetti S, Steuer S, Stelzig C, Hartwiger S, Biedert S, Schaub N, Buerge C, Potocki M, Noveanu M, Breidthardt T, Twerenbold R, Winkler K, Bingisser R, Mueller C. Early diagnosis of myocardial infarction with sensitive cardiac troponin assays. N Engl J Med. 2009;361:858–67.

51. Goodacre S, Thokala P, Carroll C, Stevens JW, Leaviss J, Al Khalaf M, Collinson P, Morris F, Evans P, Wang J. Systematic review, meta-analysis and economic modelling of diagnostic strategies for suspected acute coronary syndrome. Health Technol Assess. 2013;17:v–vi, 1–188

52. Kontos MC, Fritz LM, Anderson FP, Tatum JL, Ornato JP, Jesse RL. Impact of the troponin standard

on the prevalence of acute myocardial infarction. Am Heart J. 2003;146:446–52.

53. Kavsak PA, MacRae AR, Lustig V, Bhargava R, Vandersluis R, Palomaki GE, et al. The impact of the ESC/ACC redefinition of myocardial infarction and new sensitive troponin assays on the frequency of acute myocardial infarction. Am Heart J. 2006;152:118–25.

54. Pascual-Figal DA, Casas T, Ordonez-Llanos J, Manzano-Fernández S, Bonaque JC, Boronat M, Muñoz-Esparza C, Valdés M, Januzzi JL. Highly sensitive troponin T for risk stratification of acutely destabilized heart failure. Am Heart J. 2012;163: 1002–10.

55. Latini R, Masson S, Anand I, Missov E, Carlson M, Vago T, et al. for the Val-HeFT Investigators. Prognostic value of very low plasma concentrations of troponin T in patients with stable chronic heart failure. Circulation. 2007;116:1242–9.

56. Barlera S, Tavazzi L, Franzosi MG, Marchioli R, Raimondi E, Masson S, Urso R, Lucci D, Nicolosi GL, Maggioni AP, Tognoni G, Investigators GISSI-HF. Predictors of mortality in 6975 patients with chronic heart failure in the Gruppo Italiano per lo Studio della Streptochinasi nell'Infarto Miocardico-Heart Failure trial: proposal for a Nomogram. Circ Heart Fail. 2013;6:31–9.

57. Nagarajan V, Hernandez AV, Tang WH. Prognostic value of cardiac troponin in chronic stable heart failure: a systematic review. Heart. 2012;98:1778–86.

58. Omland T, de Lemos JA, Sabatine MS, Christophi CA, Rice MM, Jablonski KA, Tjora S, Domanski MJ, Gersh BJ, Rouleau JL, Pfeffer MA, Braunwald E, Prevention of Events with Angiotensin Converting Enzyme Inhibition (PEACE) Trial Investigators. A sensitive cardiac troponin T assay in stable coronary artery disease. N Engl J Med. 2009;361:2538–47.

59. de Lemos JA, Drazner MH, Omland T, Ayers CR, Khera A, Rohatgi A, et al. Association of troponin T detected with a highly sensitive assay and cardiac structure and mortality risk in the general population. JAMA. 2010;304:2503–12.

60. deFilippi CR, de Lemos JA, Christenson RH, Gottdiener JS, Kop WJ, Zhan M, Seliger SL. Association of serial measures of cardiac troponin T using a sensitive assay with incident heart failure and cardiovascular mortality in older adults. JAMA. 2010;304:2494–502.

61. Saunders JT, Nambi V, de Lemos JA, Chambless LE, Virani SS, Boerwinkle E, Hoogeveen RC, Liu X, Astor BC, Mosley TH, Folsom AR, Heiss G, Coresh J, Ballantyne CM. Cardiac troponin T measured by a highly sensitive assay predicts coronary heart disease, heart failure, and mortality in the atherosclerosis risk in communities study. Circulation. 2011;123:1367–76.

62. Filusch A, Giannitsis E, Katus HA, Meyer FJ. High-sensitive troponin T: a novel biomarker for prognosis and disease severity in patients with pulmonary arterial hypertension. Clin Sci (Lond). 2010;119:207–13.

Noninvasive Imaging Assessment of Coronary Heart Disease

Udo Sechtem, Heiko Mahrholdt, and Peter Ong

About Us The Robert Bosch Hospital is a charitable hospital in Stuttgart, Germany. It was founded by Robert Bosch in 1936. The hospital is supported by the Robert Bosch Foundation. The Department of Cardiology is part of the Center of Cardiovascular Medicine, which also includes the Department of Cardiac and Vascular Surgery. Noninvasive imaging is an essential aspect of managing cardiac patients and nuclear medicine examinations, echocardiography, magnetic resonance imaging, and computed tomography are performed frequently in the department. Treatment of stable and unstable coronary heart disease is frequently performed (800 PCI and more than 900 bypass operations per year). Indications for revascularization in stable patients with coronary heart disease are based on the results of ischemia testing.

Why Noninvasive Imaging in Coronary Heart Disease?

- Coronary heart disease (CHD) continues to be the most frequent cause of death in Western countries and attempts at reducing the death toll lead to high expenses for healthcare systems.

U. Sechtem (✉) · H. Mahrholdt · P. Ong
Robert-Bosch-Krankenhaus, Stuttgart, Germany
e-mail: udo.sechtem@rbk.de; heiko.mahrholdt@rbk.de;
peter.ong@rbk.de

- Testing including noninvasive imaging is frequently performed in order to detect the presence of stenotic atherosclerotic disease of the coronary arteries which is thought to be the harbinger of doom. Early noninvasive detection is felt to be the optimal way of selecting patients who might benefit from subsequent coronary angiography.
- Ultimately, the aim is early intervention in the form of coronary revascularization in addition to medical therapy, with the expectation of relieving suffering and improving prognosis. Current European and US guidelines support this approach [1–3].

Do All Patients with Angina Have to Undergo Some Form of Preselection Testing Before Invasive Coronary Angiography?

- Some form of preselection testing in patients with stable coronary artery disease before invasive coronary angiography (ICA) makes sense in order to keep the number of normal coronary angiograms low.
- However, patients with severe angina and a high clinical likelihood of severe disease (clustering of risk factors, reduced ejection fraction) may and should undergo invasive coronary angiography without hesitation. This is certainly also true for patients with known coronary artery disease and such clinical features [1, 2].

© Springer International Publishing AG, part of Springer Nature 2018
A. Myat et al. (eds.), *The Interventional Cardiology Training Manual*,
https://doi.org/10.1007/978-3-319-71635-0_3

• Patients with angina who have acute coronary syndromes (ACS) are usually sent for ICA based on current guidelines [4, 5]. However, stress imaging is also recommended before ICA in low-risk ACS patients (no troponin, no ECG changes) in order to confirm the diagnosis and perform risk stratification. In such patients stress imaging is preferred over stress ECG due to its better diagnostic performance. High-risk patients are sent to ICA [4].

Is the Stress ECG Completely Useless?

• In many situations the stress ECG is still an easy, cheap, and appropriate way of excluding relevant CHD. The following requirements need to be fulfilled:
  – Pretest probability for the presence of stenotic CHD should be reasonably low (below 50–60%). This excludes male patients and female patients older than 60 years with typical (retrosternal, elicited by exercise, stopped by rest or nitroglycerin) angina (see Table 3.1).
  – The 12-lead resting ECG should be interpretable (no ST-segment depression ≥ 1 mm, no bundle branch block, no pacemaker ECG).
  – Patients should be able to exercise adequately and reach 85% of target heart rate during exercise (i.e., 220 – age).

• These points pertain only to the diagnostic qualities of the exercise ECG not to its prognostic capabilities: irrespective of pretest probability and findings on the resting ECG, prognosis is generally good in a patient who is able to exercise to a high level of metabolic equivalents of task (METs) without angina (Duke treadmill score [6]).

Table 3.1 Clinical pretest probabilities in patients with stable chest pain symptoms

	Typical angina		Atypical angina		Non-anginal pain	
Age	Men	Women	Men	Women	Men	Women
30–39	59	28	29	10	18	5
40–49	69	37	38	14	25	8
50–59	77	47	49	20	34	12
60–69	84	58	59	28	44	17
70–79	88	68	69	37	54	24
>80	93	76	78	47	65	32

ECG electrocardiogram, *PTP* pretest probability, *SCAD* stable coronary artery disease
• Probabilities of obstructive coronary disease shown reflect the estimates for patients aged 35, 45, 55, 65, 75, and 85 years
• Groups in white boxes have a PTP <15% and hence can be managed without further testing
• Groups in blue boxes have a PTP of 15–65%. They could have an exercise ECG if feasible as the initial test. However, if local expertise and availability permit a noninvasive imaging-based test for ischemia this would be preferable given the superior diagnostic capabilities of such tests. In young patients radiation issues should be considered
• Groups in light red boxes have PTPs between 66 and 85% and hence should have a noninvasive imaging functional test for making a diagnosis of SCAD
• In groups in dark red boxes the PTP is >85% and one can assume that SCAD is present. They need risk stratification only
• Reproduced from Montalescot G et al. - 2013 ESC guidelines on the management of stable coronary artery disease. Eur Heart J 2013;34:2949–3003 with permission of the publisher

How to Select Patients for Noninvasive Stress Imaging?

- Irrespective of pretest probability, stress imaging has a higher diagnostic accuracy than the stress ECG. The main difference is the higher sensitivity of stress imaging.
- However, there is one caveat: the low sensitivity of the stress ECG was reported in studies compensating for referral bias (this is the effect of preferentially including patients with abnormal stress ECGs into angiographic verification studies and under-representation of patients with normal stress ECGs in such studies which leads to overestimation of sensitivity and underestimation of specificity) [7].
- In contrast to the stress ECG, some stress imaging studies may not be entirely free from referral bias (at least it is often not mentioned that referral bias was systematically excluded), which would also lead to overestimation of sensitivity of these tests at the cost of specificity.
- However, a recent cardiac magnetic resonance (CMR) study in which all patients irrespective of the result of CMR were rigorously also studied by coronary angiography (exclusion of referral bias) confirmed the high sensitivity of this imaging technique while specificity was maintained above 80% [8].
- Single-photon-emission computed tomography (SPECT) perfusion imaging which was used for comparison in this study showed a sensitivity of only 67% (still above the sensitivity of the stress ECG) but specificity was at 83% similar to CMR. The low sensitivity of SPECT in this study without referral bias would support the argument that some of the stress imaging studies reported somewhat too high sensitivity values.
- The higher sensitivity of stress imaging is the argument for selecting one of these diagnostic procedures in patients who have an intermediate to high pretest probability [1, 2]. If the probability of having a flow-limiting coronary stenosis is already high based on sex, age, and angina typicality a low-sensitivity technique would miss many patients who might profit from an invasive procedure.
- Other advantages of stress imaging as compared to the exercise ECG are the ability to quantify and localize areas of ischemia and the ability to provide diagnostic information even in the presence of resting ECG abnormalities.
- Another important clinical reason for selecting stress imaging is the high diagnostic accuracy of pharmacologic stress testing. This makes this form of stress imaging ideally suited for patients who are too old or physically incapable of performing physical stress up to an adequate level.
- However, exercise testing better reflects the physical capacities of the patient and higher levels of stress can be achieved in many patients when exercise is used to provoke ischemia. One also gets a better impression about the level of exercise that provokes angina in daily life plus additional information from the ECG that is always registered simultaneously.
- Therefore, exercise stress testing in combination with imaging is preferred (if possible) over pharmacological stress testing alone although the reported sensitivities and specificities are similar.
- Finally, stress imaging is the first choice in patients with previous percutaneous coronary intervention (PCI) or coronary artery bypass grafting (CABG), who often have preexisting ECG abnormalities and in whom the diagnosis of CAD is already known.
- On a more general note, the superior ability of stress imaging, compared with the exercise ECG, to localize and quantify ischemia also translates into more effective risk stratification, thus avoiding unnecessary invasive procedures [9]. This is why the 2013 ESC guidelines on the management of patients with stable coronary artery disease [1] recommend stress imaging as the first-line technique and the stress ECG only if imaging techniques are not available or too expensive.
- Stress imaging is also ideally suited to confirm or exclude ischemia in the perfusion bed of

angiographically seen intermediate coronary lesions (if fractional flow reserve—FFR—was not performed immediately). Ischemia associated with such lesions may be predictive of future events whereas the absence of ischemia can be used to define—and reassure—patients with a low cardiac risk [10].

Stress Imaging Versus Anatomic Imaging

- Noninvasive anatomic imaging of the coronary arteries has now become possible using advanced computed tomography (CT) technology [11]. The main advantages of coronary CT angiography are the following:
  - It has a superb capability of ruling out relevant CAD (sensitivity 98–99% [12]).
  - It can be quickly performed.
  - It provides additional information on the presence of coronary plaques which provides the indication for starting preventive medication [13].
- There are also downsides to the use of coronary CT angiography:
  - Specificity is not perfect and becomes rather low in patients who have a high pretest probability of disease [1]. The reason for this is that such patients frequently harbor coronary calcifications and these may lead to the false impression that the lumen is obstructed [14] (Fig. 3.1).
  - Coronary CT angiography exposes the patient to radiation and contrast media, which may be a problem in young patients, in the elderly, and those with renal dysfunction overall.
  - Coronary CT angiography does not provide adequate image quality in obese patients, those with irregular heart rhythms, or patients at a high heart rate (unless relatively high doses of radiation are applied). Table 3.2 lists factors to be considered when selecting patients for coronary CT angiography.

- Current guidelines still favor stress testing [2] (stress imaging [1]) over coronary CT angiography but this may soon change with the advent of the 2017 National Institute for Health and Care Excellence (NICE) guidelines on stable angina. Recent randomized data prove that outcomes are similar irrespective of whether functional or anatomic testing is the initial test in the workup of intermediate-risk patients with stable CHD [15]. However, patients in the CT arm had ICA more often and more revascularization procedures in this study [14].

Is CT Calcium Scoring Useful in Symptomatic Patients?

- The use of calcium scoring by CT in symptomatic patients has been intensely debated. A recent study in 868 patients with low- to intermediate-risk stable angina and a calcium score of zero showed ischemia in only 3% [16]. None of these patients had obstructive disease at angiography.
- This suggests that state-of-the-art calcium scoring which can be done at a very low radiation dose of 0.2 mSV should be performed before coronary CT angiography.
- This would allow skipping subsequent coronary CT angiography in 25% of patients and saving additional radiation [16].

Which Kind of Stress Imaging?

- There is no ideal stress imaging techniques suitable for all patients. Table 3.3 lists the advantages and disadvantages of the available techniques and Table 3.4 gives the values for sensitivity and specificity of these techniques as listed in the 2013 ESC guidelines on the management of stable coronary artery disease.
- The references on which the values in Table 3.4 are based can be found in the full text of the

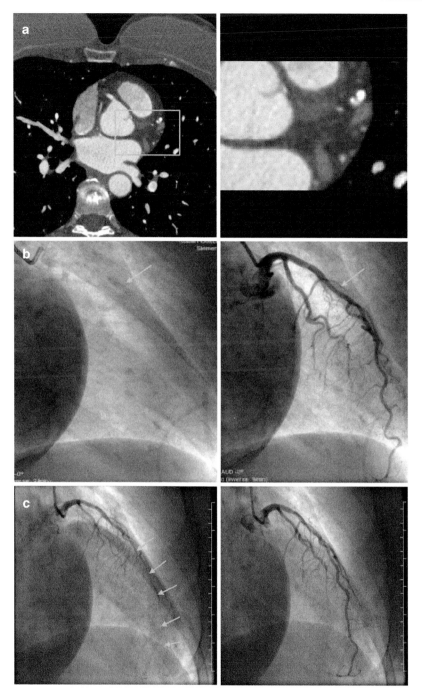

Fig. 3.1 Effect of a focal calcified plaque on the interpretation of coronary CT angiography examination. This 57-year-old woman had dyspnea when climbing three flights of stairs. She also had occasional mild resting chest pain. An exercise stress ECG was mildly abnormal (0.1 mV ST-segment depression). Her 64-line coronary CT angiogram showed focal calcification in the left anterior descending (LAD) coronary artery (Panel A with magnification inset) and was read as diagnostic of a significant stenosis in the LAD. Invasive coronary angiography was advised (Panel B). The grey shadow of linear calcification next to the LAD (yellow arrow) can be seen on the X-ray image without application of intracoronary contrast material (Panel B, left). It is evident that there is no LAD stenosis when contrast is injected (Panel B, right). Intracoronary acetylcholine testing (Panel C) demonstrated diffuse distal occlusive LAD spasm (left) associated with her usual chest oppression which, however, was now more intense. This indicates an enhanced reaction to the substance, which is often associated with clinical symptoms of microvascular dysfunction. LAD after intracoronary nitroglycerine is shown on the right (Panel C). Reproduced from Sechtem U et al. - Testing in patients with stable coronary artery disease – the debate continues. Circ J 2016;80:802–810 with permission of the publisher

Table 3.2 Patient factors considered important for optimal image quality of coronary CT angiography

No known CHD
Intermediate pretest probability up to 50%
Age <70 years
Regular heart rhythm
Low heart rate (e.g., <65 bpm), in some patients only after administration of beta-blockers
BMI <40 kg/m^2
Creatinine clearance >30 mL/kg/1.73 m^2
No known contrast allergy

BMI body mass index, *CHD* coronary heart disease, *CT* computed tomography

Table 3.3 Advantages and disadvantages of stress imaging techniques and coronary CT angiography

Technique	Advantages	Disadvantages
Echocardiography	Wide access	Echo contrast needed in patients with poor ultrasound windows
	Portability	
	No radiation	Dependent on operator skills
	Low cost	
SPECT	Wide access	Radiation
	Extensive data	
PET	Flow quantitation	Radiation
		Limited access
		High cost
CMR	High soft-tissue contrast including precise imaging of myocardial scar	Limited access in cardiology
		Contraindications
	No radiation	Functional analysis limited in arrhythmias
		Limited 3D quantification of ischemia
		High cost
Coronary CTA	High NPV in pts. with low PTP	Limited availability
		Radiation
		Assessment limited with extensive coronary calcification or previous stent implantation
		Image quality limited with arrhythmias and high heart rates that cannot be lowered beyond 60–65/min
		Low NPV in patients with high PTP

3D three-dimensional, *CMR*, cardiac magnetic resonance, *CTA* computed tomography angiography, *NPV* negative predictive value, *PET* positron-emission tomography, *PTP* pretest probability, *pts.* patients, *SPECT* single-photon-emission computed tomography

Reproduced from Montalescot G et al. - 2013 ESC guidelines on the management of stable coronary artery disease – web addenda to 2013 ESC guidelines under "Related Materials" http://www.escardio.org/Guidelines-&-Education/Clinical-Practice-Guidelines/Stable-Coronary-Artery-Disease-Management-of). With permission of the publisher

ESC guideline (in Table 12 of the guideline). It is obvious that the range of these values is very similar between stress echocardiography, stress SPECT, and stress CMR. Stress PET plays a minor role because this tech- nique is even less broadly available than stress CMR. The major players worldwide are stress echocardiography and stress SPECT.

- Stress echocardiography is the obvious choice for patients with adequate anatomy, as well as

Table 3.4 Characteristics of tests commonly used to diagnose the presence of coronary heart disease

	Diagnosis of CAD	
	Sensitivity (%)	Specificity (%)
Exercise ECG[a]	45–50	85–90
Exercise stress echocardiography	80–85	80–88
Exercise stress SPECT	73–92	63–87
Dobutamine stress echocardiography	79–83	82–86
Dobutamine stress MRI[b]	79–88	81–91
Vasodilator stress echocardiography	72–79	92–95
Vasodilator stress SPECT	90–91	75–84
Vasodilator stress MRI[b]	67–94	61–85
Coronary CTA[c]	95–99	64–83
Vasodilator stress PET	81–97	74–91

CAD coronary artery disease, *CTA* computed tomography angiography, *ECG* electrocardiogram, *MRI* magnetic resonance imaging, *PET* positron-emission tomography, *SPECT* single-photon-emission computed tomography
[a]Results without/with minimal referral bias
[b]Results obtained in populations with medium-to-high prevalence of disease without compensation for referral bias
[c]Results obtained in populations with low-to-medium prevalence of disease
Reproduced from Montalescot G et al. - 2013 ESC guidelines on the management of stable coronary artery disease. Eur Heart J 2013;34:2949–3003 with permission of the publisher

due to the availability of an experienced echocardiographer and sufficient space and manpower to perform this complex procedure in larger numbers of patients. This technique is cheap, does not expose the patient to ionizing radiation, and can be performed in many patients as an exercise stress test.

- However, interpretation of stress-induced wall motion abnormalities can be difficult, especially in the presence of preexisting wall motion abnormalities. Therefore, the use of contrast agents is advised when two or more contiguous segments in the 17 segment LV model are not well visualized at rest [17].
- The use of contrast during stress echocardiography not only enhances image quality, but also improves reader confidence and enhances accuracy for the detection of CHD.

- Myocardial perfusion scintigraphy (SPECT) is most commonly used in conjunction with technetium-99m radiopharmaceuticals as tracers. Symptom-limited physical exercise is the stress of choice.
- New SPECT cameras reduce radiation and/or acquisition times significantly [18]. In the US SPECT perfusion imaging is the most commonly used stress imaging modality whereas stress echocardiography is more prevalent in Europe. In the hands of experienced examiners both techniques yield similar results.
- Myocardial perfusion imaging using positron-emission tomography (PET) is superior to SPECT imaging for the detection of stable CHD in terms of image quality, interpretative certainty, and diagnostic accuracy [19]. It also has the unique ability to quantify blood flow in mL/min/g of myocardium, which allows detection of microvascular disease [20]. Nevertheless, PET scanners and especially cyclotron-produced radiotracers are more expensive than SPECT equipment, which limits their use in daily clinical practice.
- Stress CMR imaging is not performed with physical exercise but with pharmacological stress. If dobutamine is used as a stressor induction of wall motion abnormalities is the target. If adenosine is the stressor imbalances of perfusion are sought for.
- Stress CMR is an alternative to stress echocardiography in patients with suboptimal acoustic windows [21] or an alternative to stress SPECT for patients in whom radiation should be avoided [21].
- In a head-to-head comparison with SPECT, adenosine CMR was found to have a significantly better sensitivity in diagnosing obstructive coronary artery disease in women but specificities were similar for both techniques (both >80%) [22].

How Should Imaging Be Employed in a Patient with Suspected Stable Coronary Artery Disease?

- The guidelines of the ESC [1], the AHA guidelines [2], and the NICE guidelines [23] differ in their recommendations on the use of stress imaging in such patients. All three recommend stress testing in patients who have an intermediate pretest probability of obstructive disease.
- However, intermediate is defined in the NICE guidelines on "chest pain of recent onset" [23] as 10–90%, the ESC feel that the appropriate level is 15–85%, and the US guidelines set the level from 20 to 70%.
- All three guidelines recommend omitting testing in patients with a pretest probability below these levels. The reason is that the imperfect test characteristics of the main test employed (stress ECG, stress echocardiogram, stress SPECT) lead to a higher number of false positives than true positives at this low level of pretest probability.
- Guidelines differ in their recommendations on what to do with patients who have a pretest probability above the intermediate level. Whereas the ESC and the NICE guidelines consider the diagnosis of obstructive CHD is based just on the high pretest probability, further testing is recommended in the US guidelines. However, testing at such high pretest probabilities with the characteristics of the imperfect tests available may lead to more false negatives than true negatives with the obvious problem of underestimation of disease.
- Stress imaging is the preferred test mode in the ESC guidelines and the only recommended ischemia test in patients in the higher intermediate range of pretest probabilities. No differential recommendations are made with respect to the use of specific imaging techniques.
- In contrast to the ESC guidelines, the US guidelines restrict the use of stress imaging to patients whose resting ECG is not interpretable and those with a high pretest probability of obstructive CHD. They also favor stress echocardiography and stress SPECT over stress CMR.
- The US guidelines feel that coronary CT angiography is appropriate in patients with intermediate to high pretest probabilities.
- In contrast, the ESC guidelines advise specifically against the use of coronary CTA in patients with a pretest probability above 50% due to the frequent presence of severe calcifications.
- The only other patients in whom the US guidelines recommend coronary CT angiography are those who have contraindications to stress testing.
- In contrast, the ESC guidelines suggest coronary CT angiography as a second-line choice behind stress testing in patients with a pretest probability in the lower intermediate range. The ESC guidelines specifically add that coronary CT scans showing high global or focal calcifications should be read as "not interpretable" with respect to lesion quantification.
- The NICE guidelines chose to use cardiac CT calcium scoring as a first-line investigation in patients with a low pretest probability between 10 and 30%. In these patients, the NICE guideline advises that the absence of calcium makes obstructive CHD likely not the reason for the patient's symptoms.
- Intermediate calcium scores in these low pretest probability patients between 1 and 400 are recommended to be followed by coronary CT angiography whereas patients with high calcium scores (>400) are recommended to undergo ICA.
- Thus, the largest disparities among the three guidelines with respect to imaging for testing for the presence of obstructive CAD are in their recommendations pertaining to coronary CT.
- The flowchart of testing in patients with intermediate pretest probability as described in the ESC guidelines is shown in Fig. 3.2.

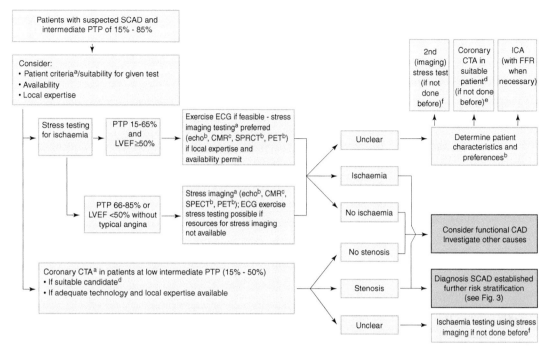

Fig. 3.2 Noninvasive testing in patients with suspected stable coronary artery disease (SCAD) and an intermediate pretest probability. *CAD* coronary artery disease, *CTA* computed tomography angiography, *CMR* cardiac magnetic resonance, *ECG* electrocardiogram, *ICA* invasive coronary angiography, *LVEF* left ventricular ejection fraction, *PET* positron-emission tomography, *PTP* pretest probability, *SCAD* stable coronary artery disease, *SPECT* single-photon-emission computed tomography. (1) Consider the age of patient versus radiation exposure. (2) In patients unable to exercise use echo or SPECT/PET with pharmacologic stress instead. (3) CMR is only performed using pharmacologic stress. (4) Patient characteristics should make a fully diagnostic coronary CTA scan highly probable. Consider result to be unclear in patients with severe diffuse or focal calcification. (5) Proceed as in lower left coronary CTA box. (6) Proceed as in stress testing for ischemia box. (7) It is not uncommon that the clinician could consider a stress test indeterminate or unclear as seen in the upper right-hand corner. In such a circumstance there are three possibilities and the decision on how to proceed further should be made together with the patient: it is justified to push for a diagnosis by using ICA but one needs to be careful to not fall victim to the oculostenotic reflex and perform PCI on any lesion of questionable significance but instead employ FFR measurements and only place a stent if this measurement is clearly abnormal. One may also switch from stress testing to coronary CT angiography in suitable patients. (8) Finally it is also a possibility to perform a second imaging stress test although this is conceptually the least attractive choice. On the other hand if the patient had coronary CT angiography as the first test and calcifications obscure the image to a degree that no judgement can be made to the degree of stenosis at this position then stress imaging is a valid potential second test (see lower right-hand corner). Reproduced from Montalescot G et al. - 2013 ESC guidelines on the management of stable coronary artery disease. Eur Heart J. 2013;34:2949–3003 with permission of the publisher

What to Do with the Result of Noninvasive Imaging Assessment?

- Improving symptoms in patients with obstructive coronary disease can be achieved by medication and/or coronary revascularization. The latter produces the desired result immediately. However, in the long term (3 years) both forms of therapy achieve similar symptomatic results (although there is approximately one-third of patients crossing over from the initially chosen medical arm to the revascularization arm) [24].

Table 3.5 Definitions of risk for various test modalities

Exercise stress ECG[a]	High risk	CV mortality >3%/year
	Intermediate risk	CV mortality between 1 and 3%/year
	Low risk	CV mortality <1%/year
Ischemia imaging	High risk	Area of ischemia >10% (>10% for SPECT; limited quantitative data for CMR—probably ≥2/16 segments with new perfusion defects or ≥3 dobutamine-induced dysfunctional segments; ≥3 segments of LV by stress echo)
	Intermediate risk	Area of ischemia between 1 and 10% or any ischemia less than high risk by CMR or stress echo
	Low risk	No ischemia
Coronary CTA[b]	High risk	Significant lesions of high-risk category (three-vessel disease with proximal stenoses, LM, and proximal anterior descending CAD)
	Intermediate rick	Significant lesion(s) in large and proximal coronary artery(ies) but not high-risk category
	Low risk	Normal coronary artery or plaques only

CAD coronary artery disease, *CMR* cardiac magnetic resonance, *CTA* computed tomography angiography, *CV* cardiovascular, *ECG* electrocardiogram, *ICA* invasive coronary angiography, *LM* left main, *PTP* pretest probability, *SPECT* single-photon-emission computed tomography

[a] From nomogram (see web addenda of the 2013 ESC guidelines on the management of stable coronary artery disease, Figure W1) or http://www.cardiology.org/tools/medcalc/duke/

[b] See Fig. 3.2; consider possible overestimation of the presence of significant multivessel disease by coronary CTA in patients with high intermediate PTP (≥50%) and/or severe diffuse or focal coronary calcifications and consider performing additional stress testing in patients without severe symptoms before ICA

Reproduced from Montalescot G et al. - 2013 ESC guidelines on the management of stable coronary artery disease. Eur Heart J 2013;34:2949–3003 with permission of the publisher

- Thus, it is largely the choice of the patient and the physician whether to choose drugs or revascularization when it comes to improvement of symptoms.
- The matter is more complicated when it comes to improvement of prognosis. However, in the absence of randomized data results from registries indicate that larger extents of ischemia or severe proximal coronary obstructions are required functionally or anatomically in order to demonstrate positive prognostic effects of revascularization [25, 26]. Death rates in patients with such large areas of ischemia or such severe proximal coronary obstructions, receiving previously suboptimal medical treatment in the 1980s and 1990s, were more than 3% annually. Only in these patients it could be shown that revascularization may improve prognosis [25, 26].
- The ESC guidelines indicate how the results of stress testing and coronary CT angiography can be translated into risk groups with different annual mortalities (Table 3.5). Consequently, they recommend revascularization for prognostic purposes only in those in the highest risk group but an invasive strategy can be chosen by the patient and the physician in patients in the intermediate-risk group (Fig. 3.3).

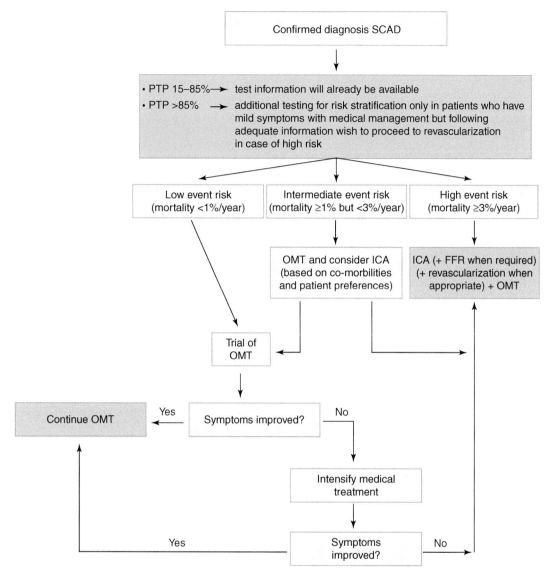

Fig. 3.3 Management based on risk determination for prognosis in patients with chest pain and suspected SCAD (for choice of test see Fig. 3.2, for definitions of event risk see Table 3.5). *ICA* invasive coronary angiography, *OMT* optimal medical therapy, *PTP* pretest probability, *SCAD* stable coronary artery disease. Reproduced from Montalescot G et al. - 2013 ESC guidelines on the management of stable coronary artery disease. Eur Heart J 2013;34:2949–3003 with permission of the publisher

Critique of Imaging in Patients with Suspected CHD

- The recent PROMISE trial randomized patients with an intermediate mean pretest probability of 50% (according to the Diamond-Forrester tables) to stress imaging or coronary CT angiography [15]. In both arms pathology was only found in about 10% of patients despite the expectation (based on pretest probability) that 50% of those should have either ischemia or anatomic stenosis. Moreover, only about 2% of these patients in both arms experienced hard events (death or myocardial infarction) during a follow-up of 2 years.
- Other findings of a similar kind [27] led to concerns about over-testing in patients with chest pain especially with respect to inappropriate use and overuse of imaging techniques [28].
- Patients who are unlikely to have high-risk CAD, clinical events, or revascularization will derive minimal benefit and value from noninvasive testing. Efforts are made to design clinical tools in order to identify such minimal risk patients for whom deferred testing may be considered [29].

Conclusion

- Preselection of patients with chest pain who are likely to derive any benefit from an invasive management strategy is highly desirable in order to avoid even more invasive coronary angiograms showing the absence of stenoses.
- The purpose of excluding relevant CHD is most elegantly served by coronary CT angiography but this approach might also lead to some overuse of imaging (if employed in patients with very low pretest probabilities).
- Stress imaging techniques are most useful in patients with known diffuse CAD in whom a normal stress test confers a good prognosis.
- In patients with an abnormal stress test who are sent to invasive coronary angiography, the angiographer has some important clues as to where to direct special attention.

Reproduced from Montalescot G et al. - 2013 ESC guidelines on the management of stable coronary artery disease. Eur Heart J 2013;34:2949–3003 with permission of the publisher.

References

1. Task Force M, Montalescot G, Sechtem U, Achenbach S, Andreotti F, Arden C, Budaj A, Bugiardini R, Crea F, Cuisset T, Di Mario C, Ferreira JR, Gersh BJ, Gitt AK, Hulot JS, Marx N, Opie LH, Pfisterer M, Prescott E, Ruschitzka F, Sabate M, Senior R, Taggart DP, van der Wall EE, Vrints CJ, Guidelines ESCCP, Zamorano JL, Achenbach S, Baumgartner H, Bax JJ, Bueno H, Dean V, Deaton C, Erol C, Fagard R, Ferrari R, Hasdai D, Hoes AW, Kirchhof P, Knuuti J, Kolh P, Lancellotti P, Linhart A, Nihoyannopoulos P, Piepoli MF, Ponikowski P, Sirnes PA, Tamargo JL, Tendera M, Torbicki A, Wijns W, Windecker S, Document R, Knuuti J, Valgimigli M, Bueno H, Claeys MJ, Donner-Banzhoff N, Erol C, Frank H, Funck-Brentano C, Gaemperli O, Gonzalez-Juanatey JR, Hamilos M, Hasdai D, Husted S, James SK, Kervinen K, Kolh P, Kristensen SD, Lancellotti P, Maggioni AP, Piepoli MF, Pries AR, Romeo F, Ryden L, Simoons ML, Sirnes PA, Steg PG, Timmis A, Wijns W, Windecker S, Yildirir A, Zamorano JL. ESC guidelines on the management of stable coronary artery disease: the task force on the management of stable coronary artery disease of the European Society of Cardiology. Eur Heart J. 2013;34:2949–3003.
2. Fihn SD, Gardin JM, Abrams J, Berra K, Blankenship JC, Dallas AP, Douglas PS, Foody JM, Gerber TC, Hinderliter AL, King SB 3rd, Kligfield PD, Krumholz HM, Kwong RY, Lim MJ, Linderbaum JA, Mack MJ, Munger MA, Prager RL, Sabik JF, Shaw LJ, Sikkema JD, Smith CR, Jr SSC Jr, Spertus JA, Williams SV, American College of Cardiology F, American Heart Association Task Force on Practice G, American College of P, American Association for Thoracic S, Preventive Cardiovascular Nurses A, Society for Cardiovascular A, Interventions, Society of Thoracic S. 2012 ACCF/AHA/ACP/AATS/PCNA/SCAI/STS guideline for the diagnosis and management of patients with stable ischemic heart disease: a report of the American College of Cardiology Foundation/American Heart Association Task Force on Practice Guidelines, and the American College of Physicians, American Association for Thoracic Surgery, Preventive Cardiovascular Nurses Association, Society for Cardiovascular Angiography and Interventions, and Society of Thoracic Surgeons. J Am Coll Cardiol. 2012;60:e44–e164.
3. Fihn SD, Blankenship JC, Alexander KP, Bittl JA, Byrne JG, Fletcher BJ, Fonarow GC, Lange RA,

Levine GN, Maddox TM, Naidu SS, Ohman EM, Smith PK. 2014 ACC/AHA/AATS/PCNA/SCAI/STS focused update of the guideline for the diagnosis and management of patients with stable ischemic heart disease: a report of the American College of Cardiology/American Heart Association Task Force on Practice Guidelines, and the American Association for Thoracic Surgery, Preventive Cardiovascular Nurses Association, Society for Cardiovascular Angiography and Interventions, and Society of Thoracic Surgeons. J Am Coll Cardiol. 2014;64:1929–49.

4. Roffi M, Patrono C, Collet JP, Mueller C, Valgimigli M, Andreotti F, Bax JJ, Borger MA, Brotons C, Chew DP, Gencer B, Hasenfuss G, Kjeldsen K, Lancellotti P, Landmesser U, Mehilli J, Mukherjee D, Storey RF, Windecker S, Baumgartner H, Gaemperli O, Achenbach S, Agewall S, Badimon L, Baigent C, Bueno H, Bugiardini R, Carerj S, Casselman F, Cuisset T, Erol C, Fitzsimons D, Halle M, Hamm C, Hildick-Smith D, Huber K, Iliodromitis E, James S, Lewis BS, Lip GY, Piepoli MF, Richter D, Rosemann T, Sechtem U, Steg PG, Vrints C, Luis Zamorano J. 2015 ESC guidelines for the management of acute coronary syndromes in patients presenting without persistent ST-segment elevation: Task Force for the Management of Acute Coronary Syndromes in Patients Presenting without Persistent ST-Segment Elevation of the European Society of Cardiology (ESC). Eur Heart J. 2016;37:267–315.

5. Amsterdam EA, Wenger NK, Brindis RG, Casey DE, Jr GTG, Holmes DR, Jr JAS, Jneid H, Kelly RF, Kontos MC, Levine GN, Liebson PR, Mukherjee D, Peterson ED, Sabatine MS, Smalling RW, Zieman SJ, American College of C, American Heart Association Task Force on Practice G, Society for Cardiovascular A, Interventions, Society of Thoracic S, American Association for Clinical C. 2014 AHA/ACC Guideline for the Management of Patients with Non-ST-Elevation Acute Coronary Syndromes: a report of the American College of Cardiology/American Heart Association Task Force on Practice Guidelines. J Am Coll Cardiol. 2014;64:e139–228.

6. Mark DB, Shaw L, Harrell FE Jr, Hlatky MA, Lee KL, Bengtson JR, McCants CB, Califf RM, Pryor DB. Prognostic value of a treadmill exercise score in outpatients with suspected coronary artery disease. N Engl J Med. 1991;325:849–53.

7. Ladapo JA, Blecker S, Elashoff MR, Federspiel JJ, Vieira DL, Sharma G, Monane M, Rosenberg S, Phelps CE, Douglas PS. Clinical implications of referral bias in the diagnostic performance of exercise testing for coronary artery disease. J Am Heart Assoc. 2013;2:e000505.

8. Greenwood JP, Maredia N, Younger JF, Brown JM, Nixon J, Everett CC, Bijsterveld P, Ridgway JP, Radjenovic A, Dickinson CJ, Ball SG, Plein S. Cardiovascular magnetic resonance and single-photon emission computed tomography for diagnosis of coronary heart disease (CE-MARC): a prospective trial. Lancet. 2012;379:453–60.

9. Chelliah R, Anantharam B, Burden L, Alhajiri A, Senior R. Independent and incremental value of stress echocardiography over clinical and stress electro-cardiographic parameters for the prediction of hard cardiac events in new-onset suspected angina with no history of coronary artery disease. Eur J Echocardiogr. 2010;11:875–82.

10. Hachamovitch R, Rozanski A, Shaw LJ, Stone GW, Thomson LE, Friedman JD, Hayes SW, Cohen I, Germano G, Berman DS. Impact of ischaemia and scar on the therapeutic benefit derived from myocardial revascularization vs. medical therapy among patients undergoing stress-rest myocardial perfusion scintigraphy. Eur Heart J. 2011;32:1012–24.

11. Bittencourt MS, Hulten EA, Veeranna V, Blankstein R. Coronary computed tomography angiography in the evaluation of chest pain of suspected cardiac origin. Circulation. 2016;133:1963–8.

12. Nielsen LH, Ortner N, Norgaard BL, Achenbach S, Leipsic J, Abdulla J. The diagnostic accuracy and outcomes after coronary computed tomography angiography vs. conventional functional testing in patients with stable angina pectoris: a systematic review and meta-analysis. Eur Heart J Cardiovasc Imaging. 2014;15:961–71.

13. Piepoli MF, Hoes AW, Agewall S, Albus C, Brotons C, Catapano AL, Cooney MT, Corra U, Cosyns B, Deaton C, Graham I, Hall MS, Hobbs FD, Lochen ML, Lollgen H, Marques-Vidal P, Perk J, Prescott E, Redon J, Richter DJ, Sattar N, Smulders Y, Tiberi M, van der Worp HB, van Dis I, Verschuren WM, Authors/Task Force M. European guidelines on cardiovascular disease prevention in clinical practice: The Sixth Joint Task Force of the European Society of Cardiology and Other Societies on Cardiovascular Disease Prevention in Clinical Practice (constituted by representatives of 10 societies and by invited experts) Developed with the special contribution of the European Association for Cardiovascular Prevention & Rehabilitation (EACPR). Eur Heart J. 2016;37:2315–81.

14. Schmidt T, Maag R, Foy AJ. Overdiagnosis of coronary artery disease detected by coronary computed tomography angiography: a teachable moment. JAMA Intern Med. 2016;176:1747–8.

15. Douglas PS, Hoffmann U, Patel MR, Mark DB, Al-Khalidi HR, Cavanaugh B, Cole J, Dolor RJ, Fordyce CB, Huang M, Khan MA, Kosinski AS, Krucoff MW, Malhotra V, Picard MH, Udelson JE, Velazquez EJ, Yow E, Cooper LS, Lee KL, Investigators P. Outcomes of anatomical versus functional testing for coronary artery disease. N Engl J Med. 2015;372:1291–300.

16. Mouden M, Timmer JR, Reiffers S, Oostdijk AH, Knollema S, Ottervanger JP, Jager PL. Coronary artery calcium scoring to exclude flow-limiting coronary artery disease in symptomatic stable patients at low or intermediate risk. Radiology. 2013;269:77–83.

17. Senior R, Becher H, Monaghan M, Agati L, Zamorano J, Vanoverschelde JL, Nihoyannopoulos P. Contrast echocardiography: evidence-based recommendations

by European Association of Echocardiography. Eur J Echocardiogr. 2009;10:194–212.

18. Imbert L, Poussier S, Franken PR, Songy B, Verger A, Morel O, Wolf D, Noel A, Karcher G, Marie PY. Compared performance of high-sensitivity cameras dedicated to myocardial perfusion SPECT: a comprehensive analysis of phantom and human images. J Nucl Med. 2012;53:1897–903.

19. Bateman TM, Heller GV, McGhie AI, Friedman JD, Case JA, Bryngelson JR, Hertenstein GK, Moutray KL, Reid K, Cullom SJ. Diagnostic accuracy of rest/stress ECG-gated Rb-82 myocardial perfusion PET: comparison with ECG-gated Tc-99m sestamibi SPECT. J Nucl Cardiol. 2006;13:24–33.

20. Taqueti VR, Shaw LJ, Cook NR, Murthy VL, Shah NR, Foster CR, Hainer J, Blankstein R, Dorbala S, Di Carli MF. Excess cardiovascular risk in women relative to men referred for coronary angiography is associated with severely impaired coronary flow reserve, not obstructive disease. Circulation. 2017;135(6):566–77.

21. Al Sayari S, Kopp S, Bremerich J. Stress cardiac MR imaging: the role of stress functional assessment and perfusion imaging in the evaluation of ischemic heart disease. Radiol Clin North Am. 2015;53: 355–67.

22. Greenwood JP, Motwani M, Maredia N, Brown JM, Everett CC, Nixon J, Bijsterveld P, Dickinson CJ, Ball SG, Plein S. Comparison of cardiovascular magnetic resonance and single-photon emission computed tomography in women with suspected coronary artery disease from the clinical evaluation of magnetic resonance imaging in coronary heart disease (CE-MARC) trial. Circulation. 2014;129:1129–38.

23. National Institute for Health and Clinical Excellence. Chest pain of recent onset. (Clinical guideline 95). http://guidance.nice.org.uk/CG95 and http://www.nice.org.uk/guidance/CG95. 2010.

24. Weintraub WS, Spertus JA, Kolm P, Maron DJ, Zhang Z, Jurkovitz C, Zhang W, Hartigan PM, Lewis C, Veledar E, Bowen J, Dunbar SB, Deaton C, Kaufman S, O'Rourke RA, Goeree R, Barnett PG, Teo KK, Boden WE, Group CTR, Mancini GB. Effect of PCI on quality of life in patients with stable coronary disease. N Engl J Med. 2008;359:677–87.

25. Hachamovitch R, Hayes SW, Friedman JD, Cohen I, Berman DS. Comparison of the short-term survival benefit associated with revascularization compared with medical therapy in patients with no prior coronary artery disease undergoing stress myocardial perfusion single photon emission computed tomography. Circulation. 2003;107:2900–7.

26. Mark DB, Nelson CL, Califf RM, Harrell FE Jr, Lee KL, Jones RH, Fortin DF, Stack RS, Glower DD, Smith LR, et al. Continuing evolution of therapy for coronary artery disease. Initial results from the era of coronary angioplasty. Circulation. 1994;89:2015–25.

27. Rozanski A, Gransar H, Hayes SW, Min J, Friedman JD, Thomson LE, Berman DS. Temporal trends in the frequency of inducible myocardial ischemia during cardiac stress testing: 1991 to 2009. J Am Coll Cardiol. 2013;61:1054–65.

28. Ladapo JA, Blecker S, Douglas PS. Physician decision making and trends in the use of cardiac stress testing in the United States: an analysis of repeated cross-sectional data. Ann Intern Med. 2014;161: 482–90.

29. Fordyce CB, Douglas PS, Roberts RS, Hoffmann U, Al-Khalidi HR, Patel MR, Granger CB, Kostis J, Mark DB, Lee KL, Udelson JE, Prospective Multicenter Imaging Study for Evaluation of Chest Pain I. Identification of patients with stable chest pain deriving minimal value from noninvasive testing: the PROMISE minimal-risk tool, a secondary analysis of a randomized clinical trial. JAMA Cardiol. 2017;2(4):400–8.

Left Heart Catheterization

4

Satpal Arri and Brian Clapp

About Us The authors are based at St Thomas' Hospital in London. This is a busy tertiary surgical center providing a primary angioplasty service to its local residents in central and south east London. The unit has an interest in complex coronary intervention and a thriving structural heart disease program. The department also has an internationally recognized productive research team with a particular interest in coronary physiology.

Introduction

The selective injection of contrast media into the right coronary artery of a middle-aged male by Mason Sones on October 30, 1958, introduced a new era in cardiovascular medicine that was to revolutionize our understanding and management of coronary disease. Two radiologists, Judkins and Amplatz, later used the Seldinger technique to gain access to the femoral artery. Independently, they designed pre-formed catheters, allowing easier intubation of the left and right coronary arteries as well as facilitating access to the left ventricle. This subsequently

S. Arri · B. Clapp (✉)
Cardiothoracic Centre, St Thomas' Hospital, Guy's and St Thomas' Hospitals NHS Foundation Trust, London, UK
e-mail: brian.clapp@gstt.nhs.uk

enabled the widespread dispersion of angiography as a diagnostic technique throughout the cardiology and radiology communities.

Noninvasive Investigations Prior to Coronary Angiography

- In patients with stable symptoms, noninvasive testing can enhance the pretest probability of finding significant coronary stenosis at the time of angiography and also provides important functional information on the extent and anatomical location of myocardial ischemia, which may guide future revascularization strategies.
- These include exercise treadmill testing (ETT), stress echocardiography, nuclear perfusion imaging, cardiac MRI, and cardiac CT.

Indications for Coronary Angiography (See Tables 4.1, 4.2, and 4.3)

- Coronary angiography is a prerequisite for coronary revascularization, and assists in clarification of cases with diagnostic uncertainty following noninvasive testing and in the assessment of other forms of cardiac disease such as valve disease or cardiomyopathy.

Table 4.1 Indications for coronary angiography

°•°Canadian cardiovascular society class III or IV angina on medical therapy
°•°High-risk criteria on noninvasive assessment
°•°Return of spontaneous circulation following cardiac arrest/pulseless ventricular tachycardia
°•°Acute coronary syndrome
°•°ST-elevation myocardial infarction—primary percutaneous coronary intervention
°•°Cardiogenic shock patients who may be candidates for revascularization
°•°Persistent hemodynamic and/or electrical instability
°•°Prior to valve surgery
°•°Unexplained cardiac arrest
°•°Prior to surgical correction of congenital heart disease
°•°Prior to cardiac transplantation

Table 4.2 Relative contraindications to coronary angiography

°•°Coagulopathy or formal anticoagulation—consider radial approach
°•°Decompensated congestive heart failure
°•°Uncontrolled hypertension
°•°Pregnancy
°•°Inability for patient cooperation
°•°Active infection
°•°Renal failure
°•°Severe contrast allergy

Table 4.3 The coronary angiogram checklist

Has consent been obtained?	
Relevant comorbidities	°•°Diabetes mellitus—last BM? °•°Renal impairment—consider IV fluids °•°Peripheral vascular disease—consider radial approach °•°Previous stroke? °•°Previous CABG—graft details, previous operation note
Recent bloods	°•°Hemoglobin °•°Platelets °•°Clotting studies °•°Renal profile
Allergies?	Consider hydrocortisone ± antihistamine for previous contrast allergy
Medications	Current anti-anginal therapy?
Dual-antiplatelet therapy (DAPT)	°•°Any bleeding issues or coagulopathy? °•°Has the patient been loaded on DAPT? °•°Any contraindications to long-term DAPT?
Height and weight	Will influence catheter selection and heparin dose
Good pulse?	Radial/femoral/ulnar Allen's test for radial access
Previous study?	°•°Previous catheters used? °•°Previous problems encountered? °•°Previous access used? °•°Previous angioplasty details?
Previous echocardiogram?	°•°What is the LV systolic function? °•°Any regional wall motion abnormality? °•°Valvular disease? °•°Dilated aortic root—will influence catheter selection
Does the patient require sedation?	Consider for all radial procedures to minimize spasm
Timeout	°•°Ensure that all staff involved are aware of the patient history, indication of procedure, comorbidity, and planned strategy °•°World Health Organization checklist
Is the team present?	An operator—to perform the procedure A cath lab nurse—to administer drugs and collect/hand over equipment A scrubbed assistant to the operator A radiographer—responsible for fluoroscopic equipment A physiologist—responsible for monitoring the ECG and cardiac pressures

- Given the small, but significant, risks and radiation exposure of diagnostic angiography careful patient selection is essential.
- Formal clinical assessment is the first and most important step in assessing patients with suspected ischemic heart disease. This includes a detailed clinical history incorporating evaluation of risk factors, thorough examination and baseline investigations including relevant blood tests (full blood count, renal profile, fasting glucose, cholesterol, and HbA1c), and an ECG.
- The sensitivity and specificity of all subsequent investigations depend on the pretest probability of coronary disease established during this process. This assessment is also key in obtaining crucial data on relevant comorbidities that may alter the safety of subsequent coronary angiography.

The Coronary Angiography Checklist

There are a number of essential patient and procedural factors to consider prior to coronary angiography. **The most important is a relevant indication for the procedure to be performed.** The remainder of the checklist can be seen in Table 4.3.

Informed Consent and Complications

- Invasive coronary angiography is not without risk although with improving technique, experience, and equipment the risk of major complications is generally quoted as less than 1 in 1000.
- The most common complication is vascular injury and bleeding that occurs in 1–2% of cases and is more common with femoral angiography compared to radial.
- Important complications that should be covered during the consenting process include contrast allergy, arrhythmia, stroke, myocardial infarction, renal impairment, radiation

injury, bleeding, vascular complication, pericardiocentesis, need for emergency coronary bypass surgery, and mortality.

Coronary Angiography via the Right Radial Artery

- The right radial artery is now the default for most contemporary operators.
- Radial coronary angiography is associated with fewer vascular and bleeding complications as well as being more comfortable for patients. Patients are able to mobilize much sooner and many units now have dedicated radial lounges.
- The left radial approach also allows easier intubation of the left internal mammary artery (LIMA) in patients with a history of previous coronary artery bypass graft (CABG) surgery.
- Access is achieved using the Seldinger technique. Following puncture with a cannula, a guide wire is passed into the artery and advanced smoothly with or without fluoroscopic guidance.
- The needle is then removed and an arterial sheath of appropriate caliber is passed over the guide wire into the arterial lumen. Finally the guide wire is withdrawn and the sheath left in position.
- For diagnostic coronary angiography, 4, 5, or 6 French diameter catheters are commonly used (1 French = 1/3 mm).
- More complex coronary intervention may require larger diameter catheters (and hence larger sheaths). Specialist hydrophilic sheaths are also now available specifically for radial access.
- Given its relatively smaller size the radial artery is susceptible to spasm. Measures to reduce the risk of spasm include adequate hydration with intravenous fluids, light sedation, and administration of intra-arterial nitrates and/or verapamil.
- When performing coronary angiography via the radial artery patients also require 2500–5000 units of heparin in order to prevent radial artery thrombosis. This can be administered

via the radial sheath or via a diagnostic catheter into the aortic root.

- Once access is gained a standard 0.38-in. 150 cm J-tipped guide wire is passed into the ascending aorta. The catheter is then passed onto the guide wire and both catheter and wire are advanced under fluoroscopic screening until the guide tip is positioned in the ascending aorta.

- The wire position is then fixed to prevent further movement and the catheter advanced over its tip. Once in the ascending aorta, the guide wire is removed and the catheter allowed to bleed back to remove any air, thrombus, or atherosclerotic debris.

- When approaching the aortic arch from the right radial artery the guide wire may select the descending aorta. In this situation using the curve of the diagnostic catheter to help direct the guide wire usually allows passage of the wire into the ascending aorta.

- Asking the patient to take a deep breath in and hold also helps in straightening the vasculature allowing the guide wire to pass down to the aortic root.

- Coronary angiography via the radial artery can be technically challenging due to the greater tortuosity that needs to be negotiated as the catheter is passed from the wrist to the aortic root.

- Significant vessel tortuosity can hinder advancement and this is usually detected by resistance to free guide wire manipulation. In this situation direct fluoroscopy is essential in identifying the position of the wire tip and excluding vessel dissection.

- Careful passage of the catheter to the point of resistance with subsequent contrast injection may allow visualization of the arterial lumen and identification of the cause of obstruction.

- Often but not always this can be overcome with the use of a hydrophilic wire such as the Terumo wire.

- It should be noted, however, that significant tortuosity can make manipulating and torqueing the catheter more difficult and sometimes transferring to femoral access is necessary.

- Following challenging guide wire passage into the aortic root, a longer (260 cm) "exchange" wire should be used during subsequent catheter exchanges.

- The extra length allows the tip of the wire to be fixed in the aortic root during catheter exchanges, thus preventing repeated guide wire passage and potential injury through difficult or diseased areas of the peripheral arterial system as well as reducing the risk of radial artery spasm.

- Once in the ascending aorta, the guide wire is removed and the catheter allowed to bleed back to remove any air, thrombus, or atherosclerotic debris.

- The catheter is then connected to the manifold assembly that is connected to a pressure transducer allowing continuous central pressure monitoring. Once connected a few milliliters of blood should be aspirated back into the manifold prior to flushing the catheter to ensure an air-free system (Fig. 4.1).

- The catheter should then be filled with 3–4 mL of contrast and advanced to intubate the coronary system.

- Many operators would advocate assessing the right coronary artery first when performing radial angiography. This is because right coronary catheters have less curve and so are less traumatic to the radial artery compared to left catheters, thus potentially reducing the risk of radial artery spam.

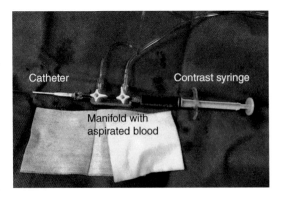

Fig. 4.1 Ensure that a few milliliters of blood are aspirated back from the catheter into the manifold prior to flushing to ensure an air-free system

- The right coronary artery should be engaged in the left anterior oblique (LAO) projection while the left coronary system should be engaged in the PA (posteroanterior) or LAO projection.
- Once at the coronary ostium operators must be diligent in ensuring that there is no ventricularization or damping of the pressure prior to a small contrast injection of 2–3 mL.
- Coronary angiography should be performed in standard views in orthogonal planes to appreciate the anatomy, visualize lesions, and serve as a road map for future revascularization or intervention.
- Non-standard views should be considered based on coronary anatomy, lesion location, and patient body habitus.
- At the end of the procedure the diagnostic catheter should be removed over the J-tipped guide wire to straighten out the curve on the catheter and thus minimize the risk of vascular injury.
- A number of devices including the TR band or Helix device can be used to achieve hemostasis once the radial sheath is removed.

Coronary Angiography via the Right Femoral Artery

- Technically easier as there are fewer bends to negotiate when advancing the catheter to the aortic root.
- Furthermore, the majority of diagnostic catheters were designed to intubate the coronary arteries from the femoral artery. In patients with a history of previous CABG, the left internal mammary artery can be intubated more easily from the femoral approach if the left radial is not directly accessed.
- The larger femoral artery is, however, associated with a greater risk of vascular injury and bleeding complications and the femoral artery should therefore be avoided in patients who are anticoagulated.
- Femoral access is achieved using the Seldinger technique as described above. Being a larger

artery the femoral artery can accommodate larger 7F and 8F sheaths that may be required for complex coronary intervention.
- Vascular complications include hematoma, pseudoaneurysm, and retroperitoneal bleeding. The femoral puncture should ideally be at the mid point of the femoral head above the femoral artery bifurcation. Usually puncture should be made 1–2 cm above the inguinal crease although we would advocate screening the groin first using an overlying metallic object such as a blade, scalpel, or scissors (see also Chap. 5).
- One should also consider real-time ultrasound-guided vascular puncture especially when introducing larger sheaths for complex interventions.
- Following vascular access a femoral angiogram should be performed by injecting contrast directly into the side arm of the sheath. This not only confirms the position of the puncture and the appropriateness of vascular closure devices at the end of the procedure, but also excludes any significant vascular complication that may have arisen.
- If the patient then becomes hypotensive during the case, at least most femoral complications have already been excluded as a potential cause with the exception of a retroperitoneal bleed.
- Once access is gained and position of the puncture and sheath confirmed, a standard 0.38-in. 150 cm J-tipped guide wire is passed into the descending aorta.
- The catheter is then passed onto the guide wire and both catheter and wire are advanced under fluoroscopic screening until the guide tip is positioned in the ascending aorta. The wire position is then fixed to prevent further movement and the catheter advanced over its tip. Once in the ascending aorta, the guide wire is removed and the catheter allowed to bleed back to remove any air, thrombus, or atherosclerotic debris.
- Passage of the guide wire within the aorta may be difficult. From the femoral route, iliofemoral atheroma or tortuosity may hinder advance-

ment and this may be detected by resistance to free guide wire manipulation. In this situation direct fluoroscopy is essential in identifying the position of the wire tip. Careful passage of the catheter to the point of resistance with subsequent contrast injection may allow visualization of the arterial lumen and identification of the cause of obstruction.

- Switching to a hydrophilic (e.g., Terumo) wire may help. For atheroma or tortuosity within the iliac system, a long sheath may be useful in protecting and straightening the area and improving catheter torque.
- Following challenging guide wire passage into the aortic root, a longer (260 cm) "exchange" wire may be used during subsequent catheter exchanges. The extra length allows the tip of the wire to be fixed in the aortic root during catheter exchanges, thus preventing repeated guide wire passage and potential injury through difficult or diseased areas of the peripheral arterial system.
- Once in the ascending aorta, the guide wire is removed and the catheter allowed to bleed back to remove any air, thrombus, or atherosclerotic debris.
- The catheter is then connected to the manifold assembly that is connected to a pressure transducer allowing continuous central pressure monitoring. Once connected a few milliliters of blood should be aspirated back into the manifold prior to flushing the catheter to ensure an air-free system (Fig. 4.1). The catheter should then be filled with 3–4 mL of contrast and advanced to intubate the coronary system.
- In stable patients it is routine practice to visualize the left coronary system first when performing femoral angiography.
- The left coronary artery should be engaged in the PA or LAO projection while the right coronary system should be engaged in the LAO projection. Following intubation of the coronary ostium operators must be diligent in ensuring that there is no ventricularization or

damping of pressure prior to a small contrast injection of 2–3 mL.

- Coronary angiography should be performed in standard views in orthogonal planes to appreciate the anatomy, visualize lesions, and serve as a road map for PCI. Nonstandard views should be considered based on coronary anatomy, lesion location, and patient body habitus.
- At the end of the procedure the diagnostic catheter should be removed over the J-tipped guide wire to straighten out the curve on the catheter and thus minimize the risk of vascular injury.
- Hemostasis can be achieved with a number of vascular closure devices such as the AngioSeal or Proglide. If these devices are contraindicated due to the position of the puncture then manual pressure is required.

Monitoring During Angiography

- During coronary angiography there should be continuous monitoring of the electrocardiogram, peripheral oxygen saturations, and invasive blood pressure—transduced from the fluid-filled catheter (Fig. 4.2).
- Full resuscitation facilities should be readily available, ideally with access to mechanical circulatory support devices if needed.

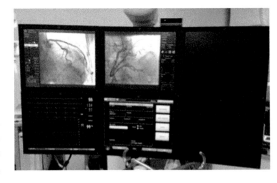

Fig. 4.2 Cardiorespiratory monitoring alongside radiographic images during coronary angiography

Catheter Selection

- Catheters usually have two curves: the primary distal curve and a secondary proximal curve. The distance between the two curves is the length of the catheter.
- Generally shorter curves are more ideal for superior takeoffs while longer curves are better for inferior takeoffs.
- Important considerations when selecting a catheter include the access site. For example a Judkins Left size 4 would be a standard choice for the left coronary system when approaching via the femoral artery whereas many operators would prefer a Judkins Left 3.5 if performing radial coronary angiography.
- The diameter of the aortic root may also influence the catheter selection—larger roots are likely to require a JL5 or larger.

Catheters for the Left Coronary System

- Engagement of the left coronary ostium is usually performed in the PA or LAO projection. The most common catheters used are the Judkins Left (usually JL4) catheters (Fig. 4.3). Larger aortic roots may require a broader hooked section at the catheter tip and alternatives include the Amplatz catheters.

Catheters for the Right Coronary System

- Engagement of the right coronary system is usually performed in the LAO projection. Once the catheter is located in the aortic root, gentle clockwise rotation is used to engage the ostium. The Judkins Right is a common first choice with the Williams (3DRC) catheter a popular alternative (Fig. 4.4).

Catheters for Saphenous Vein Grafts

- Location of vein graft ostia varies with surgical technique and aortic root anatomy.
- Right coronary vein grafts may be accessed with a Judkins Right 4, right coronary bypass (RCB), multipurpose, or Sones catheters.

Fig. 4.3 Common diagnostic catheters to study the left coronary artery

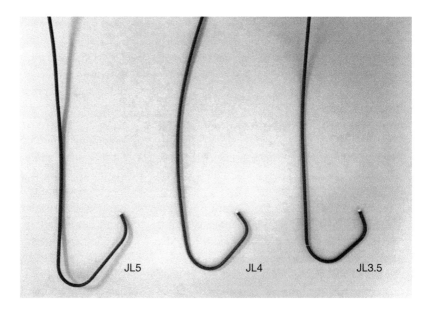

Fig. 4.4 Common diagnostic catheters to study the right coronary artery

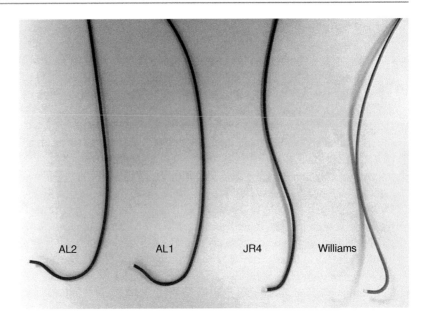

- Left coronary vein grafts may be intubated successfully with a Judkins Right 4, left coronary bypass (LCB), or Amplatz catheters.
- Aortography can facilitate the location of vein graft ostia although patent grafts are not always identified, so this should not be first line when trying to locate vein grafts.
- Care must be taken to ensure coaxial intubation of a graft as otherwise lumen patency may be underestimated—this can typically occur with a right-sided graft and ma\y be avoided with a more gentle angle catheter such as a multipurpose.

Catheters for Internal Mammary Artery

- The left internal mammary artery (LIMA) is the most common arterial conduit used for surgical revascularization.
- The LIMA is usually accessed using a Judkins Right 4 or dedicated internal mammary artery (IMA) catheter from the aortic arch into the left subclavian artery (Fig. 4.5).
- Selective intubation does carry the risk of ostial dissection and often a nonselective injection is adequate to visualize the LIMA and the territory it supplies.

- Simultaneous inflation of a left-arm blood pressure cuff to supra-systolic pressure may improve LIMA visualization during nonselective contrast injection.
- LIMA grafts that are difficult to access may be more easily approached from the left radial artery.

Radial Catheters

- The standard catheters used in femoral angiography may also be used when performing radial angiography.
- However, most operators would start with a JL3.5 as opposed to a JL4.0 when initially attempting to intubate the left coronary system.
- Furthermore, many operators advocate imaging the right coronary artery first as the catheters used to intubate the right coronary artery have less curve and are thus less likely to induce radial artery spasm compared to standard left coronary catheters.
- Specific radial catheters now also exist that allow intubation of both left and right coronary ostia without catheter exchange. These include the Kimny (guide only) and Tiger and Ikari (guide only) catheters (Fig. 4.6).

Fig. 4.5 Common diagnostic catheters used for graft studies

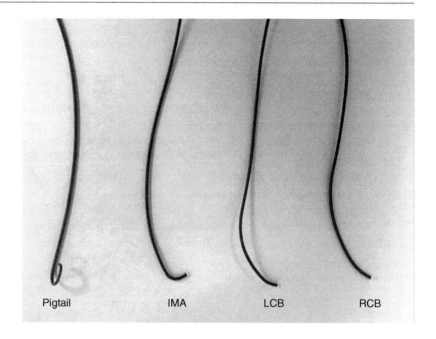

Pigtail   IMA   LCB   RCB

Fig. 4.6 Other commonly used diagnostic catheters

Most Frequently Used Dignostic Coronary Catheter Shapes

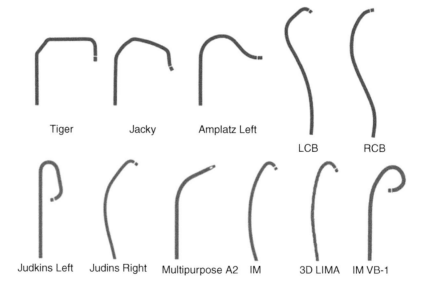

Tiger   Jacky   Amplatz Left

LCB   RCB

Judkins Left   Judins Right   Multipurpose A2   IM   3D LIMA   IM VB-1

Complications That May Arise During Catheter Engagement

- **Coronary dissection**—This potentially life-threatening complication is more likely if there is ostial disease and may result from poorly controlled intubation, especially with a catheter tip that is not coaxial to the vessel.

Subsequent high-pressure contrast injection can be potentially catastrophic.

- **Pressure damping**—This usually occurs in the presence of significant ostial disease although it can also occur on intubation of small-caliber vessels. Contrast injection reveals the extent of the disease usually with little back flow into the aortic root. Prolonged intubation can lead to obstruction of coronary flow, ischemia, and arrhythmia.

- **Conal injection and arrhythmia**—Care must be taken when intubating the right coronary artery as the catheter tip may selectively intubate the conus branch. Subsequent contrast injection can result in ventricular arrhythmia. Thus injection of a small test shot of contrast is recommended following intubation and exclusion of pressure damping.
- **Coronary spasm**—Catheter intubation can promote coronary spasm and areas of spasm can appear angiographically similar to stenotic atheromatous lesions. Spasm, however, usually resolves with intracoronary nitrates.
- **Injection of air**—Operators should be meticulous in ensuring that there is no air in the manifold system and that all catheters are flushed prior to use. Despite these measures, in the event of injecting air ensure close monitoring of the ECG and hemodynamics as the patient can deteriorate quickly. In the majority of cases there is usually only transient ECG changes and/or hemodynamic instability.

Standard Angiographic Views
(Figs. 4.7a–g and 4.8a–c)

Imaging Coronary Bypass Grafts

- Saphenous vein grafts are generally intubated in the LAO and RAO projections.
- In the LAO projection right-sided grafts are found on the left whiles in the RAO projection left-sided grafts are found on the right side.
- The left internal mammary pedicle is accessed via the left subclavian artery in the PA projection.
- Two orthogonal views are required and may include the RAO caudal and LAO cranial pro-

jections although the projection angles may vary depending on each patient's anatomy (Fig. 4.9a–c).

Coronary Aneurysm

Coronary aneurysm is seen when the vessel diameter of a coronary segment is greater than 1.5 times that of a neighboring segment. The incidence is 0.15–4.9%. It is usually associated with atherosclerotic disease although other causes include Kawasaki, previous angioplasty, inflammatory disease, trauma, and association with connective tissue disease. Treatments include observation, surgery, covered stents, and therapeutic coiling (Fig. 4.10).

Common Coronary Anomalies

- Left main coronary artery originating from right sinus of Valsalva: This may run an inter-arterial course where there is an increased risk of sudden death, or a retroaortic course, which has a favorable benign prognosis.
- Right coronary artery originating from the left sinus of Valsalva.
- Right coronary artery originating above the sinus of Valsalva or from the anterior aortic wall.
- Left anterior descending artery originating from the right sinus of Valsalva.
- Left anterior descending artery and left circumflex artery originating from separate ostia.

Left Ventriculography

Although echocardiography has largely superseded left ventriculography it can still be useful in certain settings. The image is achieved by passing a pigtail catheter over a standard J-tipped guide wire into the left ventricle. Once in the left ventricle injection of a 30–40 mL

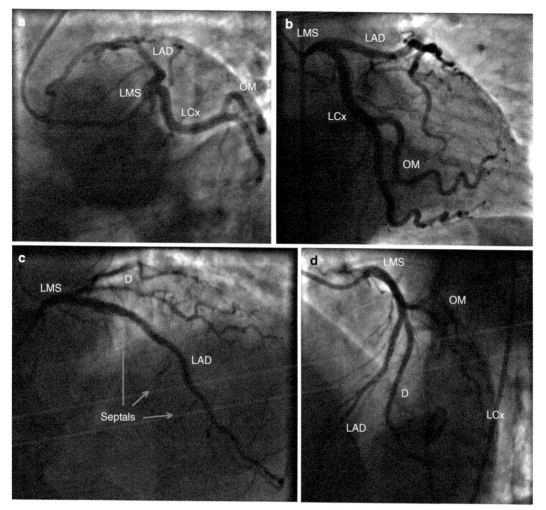

Fig. 4.7 Standard angiographic views—left coronary system. (**a**) *LAO caudal projection: 40–60° LAO and 10–30° caudal.* Commonly referred to as the "spider" view. This projection is best for visualizing the left main stem and proximal LAD/LCx bifurcation. Key: *LMS* left main stem, *LAD* left anterior descending, *LCx* left circumflex, *OM* obtuse marginal. (**b**) *RAO caudal projection: 10–20° RAO and 15–20° caudal.* Best for visualizing left main bifurcation, proximal LAD, and proximal to mid LCx. The greater separation of the LAD and LCx in this projection allows for better visualization of the OM branches of the LCx. Key: *LMS* left main stem, *LAD* left anterior descending, *LCx* left circumflex, *OM* obtuse marginal. (**c**) *RAO cranial projection: 0–10° RAO and 25–40° cranial.* Best for visualizing the proximal LAD and its diagonal branches. This view separates out the septals from the diagonals. The LCx is poorly seen in this projection. Key: *LMS* left main stem, *LAD* left anterior descending, *D* diagonal branch. (**d**) *LAO cranial projection: 30–60° LAO and 15–30° cranial.* This view is best for visualizing mid and distal LAD and the distal LCx in a left dominant system. This view also separates out the septals from the diagonals. The proximal LAD may be foreshortened in this view and overlapped by the LCx (arrow). Key: *LMS* left main stem, *LAD* left anterior descending, *LCx* left circumflex, *OM* obtuse marginal, *D* diagonal. (**e**) *PA projection: 0° lateral and 0° craniocaudal.* Many operators take their first image in a straight PA projection. This provides visualization of the left main stem ostium, proximal LAD, and Cx arteries. Key: *LMS* left main stem, *LAD* left anterior descending, *LCx* left circumflex, *PA* posteroanterior. (**f**) *PA caudal projection: 0° lateral and 20–30° caudal.* This is an alternative view for assessing the proximal LAD/LCx bifurcation, especially if the other caudal views are affected by foreshortening or overlapping vessels. Key: *LMS* left main stem, *LAD* left anterior descending, *LCx* left circumflex, *OM* obtuse marginal branch. (**g**) *PA cranial projection: 0° lateral and 30° cranial.* This is an alternative to the RAO cranial projection and is best for visualizing the proximal and mid LAD and its branches. Key: *LMS* left main stem, *LAD* left anterior descending, *D1* first diagonal branch, *RAO* right anterior oblique

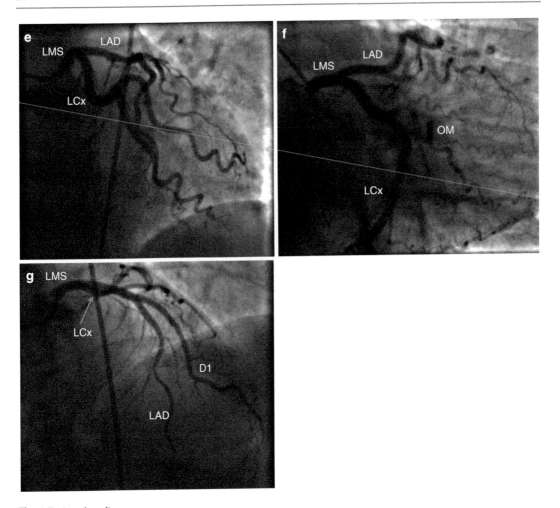

Fig. 4.7 (continued)

bolus of contrast via a mechanical pump at 10–15 mL/s allows assessment of left ventricular function and identification of any regional wall motion abnormalities. Left ventricular angiography is usually performed in the right anterior oblique projection, which also allows assessment of the degree of mitral regurgitation and demonstration of the aortic root. Crossing the aortic valve also provides key information on any gradient across the valve as is seen with aortic stenosis, although in cases of severe AS this is often avoided due to concerns of embolic stroke associated with trauma to a heavily calcified valve (Figs. 4.11 and 4.12).

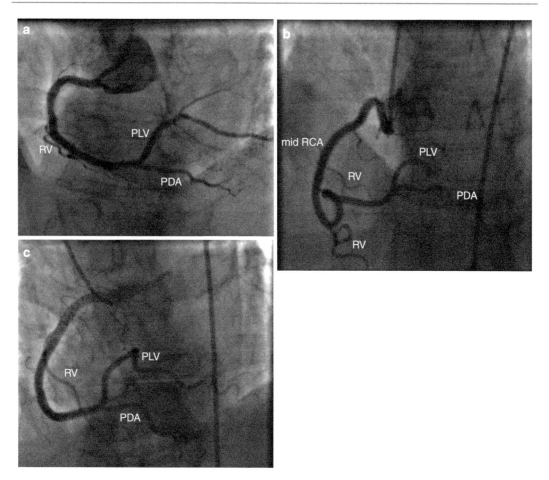

Fig. 4.8 Standard angiographic views for the right coronary system. (**a**) *LAO 30: 30° LAO*. This view is best for visualizing the ostial, proximal, and mid RCA. There is often some overlap of the distal branches. Key: *LAO* left anterior oblique, *PDA* posterior descending artery, *PLV* posterolateral ventricular branch, *RCA* right coronary artery, *RV* right ventricular branch. (**b**) *RAO 30: 30° RAO*. This projection is best for visualizing the mid RCA and PDA. The ostium and proximal RCA is often foreshort-ened in this view. Key: *RAO* right anterior oblique, *PDA* posterior descending artery, *PLV* posterolateral ventricular branch, *RCA* right coronary artery, *RV* right ventricular branch, (**c**) *PA cranial: PA and 30° cranial*. This view is best for visualizing the distal RCA bifurcation and the PDA. Key: *PA* posteroanterior, *PDA* posterior descending artery, *PL* posterolateral ventricular branch, *RCA* right coronary artery, *RV* right ventricular branch

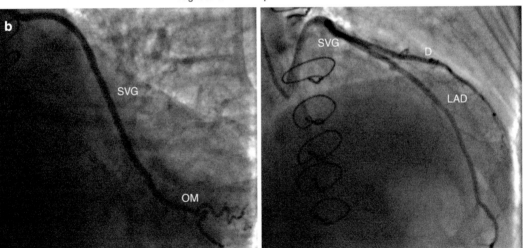

Left anterior oblique view   Postero-anterior cranial view

Right anterior oblique views

Fig. 4.9 (**a**) Standard graft study projections: saphenous vein graft (SVG) to posterior descending artery (PDA). (**b**) Standard graft study projections: saphenous vein graft (SVG) to obtuse marginal and SVG to left anterior descending (LAD) artery. (**c**) Standard graft study projections: left internal mammary artery (LIMA) graft origin (left, arrow) and anastomosis (right, arrow) with left anterior descending (LAD) artery

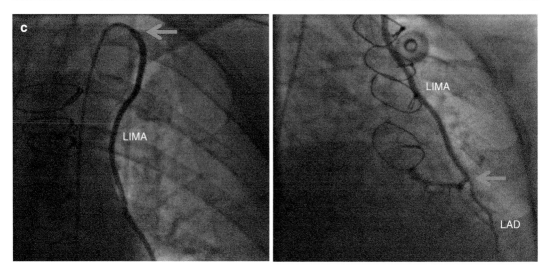

Fig. 4.9 (continued)

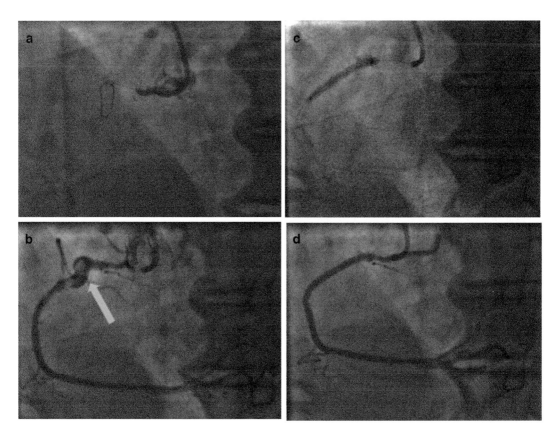

Fig. 4.10 Acute occlusion of right coronary artery (RCA) aneurysm treated by deployment of covered stent. (**a**) Acutely occluded proximal RCA with coronary wire looping around aneurysm; (**b**) restoration of coronary flow followed by positioning of covered stent across aneurysm (arrow); (**c**) inflation of covered stent balloon; (**d**) deployment of covered stent with restoration of normal coronary flow

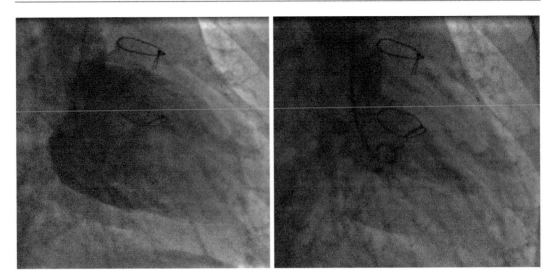

Fig. 4.11 Left ventriculography revealing overall preserved systolic function

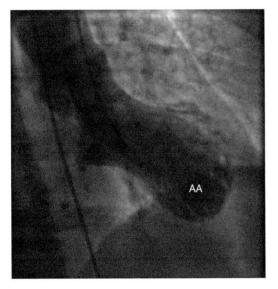

Fig. 4.12 Left ventriculography revealing an apical aneurysm (AA) consistent with Takotsubo cardiomyopathy

Aortogram

This is usually performed in the left anterior oblique projection and involves injection of 30–40 mL of contrast via a mechanical pump at 15–20 mL/s and pigtail catheter positioned in the aortic root. This allows assessment of the aortic root, ascending aorta, and arch and is particularly important in the workup of patients with significant aortic valve disease. An aortogram may also be performed when trying to locate the origins of bypass grafts (Fig. 4.13).

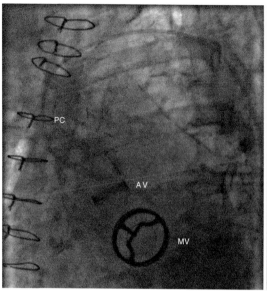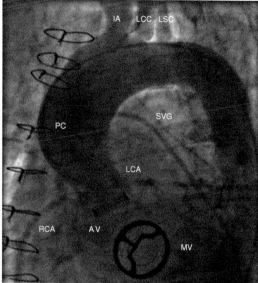

Fig. 4.13 A standard aortogram, before and after contrast injection, which allows for visualization of the aortic root, coronary ostia, aortic arch and great vessels, and origin of cardiac bypass grafts. Key: *PC* pigtail catheter, *AV* aortic valve (prosthesis), *MV* mitral valve (prosthesis), *RCA* right coronary artery, *LCA* left coronary artery, *SVG* saphenous vein graft, *IA* innominate artery (brachiocephalic trunk), *LCC* left common carotid artery, *LSC* left subclavian artery

Limitations of Coronary Angiography (See Table 4.4)

- Coronary angiography provides a two-dimensional image of a three-dimensional structure. Therefore a series of images must be obtained to allow visualization of all segments of the coronary arteries in at least two orthogonal projections.
- This is particularly relevant when assessing eccentric plaque as this may only be seen in a single projection.
- Particular attention must also be taken when assessing overlapping vessel segments as disease may be concealed.
- Significant disease may also be underestimated if coronary segments are progressing towards or away from the imaging plane as opposed to perpendicular to it—so-called foreshortening of the coronary vessel. This may also lead to underestimation of lesion length, which is problematic when planning a PCI strategy.
- These issues of overlapping segments and foreshortening are particularly relevant at bifurcation points. Here angiographic images should be obtained where the vessels are maximally divergent to ensure adequate assessment.
- Modification of standard views may be required to achieve an optimal dataset. Further information on lesion severity may require invasive techniques such as fractional flow reserve or intravascular imaging.

Table 4.4 Tips and tricks

RAO vs. LAO	If the spine and the catheter are to the right of the image, it is LAO and vice versa. If central, it is likely PA view
Cranial vs. caudal	If the diaphragm shadow can be seen on the image, it is likely a cranial view; if not it is caudal
LAD or LCx?	The circumflex is seen closer to the spine in all projections
Minimizing radial spasm	○•○Sedation ○•○IV fluids + adequate hydration ○•○Intra-arterial nitrates ○•○Verapamil ○•○Right coronary acquisition before left coronary system (especially when using radial access)
Radial loops	Significant tortuosity can usually be negotiated using a hydrophilic wire (e.g., Terumo). Subsequent passage of the diagnostic catheter usually straightens up most loops
Femoral tortuosity	Exchanging for a long sheath can help straighten out any iliofemoral tortuosity to allow better control of the diagnostic catheter
Vascular tortuosity	○–○Hydrophilic wire ○–○Stiff wire—with caution ○–○Long sheath—femoral ○–○Exchange length wire for subsequent catheter exchanges
Dedicated radial catheters	When using dedicated radial catheters such as the TIGA, engage the left coronary ostium as you would normally do. Following left coronary acquisition, disengage the catheter, advance, and rotate clockwise to engage the right coronary ostium
Grafts	○–○Know the anatomy of the grafts prior to starting the case ○–○Walk the catheter up and down in the RAO and LAO projections. For right-sided grafts the catheter tip should be pointing left in the LAO projection. For left-sided grafts the catheter tip should be pointing right in the RAO projection ○–○If known LIMA graft consider femoral or left radial approach
Catheter selection	○–○If the catheter is easily folding up—consider larger size ○–○If the catheter is pointing down into the aortic root consider a smaller catheter
Aortic stenosis	In patients with severe aortic stenosis the aorta can be very tortuous and the ostium of the RCA is often very inferior; aortic flow in valve disease may require a larger French catheter to allow adequate coronary opacification
Coronary anomalies	Always check that you have seen enough coronary arteries to supply the entire myocardial bed—are you missing another coronary?
Valves	Practice caution and be careful not to cross the aortic valve if there is active infection or significant calcific disease or with prosthetic valves

Minimizing contrast	Limited views
	  – Left coronary system—LAO caudal, RAO caudal, and PA cranial/RAO cranial
	  – Right coronary system—LAO and RAO

Poor radial pulse	Consider the left radial, ulnar, or femoral artery instead

Angiogram Interpretation

- Evaluate extent and severity of coronary calcification—ideally just prior to or soon after contrast opacification.
- Lesion quantification in at least two orthogonal views:
  - Severity
  - Calcification
  - Presence of ulceration/thrombus
  - Degree of tortuosity and angulation
  - Lesion length
  - ACC/AHA lesion classification (Table 4.5)
  - Reference vessel size
- Grading thrombolysis in myocardial infarction (TIMI) flow (Table 4.6).
- Grading TIMI myocardial perfusion blush grade (Table 4.7).
- Identifying and quantifying coronary collaterals:
  - *Grade 0*—no collateral circulation

Table 4.5 ACC/AHA lesion classification [1]

Type A lesion	Minimally complex, discrete (length <10 mm), concentric, readily accessible, non-angulated segment (<45°), smooth contour, little or no calcification, less than totally occlusive, not ostial in location, no major side branch involvement, and absence of thrombus
Type B lesion	Moderately complex, tubular (length 10–20 mm), eccentric, moderate tortuosity of proximal segment, moderately angulated segment (>45°, <90°), irregular contour, moderate or heavy calcification, total occlusions <3 months old, ostial in location, bifurcation lesions requiring double-guide wires, and some thrombus present
Type C lesion	Severely complex, diffuse (length >2 cm), excessive tortuosity of proximal segment, extremely angulated segments >90°, total occlusions >3 months old and/or bridging collaterals, inability to protect major side branches, and degenerated vein grafts with friable lesions

Table 4.6 TIMI flow grades [2]

TIMI 0 flow	Absence of any antegrade flow beyond a coronary occlusion
TIMI 1 flow	Penetration without perfusion—faint antegrade coronary flow beyond the occlusion, with incomplete filling of the distal coronary bed
TIMI 2 flow	Partial reperfusion—delayed or sluggish antegrade flow with complete filling of the distal territory
TIMI 3 flow	Complete perfusion—normal flow, which fills the distal coronary, bed completely

Table 4.7 TIMI myocardial perfusion grades [3]

Grade 0	Either minimal or no ground-glass appearance ("blush") of the myocardium in the distribution of the culprit artery
Grade 1	Dye slowly enters but fails to exit the microvasculature. Ground-glass appearance ("blush") of the myocardium in the distribution of the culprit lesion that fails to clear from the microvasculature, and dye staining is present on the next injection (approximately 30 s between injections)
Grade 2	Delayed entry and exit of dye from the microvasculature. There is the ground-glass appearance ("blush") of the myocardium that is strongly persistent at the end of the washout phase (i.e., dye is strongly persistent after three cardiac cycles of the washout phase and either does not or only minimally diminishes in intensity during washout)
Grade 3	Normal entry and exit of dye from the microvasculature. There is the ground-glass appearance ("blush") of the myocardium that clears normally, and is either gone or only mildly/moderately persistent at the end of the washout phase (i.e., dye is gone or is mildly/moderately persistent after three cardiac cycles of the washout phase and noticeably diminishes in intensity during the washout phase), similar to that in an uninvolved artery

- *Grade 1*—very weak opacification
- *Grade 2*—re-opacified segment, less dense than the feeding vessel and filling slowly
- *Grade 3*—re-opacified segment as dense as the feeding vessel and filling rapidly

References

1. Scanlon PJ, Faxon DP, Audet AM, et al. ACC/AHA guidelines for coronary angiography: executive summary and recommendations. A report of the American College of Cardiology/American Heart Association Task Force on Practice Guidelines (Committee on Coronary Angiography) developed in collaboration. Circulation. 1999;99(17):2345–57.
2. TIMI Study Group. The thrombolysis in myocardial infarction (TIMI) trial. Phase I findings. N Engl J Med. 1985;312(14):932–6. https://doi.org/10.1056/NEJM198504043121435.
3. van 't Hof AW, Liem A, Suryapranata H, Hoorntje JC, de Boer MJ, Zijlstra F. Angiographic assessment of myocardial reperfusion in patients treated with primary angioplasty for acute myocardial infarction: myocardial blush grade. Zwolle Myocardial Infarction Study Group. Circulation. 1998;97(23):2302–6.

Vascular Access for Left Heart Catheterization

5

Aditya Mandawat and Sunil V. Rao

About Us The catheterization laboratories at Duke University Medical Center and the Durham VA Medical Center serve as quaternary referral centers for invasive cardiac care for the Southeastern United States.

Introduction

- While traditionally viewed as benign when compared with nonaccess-site complications, vascular access-site complications are associated with a short- and long-term risk of morbidity or mortality as well as increased costs [1–4].
- In a study of 17,901 consecutive patients undergoing transfemoral PCI at the Mayo Clinic, Doyle et al. demonstrated that major femoral complications (including major hematoma, external bleeding, and retroperitoneal bleeding) were independently associated with a 30-day adjusted hazard ratio (HR) for a

mortality of 9.96 (95% confidence interval [95% CI]: 6.94–14.3, $p < 0.001$) [1].

- Similarly, Yatskar et al. reported that hematomas requiring transfusions were associated with an increased 1-year mortality (HR 1.65, 95% CI 1.01–2.70, $p = 0.048$) among patients undergoing PCI during the NHLBI Dynamic registry recruitment waves [2].
- While relatively uncommon, retroperitoneal bleeding remains a catastrophic vascular access-site complication, with 73.5% requiring transfusion and 10.4% dying during hospitalization [3].
- Furthermore, in an era of increasing public concern regarding healthcare costs, it is also worth noting that even after adjustments for baseline differences among patients enrolled in an economic sub-study of Gusto IIb, each moderate or severe bleeding event increased costs by $3770 and each transfusion event increased costs by $2080 [4].
- In current practice, while the risk of major bleeding is dependent on patient characteristics and to an extent the choice of antithrombotic agent, the choice of vascular access strategy (transfemoral vs. transradial) and a meticulous attention to good technique, proper equipment, and skilled operators may reduce major bleeding and thereby reduce morbidity, mortality, as well as costs.

A. Mandawat · S. V. Rao (✉)
Duke University Medical Center, Durham, NC, USA

Durham VA Medical Center, Durham, NC, USA
e-mail: aditya.mandawat@duke.edu;
sunil.rao@duke.edu

© Springer International Publishing AG, part of Springer Nature 2018
A. Myat et al. (eds.), *The Interventional Cardiology Training Manual*,
https://doi.org/10.1007/978-3-319-71635-0_5

Choosing Between the Transradial Versus Transfemoral Approaches

- As neither radial nor femoral access can be used universally, operators should become and remain proficient in both approaches.
- The essence of the radial versus femoral approach choice may be summarized as the following—for inexperienced operators, radial access is more technically challenging and is perhaps associated with more radiation exposure than femoral access, but radial access decreases patient's bleeding and vascular complications and is associated with reduced mortality in high-risk patients such as those with ST-segment elevation MI [5].
- For experienced operators, i.e., those who have overcome the transradial learning curve, radiation exposure is similar between radial and femoral access (Table 5.1).

Since its introduction, a wealth of evidence has accumulated on the risk-benefit profile of transradial access, largely in its favor:

- The first trial of radial access was the ACCESS trial, published in 1997, which randomized 900 patients undergoing elective PCI to right-sided transradial, transbrachial, or transfemoral access [6].
- Procedure duration (40, 39, and 38 min, $p = 0.603$), fluoroscopy time (13, 12, and 11 min), procedural success (respectively, 91.7%, 90.7%, and 90.7%, $p = 0.885$), and

1-month events (6.7%, 8.3%, and 5.3%, $p = 0.342$) were similar across all three groups.
- Importantly however, transradial access was associated with fewer major entry-site complications (none, 2.3%, and 2.0%, $p = 0.035$).
- The TEMPURA study, conducted between 1999 and 2001, was the first to randomize patients with ST-elevation myocardial infarction (STEMI) undergoing primary PCI to transradial versus transfemoral access [7].
- In 149 patients, reperfusion success (96.1% vs. 97.2%, $p = 0.624$) and in-hospital major adverse cardiac events (5.2% vs. 8.3%, $p = 0.444$) were similar in both groups with two patients in the transfemoral group experiencing severe bleeding.
- Expanding upon this, the RIVAL trial randomized 7021 patients with acute coronary syndromes (ACS), and specifically 1958 patients with STEMI, to transradial versus transfemoral access [8]. The primary endpoint was a composite of death, myocardial infarction (MI), stroke, or non-CABG-related major bleeding at 1 month.
- For patients without suspected or confirmed STEMI, transradial access was associated with a similar risk of the primary endpoint (3.7% vs. 4.0%, $p = 0.50$), with the caveat that transradial access appeared to be more beneficial in high-volume radial centers (1.6% vs. 3.2%, p for effect = 0.015, p for interaction = 0.021).
- Importantly, transradial access was significantly safer than transfemoral access in

Table 5.1 Femoral versus radial vascular access

Feature	Femoral	Radial
Access-site bleeding	3–4%	0–0.6%
Vascular complications	0.3–5% (AV fistula, pseudoaneurysm, retroperitoneal bleed, local hematoma)	0–0.6% (local hematoma, pseudoaneurysm)
Arterial occlusion	Rare	0.1–9%
Patient comfort	**	*****
Ambulation	2–4 h	Immediate
Procedure time[a]	Perceived shorter	Perceived longer
Estimated radiation exposure[a]	Perceived shorter	Perceived longer
Learning curve	Short	Longer
>8-F guide catheters	Feasible	Not possible

[a]Operator dependent

patients with suspected or confirmed STEMI (3.1% vs. 5.2%, p for effect = 0.026, p for interaction = 0.025), with a significant mortality benefit (1.3% vs. 3.2%, p for effect = 0.006, p for interaction = 0.001).

- These results were confirmed by the RIFLE-STEACS trial which focused only on patients with suspected or confirmed STEMI and involved only centers with an established expertise in transradial access [9]. The primary endpoint was a 30-day rate of net adverse clinical events (NACE), defined as a composite of cardiac death, MI, stroke, target vessel revascularization, and bleeding, which occurred in 13.6% of patients allocated to transradial access versus 21.0% in those allocated to transfemoral access (p = 0.003). 30-day mortality (5.2% vs. 9.2%, p = 0.020) and bleeding (7.8% vs. 12.2%, p = 0026) were lower in patients receiving transradial access.
- The STEMI-RADIAL trial randomized 707 patients referred for STEMI presenting <12 h of symptom onset [10]. The primary endpoint was the cumulative incidence of major bleeding and vascular access-site complications at 30 days.
- The primary endpoint occurred in 1.4% of the radial group versus 7.2% of the femoral group (p = 0.0028).
- The MATRIX trial randomized 8404 patients with ACS to transradial or transfemoral access [11].
- While at a pre-specified alpha of 0.025, MACE defined as death, MI, or stroke at 30 days was not statistically significant (8.8% vs. 10.3%, p = 0.0327), NACE defined as MACE or Bleeding Academic Research Consortium (BARC) non-CABG major bleeding was lower in patients receiving transradial access (9.8% vs. 11.7%, p = 0.0092).
- This difference was driven by reductions in BARC non-CABG major bleeding (1.6% vs. 2.3%, p = 0.0013) and all-cause mortality (1.6% vs. 2.2%, p = 0.045).
- The SAFE-PCI for Women trial sought to determine the effect of radial access on outcomes in 1781 women undergoing PCI using a novel registry-based randomized trial.

- Among women undergoing cardiac catheterization or PCI, radial access significantly reduced bleeding and vascular complications (0.6% vs. 1.7%, OR 3.70, 95% CI 2.14–6.40). Moreover, more women preferred radial access [12].
- Several systematic reviews have in large part confirmed the above findings, albeit increasing statistical precision as well as bolstering external validity [13, 14].
- Given this, there has been increased adoption of radial access and many centers are moving to a "radial first" approach [15] especially in high-risk populations (ACS [especially STEMI]; high bleeding risk; obese patients; octa- and nonagenarians; and women).
- Several situations however exist where transradial access may best be avoided except by highly experienced operators (Table 5.2).

Patient Preparation

- Pre-procedure planning begins with thoughtful review of a patient's chart to determine the planned objectives of the investigations or interventions, the patient's history of presenting illness, prior medical history (prior CABG anatomy, PAD, iliofemoral grafts), allergies, laboratory values (particularly those related to coagulation/hemostasis), medications (especially anticoagulants), EKG, noninvasive investigations (particularly recent stress testing), and difficulties encountered with sedation, vascular access, or navigation of the femoral or radial arteries during prior procedures.
- A physical examination focused on identifying anatomic conditions that may influence the choice of sedation or access site is mandatory. For example, a patient's inability to lay flat for several hours post-procedure due to orthopnea or preexisting spinal disease, diminished or absent pulses or bruits, or presence of arteriovenous fistulas for hemodialysis is important to note.
- In patients in whom radial access is a consideration, the utility of performing the modified

Table 5.2 Practical Hints for Patient Selection for Transradial Access from "Best Practices for Transradial Approach in Diagnostic Angiography and Intervention," Table 3–4, pg. 23

	Suitability	
	Inexperienced operators	*Experienced operators*
Ideal Situations for Transradial Access		
Acute coronary syndrome (especially ST-elevation myocardial infarction)	+/–	+/+
High bleeding risk (including anticoagulants)	++	++
Obese patients	++	++
Octogenarians	++	++
Previous bypass surgery (with single internal marnmary graft)	+/–	++
Women	+/–	++
Situations in which transradial access may best be avoided		
End-stage renal failure or dialysis	+/–	++
Known innominate/subclavian axis anomalies	– –	+
Patient is a candidate for bypass surgery in centers commonly using radial grafts	+/–	+/–
Previous bypass surgery (with bilateral internal mammary graft)	– –	+
Prior severely painful transradial access or radial spasm	– –	+/–
Pulseless cardiogenic shock	– –	+/–
Raynaud's syndrome or small artery inflammatory disease	+/–	+
Very complex or high-risk PCI (e.g., on last remaining vessel)	– –	+

++, highly recommended; +, recommended; +/-, possible; -, not recommended;--, avoid; PCI, percutaneous coronary intervention

Allen's or Barbeau's test to assess ulnar flow into the palmar arch is of unclear clinical significance.

- In the RADAR study of 203 patients undergoing elective or urgent angiography via the radial approach, thumb capillary lactate concentrations, handgrip strength, and discomfort ratings did not differ between patients with a normal, intermediate, or abnormal modified Allen's test at 1 day, 1 month, or 1 year [16].
- Furthermore, vascular recruitment as confirmed by plethysmographic readings and Doppler examination occurred in patients with intermediate or abnormal modified Allen's tests, thus preventing objective and subjective signs of hand ischemia even in patients with poor collateral circulation at baseline and loss of a previously

documented radial pulse at day 1 following catheterization.

- An assessment of periprocedural bleeding risk, which may inform the use of bleeding avoidance strategies such as bivalirudin, radial access, and in some studies vascular closure devices, is useful [17].
- Using detailed clinical data from >1,000,000 PCI procedures from the NCDR CathPCI registry, a bedside bleeding risk score using ten variables has been published with a high concordance between the risk predicted by the model and observed bleeding events:
  - STEMI
  - Age
  - BMI
  - Previous PCI
  - Chronic kidney disease
  - Shock

- Cardiac arrest within 24 h
- Female
- Hemoglobin
- PCI status [18]

- In a study of 6941 PCIs at a single healthcare system, use of the NCDR bleeding risk model was associated with an increase in bivalirudin use in patients at intermediate and high bleeding risk and decreased use in lower risk patients, leading to a reversal of the risk-treatment paradox [19].
- Patients should be given the opportunity to ask questions regarding who, what, where, when, why, and how of the planned diagnostic investigations or interventions.
- Specifically, patients should receive an explanation regarding the differences between the transradial and transfemoral approaches, with the advantages/disadvantages of performing the procedure through the anticipated approach for each individual patient discussed in detail.
- Any preferences patients have (laterality, good or bad experiences with prior access attempts) should be taken into consideration.
- Audiovisual adjuncts may increase information retention and may make patients more familiar with both the environment of the catheterization laboratory and the technical aspects of the procedure [20].
- Prior to arriving in the catheterization laboratory, all jewelry and watches should be removed from the wrist and rings should be removed from the fingers.
- Patients should have preferably two peripheral intravenous (IV) lines placed, with one ideally well away from the radial site if that is the anticipated site of access. If an IV must be placed on the side of planned radial/ulnar access, it should be placed well proximal to the wrist, ideally at or above the level of the elbow.
- For transradial/ulnar cases, hair on the wrist of interest should be removed with clippers, and consideration should be given to prepping both femoral sites in case they are needed, especially in the presence of weak radial pulses, with the potential need for hemody-

namic support, or during the learning curve for radial access.
- In the catheterization lab, it is important that both the patient and the operator feel comfortable and consequently arm preparation and positioning are of paramount importance.
- While either the left or the right wrist may be used for radial/ulnar access, the preferred access site has historically been the right radial [21]. In this case, with the patient lying supine, the arm should be maintained as close to the patient's right side as possible (radial artery running parallel to the femoral artery) in the anatomic position with the palm up.
- Hyperextension of the wrist to 30–60°, which may allow easier cannulation of the radial artery, can be achieved using a roll of gauze, a rolled-up towel, or a commercially available wrist splint.
- Extreme hyperextension of the wrist should be avoided as it may blunt the pulse and can be uncomfortable for the patient.
- To maintain this position, the arm can be immobilized with tape across the palm. In obese patients, it may be necessary to place an arm board or arm extension under the patient's mattress along the table to provide a suitable working area (Fig. 5.1).
- Since there can be ergonomic challenges to performing procedures via the left radial approach if the operator stands on the right side of the patient, optimal arm positioning is key.

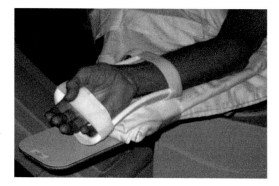

Fig. 5.1 Ideal right-arm positioning for radial artery access. Adopted from Kern, Morton J. The Interventional Cardiology Handbook, 2, 38–82

- A common approach is to prepare the left wrist in a manner analogous to that described above for right but following access raise and adduct the arm to lay in on the patient's abdomen as close to midline as possible.
- Following arm/groin preparation, one of several commercially available drapes, with pre-cut radial and femoral fenestrations, can be used to cover the patient and create a sterile field.

Radial/Ulnar Approach

Radial/Ulnar Anatomy

- Knowledge of the anatomy of the vessels of the upper extremity and aortic arch is essential for successful radial access.
- The aortic arch gives off three great vessels: the innominate on the right and the common carotid and subclavian arteries on the left.
- The innominate artery becomes the right subclavian artery after the takeoff of the right carotid artery and then the axillary artery at the lateral margin on the first rib. At the inferior border of the teres major muscle, the axillary artery continues as the brachial artery that then bifurcates in most patients into the radial and ulnar arteries below the elbow. The radial artery then continues along the lateral aspect of the forearm into the wrist where it divides into the deep and superficial palmar arches.

- The deep and superficial branches of the of the radial artery communicate with the corresponding divisions of the ulnar artery to complete the two palmar arches and provide dual-collateral blood flow to the hand in most patients. The ulnar artery begins below the bend of the elbow and reaches the ulnar side of the forearm at a point about midway between the elbow and the wrist. Then it runs along the ulnar border to the wrist and divides into two branches, which complete the two palmer arches (Fig. 5.2).
- The arm arteries may also demonstrate a variety of tortuosity and loops, particularly in patients above 75 years old, of female gender, with prior coronary artery bypass surgery, and of short stature [22].
- Most problems involve variant origins to the radial artery and anastomosis at the antecubital fossa, but problems can also occur in the brachial, axillary, and subclavian arteries.
- There are two arterial anomalies that can significantly complicate transradial or transulnar procedures. The first is the radial artery loop that often occurs at the level of the elbow (Fig. 5.3a). This is often accompanied by the recurrent radial artery, a very small caliber artery that runs parallel with the brachial artery.
- The recurrent radial artery can be large enough to accommodate the 0.035″ wire and sometimes even a 5-French or 6-French diagnostic catheter. However, the small caliber of the artery

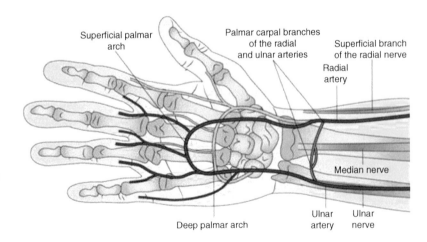

Fig. 5.2 Essential anatomy for radial artery access. Adopted from Byrne, R. A. et al. Nat. Rev. Cardiol. 10, 27–40 (2013)

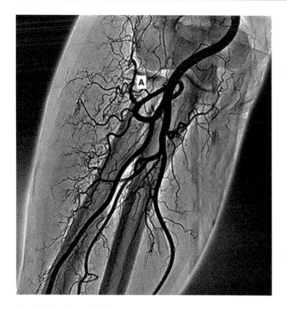

Fig. 5.3 A radial loop (A) complicating radial artery access for coronary angiography. Adopted from Rao, SV. Approaching the Post-Femoral Era for Coronary Angiography and Intervention. JACC Cardiovascular Interventions. Volume 8, Issue 4, 20 April 2015, 524–526

leads to significant difficulty in manipulating the catheter that is often interpreted as severe spasm with significant patient discomfort.

- The development of severe spasm should prompt angiography of the radial artery to identify a radial loop and presence of the recurrent radial artery. Loops can be crossed using the technique described below or the procedure can be completed using an alternative access site. The use of pre-procedure ultrasound of the radial and ulnar arteries as well as the antecubital fossa may facilitate transradial or transulnar procedures by identifying arterial anomalies prior to the procedure [23].

- The other anomaly that can complicate transradial and in this case even transulnar procedures is arteria lusoria. This congenital anomaly is when the right subclavian artery courses behind the esophagus and connects to the aorta distal to the right subclavian (Fig. 5.4). This is a relatively rare anomaly that occurs in 0.5–1.8% of patients.

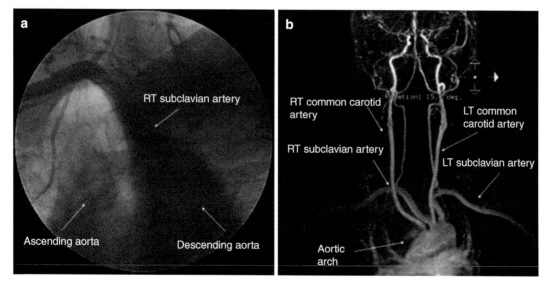

Fig. 5.4 Arteria lusoria complicating right radial artery access for coronary angiography. Adopted from Yiu, Kai-Hang. Arteria Lusoria Diagnosed by Transradial Coronary Catheterization. J Am Coll Cardiol Intv. 2010;3(8):880–881

- While the procedure can sometimes be completed using stiff Amplatz wires to facilitate entry of the catheters into the ascending aorta, it is often more straightforward to complete the case via the left radial approach or femoral approach.
- If tortuosity or loop is suspected, an angiogram of the radial or ulnar artery should be performed. Tortuosities may often be carefully crossed using a 0.025 or 0.032 hydrophilic J wire, a Wholey wire, or a 0.014 soft-tip coronary guide wire. Once the tortuous segment is crossed, the procedure may be completed in the usual fashion.
- Loops/curvatures may require downsizing of the guide wire, use of a buddy wire, straightening of the loop, or upsizing of the guide wire [24].
- In the most extreme cases, balloon-assisted tracking (BAT) may be necessary (Fig. 5.5) [25]. Balloon-assisted tracking involves minimizing the "razor effect" of the large transition between the catheter tip and the guide wire by advancing a 0.014″ coronary guide wire through the tortuous segment, protruding an angioplasty balloon halfway out of the tip of the catheter, inflating it to low pressure, and advancing the catheter-balloon assembly over the guide wire through the tortuous segment. If the patient experiences significant pain or the procedure time is significantly prolonged, consideration should be given to bailing out to either the contralateral radial artery or the femoral approach.

Left Versus Right Transradial Access

- While vessel diameters are usually comparable between right and left vessels, a difference in pulse strength and palpability can occur. Moreover, tortuosities/loops/curvatures are not always bilateral and may differ in complexity.
- The use of the left transradial approach is associated with several important anatomical and technical advantages including a shorter learning curve [26], reduced severe tortuosity of the subclavian artery [27, 28], and easier cannulation of the left internal mammary artery (LIMA) in patients with previous use of the LIMA as a coronary artery bypass [29].
- The TALENT trial randomized 1540 patients undergoing diagnostic (1467 patients) or interventional (668 patients) coronary procedures to right versus left radial access [30]. While left radial access was associated with a lower fluoroscopy time (149 s vs. 168 s, $p = 0.003$) and dose area product (107 Gy-cm^2 vs. 12.1 Gy-cm^2, $p = 0004$) in the diagnostic group (but not in the interventional cohort), subgroup analyses showed that the differences were significant only in older patients and with operators on the transradial learning curve.
- In a meta-analysis of 6840 patients from 14 randomized controlled trials, no significant differences in the rate of procedure failure of the left and right radial approaches (RR 0.98,

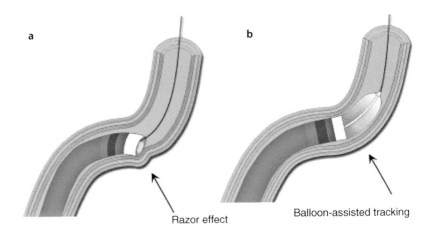

Fig. 5.5 Balloon-assisted tracking technique for tortuous radial artery anatomy. Adopted from Patel T. Balloon-assisted tracking: A must-know technique to overcome difficult anatomy during transradial approach. Catheter Cardiovasc Interv. 2014;83(2):211–20

a

b

Razor effect

Balloon-assisted tracking

95% CI 0.77–1.25, $p = 0.88$) or procedure time ($p = 0.38$) were seen [31]. Ultimately, the selection of the artery with the best radial pulse is usually advisable.

Radial Artery Access

- The course of the radial artery is identified by palpitation over several centimeters along the wrist. The ideal puncture site is 1–2 cm proximal to the bony prominence of the distal radius (radial styloid).
- Distal puncture sites (closer to the hand) risk puncture of the radial artery after its bifurcation into the deep and superficial palmar arches where it is smaller, more tortuous, and partially located below the transverse carpal ligament.
- More proximal punctures may be associated with large hematoma formation as they are more difficult to compress.
- Following a combination of low-dose opiates and benzodiazepines to minimize patient discomfort and anxiety and thereby the risk of radial artery spasm, a small amount (no more than 1 mL) of subcutaneous local anesthetic is given to raise a small wheal (Fig. 5.7, Panel A).
- It is important to avoid large amounts of lidocaine as large wheals may obscure palpation of the radial pulse and make cannulation more difficult. The course of the radial artery is then fixed between the index and middle fingers of the nondominant hand in preparation for arteriotomy.
- The use of ultrasound guidance for radial access was explored in RAUST [32]. Ultrasound guidance significantly improved first-pass success rate (64.8% vs. 43.9%, $p < 0.0001$), median number of access attempts (1.64 vs. 3.05, $p < 0.0001$), and median time to access (64 s vs. 74 s, $p < 0.0001$).
- When using a **"through-and-through" technique**, a micropuncture catheter-over-needle system is inserted with bevel up at a 45-degree angle along the direction of the radial artery until a flashback of blood is visualized. The system is then advanced until the back wall of

the artery is punctured and blood flow stops. The needle is then removed and the catheter is carefully withdrawn parallel to the skin until its tip is intraluminal as confirmed by free-flowing blood. A 0.018 or 0.025-in. guide wire with a hydrophilic coating and a straight or slightly angulated tip is gently inserted using a twirling motion. **There should be little to no resistance to wire introduction.**
- If resistance is encountered, it is important to avoid forceful introduction of maneuvers. Difficult advancement of the guide wire may be due to artery spasm, placement into a small branch vessel, tortuosity, loop, or partial embedment into the vessel wall. Fluoroscopy should be immediately used to visualize the position of the wire if resistance is met.
- In a study of 412 patients randomized to a "through-and-through" (counterpuncture) technique versus a single anterior wall puncture, access time, procedure time, and number of attempts to get access were significantly shorter with a "through-and-through" technique with no increases in the incidence of hematoma or radial artery occlusion (ROA) [33].
- Should a **single anterior wall puncture technique** of the radial artery be used (Fig. 5.6), following the initial flashback of blood, the bare metal needle is advanced slightly to ensure that the whole tip (not just the tip of the bevel) is intraluminal.
- If blood continues to flow freely, a 0.025-in. nitinol wire is advanced into the needle and the needle is removed. Notably, only metal wires should be used with bare metal needles as plastic-coated wires can be shredded if pulled back again the bevel.
- In patients with radial artery spasm caused by failed access attempts, three options exist:
  - Observation for the spasm to resolve
  - The administration of 400 mcg of sublingual nitroglycerin
  - The subcutaneous injection of 200 mcg of nitroglycerin on the medial and lateral aspects of the radial artery
- The mean time for the radial pulse to reappear was 18 ± 5, 8 ± 1, and 3 ± 1 min for observation, sublingual nitroglycerin, and subcutane-

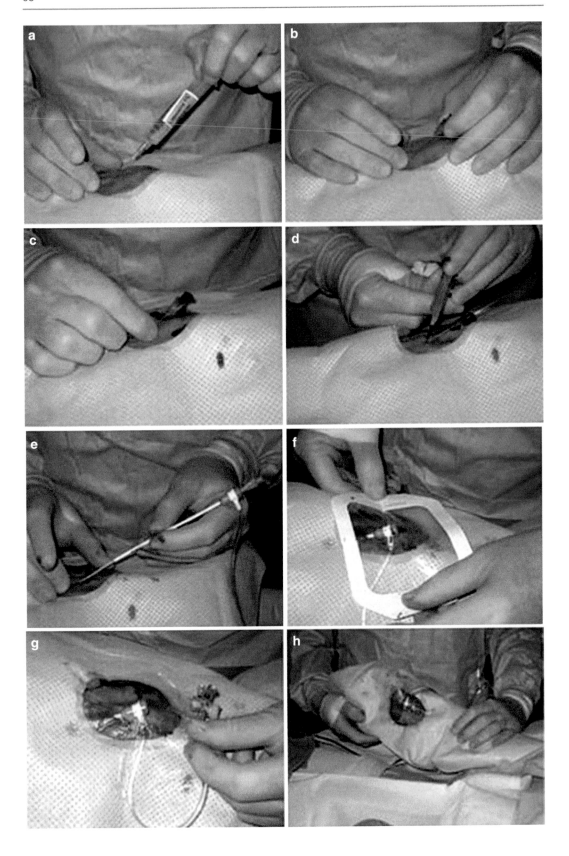

ous nitroglycerin, respectively, with the subsequent rate of successful radial cannulation 72, 90, and 100% [34].

- If the spasm is intense and irreversible, it may become necessary to switch to a completely different site altogether—ideally to the contralateral radial artery.
- Following sheath insertion over the wire, an antispasmodic cocktail should be given to reduce the risk of radial artery spasm.
- Available agents include calcium channel blockers (verapamil, diltiazem, nicardipine) or nitroglycerin. Intravenous unfractionated heparin (50–70 U/kg, up to 5000 U) should also be given at some point during the procedure to reduce the risk of radial artery occlusion (RAO) [35].

Ulnar Artery Access

- Transradial access has been the preferred approach in light of conflicting evidence for ulnar access, with Hahalis et al. reporting increased MACE and major arm vascular events with transulnar access compared with transradial access [36] but others reporting no differences [37].
- A recent meta-analysis by Dahal and colleagues of 2744 patients undergoing transulnar versus transradial access reports similar efficacy and safety except for more access attempts and increased access-site crossover with ulnar approach [38].
- Ulnar artery cannulation may however serve as a reasonable and useful alterna-

tive, especially when the radial access site is not available, at high risk of failure or complications after repeated radial catheterizations, or tortuous or anomalous radial arterial vasculature.

- Ulnar artery puncture can be more challenging because of the deeper course of the ulnar artery and lower intensity of palpable pulsations.
- Compression of the ipsilateral radial artery may improve weak or hardly palpable ulnar artery pulsations.
- Ideally, the ulnar artery should be punctured 0.5–3.0 cm proximal to the pisiform bone, where the risk of post-procedural hematoma is lower. The ulnar artery however can be punctured up to the mid-forearm as long as the pulsations can be felt.
- **However, the ulnar nerve is very close to the ulnar artery in that region, so the puncture has to be very accurate, avoiding accidental nerve damage.**
- Real-time ultrasound guidance may facilitate ulnar artery puncture.
- Following the administration of sedation and local anesthetic, either the counterpuncture or anterior wall puncture technique can be used.

Sheath Types for Radial/Ulnar Approach

- While sheath selection is often dictated by operator preference, patient anatomy, and size of the catheters planned to be employed in the

Fig. 5.6 Radial artery access for cardiac catheterization. Lidocaine is instilled at the intended site of puncture to make a small wheal (**Panel A**). Here a single anterior wall puncture technique is demonstrated with flashback of blood from the radial artery (**Panels B** and **C**). Once a guide wire is placed within the radial artery without resistance, a small cut can be made with a scalpel at the point of insertion of the introducer (**Panel D**). This is not mandatory given that most sheaths are hydrophilic and so tend to pass easily over the wire and through the skin into the radial artery without much resistance (**Panel E**). Once the sheath is in place, secure with adhesive dressing (**Panel F**), and flush with heparinized saline to confirm patency (**Panel G**). Once the sheath is secure the arm can be moved into a more comfortable position for the patient if necessary (**Panel H**). Reproduced with permission from the Cardiac Catheterization Handbook, First Edition by Kern MJ. "Radial artery access for cardiac catheterization" Page 55–97; Copyright Elsevier (1996)

procedure, sheath size should be kept as small as possible in order to minimize vascular complications.

- Furthermore, following the completion of the planned procedure, sheaths should be removed as quickly as possible as both the risk of bleeding and thrombotic complications increase with the duration of time that the sheath is left in place.
- Most commercial radial sheaths available today range from 4 to 7 Fr outer diameter and often feature a tapered edge that allows smooth insertion of the sheath through the skin and subcutaneous tissue into the artery (Fig. 5.6, Panel E).
- Furthermore, many feature a hydrophilic coating that has been shown to be associated with less patient discomfort and local pain, easy removal, and less post-procedural inflammatory reactions, particularly in the case of the small-caliber radial artery [39].
- However, rare cases of allergic reactions and noninfectious granulomas associated with the use of these sheaths have been described [40–42]. The ideal sheath length is not codified, but sheath length does not appear to affect the risk of radial artery spasm [39].
- "Slender sheaths," such as the 6 Fr GlideSheath Slender (Terumo Interventional Systems Inc.,

Somerset, NJ) that features a 6 Fr inner diameter but 5.5 Fr outer diameter, can minimize radial arterial trauma while facilitating the use of 6-French equipment [43].

- Slender sheaths are also available in 4.5F and 6.5F outer diameters that accommodate 5- and 7-French equipment, respectively.

Complications

- Up to 5% of access attempts may be associated with radial artery spasm (RAS), which is diagnosed by resistance during manipulation of intra-arterial equipment and by a patient complaining of pain in the forearm, generally without serious lasting clinical complications but often leading to procedural failure and patient discomfort.
- Independent predictors of radial artery spasm include:
  - The presence of radial artery anomalies
  - Female gender
  - Younger age
  - Diabetes
  - Anxiety
  - Multiple catheter exchanges
  - Unsuccessful access at first attempt

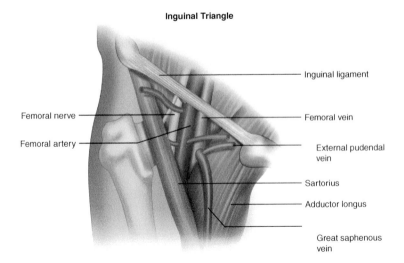

Fig. 5.7 Relevant anatomic features for femoral artery cannulation

- Pain during radial cannulation
- Radial diameter after administration of vasodilatory agents
- Operator experience [44]
- Many strategies have been developed to prevent spasm. By far the best prevention is a clear arteriotomy with a gentle and smooth technique that emphasizes minimal manipulation. It is also essential that the patient be comfortable and relaxed.
- As described above, meticulous patient preparation, low doses of opiates and benzodiazepines, and subcutaneous lidocaine may be used in combination to achieve this.
- Various antispasmodic cocktails have been tried, with the most commonly used vasodilators being diltiazem or verapamil (2.5–5.0 mg, diluted up to 15 mL with blood or saline) and nitroglycerin (100–200 mcg, diluted up to 15 mL with blood or saline).
- In a randomized trial of 150 patients undergoing transradial access, diltiazem plus nitroglycerin showed no advantage compared to nitroglycerin alone in the prevention of RAS [45]. Similarly, in a randomized trial of 406 patients by Chen et al., verapamil plus nitroglycerin was no more effective than nitroglycerin alone in the prevention of RAS [46].
- The patient should be warned of a transient burning sensation in the arm during vasodilator injection. Radial artery spasm that is refractory to pharmacological agents should prompt consideration that the catheter is in the recurrent radial artery rather than the main radial artery as described above.
- Subintimal positioning of the wire and/or a dissection plane may be seen on radial artery angiography. If this occurs, the procedure can usually proceed if the wire can be repositioned intraluminally.
- Insertion of a long radial sheath or a catheter across the dissection will tack up the intimal flap and heal the dissection by the time the procedure ends.
- Radial-brachial perforation is identified by significant resistance during manipulation of intra-arterial equipment and by a patient complaining of significant pain in the forearm,

with or without development of a large forearm hematoma. In case series, the incidence has been 0.1–1% [47, 48]. Injection of dilute contrast through the side port of an introducer sheath confirms the location and size of the perforation. **The procedure should not be abandoned.** Crossing the area of perforation with a soft-tipped 0.014″ coronary guide wire, followed by balloon-assisted tracking, will result in "internal tamponade" and sealing of the perforation. Repeat radial angiography should be performed at the end of the case to assess for any residual dissection or perforation.

- Another type of perforation involves small branches of the radial artery that are traumatized by the small profile of the access wire. These perforations result in the insidious formation of forearm hematomas that are often evident after the procedure. These hematomas should be recognized quickly and compressed gently with wrapping of the forearm.
- The most serious complication of forearm bleeding is compartment syndrome with resultant hand ischemia. While extremely rare, this requires emergent surgical fasciotomy when it occurs.
- Radial artery occlusion (RAO), estimated to occur in 1–10% of cases, is a silent complication of transradial access that can lead to permanent occlusion of the radial artery, thereby making it unusable as an access site for future catheterization or as an arterial conduit for bypass surgery.
- Risk factors for RAO include a large sheath to artery ratio, the omission of anticoagulation for diagnostic catheterizations, and radial artery spasm [35].
- Interestingly, techniques achieving patent hemostasis have been shown to significantly decrease the risk of RAO when compared with occlusive hold hemostasis [49, 50].
- In the PROPHET study, 436 patients undergoing transradial catheterization were randomized to either occlusive hold hemostasis or patent hemostasis [49]. In patients receiving patent hemostasis, RAO was decreased by 59% at 24 h and by 75% at 30 days ($p < 0.05$).

- Furthering this, the PROPHET-II study randomized 3000 patients to patent hemostasis or patent hemostasis and ipsilateral ulnar artery compression [50]. The primary endpoint, 30-day RAO, was significantly reduced in patients receiving patent hemostasis and ipsilateral ulnar artery compression compared with standard patent hemostasis (0.9% vs. 3.0%, $p = 0.0001$) without an increase in hand ischemia.
- In the case of RAO as assessed by duplex ultrasonography 3–4 h after hemostasis, 1-h ulnar artery compression can be safely used to recanalize the radial artery [51].

Femoral Approach

Femoral Anatomy

- The common femoral artery is a zone defined as that continuation of the external iliac artery that is bounded superiorly by the inguinal ligament and internal epigastric artery and inferiorly by the femoral sheath and its subsequent bifurcation into the super-ficial femoral artery and profunda femoris artery (Fig. 5.7).
- It is an ideal target for arteriotomy and sheath access because it is relatively large, less involved with atherosclerosis, and readily compressible against the underlying head of the femur [52].

Femoral Artery Access

- As compelling evidence exists that femoral arterial access complications are related to the site of puncture, appropriate femoral access technique is important to reduce complications.
- Femoral artery access should occur in the "safe zone" of the common femoral artery above the femoral artery bifurcation and below the origin of the internal epigastric artery (Fig. 5.8).
- Several methods can be used to facilitate access into the safe zone, and using the pulse to solely guide access is the least effective method. Fluoroscopic guidance was proposed as early as 1978 [53].

Fig. 5.8 Safe zone for femoral artery cannulation. Adopted from the PCR-EAPCI Textbook, Ch. 3, Figure 5.3

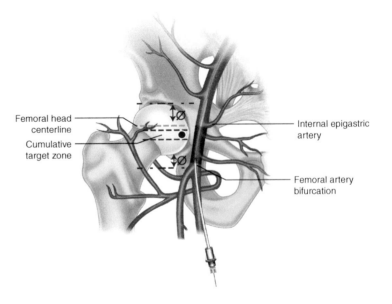

Femoral head centerline

Cumulative target zone

Internal epigastric artery

Femoral artery bifurcation

- The safe zone for arteriotomy can be identified using the femoral head. The safe zone of the common femoral artery runs between lower border of the femoral head and its midportion.
- At present, ultrasound-guided femoral access is the most evidence-based approach to facilitate safe zone arteriotomy. In a randomized trial of ultrasound guidance versus standard access technique, the use of ultrasound increased first-pass success into the safe zone and was particularly useful in patients with reduced pulses and obese patients [54].
- When obtaining transfemoral access, a single anterior wall puncture is highly desirable. An 18-gauge needle is inserted with the bevel up at a 30–45-degree angle and advanced along the direction of the femoral artery until a good, pulsatile blood flow returns.
- A 0.035 J-tip guide wire is then advanced through the needle into the femoral artery, iliac artery, and descending aorta. If resistance is felt, fluoroscopy should be immediately used to visualize the position of the wire.
- While conceptually attractive as they decrease the size of the arteriotomy by 56% and blood flow sixfold, no clear evidence exists to suggest that the routine use of micropuncture needles reduces the risk of vascular complications during transfemoral access.
- Micropuncture needles may however have a role to play in patients with access complicated by severe PAD as well as in patients with iliofemoral grafts.

Complications

- Cannulation of the femoral artery above the lowest point of the internal epigastric artery is associated with an increased risk of retroperitoneal hemorrhage due to a lack of underlying bony structures against which effective compression and tamponade may occur.
- Similarly, cannulation of the femoral artery immediately underneath the inguinal ligament may be problematic because the taut inguinal ligament prevents effective compression.

- Cannulation of the superficial femoral artery or profunda femoris artery, which lacks an underlying bony structure and scaffolding provided by the femoral sheath, is associated with an increased rate of bleeding, hematoma, arteriovenous fistula, and pseudoaneurysm.
- One of the most feared complications of transfemoral access remains retroperitoneal hemorrhage. The incidence ranges from 0.2 to 0.6% and is associated with a mortality rate from 4 to 12%.
- Predictors of retroperitoneal hemorrhage include a "high stick," large sheath size, duration and intensity of anticoagulation, and longer procedural times. The treatment of a retroperitoneal hemorrhage may include transfusion, covered-stent placement, embolization, or emergency surgery.
- The incidence of femoral artery pseudoaneurysms is <1%. In current practice, ultrasound-guided direct thrombin injection is the preferred treatment [55–57].
- Arteriovenous fistulas are rare complications associated with the inadvertent puncture of the femoral vein while attempting to cannulate the femoral artery. Treatment may include close observation (one-third of A-V fistulas close spontaneously at 1 year) [58], endovascular embolization or coiling, or open surgical repair.

Brachial Approach

Brachial Artery Access

- Transbrachial access is rarely used for left-heart catheterization in the modern era as it is more prone to complications compared with transradial or transfemoral access. This includes antecubital hematomas that may rapidly progress to compartment syndrome.
- It is usually indicated when severe PAD precludes femoral access and lack of adequate radial or ulnar artery caliber.
- Access technique is similar to femoral arterial access and manual compression should be used for hemostasis.

Hemostasis

- For radial/ulnar cases, hemostasis can be achieved by manual compression (occlusive hold hemostasis) or more commonly through the use of a specifically designed mechanical device (patent hemostasis). The preferred and recommended technique is patent hemostasis.
- For femoral arterial access, manual compression is the most commonly used. Before removing the sheath, the activated clotting time (ACT) should be <180 s for unfractionated heparin. If bivalirudin is used and the patient's kidney function is normal, the sheath can be removed 2 h after the bivalirudin infusion has been discontinued. In the presence of compromised renal function, sheath removal should be guided by the ACT.
- After sheath removal, the duration of compression varies with the French size of the catheter, with larger sheaths requiring longer compression times. A variety of assisted mechanical compression devices such as C-type clamps or the FemStop (St. Jude Medical, St. Paul, MN) are available to use as an adjunct when longer pressure application is needed.
- Vascular closure devices (VCD) have emerged as an alternative to manual/mechanical compression after transfemoral access. The data on the efficacy and safety of these devices is mixed but seems to indicate earlier patient mobilization and decreased length of stay compared with manual compression at the expense of an increased rate of complications (infection, inflammation, scarring).
- The recently completed ISAR-CLOSURE trial randomly assigned 4524 patients undergoing diagnostic coronary angiography to intravascular VCD, extravascular VCD, or manual compression [59]. The primary endpoint was access-site-related vascular complications at 30 days. The rate of the primary endpoint was 6.9% in the VCD group and 7.9% in the manual compression group ($p < 0.001$ for non-inferiority). VCD use compared with manual compression resulted in fewer large hematomas (4.8% vs. 6.8%, $p = 0.006$) and a shorter time to hemostasis.

Summary

- Attaining vascular access is among the most critical parts of the cardiac catheterization procedure and requires meticulous attention to good technique, proper equipment, and skilled operators.
- Thoughtful patient selection, including an assessment of periprocedural bleeding risk, should guide the choice of left or right transradial, transulnar, or transfemoral access.
- While the transradial and transulnar approaches are associated with significantly reduced patient's bleeding, vascular complications, and mortality when compared with transfemoral access, they may be more technically difficult for those operators still on the radial/ulnar "learning curve."
- If transfemoral access is planned, fluoroscopic and/or ultrasound guidance, smaller sheath sizes, and vascular closure devices may decrease access-site complications.

References

1. Doyle BJ, Ting HH, Bell MR, Lennon RJ, Mathew V, Singh M, et al. Major femoral bleeding complications after percutaneous coronary intervention: incidence, predictors, and impact on long-term survival among 17,901 patients treated at the Mayo Clinic from 1994 to 2005. JACC Cardiovasc Interv. 2008;1(2):202–9.
2. Yatskar L, Selzer F, Feit F, Cohen HA, Jacobs AK, Williams DO, et al. Access site hematoma requiring blood transfusion predicts mortality in patients undergoing percutaneous coronary intervention: data from the National Heart, Lung, and Blood Institute Dynamic Registry. Catheter Cardiovasc Interv. 2007;69(7):961–6.
3. Ellis SG, Bhatt D, Kapadia S, Lee D, Yen M, Whitlow PL. Correlates and outcomes of retroperitoneal hemorrhage complicating percutaneous coronary intervention. Catheter Cardiovasc Interv. 2006;67(4):541–5.
4. Rao SV, Kaul PR, Liao L, Armstrong PW, Ohman EM, Granger CB, et al. Association between bleeding, blood transfusion, and costs among patients with non–ST-segment elevation acute coronary syndromes. Am Heart J. 2008;155(2):369–74.

5. Kern MJ. Cardiac catheterization on the road less traveled navigating the radial versus femoral debate. J Am Coll Cardiol Intv. 2009;2(11):1055–6.

6. Kiemeneij F, Laarman GJ, Odekerken D, Slagboom T, van der Wieken R. A randomized comparison of percutaneous transluminal coronary angioplasty by the radial, brachial and femoral approaches: the access study. J Am Coll Cardiol. 1997;29(6):1269–75.

7. Saito S, Tanaka S, Hiroe Y, Miyashita Y, Takahashi S, Tanaka K, et al. Comparative study on transradial approach vs. transfemoral approach in primary stent implantation for patients with acute myocardial infarction: results of the test for myocardial infarction by prospective unicenter randomization for access sites (TEMPURA) trial. Catheter Cardiovasc Interv. 2003;59(1):26–33.

8. Mehta SR, Jolly SS, Cairns J, Niemela K, Rao SV, Cheema AN, et al. Effects of radial versus femoral artery access in patients with acute coronary syndromes with or without ST-segment elevation. J Am Coll Cardiol. 2012;60(24):2490–9.

9. Romagnoli E, Biondi-Zoccai G, Sciahbasi A, Politi L, Rigattieri S, Pendenza G, et al. Radial versus femoral randomized investigation in ST-segment elevation acute coronary syndrome: the RIFLE-STEACS (Radial Versus Femoral Randomized Investigation in ST-Elevation Acute Coronary Syndrome) study. J Am Coll Cardiol. 2012;60(24):2481–9.

10. Bernat I, Horak D, Stasek J, Mates M, Pesek J, Ostadal P, et al. ST-segment elevation myocardial infarction treated by radial or femoral approach in a multicenter randomized clinical trial: the STEMI-RADIAL Trial. J Am Coll Cardiol. 2014;63(10):964–72.

11. Valgimigli M, Gagnor A, Calabró P, Frigoli E, Leonardi S, Zaro T, et al. Radial versus femoral access in patients with acute coronary syndromes undergoing invasive management: a randomised multicentre trial. Lancet. 2015;385(9986):2465–76.

12. Rao SV, Hess CN, Barham B, Aberle LH, Anstrom KJ, Patel TB, et al. A registry-based randomized trial comparing radial and femoral approaches in women undergoing percutaneous coronary intervention: the SAFE-PCI for women (study of access site for enhancement of PCI for women) trial. J Am Coll Cardiol Intv. 2014;7(8):857–67.

13. Jolly SS, Amlani S, Hamon M, Yusuf S, Mehta SR. Radial versus femoral access for coronary angiography or intervention and the impact on major bleeding and ischemic events: a systematic review and meta-analysis of randomized trials. Am Heart J. 2009;157(1):132–40.

14. Bavishi C, Panwar SR, Dangas GD, Barman N, Hasan CM, Baber U, et al. Meta-analysis of radial versus femoral access for percutaneous coronary interventions in non-ST-segment elevation acute coronary syndrome. Am J Cardiol. 2016;117(2):172–8.

15. Rao SV, Ou F-S, Wang TY, Roe MT, Brindis R, Rumsfeld JS, et al. Trends in the prevalence and outcomes of radial and femoral approaches to percutaneous coronary intervention: a report from the national cardiovascular data registry. J Am Coll Cardiol Intv. 2008;1(4):379–86.

16. Valgimigli M, Campo G, Penzo C, Tebaldi M, Biscaglia S, Ferrari R. Transradial coronary catheterization and intervention across the whole spectrum of Allen test results. J Am Coll Cardiol. 2014;63(18):1833–41.

17. Marso SP, Amin AP, House JA, Kennedy KF, Spertus JA, Rao SV, et al. Association between use of bleeding avoidance strategies and risk of periprocedural bleeding among patients undergoing percutaneous coronary intervention. JAMA. 2010;303(21):2156–64.

18. Rao SV, LA MC, Spertus JA, Krone RJ, Singh M, Fitzgerald S, et al. An updated bleeding model to predict the risk of post-procedure bleeding among patients undergoing percutaneous coronary intervention: a report using an expanded bleeding definition from the National Cardiovascular Data Registry CathPCI Registry. J Am Coll Cardiol Interv. 2013;6(9):897–904.

19. Rao SC, Chhatriwalla AK, Kennedy KF, Decker CJ, Gialde E, Spertus JA, et al. Pre-procedural estimate of individualized bleeding risk impacts physicians; utilization of bivalirudin during percutaneous coronary intervention. J Am Coll Cardiol. 2013;61(18):1847–52.

20. Steffenino G, Viada E, Marengo B, Canale R. Effectiveness of video-based patient information before percutaneous cardiac interventions. J Cardiovasc Med (Hagerstown MD). 2007;8(5):348–53.

21. Bertrand OF, Rao SV, Pancholy S, Jolly SS, Rodés-Cabau J, Larose É, et al. Transradial approach for coronary angiography and interventions: results of the first international transradial practice survey. J Am Coll Cardiol Intv. 2010;3(10):1022–31.

22. Dehghani P, Mohammad A, Bajaj R, Hong T, Suen CM, Sharieff W, et al. Mechanism and predictors of failed transradial approach for percutaneous coronary interventions. J Am Coll Cardiol Intv. 2009;2(11):1057–64.

23. Kumar Chugh S, Chugh S, Chugh Y, Rao SV. Feasibility and utility of pre-procedure ultrasound imaging of the arm to facilitate transradial coronary diagnostic and interventional procedures (PRIMAFACIE-TRI). Catheter Cardiovasc Interv. 2013;82(1):64–73.

24. Lo TS, Nolan J, Fountzopoulos E, Behan M, Butler R, Hetherington SL, et al. Radial artery anomaly and its influence on transradial coronary procedural outcome. Heart. 2009;95(5):410–5.

25. Patel T, Shah S, Pancholy S, Rao S, Bertrand OF, Kwan T. Balloon-assisted tracking: a must-know technique to overcome difficult anatomy during transradial approach. Catheter Cardiovasc Interv. 2014;83(2):211–20.

26. Sciahbasi A, Romagnoli E, Trani C, Burzotta F, Pendenza G, Tommasino A, et al. Evaluation of the "learning curve" for left and right radial approach dur-

ing percutaneous coronary procedures. Am J Cardiol. 2011;108(2):185–8.

27. Kawashima O, Endoh N, Terashima M, Ito Y, Abe S, Ootomo T, et al. Effectiveness of right or left radial approach for coronary angiography. Catheter Cardiovasc Interv. 2004;61(3):333–7.

28. Norgaz T, Gorgulu S, Dagdelen S. A randomized study comparing the effectiveness of right and left radial approach for coronary angiography. Catheter Cardiovasc Interv. 2012;80(2):260–4.

29. Burzotta F, Trani C, Todaro D, Romagnoli E, Niccoli G, Ginnico F, et al. Comparison of the transradial and transfemoral approaches for coronary angiographic evaluation in patients with internal mammary artery grafts. J Cardiovasc Med (Hagerstown MD). 2008;9(3):263–6.

30. Sciahbasi A, Romagnoli E, Burzotta F, Trani C, Sarandrea A, Summaria F, et al. Transradial approach (left vs right) and procedural times during percutaneous coronary procedures: TALENT study. Am Heart J. 2011;161(1):172–9.

31. Xia SL, Zhang XB, Zhou JS, Gao X. Comparative efficacy and safety of the left versus right radial approach for percutaneous coronary procedures: a meta-analysis including 6870 patients. Braz J Med Biol Res. 2015;48(8):743–50.

32. Seto AH, Roberts JS, Abu-Fadel MS, Czak SJ, Latif F, Jain SP, et al. Real-time ultrasound guidance facilitates transradial access: RAUST (Radial Artery Access with Ultrasound Trial). J Am Coll Cardiol Interv. 2015;8(2):283–91.

33. Pancholy SB, Sanghvi KA, Patel TM. Radial artery access technique evaluation trial: randomized comparison of seldinger versus modified seldinger technique for arterial access for transradial catheterization. Catheter Cardiovasc Interv. 2012;80(2):288–91.

34. Pancholy SB, Coppola J, Patel T. Subcutaneous administration of nitroglycerin to facilitate radial artery cannulation. Catheter Cardiovasc Interv. 2006;68(3):389–91.

35. Kotowycz MA, Džavík V. Radial artery patency after transradial catheterization. Circ Cardiovasc Interv. 2012;5(1):127–33.

36. Hahalis G, Tsigkas G, Xanthopoulou I, Deftereos S, Ziakas A, Raisakis K, et al. Transulnar compared with transradial artery approach as a default strategy for coronary procedures: a randomized trial. The Transulnar or Transradial Instead of Coronary Transfemoral Angiographies Study (the AURA of ARTEMIS Study). Circ Cardiovasc Interv. 2013;6(3):252–61.

37. Aptecar E, Pernes JM, Chabane-Chaouch M, Bussy N, Catarino G, Shahmir A, et al. Transulnar versus transradial artery approach for coronary angioplasty: the PCVI-CUBA study. Catheter Cardiovasc Interv. 2006;67(5):711–20.

38. Dahal K, Rijal J, Lee J, Korr KS, Azrin M. Transulnar versus transradial access for coronary angiography or percutaneous coronary intervention: a meta-analysis

of randomized controlled trials. Catheter Cardiovasc Interv. 2016;87(5):857–65.

39. Rathore S, Stables RH, Pauriah M, Hakeem A, Mills JD, Palmer ND, et al. Impact of length and hydrophilic coating of the introducer sheath on radial artery spasm during transradial coronary intervention: a randomized study. J Am Coll Cardiol Intv. 2010;3(5):475–83.

40. Lim J, Suri A, Chua TP. Steroid-responsive sterile inflammation after transradial cardiac catheterisation using a sheath with hydrophilic coating. Heart. 2009;95(14):1202.

41. Kozak M, Adams DR, Ioffreda MD, Nickolaus MJ, Seery TJ, Chambers CE, et al. Sterile inflammation associated with transradial catheterization and hydrophilic sheaths. Catheter Cardiovasc Interv. 2003;59(2):207–13.

42. Zellner C, Yeghiazarians Y, Ports TA, Ursell P, Boyle AJ. Sterile radial artery granuloma after transradial cardiac catheterization. Cardiovasc Revasc Med. 2011;12(3):187–9.

43. Yoshimachi F, Kiemeneij F, Masutani M, Matsukage T, Takahashi A, Ikari Y. Safety and feasibility of the new 5 Fr Glidesheath Slender. Cardiovasc Interv Ther. 2016;31:38–41.

44. Jia DA, Zhou YJ, Shi DM, Liu YY, Wang JL, Liu XL, et al. Incidence and predictors of radial artery spasm during transradial coronary angiography and intervention. Chin Med J (Engl). 2010;123(7):843–7.

45. Dharma S, Shah S, Radadiya R, Vyas C, Pancholy S, Patel T. Nitroglycerin plus diltiazem versus nitroglycerin alone for spasm prophylaxis with transradial approach. J Invasive Cardiol. 2012;24(3):122–5.

46. Chen CW, Lin CL, Lin TK, Lin CD. A simple and effective regimen for prevention of radial artery spasm during coronary catheterization. Cardiology. 2006;105(1):43–7.

47. Hildick-Smith DJ, Lowe MD, Walsh JT, Ludman PF, Stephens NG, Schofield PM, et al. Coronary angiography from the radial artery—experience, complications and limitations. Int J Cardiol. 1998;64(3):231–9.

48. Calvino-Santos RA, Vazquez-Rodriguez JM, Salgado-Fernandez J, Vazquez-Gonzalez N, Perez-Fernandez R, Vazquez-Rey E, et al. Management of iatrogenic radial artery perforation. Catheter Cardiovasc Interv. 2004;61(1):74–8.

49. Pancholy S, Coppola J, Patel T, Roke-Thomas M. Prevention of radial artery occlusion-patent hemostasis evaluation trial (PROPHET study): a randomized comparison of traditional versus patency documented hemostasis after transradial catheterization. Catheter Cardiovasc Interv. 2008;72(3):335–40.

50. Pancholy SB, Bernat I, Bertrand OF, Patel TM. Prevention of radial artery occlusion after transradial catheterization: the PROPHET-II randomized trial. J Am Coll Cardiol Intv. 2016;9(19):1992–9.

51. Bernat I, Bertrand OF, Rokyta R, Kacer M, Pesek J, Koza J, et al. Efficacy and safety of transient ulnar artery compression to recanalize acute radial artery

occlusion after transradial catheterization. Am J Cardiol. 2011;107(11):1698–701.

52. Bangalore S, Bhatt DL. Femoral arterial access and closure. Circulation. 2011;124(5):e147-e56.

53. Dotter CT, Rosch J, Robinson M. Fluoroscopic guidance in femoral artery puncture. Radiology. 1978;127(1):266–7.

54. Seto AH, Abu-Fadel MS, Sparling JM, Zacharias SJ, Daly TS, Harrison AT, et al. Real-time ultrasound guidance facilitates femoral arterial access and reduces vascular complications: FAUST (femoral arterial access with ultrasound trial). J Am Coll Cardiol Intv. 2010;3(7):751–8.

55. Paulson EK, Sheafor DH, Kliewer MA, Nelson RC, Eisenberg LB, Sebastian MW, et al. Treatment of iatrogenic femoral arterial pseudoaneurysms: comparison of US-guided thrombin injection with compression repair. Radiology. 2000;215(2): 403–8.

56. La Perna L, Olin JW, Goines D, Childs MB, Ouriel K. Ultrasound-guided thrombin injection for the treatment of postcatheterization Pseudoaneurysms. Circulation. 2000;102(19):2391.

57. Webber GW, Jang J, Gustavson S, Olin JW. Contemporary management of postcatheterization pseudoaneurysms. Circulation. 2007;115(20):2666.

58. Kelm M, Perings SM, Jax T, Lauer T, Schoebel FC, Heintzen MP, et al. Incidence and clinical outcome of iatrogenic femoral arteriovenous fistulas: implications for risk stratification and treatment. J Am Coll Cardiol. 2002;40(2):291–7.

59. Schulz-Schupke S, Helde S, Gewalt S, Ibrahim T, Linhardt M, Haas K, et al. Comparison of vascular closure devices vs manual compression after femoral artery puncture: the ISAR-CLOSURE randomized clinical trial. JAMA. 2014;312(19):1981–7.

Right Heart Catheterization

Jean-Luc Vachiéry and Céline Dewachter

About Us The authors are cardiologists working in the Pulmonary Hypertension and Heart Failure Clinic in the Department of Cardiology at the Erasme Hospital, the academic institution of the Université Libre de Bruxelles in Belgium. The center hosts a specialized unit of national and international reputation, which manages patients with all forms of pulmonary vascular disorders and end-stage heart failure. Their scientific interest encompasses research from bench to bedside in pulmonary circulation and right ventricular function, with a strong emphasis on hemodynamics, physiology, and pathophysiology. Professor Vachiery is coauthor of the European Society of Cardiology and European Respiratory Society guidelines on the diagnosis and management of pulmonary hypertension.

Introduction

- Despite advances in imaging, right heart catheterization (RHC), also called pulmonary artery catheterization, is the gold standard for the assessment of the pulmonary circulation and the right ventricle in healthy and disease states. RHC is mandatory to establish the diagnosis of pulmonary hypertension (PH), to assess disease severity, and to determine prognosis and response to therapy [1, 2].
- In addition, it remains a critical tool in the assessment of patients who are candidates for heart transplantation [3] and may be considered in various cardiac disorders.
- Contrary to popular belief, the procedure is rather safe, even in advanced cases. A recent retrospective and prospective multicenter study reported a procedure-related mortality of 0.055% and morbidity of 1.1% in specialized centers of PH [4].
- RHC is a technically demanding procedure that requires meticulous attention to detail and accuracy in interpretation to obtain clinically useful information. It must always be integrated in the general assessment of a patient's condition, which includes the clinical context and imaging, in particular echocardiography.
- To obtain high-quality results and minimize the risk of complication, physicians appropriately trained in handling and interpretation of the test should perform the procedure in expert centers.

Goals, Indications, and Contraindications of Right Heart Catheterization

- RHC must be performed to establish the differential diagnosis of PH, as it provides a measurement of pulmonary pressures, right- and

J.-L. Vachiéry (✉) · C. Dewachter
Department of Cardiology, Pulmonary Vascular
Diseases and Heart Failure Clinic, CUB—Erasme
University Hospital, Brussels, Belgium
e-mail: jeanluc.vachiery@erasme.ulb.ac.be;
celine.dewachter@erasme.ulb.ac.be

© Springer International Publishing AG, part of Springer Nature 2018
A. Myat et al. (eds.), *The Interventional Cardiology Training Manual*,
https://doi.org/10.1007/978-3-319-71635-0_6

left-heart filling pressures, cardiac output, and staged oxygen saturation.
- The procedure is mandatory before embarking on a treatment for the most severe form of PH such as pulmonary arterial hypertension (PAH) and chronic thromboembolic pulmonary hypertension (CTEPH).
- In heart failure (HF), RHC is necessary in the assessment of candidates for heart transplantation and implantation of left ventricular assist devices (LVAD).
- In PH and HF, it is also commonly used to establish prognosis and monitor the efficacy of more invasive therapies.

- In the intensive care unit (ICU) setting, RHC has been in a "love-hate" relationship with intensivists. Nevertheless, recent technical advances in monitoring and clinical trials have reestablished a role for RHC in the assessment of ICU patients, especially in shock condition and in patients with suspected cardiac diseases.
- The indications of RHC are presented in Table 6.1. Although rare, there are some contraindications to the procedure (Table 6.2), both technical (center dependent) and clinical (patient dependent).

Table 6.1 Indications for right heart catheterization

Clinical scenario	Indications
Differential diagnosis	• Causes of shock (cardiogenic, hypovolemic, distributive, obstructive) • Mechanism of pulmonary edema (cardiogenic or not) • Diagnosis of pulmonary hypertension • Pericardial tamponade • Intracardiac shunts • Lymphangitic spread of tumor and fat embolism • Unexplained dyspnea in noncardiac disease (liver cirrhosis, COPD)
Guide to therapy	• Acute and chronic setting, pharmacological therapy (vasopressors, vasodilators, testing the pulmonary circulation) • Acute setting, nonpharmacological therapy (volume expansion, burns, renal failure, sepsis) • Vasoreactivity testing in PAH • Perioperative management of unstable cardiac patients undergoing cardiac and noncardiac interventions
Prognosis assessment	• Advanced heart failure prior to left ventricular assist device (LVAD) implantation and heart transplantation • Advanced chronic respiratory failure prior to lung transplantation to assess PH • Unexplained dyspnea and cardiac limitation to exercise • Severe PH, including PAH and CTEPH

Table 6.2 Contraindications for right heart catheterization

Level	Causes
Absolute	• Patient mentally unable to understand and/or undergo the procedure • Insufficient equipment and cath facility • Infection at the insertion site • Presence of a right ventricular assist device (RVAD) • Active, uncontrolled bleeding associated with established untreatable disorders of coagulation
Increased risk	• Uncontrolled congestive cardiac failure, hypertension, arrhythmias • Recent cerebral vascular accident (<1 month) • Infection/fever • Severe electrolyte and acid-base imbalance • Severe anemia • Acute gastrointestinal bleeding • Coagulopathy or on anticoagulation (international normalized ratio, INR >1.5, thrombocytopenia (platelet count <50,000/mm^3)) • Pregnancy • Uncooperative patient • Medication intoxication (i.e., digitalis, phenothiazine)

Procedure: Preparation and Insertion of Right Heart Catheter

- RHC requires prior patient's consent. In addition, it needs to be performed in an appropriate environment, which includes staff and technical facilities. In particular, blood pressure, heart rate (HR), and oxygen saturation must be monitored throughout the procedure.
- All equipment to deliver cardiorespiratory resuscitation, oxygen, and vasopressors must be available in case of shock and cardiac arrest.
- One physician can perform RHC but nursing staff (at least one) must be present throughout the procedure. The most common device used for RHC is a triple-lumen Swan-Ganz catheter. This flexible fluid-filled catheter has two pressure ports (one at the tip for pulmonary arterial pressure (PAP) measurements, and one 30 cm from the tip to allow for injection of saline and measurement of right atrial pressure (RAP)) and one closed lumen to inflate a balloon at the tip for the measurement of pulmonary artery wedge pressure (PAWP). A more rigid, non-floated, balloon-free catheter is sometimes used in the cath lab but it does not permit the measurement of cardiac output.

The following describes the step-by-step procedure to provide keys to an uneventful procedure:

- *Preparation*
  - Review of indications and contraindications
  - Patient's information and collection of informed consent
  - Decision on insertion site (jugular versus femoral, antecubital, or subclavian approach), based on patient's anatomy and physician's expertise
  - Verification of the setting, including preparation of the catheter table that should include insertion sheath, anesthetic, and pulmonary arterial catheter
- *Installation*
  - Ensure a quiet environment.
  - Place the patient in supine position, and monitor electrocardiogram (ECG), noninvasive blood pressure, and oxygen saturation.

- Insert a peripheral catheter in case of anxiety/agitation to deliver myorelaxant (midazolam).
- Deliver supplemental oxygen, if required, to aim for an arterial oxygen saturation (SaO$_2$) >90%.
- *Vascular approach—internal jugular vein*
  - Most common and easiest approach, preferable in the ICU setting
  - Low rate of complications (0.3% in PH evaluation [4]).
  - Prefer the right side for a more straightforward approach.
  - Ensure sufficient filling by slightly tilting the patient at −20°, or use ultrasonography to guide insertion.
  - Local anesthesia at the level of the clavicle part of the sternocleidomastoid muscle.
  - Puncture of the internal jugular vein, approximately three fingers above the clavicle.
  - Insertion of a guide wire, followed by a 7-F size sheath introducer.
  - Consider antecubital or subclavian approach only if the jugular vein is not accessible.
  - Femoral approach preferred in the cath lab, especially in associated left-heart procedures: However, the increasing use of the radial approach for the latter makes this less necessary.
- *Positioning of the catheter* (Fig. 6.1)
  - Either under fluoroscopic guidance or by following the pressure traces on the monitoring.
  - Inflation of the balloon in the right atrium (roughly when the catheter is inserted by 20–30 cm) with evidence of RAP tracing.
  - Further progression through the tricuspid valve in the right ventricle (a rise in systolic pressure is observed), the right ventricular outflow tract, and the main trunk of the pulmonary artery (a rise in diastolic pressure is observed).
  - Pressure decay observed in the wedge position, requiring deflation of the balloon.
  - Caveats: Inflate balloon when respiratory pressure swings; a.lways deflate balloon when pulling back; **avoid repeated deflations and inflations of the balloon in the end pulmonary arteries because of the risk of rupture of the pulmonary arteries**

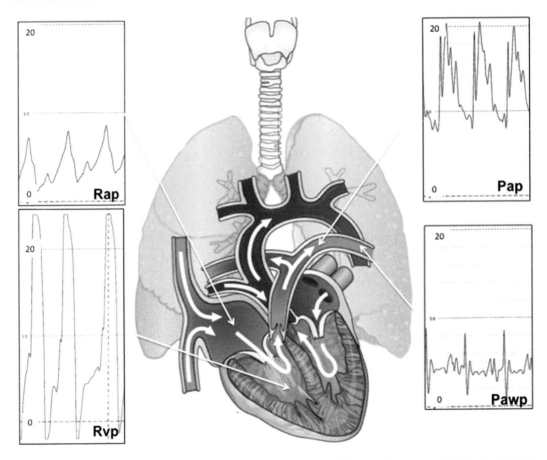

Fig. 6.1 Pressure traces collected during routine RHC. The pulmonary artery catheter is progressively advanced in the heart chambers, with the corresponding pressures. (1) Right atrial pressure (RAP); (2) right ventricular pressure (RVP); (3) pulmonary artery pressure (PAP); 4: pulmonary artery wedge pressure (PAWP)

Data Acquisition and Analysis, Measurements, and Derived Calculations

During RHC, pressures are measured with fluid-filled catheters such as a pressure difference between hydrostatic pressures at a chosen zero level and pressures in the chamber or vessel where the catheter lumen is open.

The following protocol should be followed for an optimal pressure measurement:

- **Zeroing and respiratory cycle**
  - Zero leveling of the external pressure transducer: mid-chest (half distance between the anterior sternum and the bed surface, corresponding to the left atrial level) or 5 cm below angle of Louis in a supine patient.
  - Pressure measurements at normal end expiration—or average over several respiratory cycles if marked respiratory pressure swings (in obese patients and patients with lung disease): Mean of three measurements of each pressure at end expiration.

- **Data acquisition**
  - *Pressures*
    - The following pressures must be recorded: central venous pressure (CVP), RAP equal to right ventricular end-diastolic pressure, right ventricular pressure (RVP) (systolic, diastolic, mean), pulmonary artery pres-

sure (PAP) (systolic, diastolic, mean), PAWP—a surrogate of left atrial pressure.

- Ideally, pressure should be read on paper traces at a speed of 12.5–25 mm/s for quality control. Scale must be adapted to position the pressure traces in the upper 1/3rd of the paper. Readings can also be made from screenshots if the system allows for a cursor placement in a proper position. Direct display of measures should be avoided as they may be influenced by the respiratory cycle and arrhythmias.

- *Cardiac output*
  - Several methods have been used to measure cardiac output (CO). The Fick method is considered the gold standard, by using the following: $CO = VO_2/CaO_2 - CvO_2$, where VO_2 = oxygen consumption, CaO_2 = oxygen concentration of arterial blood, and CvO_2 = oxygen concentration of mixed venous blood. To be accurate, VO_2 should be measured directly. The estimated value can lead to considerable errors.
  - The method of choice is therefore the thermodilution technique, where cardiac output is assessed after injecting 10 mL cold or room-temperature saline.

CO should be determined in triplicate with less than 10% variation.

- *Blood gas analysis*
  - In all patients, analysis of arterial (by direct arterial puncture) and mixed venous blood (by sampling blood from the tip lumen of the RHC) gases must be performed. Stepwise assessment of oxygen saturation by blood samples taken from the superior and inferior vena cava, right atrium, and pulmonary artery is needed in every patient with a pulmonary arterial oxygen saturation (mixed venous blood saturation, SvO_2) >75% and in case of suspicion of a left-to-right shunt.

- *Other data acquisition*
  - Because patients are continuously monitored, the following must be recorded: systemic arterial pressure (SAP) estimated by noninvasive blood pressure if left-heart cath is not performed at the same time, HR, and pulse oxygen saturation (SpO_2).

- *Pitfalls*
- As for any technique, RHC should be meticulously performed to avoid mistakes (Table 6.3 and Fig. 6.2).

• **Calculations and RHC report** (Fig. 6.3)

Table 6.3 Pitfalls and errors in RHC (adapted from references [1, 2, 15, 16])

Source of error	Potential error	Risk	Solution
Measurement	Catheter balloon overinflation	• False PAWP reading • Pulmonary arterial rupture	• Half inflation of the balloon • Avoid repeated inflations and deflations
	Catheter balloon underinflation	False elevation of PAWP readings	Half inflation of the balloon
	Respiratory swings	Misdiagnosis of pre- versus postcapillary PH	Average PAWP readings across respiratory cycles
	Analyzing single cycle	Potential data inaccuracy	Mean values of multiple respiratory cycles should be used
	Variation in the location of the pressure transducer	Nonuniformity of the pressure transducer setting and zero leveling	Standardized location of pressure transducer according to guideline recommendations or adoption of micromanometer-tipped catheters
Data interpretation	Failure to review traces	Data inaccuracy (measurement artifacts)	Each trace should be scrutinized to ensure that it is not affected by artifacts
Technical	Incorrectly maintained or calibrated equipment	Errors in data acquisition	Equipment maintained to a high standard and regular calibration
	Inadequate flushing of the catheter	Dampened waveforms	Adequate flushing

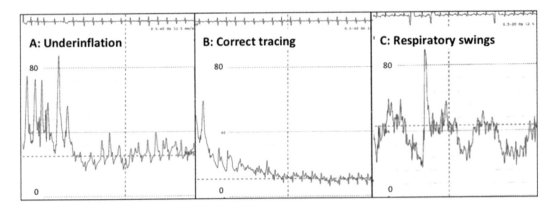

Fig. 6.2 Effect of inappropriate balloon inflation and respiratory swings on pulmonary artery wedge pressure (PAWP) reading. The pressure traces displayed in this figure were recorded in the same patient during a single RHC. The dotted line represents the placement of the cursor for meticulous measurement of PAWP. **Panel A**: The balloon is underinflated, leading to insufficient damping of the pressure and partial occlusion; PAWP is inappropriately measured at 18 mmHg. **Panel B**: The balloon is fully inflated, with a good pressure decay allowing for a correct measurement of PAWP at 7 mmHg. **Panel C**: The balloon is correctly inflated, but excessive respiratory swings are present, leading to an incorrect end-expiratory PAWP measurement >40 mmHg

Pulmonary hypertension and heart failure clinic					
Right heart catheterization - Evaluation of pulmonary hypertension					
Name:					
Folder number:					
Body surface area:					
Date:					
Indication:					
Pulmonary hypertension diagnosis:					
Vascular acces:					
Conditions	Baseline 1	Baseline 2	Baseline 3	Baseline Mean	NO 20 ppm test
Time					
Cardiac rythm, heart beat per minute					
Systemic arterial pressure, mmHg	systolic				
	diastolic				
	mean				
Pulmonary artery pressure, mmHg	systolic				
	diastolic				
	mean				
Pawp, mmHg					
Right atrial pressure, mmHg					
Transpulmonary gradient, mmHg					
Diastolic gradient, mmHg					
Arterial saturation, %					
Mixed venous saturation, %					
Cardiac output, l/min					
Cardiac index, l/min/m²					
Pulmonary vascular resistance, UW					
Compliance, mL/mmHg					
RC time, s					
Conclusions					
Doctors					

Arterial gas analysis	
pH	
PaCO2	
PaO2	
SaO2	

Fig. 6.3 Comprehensive RHC hemodynamic report

Once data are acquired, a full hemodynamic report must be generated. It must contain the following values and an interpretation of the findings:

- Pulmonary vascular resistance (PVR) = (mPAP - PAWP)/CO.
- Transpulmonary pressure gradient (TPG) = mPAP – PAWP.
- Diastolic transpulmonary gradient (DPG) = dPAP - PAWP (less affected by flow and filling pressures [5] but may not be of prognostic value [6]).
- SVR = (SAP-RAP)/CO.
- CI = CO/BSA, cardiac index (CI) corresponding to cardiac output (CO) adjusted for body surface area (BSA).
- RVSW = (mPAP-RAP) × SV (stroke volume), right ventricular stroke work.
- Other calculations may be provided (such as pulmonary arterial compliance), but their clinical relevance remains unknown.

- *PAWP or LVEDP?*
- LV end-diastolic pressure (LVEDP) measurement is needed when PAWP is unexpectedly elevated and/or inaccurate (absence of risk factors for heart failure with preserved ejection fraction (HFpEF), normal left atrial size, and absence of echocardiographic markers of elevated left ventricular filling pressures) [2].
- *Normal values for hemodynamic measurements and calculations are displayed in Table 6.4.*

Table 6.4 Normal values of variables collected during RHC (after references [2, 8])

Measurements	Mean	Limits
mPAP	13 mmHg	8–20 mmHg
PAWP	9 mmHg	5–14 mmHg
RAP	4 mmHg	0–8 mmHg
Cardiac output	6.5 L/min	4–8.3 L/min
Cardiac index	3.6 L/min/m²	2.5–4 L/min/m²
RVP	0.7 WU	0.5–2 WU

Complications Related to the Use of Pulmonary Artery Catheter

Adverse events related to RHC are rare. A large multicenter registry reported the outcome of patients undergoing RHC for the assessment of PH over a 5-year retrospective and 6-month prospective evaluation [4]. Mortality and morbidity rates were found relatively low (respectively, 0.055% and 1.1%) [4]. In most cases, complications are mild to moderate in intensity and resolve either spontaneously or after appropriate intervention.

- Major risk, associated with death, longer hospitalization, or requiring intervention:
  - Carotid artery puncture, arterial bleeding (with internal jugular vein approach)
  - Pneumothorax, hemothorax (subclavian or internal jugular vein approach)
  - Retroperitoneal hemorrhage (femoral approach)
  - Air emboli through introducers
  - Rupture of pulmonary artery
  - Tamponade
  - Lung infarction/hemoptysis
  - Arrhythmia, either atrial or ventricular
  - Transient right bundle branch block (5%), or complete heart block in patients with preexisting left bundle branch block
  - Tricuspid valve injury
- Mild-to-moderate risk, with usually no intervention and full recovery
  - Hematoma at the site of puncture
  - Transient hypotension due to vasovagal reaction
  - Catheter knotting in intracardiac chambers
  - Misplacement due to looping of the catheter inside the right atrium of the right ventricle (fluoroscopy guidance in case of doubt)
  - Infections are exceptional when the catheter is left in place <24 h (for monitoring purposes)

Most of, if not all, these risks can easily be avoided by following some "golden" rules:

- Use anatomical landmarks when inserting the introducer; if puncture is difficult, use Doppler-echo guidance.
- Advance the catheter under pressure monitoring and fluoroscopic guidance.
- Do not push the catheter too far (>50–55 cm from insertion, >15 cm from RVP to PAP).
- Avoid pushing/withdrawing the catheter in case of resistance.
- Always deflate the balloon prior to catheter withdrawal and never remove the catheter when the balloon is inflated.
- Never remove the catheter in case of hemoptysis: reinflate or leave the catheter in place and perform an angiogram.

Interpretation of Results: Pulmonary Hypertension

- *Pulmonary hypertension* is the most common indication for RHC. It is defined by a mean pulmonary arterial pressure (mPAP) $\geq$25 mmHg at rest, measured invasively [1, 2]. The clinical classification of PH identifies five groups, each sharing similar clinical, pathobiological, and outcome characteristics (Table 6.5). With roughly 80% of all causes of PH, left-heart diseases (group 2) and pulmonary disorders (group 3) represent the most common etiologies.
- In normal individuals, the upper limit of mPAP is approximately 20 mmHg [1, 7, 8]. Although the relevance of an mPAP between 21 and 24 mmHg is unclear, it may require careful follow-up in patients at risk of PAH [7].

Table 6.5 Clinical classification of pulmonary hypertension [2]

1. Pulmonary arterial hypertension	*3. PH due to lung diseases and/or hypoxia*
1.1 Idiopathic PAH 1.2 Heritable PAH 1.2.1 BMPR2 1.2.2 ALK-1, ENG, SMAD9, CAV1, KCNK3 1.2.3 Unknown 1.3 Drug and toxin induced 1.4 Associated with: 1.4.1 Connective tissue disease 1.4.2 HIV infection 1.4.3 Portal hypertension 1.4.4 Congenital heart diseases 1.4.5 SCHISTOSOMIASIS	3.1 Chronic obstructive pulmonary disease 3.2 Interstitial lung disease 3.3 Other pulmonary diseases with mixed restrictive and obstructive pattern 3.4 Sleep-disordered breathing 3.5 Alveolar hypoventilation disorders 3.6 Chronic exposure to high altitude 3.7 Developmental lung diseases
1' Pulmonary veno-occlusive disease and/or pulmonary capillary hemangiomatosis *1" Persistent pulmonary hypertension of the newborn (PPHN)*	*4. Chronic thromboembolic pulmonary hypertension (CTEPH)*
2. PH due to left-heart disease	*5. Pulmonary hypertension with unclear multifactorial mechanisms*
2.1 Left ventricular systolic dysfunction 2.2 Left ventricular diastolic dysfunction 2.3 Valvular disease 2.4 Congenital/acquired left-heart inflow/outflow tract obstruction and congenital cardiomyopathies	5.1 Hematologic disorders: chronic hemolytic anemia, myeloproliferative disorders, splenectomy 5.2 Systemic disorders: sarcoidosis, pulmonary histiocytosis, lymphangioleiomyomatosis 5.3 Metabolic disorders: glycogen storage disease, Gaucher disease, thyroid disorders 5.4 Others: tumoral obstruction, fibrosing mediastinitis, chronic renal failure, segmental PH

There is currently no approved hemodynamic definition for "PH on exercise."

- The hemodynamic definition of PH is based on the measurement of mPAP and PAWP and the calculation of PVR (Table 6.6).
  - *Precapillary PH* is defined by an mPAP ≥25 mmHg, a PAWP ≤15 mmHg, and a PVR >3 Wood units (WU).
  - *Postcapillary PH* is defined by an mPAP ≥25 mmHg and a PAWP >15 mmHg and may correspond to PH due to left-heart failure or with unclear and/or multifactorial mechanisms [1, 2].
  - Postcapillary PH is further subdivided according to the diastolic pressure gradient (DPG = dPAP-PAWP) to distinguish *isolated postcapillary PH* (IPC-PH), if the DPG <7 mmHg and/or PVR ≤3 WU, from *combined postcapillary PH* (CPC-PH), if the DPG ≥7 mmHg and/or PVR >3 WU.
- Patient with PH due to HFpEF may present with normalized PAWP when treated

Table 6.6 Hemodynamic definition of pulmonary hypertension [1]

Definition	Characteristics[1]	Clinical group(s)
PH	mPAP ≥25 mmHg	All
Precapillary PH	mPAP ≥25 mmHg PAWP ≤5 mmHg	Pulmonary arterial hypertension (group 1) PH due to lung diseases (group 3) Chronic thromboembolic PH (group 4) PH with unclear and/or multifactorial mechanisms (group 5)
Postcapillary PH Isolated postcapillary PH (IPC-PH) Combined postcapillary PH (CPC-PH)	mPAP ≥25 mmHg PAWP >15 mmHg DPG <7 mmHg and/or PVR ≤3 UW DPG ≥7 mmHg and/or PVR >3 WU [2]	PH due to left-heart diseases (group 2) PH with unclear and/or multifactorial mechanisms (group 5)

aggressively with diuretics. In addition, patients with PAH tend to present with cardiovascular comorbidities that overlap with HFpEF. Therefore, the distinction between the two conditions has major implications as PAH therapies are not approved in group 2 PH. Unmasking diastolic dysfunction is therefore critical in the assessment of patients at risk of PH due to HFpEF. An adequate measurement of PAWP is thus critical and provocative tests performed during RHC may play a role in the differential diagnosis (see below).

- RHC also plays an important role in the treatment decision for PAH, currently based on a risk-oriented strategy, which includes an invasive component. A worse prognosis is associated with a RAP >12 mmHg, a SvO_2 <60%, and a CI <2 L/min/m^2.

Provocative Pulmonary Vasoreactivity/Dynamic Testing During Right Heart Catheterization

The role of provocative testing of the pulmonary circulation has been extensively reported. However, most procedures lack standardization, definition of normal response, and validation through multicenter studies. In addition, the impact of these tests on a decision-making process and patient's outcome is frequently unclear. Despite these limitations, the following tests are/can be used in clinical practice.

- *Pulmonary vasoreactivity testing*
  RHC is part of the assessment for heart transplantation and LVAD implantation. In this setting, PH is associated with a dismal outcome, although it is not clear whether it is due to PH alone or right ventricular dysfunction found in end-stage HF. Although various vasodilators have been used (mostly in single-center studies), nitroprusside, milrinone, and enoximone are the most appropriate compounds as they act primarily by decreasing left-side filling pressures (nitroprusside) and/or by increasing CO (milrinone, enoximone). Epoprostenol and nitric oxide should be avoided as they

may further increase PAWP. Finally, there is limited evidence for the use of PDE-5 inhibitors in this context. It is generally accepted that a decrease in PVR <4–5 WU, and/or a TPG <15 mmHg with a maintained systemic pressure, would qualify a patient for surgery.

In PAH, the purpose of vasoreactivity testing is to identify calcium-channel blocker (CCB) "responders" in patients with idiopathic PAH. An acute response is defined as a decrease in mPAP below 40 mmHg and by >10 mmHg, with no change or increase in CO. Only responders can benefit from CCB therapy. Inhaled nitric oxide (10–20 parts per million) is the agent of choice as it has a short half-life and no systemic effects. Alternatively, intravenous (IV) epoprostenol (2–12 ng/kg/min) may be considered but is associated with systemic side effects (flushing, headache, nausea, hypotension). The use of other vasodilators such as nitrates, PDE-5 inhibitors, IV CCB, or iloprost should be discouraged.

• *Fluid loading test for unmasking left ventricular diastolic dysfunction*

PAWP may be reduced to <15 mmHg with diuretics in many patients with left-heart disease. In this context, the effect of an acute fluid challenge on left-heart filling pressures evaluated during RHC may help to differentiate the diagnosis between pre- and postcapillary PH [7, 9, 10]. Limited data suggest that a fluid bolus of 500 mL saline in 5–10 min is safe and may discriminate patients with precapillary PH from those with occult left ventricular diastolic dysfunction [5]. Recent studies suggest that a PAWP above 18 mmHg may be considered as an abnormal response to fluid challenge [9, 11].

• *Exercise testing to unmask left ventricular diastolic dysfunction*

Compared with fluid loading, hemodynamic measurements during exercise offer a more physiological approach to uncover left ventricular diastolic dysfunction [12–14]. The test is commonly performed in the supine position with a pedaling system attached to the catheterization table. Ideally, PAP and CO should be measured repeatedly at several levels of exercise to generate multipoint mPAP/CO relationship [8]. This approach avoids the wide individual variation of pressure and flow at a given level of workload. In healthy controls, the slope of this relationship (i.e., dynamic PVR) is between 1 and 2 WU. However, wide swings in airway and pleural pressures with exercise are associated with potential technical errors, even at low level of exercise.

Therefore, both invasive exercise testing and fluid loading require standardization and further evaluation before being recommended in routine clinical practice.

References

1. Galie N, Humbert M, Vachiery JL, Gibbs S, Lang I, Torbicki A, Simonneau G, Peacock A, Vonk Noordegraaf A, Beghetti M, Ghofrani A, Gomez Sanchez MA, Hansmann G, Klepetko W, Lancellotti P, Matucci M, McDonagh T, Pierard LA, Trindade PT, Zompatori M, Hoeper M. 2015 ESC/ERS Guidelines for the diagnosis and treatment of pulmonary hypertension: The Joint Task Force for the Diagnosis and Treatment of Pulmonary Hypertension of the European Society of Cardiology (ESC) and the European Respiratory Society (ERS): Endorsed by: Association for European Paediatric and Congenital Cardiology (AEPC), International Society for Heart and Lung Transplantation (ISHLT). Eur Respir J. 2015;46:903–75.

2. Galie N, Humbert M, Vachiery JL, Gibbs S, Lang I, Torbicki A, Simonneau G, Peacock A, Vonk Noordegraaf A, Beghetti M, Ghofrani A, Gomez Sanchez MA, Hansmann G, Klepetko W, Lancellotti P, Matucci M, McDonagh T, Pierard LA, Trindade PT, Zompatori M, Hoeper M, Aboyans V, Vaz Carneiro A, Achenbach S, Agewall S, Allanore Y, Asteggiano R, Paolo Badano L, Albert Barbera J, Bouvaist H, Bueno H, Byrne RA, Carerj S, Castro G, Erol C, Falk V, Funck-Brentano C, Gorenflo M, Granton J, Iung B, Kiely DG, Kirchhof P, Kjellstrom B, Landmesser U, Lekakis J, Lionis C, Lip GY, Orfanos SE, Park MH, Piepoli MF, Ponikowski P, Revel MP, Rigau D, Rosenkranz S, Voller H, Luis Zamorano J. 2015 ESC/ERS Guidelines for the diagnosis and treatment of pulmonary hypertension: The Joint Task Force for the Diagnosis and Treatment of Pulmonary Hypertension of the European Society of Cardiology (ESC) and the European Respiratory Society (ERS): Endorsed by: Association for European Paediatric and Congenital Cardiology (AEPC), International Society for Heart and Lung Transplantation (ISHLT). Eur Heart J. 2016;37:67–119.

3. McMurray JJ, Adamopoulos S, Anker SD, Auricchio A, Bohm M, Dickstein K, Falk V, Filippatos G, Fonseca C, Gomez-Sanchez MA, Jaarsma T, Kober L, Lip GY, Maggioni AP, Parkhomenko A, Pieske BM, Popescu BA, Ronnevik PK, Rutten FH, Schwitter J, Seferovic P, Stepinska J, Trindade PT, Voors AA, Zannad F, Zeiher A. Esc guidelines for the diagnosis and treatment of acute and chronic heart failure 2012: the task force for the diagnosis and treatment of acute and chronic heart failure 2012 of the european society of cardiology. Developed in collaboration with the heart failure association (hfa) of the esc. Eur Heart J. 2012;33:1787–847.

4. Hoeper MM, Lee SH, Voswinckel R, Palazzini M, Jais X, Marinelli A, Barst RJ, Ghofrani HA, Jing ZC, Opitz C, Seyfarth HJ, Halank M, McLaughlin V, Oudiz RJ, Ewert R, Wilkens H, Kluge S, Bremer HC, Baroke E, Rubin LJ. Complications of right heart catheterization procedures in patients with pulmonary hypertension in experienced centers. J Am Coll Cardiol. 2006;48:2546–52.

5. Naeije R, Vachiery JL, Yerly P, Vanderpool R. The transpulmonary pressure gradient for the diagnosis of pulmonary vascular disease. Eur Respir J. 2013;41:217–23.

6. Tedford RJ, Beaty CA, Mathai SC, Kolb TM, Damico R, Hassoun PM, Leary PJ, Kass DA, Shah AS. Prognostic value of the pre-transplant diastolic pulmonary artery pressure-to-pulmonary capillary wedge pressure gradient in cardiac transplant recipients with pulmonary hypertension. J Heart Lung Transplant. 2014;33:289–97.

7. Hoeper MM, Bogaard HJ, Condliffe R, Frantz R, Khanna D, Kurzyna M, Langleben D, Manes A, Satoh T, Torres F, Wilkins MR, Badesch DB. Definitions and diagnosis of pulmonary hypertension. J Am Coll Cardiol. 2013;62:D42–50.

8. Kovacs G, Berghold A, Scheidl S, Olschewski H. Pulmonary arterial pressure during rest and exercise in healthy subjects: a systematic review. Eur Respir J. 2009;34:888–94.

9. D'Alto M, Romeo E, Argiento P, Motoji Y, Correra A, Di Marco GM, Mattera Iacono A, Barracano R, D'Andrea A, Rea G, Sarubbi B, Russo MG, Naeije R. Clinical relevance of fluid challenge in patients evaluated for pulmonary hypertension. Chest. 2017;151(1):119–26.

10. Andersen MJ, Olson TP, Melenovsky V, Kane GC, Borlaug BA. Differential hemodynamic effects of exercise and volume expansion in people with and without heart failure. Circ Heart Fail. 2015;8:41–8.

11. Fujimoto N, Borlaug BA, Lewis GD, Hastings JL, Shafer KM, Bhella PS, Carrick-Ranson G, Levine BD. Hemodynamic responses to rapid saline loading: the impact of age, sex, and heart failure. Circulation. 2013;127:55–62.

12. Borlaug BA, Nishimura RA, Sorajja P, Lam CS, Redfield MM. Exercise hemodynamics enhance diagnosis of early heart failure with preserved ejection fraction. Circ Heart Fail. 2010;3:588–95.

13. Hager WD, Collins I, Tate JP, Azrin M, Foley R, Lakshminarayanan S, Rothfield NF. Exercise during cardiac catheterization distinguishes between pulmonary and left ventricular causes of dyspnea in systemic sclerosis patients. Clin Respir J. 2013;7:227–36.

14. Herve P, Lau EM, Sitbon O, Savale L, Montani D, Godinas L, Lador F, Jais X, Parent F, Gunther S, Humbert M, Simonneau G, Chemla D. Criteria for diagnosis of exercise pulmonary hypertension. Eur Respir J. 2015;46:728–37.

15. Rosenkranz S, Gibbs JS, Wachter R, De Marco T, Vonk-Noordegraaf A, Vachiery JL. Left ventricular heart failure and pulmonary hypertension. Eur Heart J. 2016;37:942–54.

16. Mehta S, Vachiery JL. Frontiers in clinical practice: pulmonary hypertension – the importance of correctly diagnosing the cause. Eur Respir Rev. 2016;25(142):372–80.

Radiation Exposure and Safety

7

Kully Sandhu, Gurbir Bhatia, and James Nolan

About Us Royal Stoke University Hospital (RSUH) is a tertiary surgical center performing both coronary and structural interventions. The Cardiac Department serves a large geographic area with a population of approximately two million. RSUH is affiliated with University Hospitals of North Midlands NHS Trust and Keele University Medical School.

RSUH was at the forefront of adopting transradial (TR) practice in the UK. Since then, it has developed a recognized TR program of teaching and research. Our center performs around 2000 percutaneous coronary interventions predominantly via the radial artery per year. Furthermore with EP studies, implantation of simple and complex pacing devices also being performed, great emphasis is placed on the importance of radiation protection.

The following highlights current issues regarding radiation safety and strategies that we employ to decrease radiation exposure.

K. Sandhu · J. Nolan (✉)
Royal Stoke University Hospital,
University Hospitals of North Midlands NHS Trust,
Stoke-On-Trent, UK
e-mail: james.nolan@uhns.nhs.uk

G. Bhatia
Royal Stoke University Hospital,
University Hospitals of North Midlands NHS Trust,
Stoke-On-Trent, UK

Birmingham Heartlands Hospital,
University Hospitals Birmingham
NHS Foundation Trust, Birmingham, UK

Introduction

Coronary angiography is a widely available diagnostic and therapeutic modality. Radiation exposure is set to increase as a result of greater complexity of coronary and structural cases now being undertaken. Therefore all cardiologists need to be aware of not only the risks of radiation but also strategies to minimize radiation exposure for both patients and catheter laboratory staff.

This chapter aims to provide a brief overview of basic radiation physics, highlight associated risks of radiation, and emphasize strategies to minimize radiation exposure.

Basic X-Ray Physics and Scatter

Basic Radiation Physics

- Coronary angiography relies on X-rays that pass through the patient before being transformed into recognizable images. X-rays are a form of ionizing radiation at the short-wavelength end of the electromagnetic spectrum.
- Typical wavelengths and frequencies are in the range of 0.01–10 nm and 30×10^{15}–30×10^{18} Hz, respectively.
- X-rays are composed of distinct packets (quanta) of energy called *photons*. The typical energy range for diagnostic X-rays is 5–150 keV.

© Springer International Publishing AG, part of Springer Nature 2018
A. Myat et al. (eds.), *The Interventional Cardiology Training Manual*,
https://doi.org/10.1007/978-3-319-71635-0_7

- X-rays are generated in a vacuum tube when accelerated electrons from a heated cathode filament collide into an anode. The collision releases energy mostly as heat. However about 1% is in the form of X-rays.
- The majority of cardiac catheter laboratories have a "*C-arm*" and a "*floating*" patient table. The C-arm consists of two components, first a radiation source and second an image receptor.
- The radiation source produces X-rays in a beam that travels through the patient to an image intensifier. The ability of X-rays to penetrate tissue is dependent on the energy of the photon but also on the atomic makeup, density, and thickness of the absorbing tissue. The image intensifier converts X-rays into images that may be stored (Fig. 7.1).

Radiation Scatter

Operators and medical staff are mainly exposed to scatter radiation rather than direct exposure. There are three types of scatter radiation:

1. Scatter radiation: This occurs from the X-rays bouncing off the patient's body and is the main source of radiation to operator and assistant.
2. Backscatter: This type of scatter radiation is created from behind the image intensifier and directed back towards the X-ray tube. To prevent backscatter lead screens are placed in front and behind the image intensifier for added protection.
3. Side scatter: Caused by objects within the catheter laboratory. To minimize side scatter modern catheter laboratories have patient table in the middle of the room with only a minimal

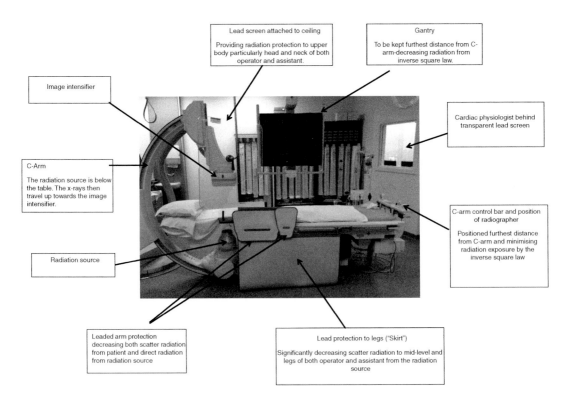

Fig. 7.1 The Royal Stoke University Hospital cardiac catheter laboratory setup

number of other objects. This isolates X-rays as much as possible and decreases side scatter.

Radiation Measures and Terminology

- We are all exposed to background radiation from the environment. However a number of common cardiac imaging modalities make use of ionizing radiation. These include noninvasive computerized tomography coronary angiography, nuclear imaging, and invasive coronary angiography (Fig. 7.2).
- Radiation dose is an important concept and determines the risk of adverse effects.

Radiation dose exposure to living tissue is expressed as "delivered energy" rather than actual radiation itself.

- There are a number of radiation measures available (Table 7.1). However the most commonly used parameters are screening time (seconds) and dose area product (DAP) ($Gy.cm^2$).

Deterministic and Stochastic Effects of Radiation

- Adverse effects are thought to be rare. However they may be higher than thought firstly due to a lack of awareness or recognition of signs or symptoms by either clinician or patient.

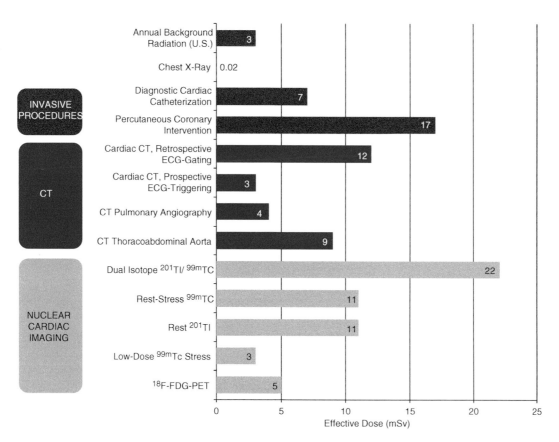

Fig. 7.2 Effective radiation doses associated with common cardiovascular imaging tests. Reproduced with permission from Meinel FG, et al. (2014) Radiation risks from cardiovascular imaging tests. *Circulation* 29;130(5):442–5. Key: *CT* computed tomography, *18F-FDG-PET* 18F-fluoro-deoxyglucose positron-emission tomography

Table 7.1 Commonly used radiation measures, definitions, and usage

Measurement	Unit	Definition	Measure	Use
Absorbed dose	Gray (Gy)	The amount of ionizing radiation deposited per unit mass	Measure of the concentration of energy absorbed in tissue	Assess the potential biological risk
Air kerma	Gray (Gy)	The dose delivered per unit mass of air	Measure of the amount of radiation energy	**K**inetic **E**nergy **R**eleased per unit **MA**ss (KERMA) of air
Dose-area-product (DAP)	Gy.cm^2	The quantity used in assessing radiation risk and is defined by the absorbed dose multiplied by the area irradiated	Dose absorbed multiplied by area irradiated	An estimate of the energy delivered to the patient and used to monitor/measure operators' procedural doses
Effective dose	Sievert (Sv)	Tissue-weighted sum of the equivalent doses in all tissues and organs. Takes into account the type of radiation and nature of each organ or tissue being irradiated	Overall calculated dose of the sum of each organ dose	Represents an estimate of stochastic risk to the staff/patient. The biological factor to convert absorbed X-ray doses (Gy) to equivalent doses (Sv) is 1
Entrance skin dose	Gray (Gy)	The absorbed dose on the skin includes backscattered radiation	Amount of radiation absorbed by skin	Assess the risk of adverse effects of radiation on skin
Equivalent dose	Sievert (Sv)	The radiation dose applied to a specific tissue or organ	Effect of radiation on a particular tissue	Measures the risk of radiation to specific organs/tissues
Fluoroscopy time	Minutes or seconds	Total fluoroscopy time used during a procedure	Time in minutes and seconds	Measure of the length of radiation time

- Secondly, there may be a latent period from radiation exposure to clinical features of excessive radiation exposure. Radiation injuries are likely to become a more common finding as a consequence of longer procedure times seen in more complex interventions.
- There are two mechanisms in which radiation may induce adverse effects. These are "deterministic" or "stochastic" effects.

Deterministic Effects

- These describe an almost linear relationship between radiation dose received and adverse effect. The higher the radiation dose the greater the adverse effect. These occur as a consequence of direct toxicity by X-rays causing cellular death or changes in biochemical response of the exposed tissue.
- Therefore deterministic adverse effects are both predictable and dose dependent.

Stochastic Effects

- These are random and may occur after a single exposure to a radiation dose. May occur as a consequence of modification(s) to DNA that may result in mutations causing cancer or heritable genetic defects. Therefore they may take several years to clinically manifest.
- Stochastic effects are probabilistic, with likelihood of adverse effect(s) proportional to the dose received.

Linear-No-Threshold Model of Radiation

- This model is derived from both deterministic and stochastic effects. This principle confers that no radiation dose is safe and greater risk of adverse effects is associated with higher radiation doses.

Adverse Effects of Radiation

Despite the beneficial use of X-ray radiation the operator must also appreciate adverse effects of ionizing radiation and methods on reducing exposure.

Adverse Effects on Skin

- The most common deterministic adverse effect is on the skin that receives the greatest dose at the beam site. Although staging procedures may allow time between procedures for the skin to repair, injury may still occur.
- Importantly there may be a lag from radiation exposure to presentation. Skin injury can manifest as erythema due to increased capillary permeability resembling mild sunburn peaking by 24 h.
- These may progress to marked erythema as a result of damage from the epidermal cell layer associated with itching and discomfort. Epilation or hair loss may occur up to a month after exposure as a consequence of depleted germinal layers of hair follicles. Epilation may be temporary but may result in only sparse hair regrowth.
- More severe injuries include ischemic dermal necrosis or skin ulceration that may be resistant to healing and require skin grafting.

Cataracts

- Cataract formation is a recognized complication of radiation exposure and occurs at the posterior subcapsular region.
- The radiation dose, and the latent period from exposure to cataract formation and subsequent visual impairment, remains unknown.
- Recently the International Commission on Radiological Protection (ICRP) has reduced the previous recommended dose threshold for cataracts to 0.5 Gy and equivalent dose limits

to 20 mSv/year (maximum of 100 mSv in a given 5-year period, with no single year exceeding 50 mSv).
- Therefore wearing protective glasses is now highly recommended.

Risk of Cancer

- The risk of cancer has been mainly derived from longitudinal studies of the survivors of the atomic bomb. These have found survivors exposed to radiation dose in the range of 5–150 mSv and mean of 40 mSv had a significantly increased risk of developing cancer.
- This is equivalent to a patient undergoing a nuclear scan, coronary angiogram, and then subsequently percutaneous coronary intervention.
- The estimated risk of cancer in men has been suggested to be 6% per Sievert. Accordingly, a coronary angiographic procedural dose of 10 mSv would be associated with a lifetime risk of cancer induction of 0.06%.
- The overall risk ranges from 0.1 to 0.24% based on complexity of intervention with the greatest risk in younger patients.

Radiation Exposure Risk to Cardiac Catheterization Laboratory Staff

- Without any radiation protection the operator receives almost the same radiation dose as patients. However with appropriate radiation protection the dose received by the operator may be significantly reduced.
- Not only is the operator exposed to radiation, but also second operators, technicians and radiographers, are exposed to 30% and 1%, respectively, of operators' dose. Historical studies have reported increased risks of cancers including leukemia and breast cancer among radiologists and radiographers. Recently, a cluster of left-sided cerebral neoplasms among interventional cardiologists has been reported.

- Therefore all cardiac catheter laboratory staff must be aware of and ensure appropriate radiation protection.

Regulatory Bodies

There are a number of regulatory bodies mandating the safe use of radiation. Regulations governing the medical use of ionizing radiation have been in existence for a number of years. These statutory legal requirements form the official code of practice for radiation exposure for patients, members of the public, and medical staff. A summary of the most important regulations follows below.

Ionising Radiations Regulations 1999 (IRR'99)

- A statutory requirement forming the official code of practice and legal requirements for the control and use of ionizing radiation in the UK enforced by the Health and Safety Executive (HSE). These UK regulations came into force in January 2000 and were based on the European Basic Safety Standards Directive produced by the International Commission on Radiological Protection.
- IRR'99 sets the maximal received annual radiation dose exposed to both staff and general public. These regulations are legal requirements of employers ensuring the safe use of ionizing radiation by appointing radiation protection supervisors and advisors.

Ionising Radiation (Medical Exposure) Regulations 2000 [IR(ME)R 2000]

- These regulations are set to ensure radiation protection of patients undergoing fluoroscopic procedures. This legal requirement requires the identification of named medical professionals involved in patient welfare.

- These regulations mandate employers to adhere to the recommended national dose reference levels (see section "The National Patient Dose Database (NPDD)"). Therefore all trainees are required to have undergone online IR(ME)R 2000 training from the Health Education England web site:
- http://www.e-lfh.org.uk/programmes/radiation-protection-for-cardiology/.

The National Patient Dose Database (NPDD)

- The National Patient Dose Database (NPDD) collates patient doses from radiographic and fluoroscopic X-ray imaging procedures from a number of hospitals in the UK.
- The Health Protection Agency (HPA) analyzes and reviews this data every 5 years and recommends national reference doses (RNRD) or more recently known as National Diagnostic Reference Levels (NDRLs).
- These tend to be based on the 75th percentile value of the distributions of mean doses observed in the NPDD. While the most commonly used parameters are mean screening time (seconds) and mean DAP ($Gy.cm^2$), several other measures are quoted. All hospitals must adhere to NDRL or local reference levels if they are lower than the NDRL.

ALARA/ALARP Principle

- The IRR'99 and IR(ME)R 2000 documents give rise to the principle of keeping the radiation dose *"as low as reasonably achievable/ practicable"*—the ALARA/ALARP principle.
- ALARA/ALARP principle provides practical tips on reducing radiation dose. Practical tips are summarized in Table 7.2.

Operator Total Radiation Dose

Every operator must have total radiation doses measured and assessed quarterly per annum. These are obtained from dosimeters worn under

Table 7.2 Summary of the strategies used at the Royal Stoke University Hospital to minimize radiation dose and exposure

Fluoroscopic considerations	Minimizing patient-to-intensifier distance decreasing patient radiation exposure and scatter radiation to catheter laboratory staff Maximizing distance of operator from X-ray source (inverse square law) Limiting fluoroscopic and more importantly cineangiographic acquisitions Collimating filters to regions of interest Minimizing magnified fluoroscopy and cineangiographic acquisitions Fluoroscopic optimization by decreasing frame rate, use of fluoroscopic image store, and replay varying angulations during lengthy procedures Minimizing or avoiding steep C-arm angulations Use of extension tube and mobile transparent screen (Figs. 7.3 and 7.4)
Shielding	Optimizing all radiation barriers and shields available within the catheter laboratory Mandating the use of all available personal lead shielding including lead aprons, glasses, thyroid and shin shields
Audit	Regular auditing of procedural doses and screening time against current regulatory body recommendations

Fig. 7.3 Mobile protective shielding. This protective shield has wheels to allow mobility and a transparent leaded screen for visualization. This allows catheter laboratory staff added protection. However full-body radiation protection must still be worn

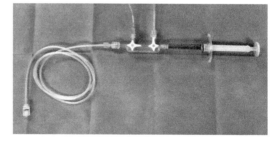

Fig. 7.4 Extension tubing. Extension lead attached to the manifold that allows the operator and assistant to stand further away from the radiation source and therefore decrease radiation exposure by the inverse square law. This extension lead is 1 m long

radiation protection apron(s), finger dosimeters, and total lens dose (TLD) from dosimeters worn on left side of the thyroid shield on the side of the operator closest to the radiation source.

Radiation Protection

Radiation protection measures may be divided into cardiac catheter laboratory and personal protective measures.

Cardiac Catheter Laboratory

All cardiac catheter laboratories have lead reinforcement shielding within the walls and lead windows to allow visualization from review rooms (Fig. 7.1).

Personal Protection

- Personal protection includes lead aprons, thyroid and shin shields, and glasses to be worn to decrease the risk of cataracts. Lead head caps have been advocated for further decreasing radiation doses to the brain. However they may not provide significantly more protection than careful use of a lead glass shield.

- A transparent lead glass shield is suspended from the ceiling and significantly reduces radiation exposure to upper body, face, and head of both operator and assistant.
- Fitted mobile lead drapes or "lead skirts" on the procedure table decrease lower limb exposure to the operator and assistant. Additional lead flaps at the operators' mid-level and side-arm flaps reduce scatter exposure to the operator and assistant.
- The use of leaded aprons on the patient's abdomen and pelvis undergoing coronary angiography via the radial artery approach is controversial. Despite being shown to reduce scatter radiation to operator an associated doubling of radiation dose to patient has been found. Therefore caution has been advised.
- A mobile leaded shield that consists of a transparent leaded screen provides further protection. This provides added protection for cardiac catheter laboratory staff (Fig. 7.3).

Factors Affecting Radiation Exposure

These can be divided into three main categories—patient, practical, and technical factors. Table 7.2 summarizes the strategies used at RSUH in reducing radiation dose and exposure. These are described below.

Patient Factors

Procedural Complexity

Higher procedural complexity (e.g., chronic total occlusions, multivessel, or graft interventions) is an independent predictor of higher radiation dose. This must be borne in mind when consenting patients.

Body Mass Index

Body mass index (BMI) was found to be an important predictor of radiation dose. Higher radiation doses are required to penetrate subcutaneous fat for satisfactory images to be formed.

Practical Factors

Inverse Square Law

Increasing the distance between operator and radiation source reduces radiation dose by a factor of $1/x^2$. In other words—doubling the distance decreases the radiation dose by a factor of 4. Therefore the operator should stand as far away from the radiation source as possible. The use of extension tubes may facilitate this by allowing both operator and assistant to stand at a considerable distance from the radiation source (Fig. 7.4).

Source-to-Image Distance

The image intensifier should be as close as possible to the patient. Minimizing source-to-image distance (*SID*) decreases radiation dose exposure to patient and scattering radiation dose to operator.

C-Arm Angulation

The radiation delivered to the patient and scattering radiation to the operator are dependent on C-arm angulation. Steeper left or right oblique projections ($\geq 60°$) and in particular left anterior oblique angulation have been found to be associated with greater radiation dose. For example using the posteroanterior caudal view instead of left anterior oblique caudal ($60°/20°$) can be associated with a 60% and 90% reduction in radiation dose received by patient and operator, respectively.

Fluoroscopy and Acquisition Time

- Coronary procedures rely on both fluoroscopy and cineangiographic acquisitions.

Fluoroscopy is used to allow the operator for appropriate positioning of catheter, wires, or stents.

- Acquisition allows archiving of diagnostic higher quality images. However acquisition is typically associated with 10–20 times greater radiation dose than fluoroscopy and may account for as much as 60–70% of the total DAP.
- Reducing acquisition has been shown to be a more effective means of reducing radiation dose than fluoroscopy. Therefore the number and length of acquisitions should be kept to a minimum.

Fluoroscopic Optimization

There have been a number of technical advances that may be used to decrease radiation doses such as pulsed fluoroscopy, image store, and frame rate.

Pulsed Fluoroscopy

This allows short rapid pulses of X-rays to be delivered rather than a continuous beam. This shortens the overall duration of X-ray radiation and may significantly decrease radiation exposure.

Fluoroscopic Image Store and Replay

Modern machines allow storage of fluoroscopic images and therefore limit the number of cineangiographic acquisitions. This is particularly useful when image quality is not essential such as during balloon inflation or deployment of stents. In patients with a low BMI, acquisition may not be required if stored fluoroscopic coronary images are of adequate quality.

Frame Rate

Decreasing fluoroscopic frame rate is associated with lower radiation dose. A study found a significant difference in operator radiation exposure between frame rates of 7.5 frames/s and standard 15 frames/s. However this may be associated with decrease in image quality. The operator should optimize the frame rate in every patient ensuring optimal image quality and lowest possible radiation dose.

Filtering and Collimation Optimization

Modern machines have, as standard, filters that exclude low-energy rays produced by the X-ray tubes. This decreases artifact but more importantly radiation dose absorbed by patient.

"Wedge" filtering is used to not only optimize image quality but also decrease radiation exposure. This should be employed for example when patient lung border or diaphragm is exposed to X-rays.

Collimation allows the operator to concentrate on a specific area of interest by reducing the image field. For example when positioning a stent the image may be *"coned"* down not only highlighting the area of interest but also significantly decreasing the size of the radiated area. This also decreases scatter to the patient as well as cardiac catheter staff.

Arterial Access Site

- RSUH was one of the first to become a predominantly TR center within the UK. Since then TR angiography has risen exponentially over the last decade.
- Initial suggestions that radial access was associated with greater radiation doses have proven unfounded; many early studies did not rigorously control several important variables such as operator experience or radiation protection.
- A sub-analysis of the multicenter RIVAL study found a modest but significant increase in fluoroscopy time in radial cases performed in low–intermediate-volume centers, but not in high-volume centers. There were no significant differences in DAP between either femoral or radial access for the entire cohort. Further sub-analysis and multivariate analysis found the highest radial volume centers and operators had the lowest radiation exposure (DAP).
- The single-center REVERE trial found no difference in air kerma or DAP in 1500 patients undergoing coronary angiography by either femoral, right, or left radial artery approach.
- With greater experience, radiation exposure is reduced for radial (but also femoral) operators.

Summary

- The importance of fluoroscopy in modern-day cardiology is well recognized. However medical staff must also appreciate the potential harm of radiation. This includes recognition of adverse effects and symptoms.
- Therefore methods limiting radiation exposure not only to patients but also to medical staff are paramount. This has led to the mandatory IR(ME)R 2000 training that all medical staff performing any fluoroscopy must undergo in the UK.
- Patient doses may be limited by reducing direct radiation exposure. However scatter radiation is the main mechanism of exposure to medical staff. The mandatory use of radiation protection suits and optimizing procedural factors decrease radiation dose to both operators and other medical staff.
- All medical staff are legally required to wear dosimeters allowing total radiation doses that are measured quarterly per annum. All hospitals are legally required to collect this information from each individual and identify any medical personal at high risk of excess radiation exposure. They also conduct regular audits comparing local radiation doses to national standards. These safety standards ensure the safe use of radiation to patients and medical staff alike.

Bibliography

Abdelaal E, Plourde G, MacHaalany J, Arsenault J, Rimac G, Dery JP, et al. Effectiveness of low rate fluoroscopy at reducing operator and patient radiation dose during transradial coronary angiography and interventions. JACC Cardiovasc Interv. 2014;7(5):567–74.

Agarwal S, Parashar A, Bajaj NS, Khan I, Ahmad I, Heupler FA Jr, et al. Relationship of beam angulation and radiation exposure in the cardiac catheterization laboratory. JACC Cardiovasc Interv. 2014;7(5):558–66.

Authors on behalf of ICRP, Stewart FA, Akleyev AV, Hauer-Jensen M, Hendry JH, Kleiman NJ, et al. ICRP publication 118: ICRP statement on tissue reactions and early and late effects of radiation in normal tissues and organs—threshold doses for tissue reactions in a radiation protection context. Ann ICRP. 2012;41(1–2):1–322.

Cantor WJ, Puley G, Natarajan MK, Dzavik V, Madan M, Fry A, et al. Radial versus femoral access for emergent percutaneous coronary intervention with adjunct glycoprotein IIb/IIIa inhibition in acute myocardial infarction—the RADIAL-AMI pilot randomized trial. Am Heart J. 2005;150(3):543–9.

Chase AJ, Fretz EB, Warburton WP, Klinke WP, Carere RG, Pi D, et al. Association of the arterial access site at angioplasty with transfusion and mortality: the M.O.R.T.A.L study (Mortality Benefit of Reduced Transfusion after percutaneous coronary intervention via the arm or leg). Heart. 2008;94(8):1019–25.

Delewi R, Hoebers LP, Ramunddal T, Henriques JP, Angeras O, Stewart J, et al. Clinical and procedural characteristics associated with higher radiation exposure during percutaneous coronary interventions and coronary angiography. Circ Cardiovasc Interv. 2013;6(5):501–6.

Hamada N, Fujimichi Y, Iwasaki T, Fujii N, Furuhashi M, Kubo E, et al. Emerging issues in radiogenic cataracts and cardiovascular disease. J Radiat Res. 2014;55(5):831–46.

Hart D, Hillier MC, Shrimpton PC. Doses to patients from radiographic and fluoroscopic x-ray imaging procedures in the UK – 2010 review. HPA-CRCE-034. 2012. http://www.hpa.org.uk/Publications/Radiation/CRCEScientificAndTechnicalReportSeries/HPACRCE034.

Jolly SS, Amlani S, Hamon M, Yusuf S, Mehta SR. Radial versus femoral access for coronary angiography or intervention and the impact on major bleeding and ischemic events: a systematic review and meta-analysis of randomized trials. Am Heart J. 2009;157(1):132–40.

Jolly SS, Cairns J, Niemela K, Steg PG, Natarajan MK, Cheema AN, et al. Effect of radial versus femoral access on radiation dose and the importance of procedural volume: a substudy of the multicenter randomized RIVAL trial. JACC Cardiovasc Interv. 2013;6(3):258–66.

Koenig TR, Wolff D, Mettler FA, Wagner LK. Skin injuries from fluoroscopically guided procedures: part 1, characteristics of radiation injury. AJR Am J Roentgenol. 2001a;177(1):3–11.

Koenig TR, Mettler FA, Wagner LK. Skin injuries from fluoroscopically guided procedures: part 2, review of 73 cases and recommendations for minimizing dose delivered to patient. AJR Am J Roentgenol. 2001b;177(1):13–20.

Kuipers G, Delewi R, Velders XL, Vis MM, van der Schaaf RJ, Koch KT, et al. Radiation exposure during percutaneous coronary interventions and coronary angiograms performed by the radial compared with the femoral route. JACC Cardiovasc Interv. 2012;5(7):752–7.

Kuon E. Radiation exposure in invasive cardiology. Heart. 2008;94(5):667–74.

Kuon E, Schmitt M, Dahm JB. Significant reduction of radiation exposure to operator and staff during cardiac interventions by analysis of radiation leakage and improved lead shielding. Am J Cardiol. 2002;89(1):44–9.

Kuon E, Birkel J, Schmitt M, Dahm JB. Radiation exposure benefit of a lead cap in invasive cardiology. Heart. 2003;89(10):1205–10.

Kuon E, Dahm JB, Empen K, Robinson DM, Reuter G, Wucherer M. Identification of less-irradiating tube angulations in invasive cardiology. J Am Coll Cardiol. 2004;44(7):1420–8.

Lange HW, von Boetticher H. Reduction of operator radiation dose by a pelvic lead shield during cardiac catheterization by radial access: comparison with femoral access. JACC Cardiovasc Interv. 2012;5(4):445–9.

Loomba RS, Rios R, Buelow M, Eagam M, Aggarwal S, Arora RR. Comparison of contrast volume, radiation dose, fluoroscopy time, and procedure time in previously published studies of rotational versus conventional coronary angiography. Am J Cardiol. 2015;116(1):43–9.

Meinel FG, Nance JW Jr, Harris BS, De Cecco CN, Costello P, Schoepf UJ. Radiation risks from cardiovascular imaging tests. Circulation. 2014;130(5):442–5.

Musallam A, Volis I, Dadaev S, Abergel E, Soni A, Yalonetsky S, et al. A randomized study comparing the use of a pelvic lead shield during trans-radial interventions: threefold decrease in radiation to the operator but double exposure to the patient. Catheter Cardiovasc Interv. 2015;85(7):1164–70.

Olcay A, Guler E, Karaca IO, Omaygenc MO, Kizilirmak F, Olgun E, et al. Comparison of fluoro and cine coronary angiography: balancing acceptable outcomes with a reduction in radiation dose. J Invasive Cardiol. 2015;27(4):199–202.

Pancholy SB, Joshi P, Shah S, Rao SV, Bertrand OF, Patel TM. Effect of vascular access site choice on radiation exposure during coronary angiography: the REVERE Trial (Randomized Evaluation of Vascular Entry Site and Radiation Exposure). JACC Cardiovasc Interv. 2015;8(9):1189–96.

Pierce DA, Preston DL. Radiation-related cancer risks at low doses among atomic bomb survivors. Radiat Res. 2000;154(2):178–86.

Plourde G, Pancholy SB, Nolan J, Jolly S, Rao SV, Amhed I, et al. Radiation exposure in relation to the arterial access site used for diagnostic coronary angiography and percutaneous coronary intervention: a systematic review and meta-analysis. Lancet. 2015;386(10009):2192–203.

Politi L, Biondi-Zoccai G, Nocetti L, Costi T, Monopoli D, Rossi R, et al. Reduction of scatter radiation during transradial percutaneous coronary angiography: a randomized trial using a lead-free radiation shield. Catheter Cardiovasc Interv. 2012;79(1):97–102.

Preston DL, Ron E, Tokuoka S, Funamoto S, Nishi N, Soda M, et al. Solid cancer incidence in atomic bomb survivors: 1958-1998. Radiat Res. 2007;168(1):1–64.

Preston DL, Shimizu Y, Pierce DA, Suyama A, Mabuchi K. Studies of mortality of atomic bomb survivors. Report 13: solid cancer and noncancer disease mortality: 1950-1997. 2003. Radiat Res. 2012;178(2):AV146–72.

Reeves RR, Ang L, Bahadorani J, Naghi J, Dominguez A, Palakodeti V, et al. Invasive cardiologists are exposed to greater left sided cranial radiation: the BRAIN Study (Brain Radiation Exposure and Attenuation During Invasive Cardiology Procedures). JACC Cardiovasc Interv. 2015;8(9):1197–206.

Roguin A, Goldstein J, Bar O, Goldstein JA. Brain and neck tumors among physicians performing interventional procedures. Am J Cardiol. 2013;111(9):1368–72.

Tsapaki V, Kottou S, Vano E, Parviainen T, Padovani R, Dowling A, et al. Correlation of patient and staff doses in interventional cardiology. Radiat Prot Dosimetry. 2005;117(1–3):26–9.

Vano E, Gonzalez L. Accreditation in radiation protection for cardiologists and interventionalists. Radiat Prot Dosimetry. 2005;117(1–3):69–73.

Vano E, Ubeda C, Leyton F, Miranda P, Gonzalez L. Staff radiation doses in interventional cardiology: correlation with patient exposure. Pediatr Cardiol. 2009;30(4):409–13.

Yoshinaga S, Mabuchi K, Sigurdson AJ, Doody MM, Ron E. Cancer risks among radiologists and radiologic technologists: review of epidemiologic studies. Radiology. 2004;233(2):313–21.

Planning Coronary Intervention: The "Golden Rules"—Patient Checklist and Troubleshooting

Sergio Buccheri and Davide Capodanno

About Us The cardiac catheterization laboratory at our hospital manages the invasive care of a wide range of cardiovascular pathological conditions, including coronary artery disease (CAD), peripheral artery disease, and structural heart disease. The center's philosophy is based on the close interplay of clinical care according to international standards, innovation, and research. Local protocols are implemented and shared between different professional figures (i.e., physicians, nurses, technicians) involved in pre-procedural, procedural, and post-procedural patients' management. A pre-procedural checklist is routinely adopted to verify the appropriateness of the indication, the correct preparation of the patient, and the absence of absolute or relative contraindications to each invasive procedure. One of the most important aspects is the implementation of a multidisciplinary Heart Team approach for the management of complex clinical cases. In keeping with guideline recommendations, the Heart Team is composed of interventional cardiologists, cardiac surgeons, clinical cardiologists, and anesthesiologists. Local meetings are regularly scheduled to discuss and select the most appropriate therapeutic strategy according to each patient's profile. Being also an academic center, clinical research is of primary importance. Whenever possible and appropriate, and after providing detailed explanations on studies' characteristics, consenting patients are enrolled in randomized controlled trials or multicenter registries. Single-center, investigator-driven observational studies are also conducted. Research is deemed as an instrument to improve daily clinical practice and overall quality of care.

Planning Coronary Intervention

Categorizing Coronary Lesions

- Discriminating coronary lesions based on their complexity has important implications for procedural planning and to predict (and prevent) the onset of procedural complications. However, the characteristics of a coronary lesion should be contextualized with the clinical presentation and patients' risk profile to get a 360° vision of PCI complexity.
- The ACC/AHA angiographic classification of coronary lesions has been largely validated and investigated in the medical literature. Coding details of this classification system are shown in Table 8.1.
- Kastrati et al. [1] investigated the prognostic value of the ACC/AHA classification system in 2944 patients undergoing PCI by dichotomization into type A/B1 and B2/C lesions

S. Buccheri · D. Capodanno (✉)
Division of Cardiology, CAST, Azienda Ospedaliero-Universitaria "Policlinico-Vittorio Emanuele", University of Catania, Catania, Italy

© Springer International Publishing AG, part of Springer Nature 2018
A. Myat et al. (eds.), *The Interventional Cardiology Training Manual*,
https://doi.org/10.1007/978-3-319-71635-0_8

Table 8.1 Characteristics of the ACC/AHA classification of coronary lesions

ACC/AHA lesion type	Characteristics
A	Discrete (<10 mm length), concentric, readily accessible, <45° angled, smooth contour, little or no calcification, less than totally occlusive, not ostial in location, no major side-branch involvement, absence of thrombus
B1	One of the following characteristics: 10–20 mm length, eccentric, moderate tortuosity of proximal segment, irregular contour, presence of thrombus, moderate or heavy calcification, moderately angulated (>45° and <90°), total occlusion <3 months, ostial lesion or bifurcation lesion requiring two guidewires
B2	Two or more of the following characteristics: 10–20 mm length, eccentric, moderate tortuosity of proximal segment, irregular contour, presence of thrombus, moderate or heavy calcification, moderately angulated (>45° and<90°), total occlusion <3 months, ostial lesion or bifurcation lesion requiring two guidewires
C	>20 mm length, excessive tortuosity of proximal segment, total occlusion >3 months, degenerated vein graft with friable lesions, inability to protect major side branches

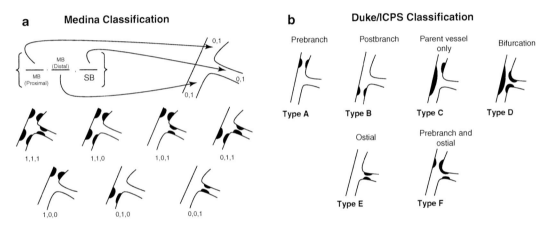

Fig. 8.1 The Medina (**a**) and the Duke/ICPS classification system (**b**) for lesions at bifurcation sites

(reflecting simple and complex anatomies, respectively). One-year event-free survival was 75.6% for patients with complex lesions and 81.1% for patients with simple lesions ($P < 0.001$) [1].

- Coronary lesions at bifurcation sites, defined as the site of junction of a main vessel with a side branch, are frequently encountered in daily clinical practice and represent a major challenge for treatment by PCI. Bifurcation sites are prone to develop and favor the progression of atherosclerotic lesions due to flow disturbances and low shear stress [2].

- The Medina classification system for bifurcations is a simple and widely used tool to categorize coronary bifurcation lesions [3]. Three components of a bifurcation are considered and scored "1" if affected by significant CAD, namely the proximal main branch, distal main branch, and side branch.

- The International Classification for Patient Safety (ICPS) classification system for bifurcation lesions is a relatively more complex system to classify lesions localized at bifurcation sites. Seven different typologies of bifurcation lesions are considered by this system [4]. Figure 8.1 graphically represents the Medina and the Duke/ICPS classification system for lesions at bifurcation sites.

- Additional potentially identifiable lesions during coronary angiography are chronic total occlusions (CTO). Up to 20% of coronary angiograms reveal the presence of a CTO [5].

- A chronic total occlusion (CTO) is defined as the absence of anterograde flow in a coronary segment. Bridging, ipsilateral, or contralateral collaterals may fill the segments distal to the occlusion.
- The total occlusion classification system and the Japanese-CTO (J-CTO) score are simple classification systems to categorize and predict the procedural complexity and the likelihood of successful revascularization in CTO PCI [6, 7].
- Parameters considered by the first system are occlusion lasting more than 3 months, presence of side branch and their size, blunt stump, presence of bridging collaterals, and occlusion length.
- The J-CTO score predicts successful wiring of a CTO within 30 min by considering the following variables: calcification, bending, blunt stump, occlusion length >20 mm, and previously failed lesion.
- Advances in the field of invasive coronary imaging with intravascular ultrasound (IVUS) and optical coherence tomography (OCT) now allow for a more detailed characterization of lesion anatomy. Coronary plaques may be classified based on the presence of necrotic core, fibro-fatty tissue, fibrous tissue, or dense calcium with IVUS imaging.
- Pathological intimal thickening, fibrotic and fibro-calcific plaques, and thick- or thin-cap fibro-atheromas can be further identifiable by IVUS-derived virtual histology [8].
- Due to its higher spatial resolution, OCT can be used for detailed measurement of cap thickness and additional identification of specific cap features including macrophage accumulation, lipid volume, microcalcifications, plaque erosion or rupture (Fig. 8.2), neovascularization, and thrombus [9].
- Invasive characterization of coronary lesions is of particular interest since some in vivo characteristics have been related to adverse clinical outcomes at follow-up. The landmark PROSPECT trial showed that the presence of a plaque burden of 70% or greater, a minimal luminal area of 4.0 mm^2 or less, and a thin-cap fibro-atheroma independently predicted the 3-year cumulative rate of major adverse cardiovascular events in non-culprit lesions at the time of PCI [11].

Plaque Rupture   Plaque Erosion

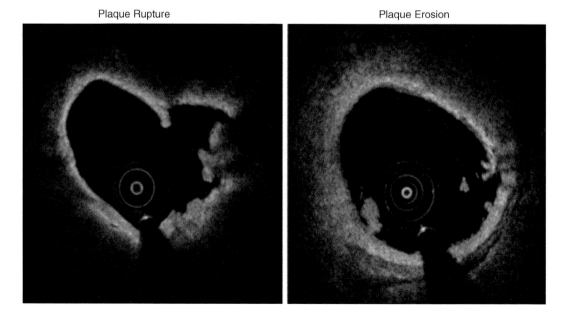

Fig. 8.2 Picture showing OCT characteristics of a ruptured and eroded plaque. Adapted with permission from Guagliumi G. et al. [10]

Quantitative Coronary Angiography

- Quantitative coronary angiography (QCA) analysis after adequate acquisition and computerized processing of coronary angiograms is a widely established tool to objectively quantify the extent and severity of CAD. Indeed, qualitative analysis based on operator visual estimation may be affected by excess in intra- and inter-observer variability.

- QCA analysis may overcome these limitations by using specific vessel edge detection algorithms that accurately identify the dimensions and course of the coronary vessels, thus providing operator-independent and objective measures of coronary anatomy [12].

- Accurate measurements of vessel stenosis may avoid unnecessary interventions in non-significant lesions or may improve PCI results by providing accurate measures for proper stent selection.

- Conventional 2D-QCA is based on the computerized analysis of two-dimensional cine angiograms. Recently, 3D-QCA tools allow for reconstruction of 3D rendered views from multiple angiographic X-ray projections; this is particularly useful to reduce potential errors of 2D-QCA such as foreshortening and out-of-plane magnification errors [13]. Moreover, 3D-QCA may be of particular value in specific anatomical contexts, like diseased coronary bifurcations, where a detailed reconstruction of spatial disease is crucial to plan PCI by selecting the most appropriate technique.

- The first step to performing a reliable and reproducible QCA depends on the performance of high-quality coronary angiography. It is of fundamental importance to select at least two projections that are orthogonal with the segment of interest to avoid foreshortening. In addition, overlap of anatomic structures or angiographic catheters along the vessel course should be avoided. It is also important to include the proximal part of the angiographic catheter in the acquisition since the catheter is used for calibration of sizing.

- Some additional tricks could improve the quality of QCA, such as cine angiogram acquisition during inspiration to increase the distinction between contrast-filled vessels and the background of image and the injection of intracoronary nitroglycerine to resolve vasospasm [14].

- After selection of the end-diastolic frame in a clear, non-foreshortened view and after proper calibration of the catheter, the QCA software allows for the measurement of different parameters (Table 8.2) by automatic vessel edge detection algorithms.

- QCA measurements can also be integrated and defined by quantitative IVUS analysis (diameters and areas, lesion length) before stent placement. Indeed, IVUS-guided PCI has the potential to highlight some adverse plaque features before (i.e., heavy calcification, high thrombotic burden) and after stent implantation (i.e., edge dissection, incomplete stent apposition) that may prevent and reduce immediate and long-term adverse events following PCI.

Table 8.2 Quantitative coronary angiography parameters

Parameters	Description
Minimal luminal diameter (MLD)	The smallest lumen diameter in the segment of interest
Reference vessel diameter (RVD)	The averaged diameter of the coronary vessel assumed without atherosclerotic disease
Lesion length	Length of the stenosis between two points (shoulders) where the diseased coronary margins change direction with the normal subsegment
Acute gain	Post-procedural MLD—pre-procedural MLD
Late loss	Post-procedural MLD—MLD at follow-up
Diameter stenosis (DS)	(RVD-MLD)/RVD
Binary restenosis	DS >50% at follow-up coronary angiography in the treated segment

Adapted from Tomasello et al. [14]

Determinants of Risk and Prognostic Indexes

- Clinical risk defines the probability or the potential hazard of complications or adverse outcomes following a therapeutic intervention. Categorization and estimation of a patient's clinical risk profile are often challenging due to the stochastic and time-varying nature of risk [15]. Indeed, several factors, including clinical, procedural, and technique-related variables, may potentially jeopardize the clinical outcomes (Table 8.3).
- Risk scores may represent helpful clinical aids to properly categorize and predict patients' risk. Indeed, risk scores are obtained with mathematical models that, by weighting and integrating the hazard conferred by specific pre-procedural clinical characteristics, estimate the risk for procedural complications or adverse outcomes.
- Beyond risk score assessment, a careful evaluation of some simple pre-procedural parameters is of primary importance to preserve safety:
  - Blood parameters (hemoglobin levels, platelet count, coagulation status, renal function)
  - Hypersensitivity to drugs or contrast medium

Table 8.3 Variables potentially affecting clinical outcomes in patients undergoing PCI

Clinical	Procedural	Technical
Diabetes	Acute coronary syndrome	Calcified lesions
Chronic renal insufficiency	Hemodynamic instability	Diffused coronary involvement
Chronic obstructive pulmonary disease	Low left ventricular ejection fraction	Chronic total occlusions
Advanced age	Significant areas of myocardium at jeopardy	PCI in diseased grafts
High bleeding risk	NA	Last remaining vessel

- Previous vascular interventions or complications at access sites
- Antithrombotic therapy at the time of the intervention (dual-antiplatelet therapy, single-antiplatelet agent, chronic oral anticoagulant)
- Patent venous access for administration of fluids or drugs in case of complications

Myocardium at Risk Scores

- Myocardium at risk scores are useful tools to estimate the amount of myocardium jeopardized by underling CAD. Such scores introduce a weighting factor for coronary lesions in relation to their location in the coronary tree. The weighting factor is attributed in relationship to the extent of blood supplied to the myocardium. Indeed, the concept that the amount of myocardium jeopardized could represent a prognostic determinant in patients undergoing revascularization is straightforward but challenging to define numerically.
- Among different myocardium at risk scores, three principal scores have been more extensively investigated and validated in the literature, including the Jeopardy score from Duke University, the Myocardial Jeopardy Index from the Bypass Angioplasty Revascularization Investigation (BARI) trial, and the Alberta Provincial Project for Outcome Assessment in Coronary Heart Disease (APPROACH score) [16].
- The Duke Jeopardy score subdivides the coronary tree into six arterial segments, namely the left anterior descending, major anterolateral (diagonal) branch, first major septal perforator branch, circumflex artery, major marginal branch, and posterior descending artery. Two points are assigned for each diseased coronary segment (defined as a diameter reduction ≥75%) and no points are given to the right coronary artery in patients with left dominance.

- In the Myocardial Jeopardy Index from the BARI trial, the terminal portion of the left anterior descending, left circumflex, and right coronary arteries as well as the terminal portion of major branches (diagonals, obtuse marginals, posterior descending, and posterolateral branches) are assigned a score between 0 and 3 based on vessel length/diameter. A score of 0 is attributed to insignificant or inconspicuous arteries while a score of 3 is conferred to large arteries (i.e., extending more than two-thirds of the base-to-apex distance). Septal branches are arbitrarily assigned a maximum total score of 3. All segmental scores affected by CAD (≥50% stenosis) are summed and divided by the total score to calculate the jeopardized myocardium subtended by CAD.

- The APPROACH score estimates the myocardium at risk by dividing the left ventricle into regions at jeopardy on the basis of the myocardium perfused by each coronary artery as identified in pathological studies in humans (Fig. 8.3).

- The external validation of the above-described scores has been performed in a large unselected cohort of >20,000 patients [16]. All the three myocardium at risk scores showed good predictive ability for the estimation of 1-year mortality. The APPROACH score performed slightly better in patients undergoing PCI or medically treated. The BARI and APPROACH scores have also been validated in the setting of acute myocardial infarction. Both scores were significantly related to the infarct transmurality and infarct endocardial surface area as assessed by cardiac magnetic resonance imaging [17].

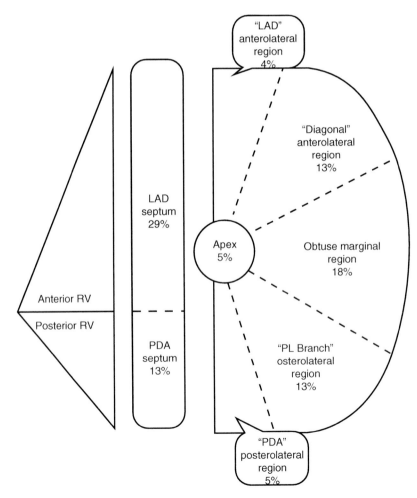

Fig. 8.3 The APPROACH score for the quantification of myocardium at risk. Reprinted with permission from Graham MM et al. [16]

EuroScore, SYNTAX, and SYNTAX II Scores

- The European System for Cardiac Operative Risk Evaluation (EuroSCORE) is a multiparametric risk score that was originally conceived to estimate the risk of operative mortality in patients undergoing cardiac surgery. The score was derived from a large cohort of 19,030 adult patients undergoing cardiac surgery (63.6% undergoing isolated coronary surgery and 29.8% valve operations) at 132 surgical centers in 8 European states [18]. Overall, in-hospital mortality was 4.8% in the study cohort.

- Independent predictors of mortality among several explored clinical parameters were identified by multivariate logistic regression analysis and were integrated into a simple integer and additive risk score. Subsequently, a different and more sophisticated way to obtain the risk estimate (logistic EuroSCORE, calculated by resolving the original equations) has been introduced [19].

- Finally, in 2011, a new version of the score (EuroSCORE II) has been introduced to update the previous models. The EuroSCORE II was derived from 22,381 consecutive patients undergoing major cardiac surgery in 154 hospitals in 43 countries between May and July 2010, reflecting a more contemporary dataset [20]. In the validation cohort, the EuroSCORE II was well calibrated and showed good discrimination. An online and user-friendly calculator of the score has been provided at http://euroscore.org/calc.html.

- Being derived and validated from surgical series, the EuroSCORE underwent subsequent validation in patients treated with PCI confirming the good discrimination and predictive performance in large series of patients undergoing percutaneous revascularization [21–23].

- The SYNergy between percutaneous coronary intervention with TAXus and cardiac surgery (SYNTAX) score is an a priori-defined angiographic tool that attempts to numerically quantify the complexity and burden of coronary artery disease.

- The SYNTAX score was firstly introduced in the landmark SYNTAX trial and is endorsed by international guidelines to guide the clinical decision-making between PCI and coronary artery bypass grafting (CABG) [24]. International guidelines recommendations [25, 26] based on the SYNTAX score are summarized in Table 8.4.

Table 8.4 International guidelines recommendations for PCI as revascularization strategy based on SYNTAX score

European guidelines	Class	LoE	ACC/AHA/SCAI guidelines	Class	LoE
Left main disease with a SYNTAX score ≤22	I	B	Anatomy at low risk of PCI procedural complications (i.e., low SYNTAX score ≤22, ostial or trunk ULMCA CAD) and increased clinical risk of adverse surgical outcomes (i.e., STS-predicted risk of operative mortality ≥5%)	IIa	B
Left main disease with a SYNTAX score 23–32	IIa	B	It is reasonable to choose CABG over PCI to improve symptoms in patients with complex three-vessel CAD (e.g., SYNTAX score >22), with or without involvement of the proximal LAD artery	IIa	B
Left main disease with a SYNTAX score >32	III	B	Anatomy at low to intermediate risk of PCI procedural complications (i.e., low-intermediate SYNTAX score <33, bifurcation ULMCA CAD) and increased clinical risk of adverse surgical outcomes (i.e., STS-predicted risk of operative mortality ≥2%)	NA	NA
Three-vessel disease with a SYNTAX score ≤22	I	B	NA	NA	NA
Left main disease with a SYNTAX score 23–32	III	B	NA	NA	NA
Left main disease with a SYNTAX score >32	III	B	NA	NA	NA

- For the score calculation, different anatomical and pathological characteristics are taken into account. The anatomical location of a lesion and, consequently, the extent of blood supplied to the myocardium are weighted.
- Further characteristics, including coronary disease involving bifurcations (according to Medina classification) or trifurcations, angiographic characterization according to ACC/AHA classification, and CTO characteristics (duration, length, blunt stump, presence of bridging collaterals or side branch), are identified.
- Finally, presence of aorto-ostial lesions, severe tortuosity, lesion length >20 mm, heavy calcification, thrombus, and diffuse or small-vessel disease are graded to refine and obtain the final score.
- A simple online calculator of the score is available at http://www.syntaxscore.com/calculator/start.htm.
- Two simple rules must be taken into account when interventionalists focus on the calculation of the score. First, only coronary segments with atheromatous disease determining a stenosis ≥50% in vessels ≥1.5 mm must be considered and scored. Sequential lesions must be considered as separate only if the distance among them is more than 3 vessel reference diameters apart.
- Despite being adopted in daily clinical practice on the basis of extensive clinical research and guideline endorsement, the SYNTAX score has some principal limitations. First, calculation of the score relies on the quality of angiograms and sometimes may become time consuming such as in complex coronary anatomies.
- The moderate reproducibility, both in terms of intra- and inter-observer variability, affects the consistency and clinical credibility of the score.
- Finally, being a pure angiographic tool without integration of clinical variables with prognostic impact in patients undergoing either percutaneous or surgical revascularization, the

score may suffer from poor calibration. In addition, the SYNTAX score does not account for clinical presentation (i.e., acute coronary syndrome) or the extent of inducible ischemia/vitality of myocardium.
- To overcome some of these limitations, different derived scores have been developed and introduced by integrating the anatomical SYNTAX score with clinical variables and functional parameters (Fig. 8.4, Table 8.5).
- Among combined (clinical and angiographic) scores, the SYNTAX II score [32] represents one of the latest tools to guide the individualized decision-making process between CABG and PCI in patients with complex CAD. The score is built on the integration of both the anatomical SYNTAX score and clinical variables affecting mortality in CABG- versus PCI-treated patients or vice versa (interaction terms).
- The score was derived using a Cox proportional hazards model in patients enrolled in the SYNTAX trial ($n = 1800$) and was externally validated in the DELTA registry ($n = 2891$).
- Eight clinical variables are considered in the calculation of the score, including age, creatinine clearance, left ventricular ejection fraction (LVEF), presence of unprotected left main CAD, peripheral vascular disease, female sex, and chronic obstructive pulmonary disease.
- Nomograms of the score have been developed to simplify the calculation and bedside application of the score (Fig. 8.5). An online calculator is also available at http://www.syntaxscore.com/calculator/start.htm.
- Beyond statistical performance, the meaningful message coming from the development of the SYNTAX II score is that to achieve similar mortality after revascularization with either CABG or PCI, the threshold value of the SYNTAX score to select the most appropriate revascularization strategy may vary according to the clinical and anatomical characteristics of patients (i.e., lower anatomical SYNTAX

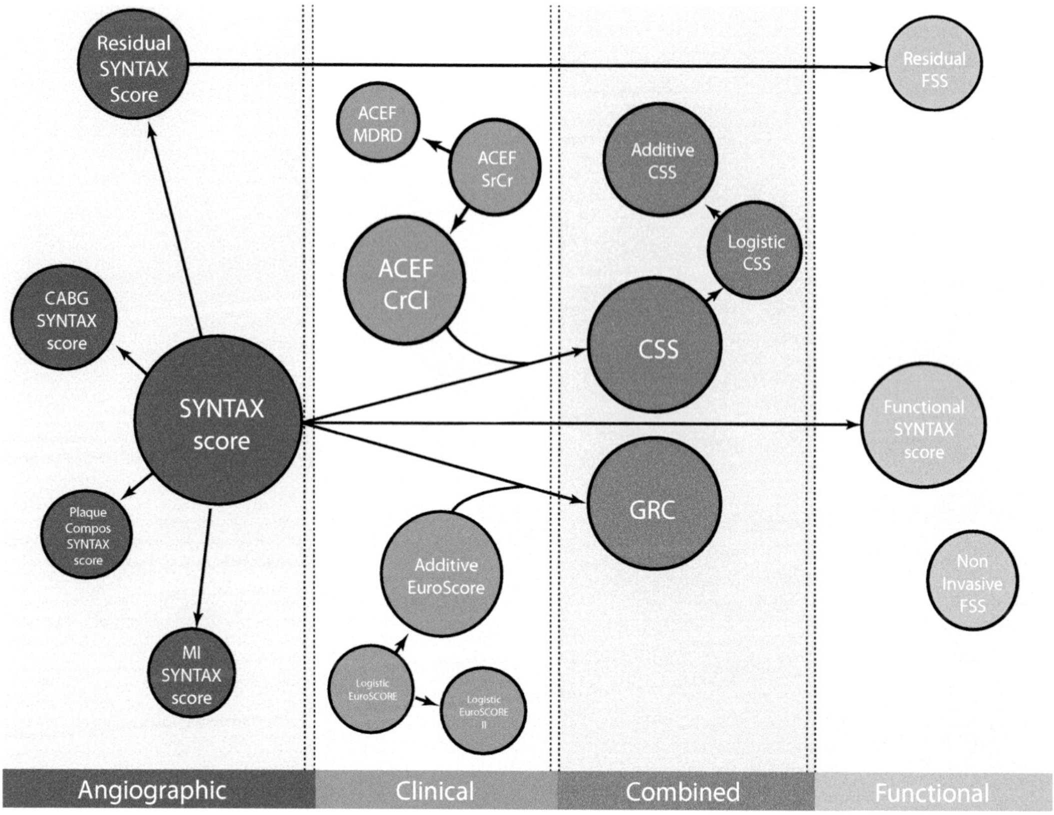

Fig. 8.4 Integration of the anatomical SYNTAX score with clinical and functional parameters. Reprinted with permission from Capodanno et al. [27]. Abbreviations: *ACEF* age, creatinine, ejection fraction, *CABG* coronary artery bypass grafting, *Compos* compositional, *CrCl* cre- atinine clearance, *CSS* clinical SYNTAX score, *FSS* functional SYNTAX score, *GRC* global risk classification, *MI* myocardial infarction, *MDRD* modification of diet in renal disease, *SrCr* serum creatinine, *SYNTAX* SYNergy between PCI with TAXus and cardiac surgery

Table 8.5 Summary of integrative scores of the anatomic SYNTAX score with clinical variable

Score	Year	Components	Objective
Functional SYNTAX score[28]	2011	Anatomic + FFR	As SYNTAX score but based on hemodynamically significant lesions
Global risk score[29]	2010	SYNTAX score + EuroSCORE	To identify a low-risk group with comparable outcomes to CABG and PCI in left main and 3VD patients
Clinical SYNTAX score[30]	2010	SYNTAX score × ACEF score	To improve the predictive power of the SYNTAX score by identifying PCI-treated patients at high risk
Logistic Clinical SYNTAX score[31]	2011	SYNTAX score + ACEF score	To improve the predictive power of the SYNTAX score predicting 1-year clinical outcomes in PCI-treated patients irrespective of the clinical presentation
SYNTAX score II [32]	2012	SYNTAX score + clinical variables	Decision-making for PCI vs. CABG

Key: *FFR* fractional flow reserve, *ACEF* age, creatinine, ejection fraction, *PCI* percutaneous coronary intervention, *CABG* coronary artery bypass grafting, *3VD* three-vessel disease

Fig. 8.5 SYNTAX score II nomograms. Reprinted with permission from Farooq et al. [32]. Abbreviations: *CrCl* creatinine clearance, *LVEF* left ventricular ejection fraction, *COPD* chronic obstructive pulmonary disease, *PVD* peripheral vascular disease

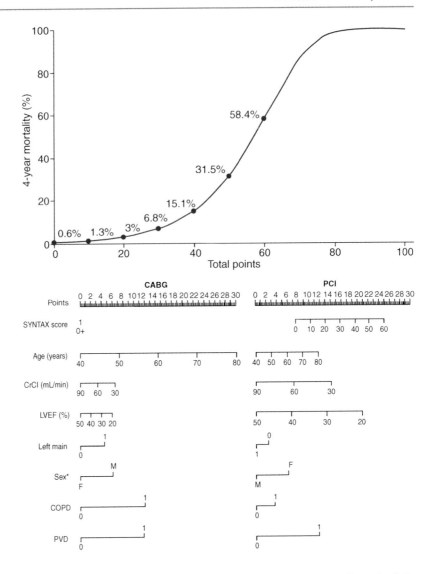

score in older patients). Therefore, when evaluating the complexity of CAD and selecting a subsequent revascularization strategy, patients' clinical profile must be carefully evaluated since it represents a strong determinant of prognosis in concert with the anatomical complexity as evaluated with the SYNTAX score.

High-Risk PCI and Supportive Measures

• Categorization and definition of high risk in patients undergoing PCI remain elusive.

Investigators and clinical researchers, both in observational studies and randomized trials, often used disparate definitions of high-risk PCI reflecting the lack of a common, standardized, and widely accepted definition [33].

• The Complex and Higher-Risk Indicated Patients (CHIP) initiative is aiming at prospectively identifying higher risk patients undergoing PCI who potentially have the most to gain from timely performed PCI (Ajay J. Kirtane, Slide Presentation, 2015, CHIP meeting).

• In a paradigmatic example, performing high-risk PCI has been compared to an attempt to repair a damaged car engine while it is turned on and the car is trying to slowly move from a steep cliff into the ocean at its base [34]. Beyond this analogy, a high-risk PCI patient could be identified in the presence of reduced cardiac reserve and limited ability to withstand arrhythmias, transient occlusion of coronary arteries, or distal embolization of atherogenic material.

- In this scenario, cardiogenic shock at presentation and large areas of myocardium at jeopardy are two hallmark features of patients undergoing high-risk PCI. Data from the large CathPCI Registry (1,208,137 PCI procedures at 1252 US hospitals) clearly showed that clinical acuity (i.e., presence of cardiogenic shock or procedure urgency) is a strong determinant of in-hospital mortality [35].
- Moreover, presence of a CTO, subacute stent thrombosis, and left main lesion location were identified as significant angiographic predictors of short-term mortality. Interestingly, the large CathPCI database has been used to develop a risk model that is able to predict short-term mortality following PCI. The correct identification of risk is crucial since adequate supportive measures could be adopted in the high-risk PCI context like mechanical support of cardiac function.
- Results of randomized trials exploring the prophylactic use of mechanical supportive strategies (i.e., intra-aortic balloon pump, Impella, and TandemHeart devices) in high-risk PCI context have been equivocal (Table 8.6). This is probably a consequence of poor study design with underpowered sample size, inaccurate and varying definitions of high-risk patients, and limited follow-up to assess and identify differences in hard clinical endpoints like mortality.

Table 8.6 Characteristics of randomized studies investigating hemodynamic supportive strategies in high-risk PCI patients

Study	Intervention	*No.* of patients	Definition of high risk	Results
Balloon pump-assisted coronary intervention study-1 [36]	IABP vs. no IABP	301	Left ventricular ejection fraction of <30%, and a large amount of myocardium at risk from extensive coronary artery disease categorized with the BCIS-1 jeopardy score (a modification of the Duke jeopardy score) ≥ 8	Similar rates of MACCEs (15.2% elective IABP vs. 16.0% no planned IABP, $p = 0.85$) at hospital discharge or 28 days after PCI. Peri-procedural complications (hypotension) more frequent in the no-planned IABP group. At 5 years, significant survival advantage identified in elective IABP group (HR: 0.66, 95% CI: 0.44–0.98, $p = 0.039$)
Intra-aortic balloon pump in cardiogenic shock II [37]	IABP vs. no IABP	600	AMI (with or without ST-segment elevation) complicated by CS (SBP <90 mmHg for more than 30 min or needed infusion of catecholamines, had clinical signs of pulmonary congestion and had impaired end-organ perfusion) with planned revascularization	No difference in 30-day mortality (RR with IABP, 0.96; 95% CI, 0.79 to 1.17; $P = 0.69$). No differences in time to hemodynamic stabilization, length of stay in the intensive care unit, serum lactate levels, dose and duration of catecholamine therapy, and renal function

(continued)

Table 8.6 (continued)

Study	Intervention	No. of patients	Definition of high risk	Results
Efficacy study of LV assist device to treat patients with cardiogenic shock [38]	Impella vs. IABP	25	Hypotension (SBP <90 mmHg) and a HR >90 beats/min or the need for inotropic drugs to maintain a SBP >90 mmHg and end-organ hypoperfusion or pulmonary edema. Hemodynamic criteria were either a CI of no more than 2.2 L/min/m² and a PCWP >15 mmHg or an angiographically measured LVEF <30% and LVEDP >20 mm Hg. The onset of shock had to be within 24 h	Significant augmentation of cardiac index with Impella but no improvements in 30-day mortality
PROTECT II trial [39]	Impella vs. IABP	452 (enrollment stopped early for futility)	Non-emergent PCI on an unprotected left main or emergent PCI on an unprotected left main or last patent coronary vessel with a LVEF ≤35%, three-vessel disease with LVEF ≤30%	30-day MAEs were not different between groups: 35.1% for Impella 2.5 vs. 40.1% for IABP, $P = 0.227$ at 90 days, a strong trend toward decreased MAE was observed in Impella 2.5-supported patients compared to IABP: 40.6% vs. 49.3%, $P = 0.066$ in ITT and 40.0% vs. 51.0%, $P = 0.023$ in PP populations, respectively
Thiele et al. [40]	Tandem Heart vs. IABP	41	Patients in CS (persistent SBP <90 mmHg or vasopressors required to maintain blood pressure >90 mmHg); evidence of end-organ failure; PCWP >15 mmHg and CI <2.1 L/min/m² after AMI with intended PCI of the infarcted artery	Significant improvement in hemodynamic and metabolic variables, 30-day mortality was similar (45% vs. 43%, log-rank, $P = 0.86$)

Key: *IABP* intra-aortic balloon pump, *MACCE* major adverse cardiovascular and cerebrovascular events, *PCI* percutaneous coronary intervention, *AMI* acute myocardial infarction, *SBP* systolic blood pressure, *RR* relative risk, *LVEF* left ventricular ejection fraction, *HR* heart rate, *PCWP* pulmonary capillary wedge pressure, *MAE* major adverse events, *ITT* intention to treat, *PP* per protocol, *CS* cardiogenic shock, *CI* cardiac index

• Accordingly, current European and American guidelines conferred an intermediate class of indication (class IIa or IIb) for the use of invasive supportive devices in the setting of high-risk PCI.

Conclusions

Several clinical and hemodynamic variables potentially factor in the immediate post-procedural and long-term outcome following PCI. The proper identification and definition of risk is a crucial prerequisite to implement adequate supportive measures and potentially avoid procedural complications.

References

1. Kastrati A, Schömig A, Elezi S, Dirschinger J, Mehilli J, Schühlen H, Blasini R, Neumann FJ. Prognostic value of the modified American college of Cardiology/American heart association stenosis morphology classification for long-term angiographic and clinical outcome after coronary stent placement. Circulation. 1999;100(12):1285–90.
2. Nakazawa G, Yazdani SK, Finn AV, Vorpahl M, Kolodgie FD, Virmani R. Pathological findings at bifurcation lesions: the impact of flow distribution on atherosclerosis and arterial healing after stent implantation. J Am Coll Cardiol. 2010;55(16):1679–87. https://doi.org/10.1016/j.jacc.2010.01.021.

3. Medina A, Suárez de Lezo J, Pan M. A new classification of coronary bifurcation lesions. Rev Esp Cardiol. 2006;59(2):183.
4. Popma J, Leon M, Topol EJ. Atlas of interventional cardiology. Philadelphia, PA: Saunders; 1994.
5. Strauss BH, Shuvy M, Wijeysundera HC. Revascularization of chronic total occlusions: time to reconsider? J Am Coll Cardiol. 2014;64(12):1281–9. https://doi.org/10.1016/j.jacc.2014.06.1181.
6. Hamburger JN, Serruys PW, Scabra-Gomes R, Simon R, Koolen JJ, Fleck E, Mathey D, Sievert H, Rutsch W, Buchwald A, Marco J, Al-Kasab SM, Pizulli L, Hamm C, Corcos T, Reifart N, Hanrath P, Taeymans Y. Recanalization of total coronary occlusions using a laser guide wire (the European TOTAL Surveillance Study). Am J Cardiol. 1997;80(11):1419–23.
7. Morino Y, Abe M, Morimoto T, Kimura T, Hayashi Y, Muramatsu T, Ochiai M, Noguchi Y, Kato K, Shibata Y, Hiasa Y, Doi O, Yamashita T, Hinohara T, Tanaka H, Mitsudo K, J-CTO Registry Investigators. Predicting successful guidewire crossing through chronic total occlusion of native coronary lesions within 30 minutes: the J-CTO (Multicenter CTO Registry in Japan) score as a difficulty grading and time assessment tool. JACC Cardiovasc Interv. 2011;4(2):213–21. https://doi.org/10.1016/j.jcin.2010.09.024.
8. Sinclair H, Veerasamy M, Bourantas C, Egred M, Nair A, Calvert PA, Brugaletta S, Mintz GS, Kunadian V. The role of virtual histology intravascular ultrasound in the identification of coronary artery plaque vulnerability in acute coronary syndromes. Cardiol Rev. 2016;24(6):303–9.
9. Koskinas KC, Ughi GJ, Windecker S, Tearney GJ, Räber L. Intracoronary imaging of coronary atherosclerosis: validation for diagnosis, prognosis and treatment. Eur Heart J. 2016;37(6):524–35a-c. https://doi.org/10.1093/eurheartj/ehv642.
10. Guagliumi G, Capodanno D, Saia F, Musumeci G, Tarantini G, Garbo R, Tumminello G, Sirbu V, Coccato M, Fineschi M, Trani C, De Benedictis M, Limbruno U, De Luca L, Niccoli G, Bezerra H, Ladich E, Costa M, Biondi Zoccai G, Virmani R, Trial Investigators OCTAVIA. Mechanisms of atherothrombosis and vascular response to primary percutaneous coronary intervention in women versus men with acute myocardial infarction: results of the OCTAVIA study. JACC Cardiovasc Interv. 2014;7(9):958–68. https://doi.org/10.1016/j.jcin.2014.05.011.
11. Stone GW, Maehara A, Lansky AJ, de Bruyne B, Cristea E, Mintz GS, Mehran R, McPherson J, Farhat N, Marso SP, Parise H, Templin B, White R, Zhang Z, Serruys PW, PROSPECT Investigators. A prospective natural-history study of coronary atherosclerosis. N Engl J Med. 2011 Jan 20;364(3):226–35. https://doi.org/10.1056/NEJMoa1002358.
12. Garrone P, Biondi-Zoccai G, Salvetti I, Sina N, Sheiban I, Stella PR, Agostoni P. Quantitative coronary angiography in the current era: principles and applications. J Interv Cardiol. 2009;22(6):527–36. https://doi.org/10.1111/j.1540-8183.2009.00491.x.
13. Pantos I, Efstathopoulos EP, Katritsis DG. Two and three-dimensional quantitative coronary angiography. Cardiol Clin. 2009;27(3):491–502. https://doi.org/10.1016/j.ccl.2009.03.008.
14. Tomasello SD, Costanzo L, Galassi AR. Quantitative coronary angiography in the interventional cardiology. In: Kiraç SF, editor. Chapter book in "Advances in the Diagnosis of Coronary Atherosclerosis". London: InTech; 2011. ISBN 978-953-307-286-9.
15. Capodanno D. Beyond the SYNTAX score—advantages and limitations of other risk assessment systems in left main percutaneous coronary intervention. Circ J. 2013;77(5):1131–8.
16. Graham MM, Faris PD, Ghali WA, Galbraith PD, Norris CM, Badry JT, Mitchell LB, Curtis MJ, Knudtson ML, APPROACH Investigators (Alberta Provincial Project for Outcome Assessment in Coronary Heart Disease. Validation of three myocardial jeopardy scores in a population-based cardiac catheterization cohort. Am Heart J. 2001;142(2):254–61.
17. Ortiz-Pérez JT, Meyers SN, Lee DC, Kansal P, Klocke FJ, Holly TA, Davidson CJ, Bonow RO, Wu E. Angiographic estimates of myocardium at risk during acute myocardial infarction: validation study using cardiac magnetic resonance imaging. Eur Heart J. 2007;28(14):1750–8.
18. Nashef SA, Roques F, Michel P, Gauducheau E, Lemeshow S, Salamon R. European system for cardiac operative risk evaluation (EuroSCORE). Eur J Cardiothorac Surg. 1999 Jul;16(1):9–13.
19. Roques F, Michel P, Goldstone AR, Nashef SA. The logistic EuroSCORE. Eur Heart J. 2003;24(9):882–3.
20. Nashef SA, Roques F, Sharples LD, Nilsson J, Smith C, Goldstone AR, Lockowandt U. EuroSCORE II. Eur J Cardiothorac Surg. 2012;41(4):734–44.; discussion 744-5. https://doi.org/10.1093/ejcts/ezs043.
21. Romagnoli E, Burzotta F, Trani C, Siviglia M, Biondi-Zoccai GG, Niccoli G, Leone AM, Porto I, Mazzari MA, Mongiardo R, Rebuzzi AG, Schiavoni G, Crea F. EuroSCORE as predictor of in-hospital mortality after percutaneous coronary intervention. Heart. 2009;95(1):43–8. https://doi.org/10.1136/hrt.2007.134114.
22. Schwietz T, Spyridopoulos I, Pfeiffer S, Laskowski R, Palm S, DE Rosa S, Jens K, Zeiher AM, Schächinger V, Fichtlscherer S, Lehmann R. Risk stratification following complex PCI: clinical versus anatomical risk stratification including "post PCI residual SYNTAX-score" as quantification of incomplete revascularization. J Interv Cardiol. 2013;26(1):29–37. https://doi.org/10.1111/j.1540-8183.2013.12014.x.
23. Capodanno D, Dipasqua F, Marcantoni C, Ministeri M, Zanoli L, Rastelli S, Romano G, Sanfilippo M, Tamburino C. EuroSCORE II versus additive and logistic EuroSCORE in patients undergoing percutaneous coronary intervention. Am J Cardiol. 2013;112(3):323–9. https://doi.org/10.1016/j.amjcard.2013.03.032.
24. Serruys PW, Morice MC, Kappetein AP, Colombo A, Holmes DR, Mack MJ, Ståhle E, Feldman TE, van den

Brand M, Bass EJ, Van Dyck N, Leadley K, Dawkins KD, Mohr FW, Investigators SYNTAX. Percutaneous coronary intervention versus coronary-artery bypass grafting for severe coronary artery disease. N Engl J Med. 2009;360(10):961–72. https://doi.org/10.1056/NEJMoa0804626.

25. Authors/Task Force members, Windecker S, Kolh P, Alfonso F, Collet JP, Cremer J, Falk V, Filippatos G, Hamm C, Head SJ, Jüni P, Kappetein AP, Kastrati A, Knuuti J, Landmesser U, Laufer G, Neumann FJ, Richter DJ, Schauerte P, Sousa Uva M, Stefanini GG, Taggart DP, Torracca L, Valgimigli M, Wijns W, Witkowski A. 2014 ESC/EACTS Guidelines on myocardial revascularization: The Task Force on Myocardial Revascularization of the European Society of Cardiology (ESC) and the European Association for Cardio-Thoracic Surgery (EACTS) Developed with the special contribution of the European Association of Percutaneous Cardiovascular Interventions (EAPCI). Eur Heart J. 2014;35(37):2541–619. https://doi.org/10.1093/eurheartj/ehu278.

26. Levine GN, Bates ER, Blankenship JC, Bailey SR, Bittl JA, Cercek B, Chambers CE, Ellis SG, Guyton RA, Hollenberg SM, Khot UN, Lange RA, Mauri L, Mehran R, Moussa ID, Mukherjee D, Nallamothu BK, Ting HH; American College of Cardiology Foundation; American Heart Association Task Force on Practice Guidelines; Society for Cardiovascular Angiography and Interventions. 2011 ACCF/AHA/SCAI Guideline for Percutaneous Coronary Intervention. A report of the American College of Cardiology Foundation/American Heart Association Task Force on Practice Guidelines and the Society for Cardiovascular Angiography and Interventions. J Am Coll Cardiol. 2011;58(24):e44-122. doi: https://doi.org/10.1016/j.jacc.2011.08.007.

27. Capodanno D. Lost in calculation: the clinical SYNTAX score goes logistic. Eur Heart J. 2012;33(24):3008–10. https://doi.org/10.1093/eurheartj/ehs346.

28. Nam CW, Mangiacapra F, Entjes R, Chung IS, Sels JW, Tonino PA, De Bruyne B, Pijls NH, Fearon WF, Study Investigators FAME. Functional SYNTAX score for risk assessment in multivessel coronary artery disease. J Am Coll Cardiol. 2011;58(12):1211–8. https://doi.org/10.1016/j.jacc.2011.06.020.

29. Capodanno D, Caggegi A, Miano M, et al. Global risk classification and clinical SYNTAX (synergy between percutaneous coronary intervention with TAXUS and cardiac surgery) score in patients undergoing percutaneous or surgical left main revascularization. J Am Coll Cardiol Intv. 2011;4:287–97.

30. Serruys PW, Farooq V, Vranckx P, et al. A global risk approach to identify patients with left main or 3-vessel disease who could safely and efficaciously be treated with percutaneous coronary intervention: the SYNTAX Trial at 3 years. JACC Cardiovasc Interv. 2012;5:606–17.

31. Farooq V, Vergouwe Y, Raber L, et al. Combined anatomical and clinical factors for the long-term risk stratification of patients undergoing percutaneous coronary intervention: the logistic clinical SYNTAX Score. Eur Heart J. 2012;33:3098–104.

32. Farooq V, van Klaveren D, Steyerberg EW, et al. Anatomical and clinical characteristics to guide decision making between coronary artery bypass surgery and percutaneous coronary intervention for individual patients: development and validation of SYNTAX Score II. Lancet. 2013;381:639–50.

33. Myat A, Patel N, Tehrani S, Banning AP, Redwood SR, Bhatt DL. Percutaneous circulatory assist devices for high-risk coronary intervention. JACC Cardiovasc Interv. 2015;8(2):229–44. https://doi.org/10.1016/j.jcin.2014.07.030.

34. O'Neill WW. What is high-risk PCI, and how do you safely perform it? J Invasive Cardiol. 2011;23(10):425–6.

35. Brennan JM, Curtis JP, Dai D, Fitzgerald S, Khandelwal AK, Spertus JA, Rao SV, Singh M, Shaw RE, Ho KK, Krone RJ, Weintraub WS, Weaver WD, Peterson ED, National Cardiovascular Data Registry. Enhanced mortality risk prediction with a focus on high-risk percutaneous coronary intervention: results from 1,208,137 procedures in the NCDR (National Cardiovascular Data Registry). JACC Cardiovasc Interv. 2013;6(8):790–9. https://doi.org/10.1016/j.jcin.2013.03.020.

36. Perera D, Stables R, Thomas M, Booth J, Pitt M, Blackman D, de Belder A, Redwood S, BCIS-1 Investigators. Elective intra-aortic balloon counterpulsation during high-risk percutaneous coronary intervention: a randomized controlled trial. JAMA. 2010;304(8):867–74. https://doi.org/10.1001/jama.2010.1190.

37. Thiele H, Zeymer U, Neumann FJ, Ferenc M, Olbrich HG, Hausleiter J, de Waha A, Richardt G, Hennersdorf M, Empen K, Fuernau G, Desch S, Eitel I, Hambrecht R, Lauer B, Böhm M, Ebelt H, Schneider S, Werdan K, Schuler G, Intraaortic Balloon Pump in cardiogenic shock II (IABP-SHOCK II) trial investigators. Intra-aortic balloon counterpulsation in acute myocardial infarction complicated by cardiogenic shock (IABP-SHOCK II): final 12 month results of a randomised, open-label trial. Lancet. 2013;382(9905):1638–45. https://doi.org/10.1016/S0140-6736(13)61783-3.

38. Seyfarth M, Sibbing D, Bauer I, Fröhlich G, Bott-Flügel L, Byrne R, Dirschinger J, Kastrati A, Schömig A. A randomized clinical trial to evaluate the safety and efficacy of a percutaneous left ventricular assist device versus intra-aortic balloon pumping for treatment of cardiogenic shock caused by myocardial infarction. J Am Coll Cardiol. 2008;52(19):1584–8. https://doi.org/10.1016/j.jacc.2008.05.065.

39. O'Neill WW, Kleiman NS, Moses J, Henriques JP, Dixon S, Massaro J, Palacios I, Maini B, Mulukutla

S, Dzavík V, Popma J, Douglas PS, Ohman M. A prospective, randomized clinical trial of hemodynamic support with Impella 2.5 versus intra-aortic balloon pump in patients undergoing high-risk percutaneous coronary intervention: the PROTECT II study. Circulation. 2012;126(14):1717–27. https://doi.org/10.1161/CIRCULATIONAHA.112.098194.

40. Thiele H, Sick P, Boudriot E, Diederich KW, Hambrecht R, Niebauer J, Schuler G. Randomized comparison of intra-aortic balloon support with a percutaneous left ventricular assist device in patients with revascularized acute myocardial infarction complicated by cardiogenic shock. Eur Heart J. 2005;26(13):1276–83.

Guide Catheters: Selection, Support, Extension and Guide Wire Selection

9

Murugapathy Veerasamy and Nicholas D. Palmer

About Us The Liverpool Heart and Chest Hospital provides tertiary cardiac care services to a population of 2.8 million in the North-West of England. It is one of only two stand-alone cardiothoracic centers in the United Kingdom and provides high-quality and comprehensive care as exemplified by our recent outstanding Care Quality Commission rating. The center is one of the largest interventional centers in the United Kingdom providing coronary and structural interventions. About 2500 percutaneous coronary interventions are performed annually, of which 900 are primary PCI. The unique daycare PCI lounge concept has nationwide recognition for excellence in the treatment of elective and ACS patients. The center offers high-quality heart and aortic surgery and has an established reputation as a leader in cardiovascular research.

Guide Catheters

- Guide catheters are the conduits through which devices essential for percutaneous coronary intervention (PCI) can be introduced into the coronary artery. Their primary role is to provide adequate support for the procedure and enable delivery of equipment with simultaneous contrast injection and pressure monitoring.
- The ideal guide catheter should have the following features [1]:
  - Strength
  - Atraumatic support
  - Kink resistance
  - 1:1 torque
  - Flexibility
  - Device compatibility
  - Large lumen
  - Lubricity
- Though not all of these features can be obtained in a single guide catheter due to competing dynamics, most of these are achieved by the three-layered structure made of inner lumen (polytetrafluoroethylene—PTFE), a middle layer of braided steel matrix, and an outer jacket made of soft nylon elastomer (Fig. 9.1).
- The middle and outer layers provide the torque and support while the inner layer provides minimal resistance and friction for the passage of devices.

M. Veerasamy
Cardiothoracic Centre, Freeman Hospital,
Newcastle-upon-Tyne, UK
e-mail: murugapathy.veerasamy@unch.nhs.uk

N. D. Palmer (✉)
Department of Cardiology, Liverpool Heart
and Chest Hospital, Liverpool, UK
e-mail: Nick.Palmer@lhch.nhs.uk

© Springer International Publishing AG, part of Springer Nature 2018
A. Myat et al. (eds.), *The Interventional Cardiology Training Manual*,
https://doi.org/10.1007/978-3-319-71635-0_9

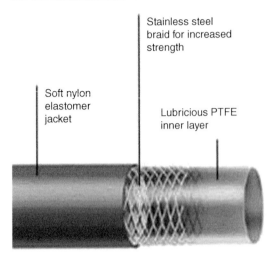

Stainless steel braid for increased strength

Soft nylon elastomer jacket

Lubricious PTFE inner layer

Fig. 9.1 Guide catheter structure

Table 9.1 Common guide catheters and degree of support provided

Target vessel	Increasing support		
	+	++	+++
LAD	JL 3.5/4.0	Q 3.5/4.0	XBU 3.5/4.0
		AL2.0	EBU 3.5/4.0
LCx	JL 3.5/4.0	AL 2.0	XBU 3.5/4.0
			EBU 3.5/4.0
			Mach KL 4.0
RCA	JR 4.0	AR 1.0/2.0	AL 1.0/2.0
			Q 4.0

Guide Catheter Support

Backup Support (Table 9.1)

- This is the ability of the guide catheter to provide a stable position to easily advance the interventional equipment to the desired location in the coronary artery. This is divided into *passive* and *active* support.
- As the name implies passive support is provided by the curve and shape of the catheter, properties of the shaft and tip at the ostium, and minimal manipulation of the catheter. For optimal passive support the curve of the catheter must match the size of the aortic root (Fig. 9.2).
- Active support is obtained from the aortic root with active manipulation of the catheter to engage (deep-seat) the catheter into the desired coronary artery (Fig. 9.3) [2]. This increases the risk of catheter-induced coronary dissection especially when the ostium or proximal coronary artery is diseased.
- In addition to the potential risk of coronary dissection this also increases prolonged coronary ischemia when there is pressure damping due to disease at the coronary ostium.

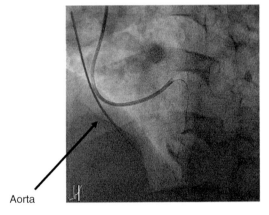

Aorta

Fig. 9.2 Passive support for LCA PCI

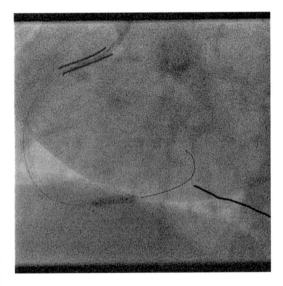

Fig. 9.3 Active support for RCA PCI

Guide Catheter Selection

- Guide catheters come in numerous shapes and sizes. In addition guide catheters are available in sheathless form and with side holes.
- "A battle is won easier based on the weapon used"; hence up-front selection of an appropriate guide catheter makes a PCI procedure simpler and quicker. This reduces the volume of contrast and radiation exposure and increases efficiency in the catheterization laboratory.
- The choice of guide catheter depends on the access site, coronary artery treated, complexity of the coronary lesion, and technique used for PCI.
- The majority of procedures can be done using the common catheter shapes. The key aim of guide catheter selection is support for delivering the PCI equipment where needed in the coronary artery.
- Irrespective of the choice of guide catheter, the tip should be coaxial in the coronary lumen to avoid catheter-induced trauma to the coronary artery. Coaxial alignment improves support in delivering the equipment.
- Experienced operators are able to manipulate the guide catheter position and shape and depth of intubation to maximize support in more complex cases.

Sizes

- The workhorse guide catheter size is 6F. For simple PCI in radial procedures 5F catheters can be used to help reduce radial spasm. For complex PCI 7F or 8F sizes may be necessary.

Sheathless Guides

- These are used in radial access procedures and have the advantage of avoiding the use of an introducer sheath. This enables the passage of a guide catheter with a larger inner lumen contained within a smaller outer lumen.

- For instance a sheathless catheter with an inner lumen of 7F has an outer lumen of less than or equal to 6F; that is, a larger lumen catheter can be used for complex PCI with no increase in trauma to the radial puncture site [3].

Anatomic Considerations

Access Site: Radial Access

- For the left coronary artery (LCA) with similar aortic root size, a catheter, which is 0.5 cm shorter than the ones used in the femoral artery, is preferred from the right radial artery (JL3.5, XBU 3.5, Q4).
- From the left radial artery access, similar sizes as used in femoral access are preferred (JL4, XBU4).
- For most right coronary artery RCA interventions a Judkins R4 is favored.
- When maximal support is anticipated Amplatz catheters are the preferred option.
- One of the considerations in radial access is the risk of radial artery spasm, especially in females, which can be reduced by the up-front use of a longer sheath and the use of a radial vasodilator cocktail (verapamil and glyceryl trinitrate).

Access Site: Femoral Access

- From the femoral route, for the LCA the standard catheters are Q4 and XBU4 when more support is needed and JL4 when lesser support is needed.
- For RCA interventions JR4 is insufficient in most of the cases. AL1 catheters are used when more support is required. Iliac artery tortuosity and calcification can make torque transmission difficult.
- Difficulty in torqueing can be overcome by catheter manipulation with a 0.038 guide wire in the catheter and occasionally braided and stiffer long sheaths are required to straighten iliac tortuosity.

Coronary Anatomy

- Aortic root size needs to be taken into account in choosing the curve of the catheter. Larger curves are needed in a dilated ascending root.
- A crude way of deciding on the curve is from the height of the patient. Smaller curves are needed in shorter patients (LCA: Q3.5, EBU3.5, or XBU3.5, RCA: AL0.75) as the aortic root is narrower.
- An anomalous anterior origin of the RCA can be reached with an AL1 catheter and this is also helpful to find an anomalous origin of the circumflex from the right coronary sinus.
- Short left main stems or separate origins of the left anterior descending and circumflex can be separately engaged by manipulating the catheter to selectively engage the LAD or circumflex arteries.

Grafts

- Though right coronary bypass and left coronary bypass (RCB, LCB) catheters can be used for grafts it is often easier with Amplatz guide catheters (AL1, AL2).
- For internal mammary artery grafts, an IM guide catheter is preferred.

PCI Techniques

- Larger lumen catheters should always be considered for complex PCI.
- In bifurcation PCI a two-stent strategy is often easier to perform using a 7F guide catheter. However, with experience most provisional side branch stenting cases can be done with 6F guide catheters.
- PCI of chronic total occlusions generally requires 7F or 8F catheters for stability, support, and passage of multiple items of PCI equipment especially when the retrograde approach is utilized.

Buddy Wire

- Despite the selection of the best possible GC, support is sometimes poor while delivering equipment.
- The use of a second coronary angioplasty wire to facilitate passage of equipment (mainly stent and sometimes balloons) to the desired location is called the "buddy wire technique."
- With this technique we use a stiffer wire along with the "workhorse" wire, as this helps to track the device by decreasing any wire bias and reducing angulation and tortuosity.

Anchor Balloon

- In this technique a wire is placed in a branch artery and an appropriately sized balloon is inflated in the branch, which increases support by stabilizing the guide catheter (Fig. 9.4) [4].
- This technique is used by experienced operators in the main for CTO-PCI procedures, especially when a lot of force is required to make a channel through the proximal cap.

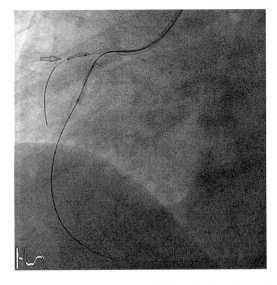

Fig. 9.4 Anchor balloon. Size 2.5 mm balloon (arrow) placed in RCA side branch to improve backup support for device crossing

- Rarely, this technique can be used with the balloon inflated in the target vessel lesion for countertraction and the stent is then delivered into the same location.
- Once the stent is delivered to the desired location the anchor balloon should be deflated and withdrawn into the catheter, to avoid jailing the balloon behind the stent.
- We recommend these techniques only for experienced operators.

Guide Catheter Extensions

- Over recent years guide extension catheters (GEC) have been established as useful adjuncts to resolve the problem of balloon or stent delivery in heavily calcified or tortuous coronary arteries.
- They have also helped overcome certain difficulties in the retrograde approach to PCI for chronic total occlusion.
- These catheters are coaxial, monorail guide catheter extensions, which are delivered through the standard guide catheter on the angioplasty guide wire.
- They enable coaxial alignment and distal placement for delivery of devices as well as selective delivery of contrast.
- Three main products are available:
  - GuideLiner (Vascular Solutions)
  - Guidezilla (Boston Scientific)
  - Guidion catheter (Acrostak)
- The design characteristics are similar. A 25 cm guide extension comprises three layers: PTFE, stainless steel coil, and an outer silicone coating for lubricity. This is attached to a stainless steel pusher.
- Radiopaque markers are set 2–3 mm from the catheter tip and proximally. The guide extension catheter is advanced over the wire through the hemostatic valve serving as an extension to the guide catheter for extra backup and deep guide engagement.
- Unlike other guide extensions such as the Heartrail "mother-and-child" catheter the working length of balloons and stents is not reduced such that distal coronary lesions can be reached and treated.
- Difficulties can be encountered when advancing the catheter through calcified and tortuous vessels. This difficulty can often be overcome by inflating a balloon in the most distal lesion to act as an anchor enabling the guide extension to pass smoothly into the distal vessel (Fig. 9.5).
- The stent procedure can be completed in the conventional way with gradual withdrawal of the guide extension as stents are placed more proximally. On completion of the case the guide extension catheter is removed in the same way as a monorail balloon or stent catheter system.
- Every time a catheter is used for deep intubation of a coronary vessel, regardless of how soft the tip is, there remains a risk of dissection of the ostium and/or the proximal aspect of the vessel. It is no different with guide extension catheters with reported dissection rates of 0.5–1%.
- Particular caution needs to be exercised in the setting of an anomalous origin of a vessel and in the setting of a diffusely diseased proximal segment. The GEC is less likely to dissect the coronary ostia than a guiding catheter because of the lack of a primary curve and the provision of atraumatic support.
- A drawback of this device is the potential for stents to get caught on the metal collar of the device. This can damage the stent and may even cause it to shear off if not recognized.
- If resistance is encountered the stent should not be pushed further but instead withdrawn and inspected for damage to its integrity.
- Wire wrap is another important consideration while using this device. When two wires are used in a coronary intervention, the GEC should be advanced only over the primary wire as the secondary wires may wrap around it and prevent advancement of devices.

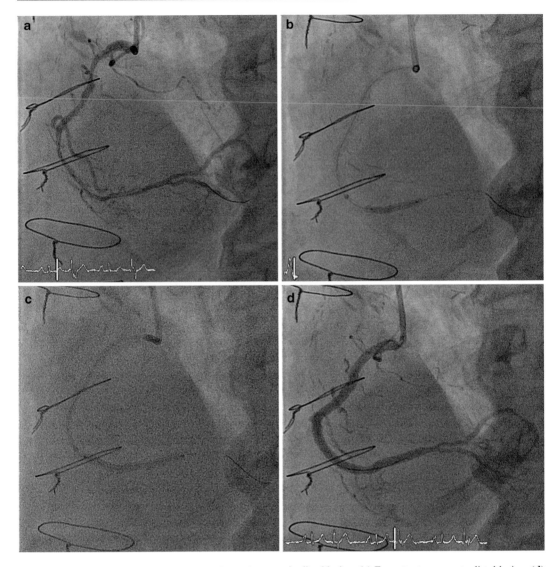

Fig. 9.5 Case example of use of guide extension catheter. (**a**) RCA CTO opened by antegrade wiring and POBA. (**b**) GuideLiner catheter advancement requires balloon anchor in distal lesion. (**c**) Easy stent passage to distal lesion. (**d**) Final angiographic result

Considerations in Complex PCI

Shape of Catheter

- **LMS PCI**—for ostial/proximal LMS PCI JL3.5/JL4.0 is used to assist withdrawal of the catheter to stent the ostium.
- **Tortuous or calcific RCA**—AL1 catheter provides the best support but a JR 4.0 can be better manipulated to be "deep-throated" into the vessel.

- **Tortuous or calcific LAD/LCx**—XBU3.5/XBU4.0

Size of Catheter

- **Rotational atherectomy**
  - 6F for 1.25 or 1.5 mm burr
  - 7F for 1.75 mm burr
  - 8F for 2.0 or 2.25 mm burr

- **Bifurcation PCI**
  - Complex bifurcation PCI with a two-stent strategy—can be performed with 6F but ideal procedure planning should consider 7F catheters.

- **CTO PCI**
  - 7F or 8F for better support as needed especially when a retrograde approach is planned.

Coronary Guide Wires

- Successful percutaneous coronary intervention always starts with the use of a coronary guide wire, which supports advancement of balloons and stents through the coronary vasculature.
- The basic functions of a guide wire are (Table 9.2):
  - To track through the vessel
  - To cross the lesion targeted for PCI without causing disruption
  - To provide support for interventional devices

Table 9.2 Essential characteristics of angioplasty guide wires [5]

Characteristics	Definition
Torque control	Proximal rotational force applied transmits efficiently and predictably to the distal end of the wire
Trackability	The wire follows the tip around bends and tortuosity with no kinking or prolapse
Flexibility	Degree of bending produced with direct pressure
Prolapse tendency	Tendency of the wire shaft to loop into adjacent branches
Steerability	Ability of the wire tip to negotiate tortuosity
Radiopacity	Visibility of the wire and tip under fluoroscopy
Tactile feedback	Sensation of distal tip movement at the proximal end
Crossing	Ability to cross a lesion
Support	Ability to support the passage of PCI devices

- The basic structure of a standard angioplasty guide wire is the presence of an inner core that extends through the shaft of the wire from proximal to distal part, which gives stability and steerability to the wire by transmitting rotatory forces to the tapered distal tip.
- The core material can be comprised of stainless steel or nitinol. The advantage of stainless steel is that it provides excellent support with better transmission of both pushing and torqueing characteristics.
- However in general, stainless steel wires are less flexible and tend to be more susceptible to kinking through excessive force.
- Nitinol wires have excellent flexibility with better durability but in general tend to be less torquable.
- A larger core allows better torque but at the expense of flexibility. The core tends to be tapered from proximal to distal end. The length and number of segmental tapers influence the flexibility of the wire.
- The angioplasty wire tip has various designs comprising the core which extends all the way to the tip and enables precise steering and tip control or a shaping ribbon design where the core stops just short of the distal tip and allows better flexibility but less torque control.
- There are various coatings designed to reduce friction through tortuous coronary anatomy as well as improve deliverability of interventional equipment.
- Hydrophilic coatings are lubricious and allow greater trackability although the downside is a greater risk of subintimal tracking causing dissection as well as coronary artery perforation. More experienced operators generally should use these wires.
- Hydrophobic coatings produce greater friction across the coronary artery segment and can give greater support and stability.
- There are various classifications of guide wires that can be used according to tip flexibility (floppy, intermediate, or standard), level of support (light, moderate, and extra support), and degree of coating. The common wire selections used for each of these classifications are demonstrated in Table 9.3.

Table 9.3 Classification of guide wires (examples)

By tip flexibility

Floppy	Intermediate	Standard
Asahi Sion blue	Hi-Torque Intermediate (Abbott)	ChoiCE Standard (Boston)
ChoiCE Floppy (Boston)	Miracle Bros 3 & 6	Pilot 200 (Abbott)
Balance middleweight (Abbott)	Fielder XT (Asahi)	Progress 80 (Abbott)
Fielder FC (Asahi)	Progress 40 (Abbott)	Miracle 9 (Asahi)
Pilot 50 (Abbott)	Cross-It 200 XT (Abbott)	
	Pilot 150 (Abbott)	

By support

Light	Moderate	Extra
Asahi Sion blue	Hi-Torque Balance Middleweight	ChoiCE ES (Boston)
ChoiCE Floppy (Boston)	(Abbott)	Pilot 200 (Abbott)
Pilot 50 (Abbott)	PT Graphix (Boston)	Asahi Grand Slam
Hi-Torque Floppy (Abbott)		Whisper ES (Abbott)

By tip load (proportional to penetration power)

Guide wire	Manufacturer	Tip load (g)	Tip characteristics (inches)
Sion blue	Asahi	0.5	0.014
Fielder XT	Asahi	1.2	0.009
Pilot 50	Abbott	1.5	0.014
MiracleBros 3	Asahi	3.5	0.0125
Pilot 200	Abbott	5.0	0.014
MiracleBros 6	Asahi	8.8	0.0125
Progress 80	Abbott	9.7	0.012
Confianza Pro 12	Asahi	12.4	0.009
Progress 200T	Abbott	13.0	0.012

- Selection of guide wire is largely based on lesion morphology and complexity and devices to be used. However when numerous guide wires in each classification are available in reality it is often operator experience and preference which determines the wire selection.
- For new interventionalists it is better to become familiar with a limited number of wires in each classification and to develop the appropriate skills to manipulate such wires in different coronary lesions and anatomies.

Specific Guide Wire Selection

- **Left main PCI**: Often the choice of guide wire is not essential other than having one that provides appropriate support. Usually a fairly soft-tipped wire (Asahi Sion Blue or Hi-Torque Balance Middleweight) is appropriate.
- **Bifurcation PCI**: Normal workhorse guide wires (Sion Blue, Balance Middleweight, or Choice Floppy) usually suffice and are appropriate for safe negotiation of the main vessel and side branch. These usually provide sufficient support for deployment of devices. Sometimes it is necessary to escalate the wire selection to provide greater penetration through the stent struts into a side branch and a hydrophilic coating to reduce friction, e.g., Pilot 50. These wires are more at risk of vessel dissection and lesion disruption but have greater success in cannulating vessels.
- **Tortuous and calcified lesions**: A floppy guide wire is usually most appropriate to negotiate the tortuous or calcified segment. Selecting a wire with good 1:1 torque for negotiation of very angulated segments is essential and sometimes a hydrophilic coating is beneficial to enable movement of the wire into the distal vessel against the frictional forces created by the tortuosity and calcification. It is sometimes necessary to use a more supportive wire (High Torque Floppy Extra Support or Whisper Extra Support) to enable

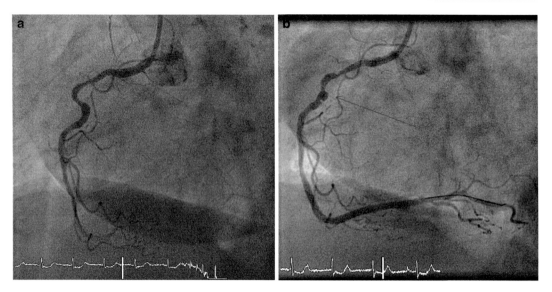

Fig. 9.6 (**a**) RCA CTO—tortuous proximal segment. (**b**) CTO reopened and stented. Stiff angioplasty guide wire creates pseudo stenosis (arrow) in proximal vessel

device delivery. Sometimes this is undertaken in a buddy wire technique to help straighten the vessel [6]. Occasionally the softer wire needs to be exchanged for an extra support using a microcatheter. It should be noted that the vessel wall straightening can create pseudo stenosis and may traumatize the vessels due to cheese wiring of the acute angulations and associated atheroma (Fig. 9.6).

Chronic Total Occlusion PCI

- A wide range of wires are available for this complex procedure [7].
- These range from simple wires for antegrade wire escalation techniques (Fielder XT, Miracle 6, Gaia Wire Series).
- More penetrative wires used for subintimal tracking are frequently required for antegrade dissection reentry techniques (Pilot 200, Gaia Wire Series, Confianza Miracle 9, Confianza Pro 12, Progress 200).
- These wires help to penetrate the proximal cap and/or enable wire tracking through into a dissection plane.
- Wire exchange is important in these techniques via a microcatheter to ensure that the

correct wire is selected for each stage of the CTO procedure.

- More advanced super-stiff wires are used for reentry from the subintimal space to the true lumen (Stingray wire). Experienced operators who are trained in this very specialized technique should only use these wires.
- The retrograde approach to CTO involves the use of relatively floppy but highly torquable wires (Asahi Sion, Fielder XT, Fielder FC) supported by specialist microcatheters (Corsair, Turnpike) to negotiate epicardial and septal collaterals and attain the distal vessel. Exchanging to more penetrative wires to cross the distal cap is often required.
- Specialist guide wires in this area also include those used for externalization following a successful retrograde crossing (Asahi RG3). Again these are for specialist use by experienced operators.

Advancing a Guide Wire

- Firstly selection of the appropriate angiographic view to visualize the target vessel is essential.
- Before inserting the wire it is important to consider the tortuosity of the vessel ostium,

proximal segments, and lesion to enable the appropriate tip shape to be fashioned to enable negotiation around the various bends.

- Often a conventional 45° tip bend is appropriate and occasionally secondary bends or more shallow bends can be used depending on the angulation of a lesion or whether the wire is required to be more penetrative such as when crossing a chronic occlusion. Tip shaping is a technique that improves with experience.
- Good knowledge of how to change angiographic views as one negotiates the wire down the vessel is important, for instance switching from an LAO caudal view to enter the ostium of the LAD to an RAO cranial view to enable passage of the guide wire into the distal LAD safely.

Technical Tips and Tricks

- In very tortuous coronary anatomy often the use of a microcatheter will reduce frictional forces on the wire and enable better torquability to gain the distal vessel. This can also be achieved with the balloon catheter.
- Use of a stiffer wire and a double angulation on the wire tip can often help negotiate around tortuous vessels and prevent prolapse into adjacent vessels.
- When crossing a freshly deployed stent, migration of the wire behind a stent strut can be prevented by creation of a large tip bend, which will facilitate the formulation of a loop through the stented segment.
- Enhanced support for lesion penetration with a guide wire can be achieved through deeper guide penetration. Use of guide extension catheters or an anchor balloon in an appropriate side branch will also enhance backup support to enable wires to cross tougher lesions such as in CTO-PCI.

Conclusion

- Selection of the appropriate guide catheter and angioplasty guide wire for a PCI pro-

cedure requires assessment of the vessel and lesion to be approached and a good level of understanding of the capabilities of the range of catheters and wires available.

- For most PCI procedures acquiring the skills to manipulate the guide catheter for improved support is an important part of the learning curve.
- Furthermore it is advised that trainees gain a good knowledge of the classification of guide wires and, through undertaking PCI, learn their handling characteristics and strengths.
- It is best to gain experience with a few popular wires. For more complex PCI appropriate skill sets have to be obtained to enable operators to safely use more aggressive guide support and wiring techniques.

References

1. Paradis J-M, Rinfret S. Guide catheter selection, manipulation, and support augmentation for PCI. In: Textbook of cardiovascular intervention. London: Springer; 2014. https://doi.org/10.1007/978-1-4471-4528-8_7.
2. Von Sohsten R, Oz R, Marone G, McCormick DJ. Deep intubation of 6 French guiding catheters for transradial coronary interventions. J Invasive Cardiol. 1998;10(4):198–202.
3. From AM, Gulati R, Prasad A, Rihal CS. Sheathless transradial intervention using standard guide catheters. Catheter Cardiovasc Interv. 2010;76(7):911–6.
4. Hirokami M, Saito S, Muto H. Anchoring technique to improve guiding catheter support in coronary angioplasty of chronic total occlusions. Catheter Cardiovasc Interv. 2006;67(3):366–71.
5. Toth GG, Yamane M, Heyndrickx GR. How to select a guidewire: technical features and key characteristics. Heart. 2015;101(8):645–52. https://doi.org/10.1136/heartjnl-2013-304243.
6. Rigattieri S, Hamon M, Grollier G. The buddy wire technique is useful in transradial coronary stenting of complex, calcified lesions: report of three cases. J Invasive Cardiol. 2005;17(7):376–7.
7. Britakis ES, Grantham JA, Thompson C, et al. A percutaneous treatment algorithm for crossing coronary chronic total occlusions. J Am Coll Cardiol Intv. 2012;5(4):367–79. https://doi.org/10.1016/j.jcin.2012.02.006.

Balloon Technology

George A. Stouffer

About Us UNC Health Care is a not-for-profit medical system owned by the State of North Carolina and based in Chapel Hill, North Carolina, at the University of North Carolina. It provides services to tens of thousands of patients each year from all over North Carolina. UNC Health Care consists of UNC Medical Center in Chapel Hill, Rex Healthcare in Raleigh, Chatham Hospital in Siler City, High Point Regional Health, Caldwell Memorial Hospital, Johnston Health, Pardee Hospital, Nash Health Care, Hillsborough Hospital, Wayne Memorial Hospital, and UNC Lenoir Health Care. UNC is the 11th largest research university in the United States and the School of Medicine is in the top 10 in number of grants received. McAllister Heart Institute is the home of cardiovascular research at UNC and includes >70 investigators.

History

Charles Dotter MD is generally credited with performing the first percutaneous transluminal angioplasty. On January 16, 1964, Dr. Dotter was a vascular radiologist at the University of Oregon and used multiple catheters of increasing diame-

G. A. Stouffer
University of North Carolina Hospitals Heart and Vascular Centre, Chapel Hill, NC, USA
e-mail: rick_stouffer@med.unc.edu

ter to open a superficial femoral artery stenosis in an 82-year-old woman with critical limb ischemia. The procedure was successful and she was able to live independently for the remaining two and a half years of her life.

The use of a balloon to perform angioplasty was pioneered by Andreas Gruentzig MD. He performed the first balloon angioplasty procedure in a femoral artery in 1974 at the University Hospital in Zurich, Switzerland. He subsequently performed the first coronary artery balloon angioplasty in September 1977. Using a balloon catheter that he made in his kitchen, he successfully opened a severe stenosis in the proximal left anterior descending coronary artery in a 38-year-old man.

Evolution of Balloon Technology

- The first angioplasty balloons were made from polyvinyl chloride (PVC) and were thicker and burst at lower pressures than balloons available today.
- The next generation of balloons were made from a polymer known as cross-linked polyethylene (PE) followed by the use of polyethylene terephthalate (PET) to develop high-pressure balloons.
- Nylon balloons were developed in the late 1980s as a compromise between the strength of PET and the flexibility of PE. Polyurethane

© Springer International Publishing AG, part of Springer Nature 2018
A. Myat et al. (eds.), *The Interventional Cardiology Training Manual*,
https://doi.org/10.1007/978-3-319-71635-0_10

balloons were developed in the 1990s. Key requirements of angioplasty balloons are radial strength and flexibility and today most interventional balloons are made from either PE, PET, polyolefin copolymer, or nylon.

- Nylon balloons are softer and more flexible than PET balloons but the strength of PET enables ultrathin-walled balloons, ranging from 5 to 50 μm (0.0002" to 0.002"), with extremely low profiles.
- Several different delivery techniques for balloon catheter designs have been used over the years. The first balloons were on a fixed wire catheter in which the balloon and wire were linked. This system was stiff and made it difficult to access distal or tortuous parts of the coronary anatomy.
- Next, over-the-wire balloon catheters were developed which enabled the balloon to be tracked over a thin (0.014 in. in diameter), steerable coronary guide wire, which was placed through the lesion and into the distal portion of a coronary artery.
- Over-the-wire balloon catheters have two lumens that extend throughout the length of the catheter, one for the wire and the other to inflate the balloon.
- More recently, rapid-exchange (monorail) catheters have been developed in which the guide wire lumen extends only a relatively short distance from the tip of the balloon.
- These catheters facilitate balloon exchanges, enable a single operator to perform exchanges, and thus improve the efficiency of the procedure.
- In order to enhance visibility during balloon placement in the artery, the vast majority of balloons have radio-opaque markers on the edges while smaller balloons (≤1.5 mm) may have a single marker in the middle of the balloon.
- Balloon technology is not evolving as rapidly as in the past but ongoing efforts aim at:
  - Increasing balloon flexibility to facilitate advancement through tortuous vascular segments
  - Increasing shaft stiffness to facilitate advancement through tightly stenotic areas
  - Improving the transition at the balloon catheter tip to allow access to complete or subtotal occlusions
  - Decreasing the diameter of the uninflated balloon to facilitate advancement through tightly stenotic areas
  - Increasing rated burst pressure to facilitate stent deployment and minimizing longitudinal and radial growth

Technique of Balloon Use and Important Balloon Catheter Parameters

- The balloon is tightly wrapped around a catheter shaft to minimize its profile.
- The angioplasty guide wire is advanced into the coronary artery, and passed through the stenosis and into the distal vessel (Fig. 10.1).
- The balloon is inserted over the wire into the narrowed section of the artery under fluoroscopic guidance.
- Position is confirmed, generally using fluoroscopy and contrast dye, and then the balloon is inflated, typically with a radiopaque solution of a 50/50 mixture of contrast and saline.
- A balloon inflation device (indeflator) is used to inflate the balloon, which allows delivery of a controlled amount of pressure.
- A pressure gauge mounted on the indeflator allows the operator to carefully control the pressure inside the balloon, usually at a range of 2–20 atmosphere (ATM).
- After inflation, a negative pressure is applied on the indeflator to create a vacuum, which removes the contrast/saline mixture and minimizes the profile of the balloon prior to retraction.
- Most balloon catheters currently in use to dilate atherosclerotic arteries utilize thin-walled, high-pressure, low-elasticity balloons, which are designed to apply a predictable amount of radial force with minimal elongation.
- They are designed to have consistent performance characteristics (diameter vs. pressure) during at least 20 inflation-deflation cycles and to burst at a rate of less than 1 in 1000 balloons.
- Radial stress of a balloon can be calculated from the following formula:
  - Radial stress = (pressure × diameter) divided by (2 × thickness)

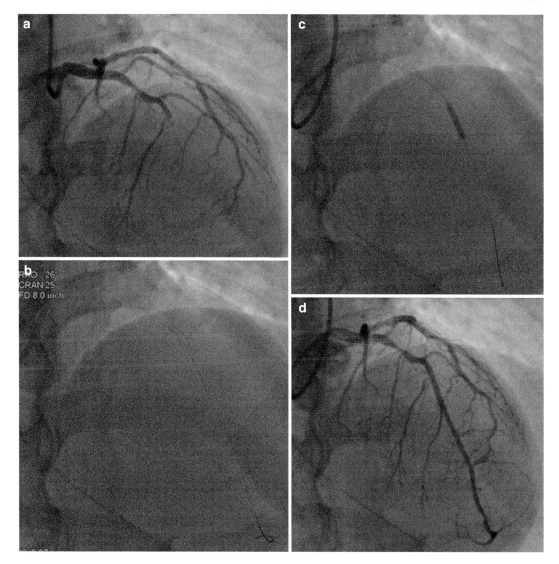

Fig. 10.1 Images from a 58-year-old male with anterior STEMI. Angiographic images showing mid-LAD occlusion (**a**), passage of angioplasty guide wire through the occlusion and into the distal LAD (**b**), inflation of 2.5 mm × 12 mm balloon at the site of occlusion (**c**), and final angiogram after stent deployment (**d**)

Glossary of Terms

- **Balloon diameter**: Inflated balloon diameter measured at a specified (nominal) pressure (Fig. 10.2).
- **Balloon length**: Working length of the balloon (generally the distance between the radio-opaque markers).
- **Balloon pressures**: Rated pressures for angioplasty balloons are typically in the range of

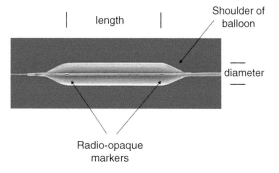

Fig. 10.2 Schematic of angioplasty balloon

2–20 ATM (32 to 320 psi) depending on the size and the material.

- **Nominal pressure**: The amount of pressure needed to inflate a balloon to the nominal diameter (diameter on the label).
- **Burst pressure**: Average pressure required to rupture a balloon, usually measured at body temperature.
- **Rated burst pressure (RBP)**: The pressure at which 99.9% of balloons will not rupture with 95% confidence.
- **Balloon crossing profile**: Maximum diameter of the balloon when mounted on a catheter in its deflated and wrapped condition or the smallest hole which the uninflated balloon catheter can pass through.
- **Balloon compliance**: Change in balloon diameter as a function of inflation pressure. A noncompliant high-pressure balloon might expand only 5–10% when inflated to the rated burst pressure while a compliant balloon might stretch 18–30%.
- **Shaft length**: The length of the shaft on which the balloon is mounted. Must be long enough to deliver the balloon to the narrowed area from the point of entry into the arterial system.

Types of Balloon Catheters for Vascular Interventions

- **Compliant balloons**: Larger change in diameter with increasing pressures (>10%). Balloons grow in areas of least resistance as pressure is increased and thus may overexpand in areas of relatively normal vessel including proximal and distal to the lesion (i.e., "dogboning"). More flexible and higher rates of crossing success compared to stiffer balloons.
- **Semi-compliant balloons**: Compliance (8–10% growth) is intermediate between compliant and noncompliant balloons. Frequently used for pre-dilation of an atherosclerotic lesion. These balloons generally have a nominal pressure of 6–8 ATM, with RBP of 12–14 ATM.
- **Noncompliant balloons**: Little change in volume with incremental increases in pressure (~4–6% growth within the working range when inflated). More force is exerted against a lesion at a given inflation pressure than semi-compliant balloons, including stent delivery balloons. Usually made with PET. Frequently used for stent post-dilation. These balloons generally have a nominal pressure of 10–12 ATM, with RBP of 18–20 ATM.
- **Super high-pressure noncompliant balloon**: The OPN super high-pressure balloon (SIS Medical, Frauenfeld, Switzerland) is a twin-layer noncompliant balloon with an RBP of 35 atmospheres used to dilate stents or lesions where 20 atmospheres proves to be insufficient. It can be used in highly calcified or undilatable lesions, in-stent restenosis (ISR), and combination with rotablation. It has also been used for pre- and postdilation in combination with bioresorbable vascular scaffolds (BVS). Note that all balloon lengths for the OPN are measured between the inside edge of each platinum marker (Fig. 10.3).

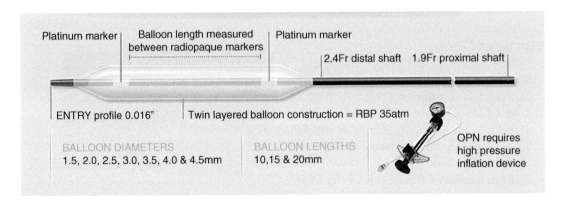

Fig. 10.3 OPN super-high-pressure balloon. This balloon has a twin-layer technology with ultralow compliance. Reproduced with permission from Vascular Perspectives

- **Stent delivery balloons**: Mostly semi-compliant or noncompliant balloons.
- **Drug-eluting balloons**: These balloons deliver an anti-restenotic agent, primarily paclitaxel, to the site of balloon angioplasty. Methodologies to load the drug on the balloon surface include spraying, dipping, and/or use of nanoparticles. The rate of release of the drug into the vessel wall during inflation, and retention of the drug within the vascular wall for sufficient time to inhibit the restenotic process, is crucial. The strong lipophilic nature of paclitaxel enables longer retention in the vessel wall. These are conventional semi-compliant balloons, usually inflated at nominal pressures, with a specific minimal inflation time.
- **Cutting balloon**: The Cutting Balloon (Boston Scientific Corporation, Natick, MA, USA) was first developed in the mid-1980s and is composed of a conventional balloon catheter with 3–4 atherotomes (razor blades) attached to the surface. The Cutting Balloon is primarily used for focal calcified lesions, ostial lesions, and ISR (Fig. 10.4).

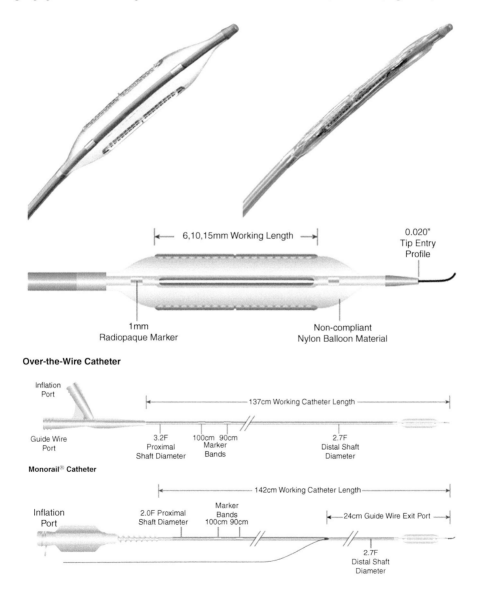

Fig. 10.4 The Flextome™ Cutting Balloon dilatation device. Reproduced with permission from Boston Scientific

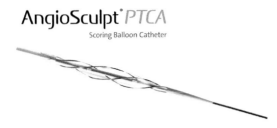

AngioSculpt *PTCA*

Scoring Balloon Catheter

Fig. 10.5 The AngioSculpt scoring balloon catheter. Reproduced with permission from Spectranetics

- **Scoring balloon**: The AngioSculpt Scoring Balloon Catheter (Spectranetics, Colorado Springs, CO, USA) was developed in 2003 and features a nitinol mesh (scoring element) encircling a semi-compliant balloon (Fig. 10.5).

Use of Balloons

Dilation of an Atherosclerotic Plaque

- Balloon angioplasty is frequently used to pre-dilate a coronary lesion prior to stent implantation and occasionally used as a stand-alone therapy (known as plain old balloon angioplasty, POBA).
- Typical sizes of balloons for coronary angioplasty range in size from 1.5 to 4.5 mm in diameter. Larger balloons are used for peripheral vascular percutaneous transluminal angioplasty (PTA), with sizes ranging from 4 to 12 mm in diameter.
- Mechanisms responsible for lumen enlargement after balloon angioplasty of an atheromatous plaque include plaque fracturing and compression and overstretching of the vessel wall with partial disruption of the intimal plaque, media, and adventitia.
- These result in enlargement of the outer diameter of the vessel and axial redistribution of plaque material. Both balloon angioplasty and stent implantation elicit a number of changes in the vessel wall including adherence of platelets and fibrin to the site within minutes of vessel injury.
- Within hours to days, inflammatory cells infiltrate the site, and vascular smooth muscle cells migrate from the media to the intima. The vascular smooth muscle cells proliferate and produce extracellular matrix. Over a period of weeks, endothelial cells colonize the surface of the lumen and regain their normal function.
- The vessel then begins to "remodel" over a period of weeks to months which can result in either a decrease in lumen diameter (negative remodeling) or an increase in lumen diameter (positive remodeling). The amount of late loss in lumen diameter is dependent on the amount of neointimal proliferation and extracellular matrix production and the degree of remodeling. After 6 months, the repair process stabilizes and the risk of restenosis decreases significantly.

Drug Delivery

- Balloons can be coated with medications, which enables localized delivery. The primary use is at the time of angioplasty to reduce the risk of restenosis. Transfer of the drug from the surface of the balloon to the artery wall occurs when the balloon is inflated.
- In contrast to drug-eluting stents in which the drug is present for weeks on the surface of the stent, drug-coated balloons rely on the rapid transfer of a medication into the artery wall with the expectation of a durable biological effect.
- Most of the drug-coated balloons use paclitaxel, which is characterized by prolonged tissue retention rates. Studies have shown that a short exposure to the drug results in structural modification of the smooth muscle cell cytoskeleton for at least 14 days.
- Theoretical advantages of drug-coated balloons in comparison to DES include the following:
  - There is no metallic implant and no residual polymer.
  - Greater drug delivery per square millimeter of balloon surface compared with DES, which may translate to greater therapeutic efficacy.

– Can be used in areas where DES are difficult to deploy such as bifurcation lesions or
ostial lesions.

• Other, less frequently used methods to locally
deliver medications include infusion catheters, infusion balloons, or isolation of the
treated area by inflation of balloons proximal
and distal to the lesion. This interrupts blood
flow and enables distillation of a medication
between the two balloons. Infusion balloons
are made from PET balloon with the formation of thousands of micropores in sizes ranging from submicron to a few microns in
diameter.

Stent Delivery

• Balloons are commonly used to deploy intravascular stents. The stent is crimped on the
balloon, which enables passage into the stenotic artery. Inflation of the balloon expands
the stent and forces it into the arterial wall.

Post-stent Dilation

• Stents are frequently under-expanded when
deployed using the stent delivery system.
• The use of high-pressure, noncompliant balloons has been shown to enhance stent expansion, especially in fibrotic and calcified
lesions.
• Kissing balloons (simultaneous inflation of
two balloons) are frequently used when placing stents into both branches of a bifurcation
(Fig. 10.6).

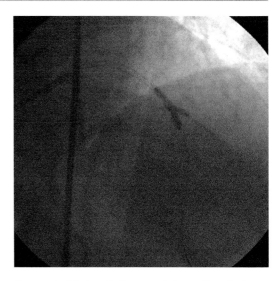

Fig. 10.6 Kissing balloon technique. Two balloons,
which are simultaneously inflated in the LAD and diagonal, are shown

Balloons for Nonvascular Uses

• Balloons are frequently used in cardiovascular
disease states for indications unrelated to the
vasculature.
• Valvuloplasty is a procedure in which a balloon is used to dilate a stenotic valve (primarily pulmonic, mitral, or aortic) (Fig. 10.7).
Balloons are also used to deploy aortic valve
and pulmonic valve stents.
• Low-pressure balloons are also used to size
atrial septal defects. Sizing balloons are low-
pressure, elastomeric balloon typically made
of latex or silicone.

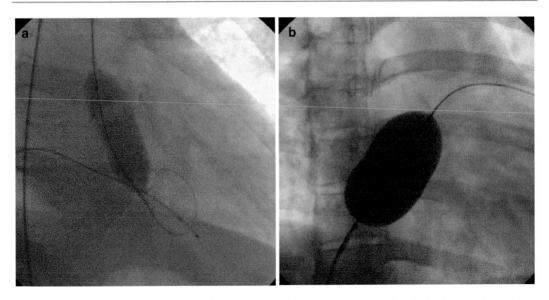

Fig. 10.7 Nonvascular uses of balloons. Balloons can be used for valvuloplasty (aortic valvuloplasty) in (**a**) and atrial septal defect (ASD) sizing (**b**) for percutaneous closure

Stent Technology

11

Raffaele Piccolo and Stephan Windecker

About Us The Department of Cardiology at the Swiss Cardiovascular Center Bern is a tertiary care facility in the setting of one of the five university hospitals in Switzerland. The catchment area is approximately one million people in the canton of Bern and surrounding cantons.

The Department of Cardiology has divisions of invasive cardiology, electrophysiology, heart failure including heart transplantation and assist devices, pediatric and grown-up congenital heart disease, cardiac imaging, preventive cardiology, and arterial hypertension.

On an annual basis, more than 5000 cardiac catheterization procedures, 2500 PCIs, 300 TAVI, and 75 MitraClip procedures are performed.

Our clinical research topics of interest include:

1. Intracoronary imaging for atherosclerosis and lipid-lowering therapy
2. Intracoronary devices—stents and scaffolds
3. Transcatheter aortic, mitral, and tricuspid devices for treatment of valvular heart disease
4. Antithrombotic therapy

Brief History of Stent Evolution

- In 2017, percutaneous coronary intervention (PCI) entered its 40th anniversary since the first balloon angioplasty performed by Andreas Grüntzig in 1977. Since then, the safety and efficacy of the procedure have continuously improved and PCI currently represents the preferred myocardial revascularization modality, owing to its life-saving features, among patients with acute coronary syndromes (ACS) and rivalling outcomes compared with coronary artery bypass grafting (CABG) among patients with multivessel and left main disease.
- Coronary stents have remarkably improved the safety profile of PCI by reducing the risk of acute closure related to coronary dissection [1] and the need for emergent CABG [2].
- The word "stent" was coined in 1916 by Jan F. Esser, a Dutch plastic surgeon, and referred to a dental impression compound developed formerly by Charles Thomas Stent.
- The first vascular stent was developed and implanted in 1968 by Charles Dotter in a canine popliteal artery [3]. The application to the coronary vasculature derived from discussions between two Swedish expatriates Hans Wallsten, an engineer, and Ake Senning, the chief cardiac surgeon, collaborating with Andreas Grüntzig during the first coronary angioplasty procedures in Zurich.

R. Piccolo · S. Windecker (✉)
Department of Cardiology, Bern University Hospital, University of Bern, Bern, Switzerland
e-mail: raffaele.piccolo@insel.ch; Stephan.Windecker@insel.ch

© Springer International Publishing AG, part of Springer Nature 2018
A. Myat et al. (eds.), *The Interventional Cardiology Training Manual*,
https://doi.org/10.1007/978-3-319-71635-0_11

- The first coronary stent (Wallstent) was self-expanding and developed by Medinvent in cooperation with Ulrich Sigwart. It was implanted for the first time in March 1986 by Jacques Puel (Toulouse, France) in a 63-year-old male suffering from restenosis after balloon angioplasty of the left anterior descending artery.
- The first bailout stenting was performed by Ulrich Sigwart during a live course (Lausanne, Switzerland) in June 1986 in a 50-year-old female suffering from occlusive dissection of the left anterior descending artery after balloon angioplasty.
- Shortly after these successful procedures, an unanticipated bane of stent implantation emerged: stent thrombosis. To limit this serious complication, aggressive anticoagulant regimens and dedicated implantation strategies were introduced.
- In June 1993, the US Food and Drug Administration (FDA) approved the first coronary stent, the Gianturco-Roubin stent, which was a balloon-expandable and coil-type stent, manufactured from a single strand of stainless steel wire [4].
- In August 1994, the FDA approved another coronary stent, the Palmaz-Schatz stent, which represented the first tubular slotted balloon-expandable stent. At that time, the stents were crimped on the coronary angioplasty balloon by the interventional cardiologists, a method that was prone to stent loss.
- The widespread acceptance of coronary artery stenting emerged after the results of the Belgian Netherlands STENT (BENESTENT) [5] and the Stent Restenosis Study (STRESS) [6] trials, which showed superiority of coronary stents compared with balloon angioplasty in reducing the risk of restenosis and the need for repeat revascularization.
- Since then, tremendous progress has been made in improving stent material, design, and processing, resulting in superior deliverability and procedural success.
- The improved results with coronary artery stenting over time were also related to expansion of the indications for stent implantation

and insight that dual-antiplatelet therapy (instead of oral anticoagulation) lowered both the incidence of stent thrombosis and hemorrhagic complications.
- On the basis of their efficacy, coronary artery stents have emerged as the preferred tool for PCI and are currently deployed in more than 90% of procedures [7].

Drug-Eluting Stents

- Drug-eluting stents (DES) were introduced into clinical practice more than 10 years ago. DES deliver site-specific, controlled release of therapeutic agents.
- Initially, heparin had been used as a stent coating in an attempt to reduce the thrombogenic potential and risk of acute/subacute stent thrombosis but its use has then been abandoned due to futility [8].
- Sirolimus-eluting stents (SES) were first implanted in 2001 and subsequently became the first DES that significantly reduced the risk of restenosis inherent to bare-metal stents (BMS).
- This was followed by paclitaxel-eluting stents (PES), which also consistently reduced the rate of restenosis and the need for repeat revascularization procedures compared with BMS.
- Both of these early-generation stents are no longer used in clinical practice and have been superseded by new-generation DES featuring lower drug loads, thinner stent struts, and more biocompatible or biodegradable polymers that have been shown to considerably improve the safety profile of DES (Fig. 11.1).
- Currently available DES are characterized by three principal components that can be modified separately (Fig. 11.2) [9]:
  - The drug: an antiproliferative agent that inhibits neointimal hyperplasia.
  - The platform: metallic stents or fully bioresorbable scaffolds.
  - The polymer: a permanent (durable) or biodegradable polymer that represents the vehicle for drug delivery and can be

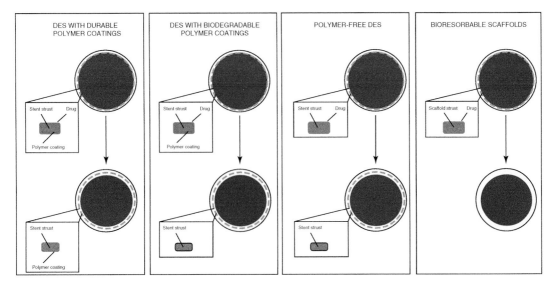

Fig. 11.1 Schematic representation of coronary stent technologies. From left to right: drug-eluting stents (DES) with durable polymer coatings, DES with biodegradable polymer coatings, polymer-free DES, and bioresorbable scaffolds. The top panels summarize the features of the coronary cross section and stent cross sections at the time of implantation, whereas the bottom panel shows the same features after the completion of drug release. In the coronary cross section, the vessel lumen is displayed in red, the intima in yellow, and the stent struts in grey. Reproduced with permission from Stefanini GG et al. Heart 2014;100:1051–1061

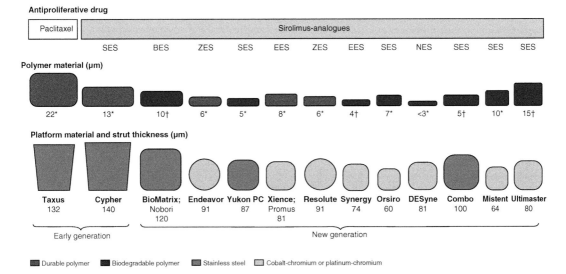

Fig. 11.2 Type and composition of available metallic drug-eluting stents. Taxus and Cypher represent early-generation DES. All other devices are regarded as new-generation DES, which were developed featuring thinner stent struts, more biocompatible or biodegradable polymers, and different antiproliferative drugs to Taxus and Cypher. Boston Scientific (Marlborough, MA, USA) makes Taxus, Promus, and Synergy. Cordis (East Bridgewater, NJ, USA) makes Cypher. Biosensors International Ltd. (Jalan Tukang, Singapore) makes BioMatrix. Terumo (Tokyo, Japan) makes Nobori and Ultimaster. Medtronic (Minneapolis, MN, USA) makes Endeavor and Resolute. Translumina (Hechingen, Germany) makes Yukon PC. Abbott Vascular (Santa Clara, CA, USA) makes Xience. Biotronik (Berlin, Germany) makes Orsiro. Elixir Medical Corporation (Sunnyvale, CA, USA) makes DESyne. Orbus Neich (Hong Kong, China) makes Combo. Micell Technologies (Durham NC, USA) makes MiStent. Key: *SES* sirolimus-eluting stent, *BES* biolimus-eluting stent, *ZES* zotarolimus-eluting stent, *EES* everolimus-eluting stent. *Circumferential coating. †Abluminal coating. Reproduced with permission from Piccolo R. et al. Lancet. 2015;386:702–713

modulated to alter the kinetic of drug release. Polymer might also be absent and more recently polymer-free DES have also been developed and tested in clinical trials.

Antiproliferative Drugs

- The role of the antiproliferative drug is to limit neointimal hyperplasia and restenosis and the ideal agent should feature the following properties:
  - Wide therapeutic window
  - Low inflammatory potential
  - Selectivity for smooth muscle cell proliferation without toxicity to the medial and adventitial cell layers
  - Promotion of re-endothelialization
- The efficacy of candidate drugs is not only dependent on biological activity in vitro but also determined by local pharmacokinetics and physicochemical drug properties.
- Drug distribution is mediated by stent strut configuration and balance between convective and diffusive forces [10].
- Hydrophilic drugs such as heparin readily permeate into tissue but are also rapidly cleared. In contrast, lipophilic agents such as paclitaxel or limus analogues are water insoluble and bind to hydrophobic sites in the arterial wall.
- Although both hydrophilic and hydrophobic drugs show large spatial concentration gradients in the arterial wall, lipophilic agents distribute better and more homogenously into the arterial wall than hydrophilic drugs.
- To date, immunosuppressive (*limus family*) and antiproliferative (paclitaxel) drugs are used, with analogues of the *limus family* representing the preferred agents in new-generation DES.

Limus Analogues
- Antiproliferative agents of the *limus family* bind to the intracellular receptor FKBP-12 (FK506-binding protein, molecular mass 12 kDa), a ubiquitously expressed and well-preserved protein throughout eukaryotic phy-

logeny, and include (1) sirolimus, (2) everolimus, (3) zotarolimus, (4) biolimus, (5) novolimus, (6) myolimus, (7) pimecrolimus, and (8) tacrolimus [11].
- The first six agents—sirolimus, everolimus, zotarolimus, biolimus-A9, novolimus, and myolimus—affect cell cycle regulation by inhibiting a phosphoinositide 3-kinase termed mammalian target of rapamycin (mTOR).
- In contrast, tacrolimus and pimecrolimus (FK506)-FKBP12 complex inhibit the phosphatase calcineurin and have no antiproliferative or antimigratory effects on vascular smooth muscle cells.
- The inhibition of calcineurin by the FK506-FKBP12 complex as well as the cyclophilin-cyclosporin A complex prevents the activation of T-lymphocytes by inhibiting the transcription of cytokines such as interleukin-2.
- Vascular smooth muscle cells usually remain in the G_0 phase of the cell cycle and proliferate at low indices (<0.05%), unless stimulated by vascular injury, when they may reenter the cell cycle at the G_1 phase and advance to the S phase.
- The cell cycle is regulated by the interaction between cyclins, cyclin-dependent kinases (CDKs), and cyclin-dependent kinase inhibitors (CDKIs) within the cell nucleus.
- Antiproliferative -limus drug analogues arrest the cell cycle at the transition from the G_1 phase to the S phase by preventing the downregulation of the CDKp27^{kip1} and phosphorylation of the protein product of the retinoblastoma gene (pRB).
- The CDKI p27^{kip1}, the essential CDKI for the mechanism of action of -limus analogues, prevents CDK activation and retinoblastoma protein (pRB) phosphorylation by inhibiting the serine/threonine kinase p70S6, and hence arrests the cell cycle at the transition from the G_1 phase to the S phase. As a result it exerts cytostatic rather than cytotoxic effects.
- Levels of CDKI p27^{kip1} are high in quiescent cells and may be downregulated by mitogenic stimuli [12]. Inactivation of pRb, another regulator of cell cycle progression, by

phosphorylation leads to progression of the cell cycle from the G_1 to S phase.

- Upregulation of FKBP-12, the intracellular binding protein for sirolimus, was demonstrated in neointimal tissue from patients with in-stent restenosis, and provides a rationale for the use of these compounds in the prevention of neointimal hyperplasia [13].
- The following antiproliferative agents are the most commonly used in currently available DES:
  - Sirolimus was first isolated from bacteria discovered on Easter Island and derived its historical name rapamycin from the indigenous name of the Island (Rapa Nui). The highly lipophilic macrocyclic lactone ($C_{56}H_{89}NO_{14}$, molecular weight 914 Da) was the first antiproliferative agent to be used with DES and is characterized by rapid absorption ($t_{max} < 2$ h), low systemic bioavailability (15%), and high intra- and intersubject variability in oral dose clearance.
  - Everolimus is a sirolimus derivative in which the hydroxyl group at position C40 of sirolimus has been alkylated with a 2-hydroxyethyl group. It is slightly more lipophilic than sirolimus and more rapidly absorbed into the arterial wall. Although binding of everolimus to the FKBP-12 domain is threefold and immunosuppressive activity in vitro two- to fivefold lower than with sirolimus, oral everolimus proved at least as potent as sirolimus in models of autoimmune disease and heart transplantation.
  - Zotarolimus is another sirolimus analogue in which the C40 position is modified by a tetrazole ring resulting in a shorter circulating half-life of the drug. Although the binding affinity to the FKBP 12 domain for zotarolimus and sirolimus is similar and the antiproliferative activities of zotarolimus are also comparable to those of sirolimus, the immunosuppressive activity in vivo is three- to fourfold lower.
  - Biolimus-A9 ($CH_{55}H_{87}NO_{14}$, molecular weight 986 Da) is another sirolimus deriva-

tive characterized by a high lipophilicity, resulting from modification of the hydroxylate position C40 of sirolimus by an ethoxyethyl group. The rationale for the ethoxyethyl group was to increase lipophilicity and, in turn, uptake by the coronary vessel.

Non-limus Analogues

- Paclitaxel stabilizes polymerized microtubules and enhances microtubule assembly, forming numerous unorganized and decentralized microtubules inside the cytoplasm. As a result, cell replication is inhibited and this effect is seen predominantly in the G_0/G_1 and G_2/M phases of the cell cycle. Paclitaxel was shown to effectively inhibit vascular smooth muscle cell migration and proliferation.
- Currently paclitaxel is mainly used as an antiproliferative agent in drug-eluting balloons in view of its lower efficacy compared with limus agents when used for coronary stents.

Metallic DES Composition (See Table 11.1)

- Stainless steel (316L) has been the most frequently used alloy for coronary stents in the past due to its excellent processing characteristics, sufficient radial force, and low elastic recoil (<5%).
- As a stent material, stainless steel has limitations, including limited radio-opacity, reduced flexibility, and a relatively high nickel content, which have been linked to an increased risk of restenosis due to allergic reactions [14].
- Cobalt-chrome (L605 CoCr) alloys have emerged more recently as an alternative and constitute the most frequently used stent material today. L605 CoCr is stronger and more radio-opaque and contains less nickel than 316L stainless steel.
- L605 CoCr stents have greater radiographic visibility, and thinner struts (with no compromise to radial strength), thereby providing improved deliverability compared with 316L stainless steel stents. Historical data from

Table 11.1 Specifications of the FDA-approved metallic drug-eluting stents

Stent	Drug (concentration)	Drug mechanism	Polymer	Polymer thickness (μm)	Release kinetics (days)	Metal	Geometry	Strut thickness (μm)
CYPHER	Sirolimus (140 μg/cm²)	Inhibits mTOR Cytostatic	Polyethylene co-vinyl acetate and PBMA	12.6	80% (28)	SS	Closed cell	140
TAXUS Express	Paclitaxel (100 μg/cm²)	Microtubule inhibitor Cell cycle arrest in G0/G1 and G2/M	Poly(styrene-b-isobutylene-b-styrene)	16	<10% (28)	SS	Open cell	132
TAXUS Liberté	Paclitaxel (100 μg/cm²)	Microtubule inhibitor Cell cycle arrest in G0/G1 and G2/M	Poly(styrene-b-isobutylene-b-styrene)	16	<10% (28)	SS	Hybrid	97
TAXUS Element	Paclitaxel (100 μg/cm²)	Microtubule inhibitor Cell cycle arrest in G0/G1 and G2/M	Poly(styrene-b-isobutylene-b-styrene)	15	<10% (90)	PtCr	Open cell	81
Endeavor ZES	Zotarolimus (100 μg/cm²)	Inhibits mTOR Cytostatic	Phosphorylcholine	4.1	95% (14)	CoCr	Open cell	91
Resolute ZES	Zotarolimus (10 μg/mm)	Inhibits mTOR Cytostatic	Biolinx	4.1	85% (60)	CoCr	Open cell	91
Xience EES	Everolimus (100 μg/cm²)	Inhibits mTOR Cytostatic	PBMA and PVDF-HFP	7	80% (90)	CoCr	Open cell	81
Promus EES	Everolimus (100 μg/cm²)	Inhibits mTOR Cytostatic	PBMA and PVDF-HFP	7	80% (90)	PtCr	Open cell	81

CoCr cobalt-chromium, *mTOR* mechanistic target of rapamycin, *PBMA* poly(butyl methacrylate), *PtCr* platinum-chromium, *PVDF:HFP* poly(vinylidene fluoride-co-hexafluoropropylene), *SS* stainless steel

stainless steel stents suggest that a reduction in strut thickness may be associated with lower rates of restenosis and repeat revascularization [15, 16]. However, assessment of neointimal hyperplasia by late lumen loss reveals no superiority of cobalt-chrome stents.

- Experimental data suggests that strut thickness is positively correlated with the propensity for thrombus formation and may therefore impact the risk of stent thrombosis [17].
- More recently, platinum alloys were introduced, offering several distinct advantages over conventional stent materials. Platinum is two times denser than iron or cobalt, malleable, corrosion resistant, fracture resistant, and fully incorporated into the platinum-chromium alloy.
- Consequently, the platinum-chromium stent offers the advantage of increased radio-opacity and thinner stent struts. Importantly, initial benchmark studies indicated that, despite these thinner struts, the platinum-chromium alloy stent had better radial strength, lower acute recoil, and better vessel conformability compared to conventional stent platforms. Moreover, the nickel content is reduced when compared with 316L stainless steel, thus reducing the risk of allergic reactions. Notwithstanding, this alloy is only present in a few available platforms.

Durable Polymer DES

Early-Generation DES

- The Cypher sirolimus-eluting stent (SES) (Cordis Corporation, Warren, NJ, USA) was the first DES to receive FDA approval in 2003. It consisted of sirolimus in a concentration of 140 $\mu g/cm^2$ incorporated in an amalgam of two biostable polymers, with the polymer/drug matrix then applied onto the tubular 316L stainless steel BX Velocity stent.
- The Cypher SES proved effective in suppressing neointimal proliferation, resulting in a relevant decrease in the risk of restenosis and need for repeat revascularization compared with BMS.

- However, long-term follow-up studies demonstrated some catchup in terms of late restenosis, and, more importantly, a significant increase in the risk of very late stent thrombosis, particularly in more complex lesion and patient subsets.
- The TAXUS paclitaxel-eluting stent (Boston Scientific, Natick, MA, USA) was the second DES to receive the FDA approval in 2003. Although more effective than BMS, direct and indirect comparisons showed a lower efficacy profile of paclitaxel-eluting stents compared with the Cypher SES.
- Similarly to the Cypher SES, the use of paclitaxel-eluting stents was associated with a higher risk of very late stent thrombosis compared with BMS.

New-Generation DES

- New-generation DES commonly feature limus analogues, thinner stent struts, and lower drug loads compared with earlier devices.
- The Xience EES (Xience V or Xience Prime or Xience Xpedition: Abbott Vascular, Santa Clara, CA, USA) has a strut thickness of 81 μm, and is coated with a 7.6 μm thick, durable, copolymer of polyvinylidene fluoride-co-hexafluoropropylene (PVDF-HFP), and poly n-butyl methacrylate (PBMA), which facilitates elution of everolimus over 120 days. The EES is loaded with 1 $\mu g/mm^2$ of everolimus.
- So far, the Xience EES represents the new-generation DES that has been most frequently investigated in randomized clinical trials and has been used as the control arm in numerous non-inferiority trials investigating newer generation DES.
- In a meta-analysis of 5 randomized trials including 4896 patients, the Xience EES compared with BMS was associated with a significant reduction in the risk of cardiac mortality (HR 0.67, 95% CI 0.49–0.91, $p = 0.01$), myocardial infarction (HR 0.71, 95% CI 0.55–0.92, $p = 0.01$), definite stent thrombosis (HR 0.41, 95% CI 0.22–0.76, $p = 0.005$), and target-vessel revascularization (HR 0.29, 95% CI 0.20–0.41, $p < 0.001$) at a median follow-up of 2 years [18].

- Moreover, a reduction in the risk of mortality favoring EES over BMS (HR 0.81, 95% CI 0.64–1.00), PES (HR 0.81, 95% CI 0.68–1.00), and SES (HR 0.70, 95% CI 0.70–1.00) has been reported in a network meta-analysis of 51 trials (n = 52,158) [19]. The safety profile of the Xience EES has been consistently reported in another large network meta-analysis of 113 trials with 90,584 patients showing that EES were associated with the lowest risk of stent thrombosis compared with all other stents at all times after stent implantation [20].
- The use of Xience EES among patients with ST-segment-elevation myocardial infarction has been investigated in the EXAMINATION trial. At 5-year follow-up, the study reported a significant reduction in the risk of the primary composite endpoint of all-cause death, any myocardial infarction, or any revascularization favoring EES over BMS (HR 0.80, 95% CI 0.65–0.98, p = 0.033) [21].
- A pooled analysis of SPIRIT II, III, and IV and COMPARE trials showed similar performance of the Xience EES compared with paclitaxel-eluting stents in diabetic patients [22].
- The TUXEDO trial comparing Xience EES with paclitaxel-eluting stents among 1830 diabetic patients demonstrated the superiority of the EES with a significant reduction in the risk of target-lesion failure, as well as myocardial infarction, definite stent thrombosis, and target-lesion revascularization [23].
- The Resolute zotarolimus-eluting stent (R-ZES, Medtronic, Inc., Minneapolis, MN, USA) is based on the Driver stent platform with a strut thickness of 91 μm made of cobalt-chromium alloy and releases zotarolimus with a concentration of approximately 1.6 μg/mm² stent surface area.
- The R-ZES features the BioLinx polymer consisting of three polymers: a hydrophilic C19 polymer, water-soluble polyvinylpyrrolidone (PVP), and a hydrophobic C10 polymer.
- Compared with the original Endeavor stent, the R-ZES allows for a more delayed release of the same zotarolimus concentration, with approximately 50% of the drug released during the first 7 days, and 85% of the drug released at 60 days after stent implantation.
- Five randomized trials, including a total of 9899 patients, evaluated the efficacy and safety of R-ZES compared with EES. A pooled meta-analysis of these trials at longest available follow-up reported a similar risk of target-vessel revascularization (risk ratio, RR, 1.06, 95% CI, 0.90–1.24, p = 0.50), definite or probable stent thrombosis (RR, 1.26, 95% CI, 0.86–1.85, p = 0.24), cardiac death (RR, 1.01; 95% CI, 0.79–1.30; p = 0.91), and target-vessel myocardial infarction (RR, 1.10, 95% CI, 0.89–1.36, p = 0.39). Moreover, R-ZES and EES had similar risks of late definite or probable very late stent thrombosis (RR, 1.06, 95% CI, 0.53–2.11, p = 0.87) [24].
- The PROMUS Element stent (Boston Scientific, Natick, MA, USA) has a platinum-chromium platform, a PBMA primer coating, and a PVDF-HFP polymer and is loaded with 1 μg/mm² of everolimus, 80% of which is eluted within 90 days of stent implantation.
- Three randomized studies demonstrated non-inferiority of the Promus Element EES compared with the Xience V EES (PLATINUM trial, n = 1532) and R-ZES (DUTCH PEERS, n = 1811; HOST-ASSURE, n = 3755).

Biodegradable Polymer DES

Polymer Composition

- Durable polymer coatings permanently reside on the stent surface beyond the time period of drug elution and have been identified as potential triggers of delayed arterial healing and stent strut endothelialization.
- To overcome these shortcomings, biodegradable polymers, which degrade over time, have been developed. Most biodegradable polymers used for coronary devices consist of polylactic acid isoforms or polyglycolic acid:
  - Poly-L-lactic acid (PLLA), which contains only the L-isomer

- Poly-D-lactic acid (PDLA), which contains only the D-isomer
- Poly-D,L-lactic acid (PDLLA), which contains a mixture of the L- and D-isomers
- Poly-lactic co-glycolic acid (PLGA), which contains a combination of lactic acid monomers and glycolic acid monomers

- During the degradation process, cleavage of covalent bonds between repeating units occurs and the long backbones break into smaller oligomers or monomers by means of hydrolysis. Macrophages phagocytose the resulting inert monomers (lactic acid for PLLA, PDLA, PDLLA; lactic acid and glycolic acid for PLGA), which are eventually metabolized to carbon dioxide and water through the Krebs cycle.

Clinical Data of Biodegradable Polymer DES

- Biodegradable polymer, biolimus-eluting stents (BES) include the Nobori BES (Terumo, Tokyo, Japan) and the BioMatrix BES (Biosensors, Morges, Switzerland). Both BES are made in 316L stainless steel, resulting in relatively thick struts (120 μm), and elute the drug from an abluminal matrix of biolimus and PLA (15.6 μg each 1 mm stent length in 1:1 ratio).
- In addition to the delivery system and balloon, the two BES differ in relation to the stent-coating process: the BioMatrix BES is coated by an automated autopipette proprietary technology, whereas the Nobori BES uses spray coating. Moreover, Nobori BES and previous iterations of BioMatrix BES (BioMatrix and BioMatrix II) present a nonbiodegradable base coat of parylene C (2 μm) that is used to connect the biolimus/PLA matrix to the stent surface, while the BioMatrix Flex BES does not contain parylene C.
- Recently, a further iteration in BES technology has been achieved with the BioMatrix alpha, which presents a CoCr platform instead of the stainless steel featuring all other BES.
- Three randomized trials investigated the efficacy and safety of the BioMatrix BES: the LEADERS, the COMFORTABLE-AMI, and the SORT-OUT VI trials.

- The LEADERS (n = 1707) compared the BioMatrix BES with the Cypher SES. At 5-year follow-up, there was a trend toward a reduction in the primary endpoint of cardiac death, myocardial infarction, or clinically indicated target-vessel revascularization favoring the BioMatrix BES (22.3% vs. 26.1%, p = 0.069). Moreover, there was a significant reduction in the risk of very late stent thrombosis among patients allocated to BioMatrix BES versus SES (0.7% vs. 2.5%, p = 0.003) [25].
- The COMFORTABLE-AMI trial (n = 1161) compared the BioMatrix BES versus BMS among patients with ST-segment-elevation myocardial infarction. At 5-year follow-up, the trial showed greater than 40% relative risk reduction in the primary composite endpoint of cardiac death, target-vessel myocardial infarction, or ischemia-driven target-lesion revascularization (8.6% vs. 14.9%, p = 0.001). This benefit was mainly related to the prevention of target-vessel myocardial infarction (2.2% vs. 5.0%, p = 0.02) and target-lesion revascularization (4.4% vs. 10.4%, p < 0.001) associated with BioMatrix BES implantation [26].
- The SORT-OUT VI trial (n = 2999) compared the BioMatrix BES with the R-ZES in an all-comer patient population and showed non-inferiority between the two new-generation DES at 1-year follow-up [27].
- The clinical performance of the Nobori BES has been mainly investigated in four randomized clinical trials: the SORT OUT V, the COMPARE II, the NEXT, and the SORT OUT VII trials.
- The SORT OUT V trial (n = 2468) randomly assigned all-comer patients undergoing PCI to Nobori BES or Cypher SES. At 1-year follow-up, the study demonstrated non-inferiority of the Nobori BES with regard to the primary endpoint of cardiac death, myocardial infarction, definite stent thrombosis, or target-vessel revascularization. However, definite stent thrombosis was significantly increased among patients allocated to Nobori BES versus SES (0.7% vs. 0.2%, p = 0.034). Nevertheless, at 3-year follow-up, the cumulative rate of stent

thrombosis did not differ between the two study arms (1.4% vs. 1.0%, $p = 0.45$) [28].

- The COMPARE II ($n = 2707$) and the NEXT ($n = 3235$) trials compared the Nobori BES with the Xience EES in all-comer patients undergoing PCI and both studies showed the non-inferiority of the Nobori BES at 1 year. At 3 years follow-up, there was no significant difference in the safety and efficacy between the Nobori BES and Xience EES in both studies [29, 30].

- The SORT OUT VII trial ($n = 2525$) compared the Nobori BES with the Orsiro SES (see next paragraph).

- The Orsiro SES (Biotronik AG, Bülach, Switzerland) combines a biodegradable PLLA polymer with an ultrathin strut cobalt-chromium platform (60 μm for stent diameters up to 3.0 mm, 80 μm for stent diameters >3.0 mm). Sirolimus is eluted over a period of approximately 100 days. The polymer matrix has an asymmetric design that allows for the release of a greater drug dose on the abluminal than luminal side.

- Four randomized studies have investigated the efficacy and safety of Orsiro SES: the BIOFLOW-II, the BIOSCIENCE, the SORT-OUT VII, and the BIORESORT trials.

- The BIOFLOW-II trial ($n = 452$) showed angiographic non-inferiority of Orsiro SES compared with EES in terms of in-stent late loss at 9 months (0.10 ± 0.32 vs. 0.11 ± 0.29 mm, p for non-inferiority <0.001) [31].

- The BIOSCIENCE trial ($n = 2119$) demonstrated the non-inferiority of Orsiro SES compared with Xience EES for the primary endpoint target-lesion failure at 12 months (6.5% vs. 6.6%, p for non-inferiority <0.004). There was a significant interaction for the primary endpoint favoring the use of Orsiro SES in patients with ST-segment-elevation myocardial infarction. At 2-year follow-up, the primary endpoint occurred at a comparable rate in the Orsiro SES and EES groups (10.5% vs. 10.4%, $p = 0.987$), with a sustained benefit in the subgroup of patients with acute myocardial infarction [32].

- The SORT OUT VII trial ($n = 2525$) showed the non-inferiority of Orsiro SES compared with the Nobori BES among all-comer patients undergoing PCI at 12-month follow-up (3.8% vs. 4.6%, p for non-inferiority <0.004). There was a lower rate of definite stent thrombosis among patients randomized to Orsiro SES (0.4% vs. 1.2%, $p = 0.03$).

- The BIORESORT trial ($n = 3514$) showed the non-inferiority of the Orsiro SES compared with the R-ZES with respect to the primary endpoint of target-vessel failure (5% vs. 5%, p for non-inferiority <0.001) [33]. The finding of a lower stent thrombogenicity of the Orsiro SES has been corroborated by a network meta-analysis of 147 trials ($n = 126,526$) showing a lower risk of stent thrombosis with the Orsiro SES compared with Cypher SES and BES [34].

- The Ultimaster SES (Terumo Corporation, Tokyo, Japan) is made of a cobalt-chromium platform with thin struts (80 μm), open-cell design, and a biodegradable polymer (PDLLA and polycaprolactone) applied to the abluminal side. The polymer elutes the drug sirolimus (3.9 μg/mm stent length), which degrades during a period of 3–4 months. At variance with other biodegradable polymer DES, the Ultimaster SES features a biodegradable gradient coating, whereby the drug and polymer coating is not present on the stent areas experiencing the highest physical stress—this feature may reduce the risk of polymer cracking and delamination.

- The CENTURY II trial ($n = 1119$) showed the non-inferiority of Ultimaster SES compared with EES, with freedom from the primary endpoint of cardiac death, target-vessel myocardial infarction, and target-lesion revascularization in 95.6% and 95.1% of patients allocated to Ultimaster SES and EES (p for non-inferiority <0.001). The composite of cardiac death and myocardial infarction rate was 2.9% and 3.8% ($p = 0.40$) and target-vessel revascularization was 4.5% with Ultimaster SES and 4.2% with PP-EES ($p = 0.77$). The rate of stent thrombosis was 0.9% in both arms [35].

- The SYNERGY stent (Boston Scientific Corporation, Marlborough, MA, USA) is a thin-strut (74–81 μm), platinum-chromium metal alloy platform with an abluminal PLGA polymer, which elutes everolimus (100 μg/cm^2).
- Three randomized trials have evaluated the angiographic and clinical performance of the SYNERGY EES: the EVOLVE I, EVOLVE II, and BIORESORT trials.
- The EVOLVE I trial ($n = 291$) found the SYNERGY EES to be non-inferior to the Promus EES for the angiographic endpoint of in-stent late lumen loss at 6 months (0.15 ± 0.34 mm for PROMUS Element, 0.10 ± 0.25 mm for SYNERGY, and 0.13 ± 0.26 mm for SYNERGY half; p for non-inferiority <0.001 for all comparisons).
- The EVOLVE II included 1684 patients undergoing PCI for stable coronary artery disease or non-ST-segment-elevation acute coronary syndrome randomized to SYNERGY EES or Promus Element EES. At 12 months, the trial demonstrated non-inferiority of two devices with respect to the primary endpoint of cardiac death, target-vessel myocardial infarction, and ischemia-driven target-lesion revascularization (6.7% vs. 6.5%, p for non-inferiority = 0.0005).
- The SYNERGY EES compared with Promus EES had a similar rate of target-lesion revascularization (2.6% vs. 1.7%, $p = 0.21$) and definite or probable stent thrombosis (0.4% vs. 0.6%, $p = 0.50$) [36].
- The BIORESORT trial, which featured a 1:1:1 randomization scheme, demonstrated non-inferiority between the SYNERGY EES and R-ZES with respect to the primary endpoint of target-vessel failure (5% vs. 5%, p for non-inferiority <0.001), in addition to the already mentioned non-inferiority between the Orsiro SES and R-ZES [33].
- The MiStent (Micell Technologies, Durham, NC, USA) is a cobalt-chromium, thin-strut (64 μm), PLGA-based, sirolimus-eluting stent. PLGA carries a crystalline form of sirolimus. The PLGA/sirolimus combination is eliminated from the stent within 45–60 days

and PLGA is fully absorbed within 90 days. Crystalline sirolimus remains in the tissue and continues to elute the drug into the surrounding tissue for up to 9 months.
- The DESSOLVE II trial (2:1) reported superiority for in-stent late lumen loss at 9 months for the MiStent compared with E-ZES (0.27 ± 0.46 mm vs. 0.58 ± 0.41 mm, $p < 0.001$). At 2-year follow-up, the primary endpoint of all-cause death, any myocardial infarction, and clinically driven target-vessel revascularization was 6.7% in the MiStent group and 13.3% in the E-ZES group ($p = 0.17$) [37].
- The Tivoli SES (EssenTech, Beijing, China) is a thin-strut (80 μm), cobalt-chromium metal platform with a PLGA polymer, which elutes sirolimus (8 μg/mm). Approximately 75% of the sirolimus is eluted at 28 days.
- The I-LOVE-IT 2 trial ($n = 2737$) reported the non-inferiority for the primary endpoint target-lesion failure at 12 months between the Tivoli SES and the durable polymer Firebird SES (6.3% vs. 6.1%, p for non-inferiority = 0.002) [38].
- The Combo stent (OrbusNeich Medical, Ft. Lauderdale, FL, USA) is a 100 μm thick stainless steel stent covered abluminally with a biodegradable polymer matrix allowing a controlled release of sirolimus. An additional circumferential layer of anti-CD34 antibodies is applied on the stent struts on top of the polymer aiming to accelerate endothelial coverage.
- The Combo stent was tested in the REMEDEE trial, an angiographic non-inferiority study, comparing the in-stent late loss at nine 9 months between the Combo stent and the Taxus Liberté PES in a total of 183 patients (2:1 randomization). The primary endpoint was met with an in-stent late loss amounting to 0.39 ± 0.45 mm in the Combo compared with 0.44 ± 0.56 mm in the Taxus Liberté stent group (p for non-inferiority =0.0012) [39].

Polymer-Free DES
- Polymer-free DES have been developed through both physical and chemical methods,

mainly consisting of creating pores and reservoirs or by coating the stent with a porous inorganic material.

- The Yukon SES (Translumina, GmbH, Hechingen, Germany) presents a specifically designed surface with micropores (2 μm deep) wherein the antiproliferative agent sirolimus is deposited. The Yukon Choice has a stainless steel platform, while the Yukon Chrome is made of cobalt-chromium alloy.

- A pooled analysis of the ISAR-TEST and LIPSIA Yukon trials ($n = 682$) comparing polymer-free Yukon SES with PES reported a similar in-stent late loss (0.53 mm vs. 0.46 mm, $p = 0.15$), with a comparable risk of target-lesion revascularization (13.6% vs. 13.7%, $p = 0.93$), and death or myocardial infarction (12.4% vs. 12.6%, $p = 0.71$) [40].

- The Biofreedom BES (Biosensors International Pte Ltd., Singapore) is made of stainless steel with a strut thickness of 112 μm and a microstructured, polymer-free surface alteration at the abluminal stent side. The investigation of drug-release kinetics revealed that >90% of the drug is released within 50 h with biolimus detectable in neointima and myocardium surrounding stent struts at 28 days.

- In the LEADERS FREE trial, a total of 2466 patients at high risk for bleeding were randomized to the Biofreedom BES or BMS. Elderly patients (≥75 years) and an indication for oral anticoagulation after PCI were the two most common criteria to qualify for high-risk bleeding status. All patients received 1 month of dual-antiplatelet therapy. At 390 days, the rate of the primary safety endpoint, a composite of cardiac death, myocardial infarction, or stent thrombosis, was significantly reduced with the Biofreedom BES (9.4% vs. 12.9%, $p = 0.005$). Moreover, Biofreedom BES was associated with a lower risk of target-lesion revascularization (5.1% vs. 9.8%, $p < 0.001$) [41]. At 2 years, the difference in the primary safety (12.6% vs. 15.3%, $p = 0.039$) and efficacy (6.8% vs. 12.0%, $p < 0.001$) endpoint was still significant [42].

Reservoir Technology Applied to DES

- A third option for drug release is modification of stent design by providing laser-cut reservoirs within stent struts, the so-called reservoir technology. Each strut may contain several reservoirs, which can be located abluminally or luminally, or feature an entire hole.

- The Amphilimus-eluting stent (Cre8, Alvimedica, Istanbul, Turkey) is made of a cobalt-chromium alloy with 80 μm strut thickness and has an ultrathin (0.3 μm) passive carbon coating. The Cre8 does not have polymer, and the antiproliferative drug (sirolimus, 90 μg/cm^2) is loaded into reservoirs on the stent's abluminal surface.

- The sirolimus is formulated with a mixture of long-chain fatty acids (so-called amphilimus) to act as a carrier and to control the drug release. Thus, 65–70% of the drug is released within the first 30 days, and the remainder is completely eluted by 90 days.

- In the NEXT trial ($n = 323$), the Cre8 stent demonstrated both non-inferiority and superiority for the primary endpoint of in-stent late loss compared with PES (0.14 ± 0.36 mm vs. 0.34 ± 0.40 mm, p for non-inferiority <0.0001, p for superiority <0.0001), with comparable clinical event rates at 12 months [43].

- In the RESERVOIR trial, which was conducted in patients with diabetes mellitus ($n = 112$), the Cre8 stent was non-inferior to EES for the primary endpoint of neointimal volume obstruction assessed by optical coherence tomography at 9-month follow-up (11.97 ± 5.94% vs. 16.11 ± 18.18%, p for non-inferiority = 0.0003) [44].

- The drug-filled stent (DFS, Medtronic, Santa Rosa, CA, USA) is a novel polymer-free DES technology that features a novel tri-layer wire design, which allows the inner sacrificial layer to become a lumen continuously coated with drug.

- The drug (sirolimus) is contained on the inside of the stent and is released from a single continuous inner lumen through multiple laser-drilled holes on the abluminal side (outer surface) of the stent.

- Drug elution is controlled and sustained through passive diffusion via direct interaction with the vessel wall with an elution profile comparable to durable polymer DES. Preliminary results of the RevElution study showed excellent strut coverage and low occurrence of malapposition among 14 patients undergoing optical coherence tomography at 1-month follow-up [45].

Clinical Indications for Coronary Artery Stents

- The advent of BMS resolved the issue of threatening or abrupt vessel closure following balloon angioplasty, thus eliminating the need for standby surgical backup.
- Subsequently, DES with release of antiproliferative drugs during the first months after implantation successfully addressed the problem of restenosis inherent to BMS due to potent suppression of neointimal hyperplasia.
- A relevant shortcoming of early-generation DES was a delayed healing response of the stented coronary vessel that was associated with a small but notable increase in late thrombotic events. Refinements in new-generation DES resulted not only in a significant reduction in the risk of stent thrombosis compared with BMS and early-generation DES during long-term follow-up, but also in improved efficacy (lower risk of repeat revascularization) and potentially safety (lower risk of death and myocardial infarction).
- Accordingly, new-generation DES represent the standard of care among patients undergoing PCI and are indicated in almost all patient and lesion subsets [46]. Fig. 11.3 summarizes the results of a systematic review of 158 randomized trials by showing clinical outcomes at 9–12 months with BMS, early-generation DES, and new-generation DES [47].

Treatment of Abrupt or Threatened Closure After Balloon Angioplasty

- Coronary stents effectively scaffold coronary dissections complicating balloon angioplasty, and the availability of stents has nearly eliminated the need for emergency CABG (<1% of all PCI procedures).
- The initial approval of coronary stents for this "bailout" indication was based on a multicenter registry of patients with angioplasty complications who were treated with the Gianturco-Roubin II stent [4].

Stable Coronary Artery Disease

- A recent network meta-analysis (100 trials with 93,553 patients) comparing revascularization by means of CABG and several PCI techniques compared with medical therapy found that CABG and new-generation DES (EES: 0.75, 0.59–0.96; R-ZES: 0.65, 0.42–1.00)—but not balloon angioplasty, BMS, or early-generation DES—were associated with improved survival compared with a strategy of initial medical treatment.
- Similarly, the risk of myocardial infarction was lower with CABG and new-generation DES, an observation confirmed by other studies [48].

Acute Coronary Syndromes

- Current guidelines indicate new-generation DES as the coronary devices of choice for patients with ACS undergoing PCI [46, 49]. Several meta-analyses of randomized trials comparing early-generation DES with BMS in patients undergoing primary PCI consistently showed that the benefits of early-generation DES, such as a reduction in the risk of target-vessel revascularization and a trend toward less definite stent thrombosis, were offset in subsequent years by an increase in the risk of very late stent thrombosis [50–52].

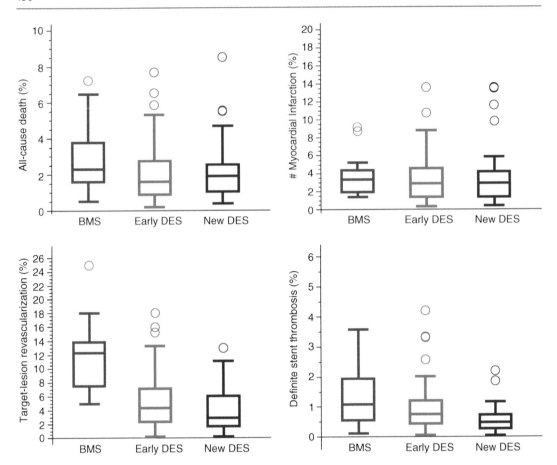

Fig. 11.3 Clinical outcomes with bare-metal stents (BMS), early-generation drug-eluting stents (DES), and new-generation DES. Clinical outcomes at 9–12 months: median rates per 100 person-years. Median rates and interquartile range per 100 person-years for the clinical endpoints all-cause death, myocardial infarction, target-lesion revascularization, and definite stent thrombosis. Reproduced with permission from Byrne RA et al. Eur Heart J. 2015;36:2608–2620

- Two main trials supported the benefit of new-generation DES over BMS in patients undergoing primary PCI: the COMFORTABLE-AMI ($n = 1161$) and EXAMINATION ($n = 1498$) [53, 54]. A pooled analysis of these two trials reported a significant reduction with new-generation DES in the risk of target-lesion revascularization (RR 0.33, 95% CI 0.20–0.52, $p < 0.0001$), target-vessel reinfarction (RR 0.36, 95% CI 0.14–0.92, $p = 0.03$), and definite stent thrombosis (RR 0.35, 95% CI 0.16–0.75, $p = 0.006$) [55].
- The 5-year follow-up data of the EXAMINATION trial showed a significant reduction in the risk of patient-oriented outcomes of all-cause death, any myocardial infarction, or any revascularization favoring

EES compared with BMS (HR 0.80, 95% CI 0.65–0.98, $p = 0.033$) [21].

Diabetes Mellitus (See Also Chap. 21)

- Diabetic patients undergoing PCI incur higher rates of restenosis and stent thrombosis following PCI. An alleged benefit of PES in diabetic patients was observed in a pooled analysis of the SPIRIT II, III, and IV and COMPARE trials with a significant interaction for the treatment effect of EES versus PES according to diabetic status with respect to myocardial infarction ($p = 0.01$), stent thrombosis ($p = 0.0006$), and target-lesion revascularization ($p = 0.02$) [22].

- However, in a network meta-analysis of 42 randomized trials that compared various stents and included 22,844 patient-years of follow-up of patients with diabetes, EES as compared with other DES and BMS were found to be the most effective and safe stents, and they had a high probability of being associated with the lowest rate of restenosis, myocardial infarction, and stent thrombosis [56].
- More recently, the TUXEDO trial randomized 1830 diabetic patients to EES vs. PES [23]. At 1-year follow-up, EES were associated with a lower rate of the primary endpoint of target-vessel failure (2.9% vs. 5.6%, $p = 0.005$), along with a significant reduction in spontaneous myocardial infarction (1.2% vs. 3.2%, $p = 0.004$), stent thrombosis (0.4% vs. 2.1%, $p = 0.002$), and target-vessel revascularization (1.2% vs. 3.4%, $p = 0.002$) [23].
- In aggregate, these findings support the use of new-generation DES among patients with diabetes.

In-Stent Restenosis (See Also Chap. 31)

- Although the use of coronary stents for the treatment of in-stent restenosis invariably introduces a new stent layer, new-generation DES are highly effective in the treatment of this lesion subset.
- A network meta-analysis of 27 trials with 5923 patients reported a significant reduction in the diameter stenosis at angiographic follow-up with EES compared with drug-coated balloons (-9.0%, 95% CI -15.8% to -2.2%) [57].
- The angiographic effectiveness of new-generation DES was particularly evident for the comparison of EES versus balloon angioplasty (-24.2%, 95% CI -32.2% to -16.4%) [57].

Complex Coronary Lesions

- The likelihood of treatment failure after PCI directly correlates with the complexity of coronary artery disease. Therefore, the treatment effect of new-generation DES may be camou-

flaged by the overriding effect of underlying coronary artery disease.
- Nonetheless, a pooled analysis of four trials ($n = 6081$) showed that the efficacy and safety of new-generation over early-generation DES not only are preserved across the spectrum of disease, but are also even more evident in patients with increased SYNTAX score [58].

Left Main Disease (See Also Chap. 27)

- Relevant unprotected left main disease is observed in 5–7% of patients undergoing coronary angiography. Although no direct randomized trials have compared new-generation with early-generation DES in this setting, the use of DES is recommended over BMS.
- In the ISAR-LEFT-MAIN 2 trial, patients with left main disease were randomized to R-ZES ($n = 324$) or EES ($n = 326$). At 1 year, the composite of death, myocardial infarction, or target-vessel revascularization was not significantly different between R-ZES and EES (17.5% vs. 14.3%, $p = 0.25$) [59].
- The safety and efficacy profile of PCI with EES in the treatment of left main disease compared with CABG has been recently confirmed in the EXCEL trial, in which PCI with EES was non-inferior to CABG with respect to the primary composite endpoint of death, stroke, or myocardial infarction at 3-year follow-up [60]. Moreover, the use of EES was associated with a very low rate of stent thrombosis (0.7%) at 3 years [60].
- In contrast, the NOBLE trial found a higher rate of definite stent thrombosis (3%) at 5-year follow-up among patients predominantly (90%) treated with the BioMatrix BES [61]. Overall, this trial failed to show non-inferiority between PCI and CABG for the treatment of left main disease [61].

Chronic Total Occlusions (See Also Chap. 28)

- The percutaneous treatment of CTO is challenged by failure to cross the lesion and restenosis. A meta-analysis of five randomized trials ($n = 1077$) comparing new-generation with early-generation DES in patients undergoing PCI of CTO lesions found a lower risk of death (OR 0.37, 95% CI 0.15–0.91, $p = 0.03$) and target-vessel revascularization (OR 0.59, 95% CI 0.40–0.87, $p = 0.007$) associated with newer devices [62].

Saphenous Vein Grafts (See Also Chap. 30)

- Saphenous vein graft stenosis after CABG may ensue in up to 50% of patients at year 5. PCI of vein graft stenoses accounts for about 6% of total PCI volume.
- The ISAR-CABG trial ($n = 610$) showed a significant reduction in the risk of the primary endpoint of death, myocardial infarction, or target-lesion revascularization at 1 year with DES compared with BMS (15% vs. 22%, $p = 0.02$), mainly driven by a lower rate of target-lesion revascularization (7% vs. 13%, $p = 0.01$) [63].
- A retrospective analysis including 2471 patients undergoing PCI of saphenous vein grafts reported a similar rate of procedural complications with DES and BMS, but a lower risk of long-term mortality with DES (HR 0.72, 95% CI 0.57–0.89) [64].

Bioresorbable Vascular Scaffolds

- The introduction of bioresorbable vascular scaffolds (BRS), which provide transient vessel support with drug delivery capability, has represented a further iteration in the field of coronary devices with the potential to overcome the limitations of permanent metallic stents [65].
- The concept of BRS is not entirely novel to the field of interventional cardiology since a first clinical description of a fully biodegradable device—the Igaki-Tamai stent (Kyoto Medical Planning Co., Ltd., Kyoto, Japan)—traces back to the early years of the twenty-first century [66].
- There are two main potential advantages of BRS:
  - The reduction of late complications related to permanent implants (i.e., very late stent thrombosis, neoatherosclerosis, late catchup phenomenon, aneurysm formation)
  - The restoration of anatomical and physiological properties in the coronary vessel (permanent side-branch occlusion, vessel vasomotion, adaptive shear stress, late luminal enlargement, and late positive remodeling)

Scaffold Composition

Current BRS are made of either a polymer or a bioresorbable metal alloy. The scaffold composition is of great importance as it entails different chemical compositions, mechanical properties, and subsequent resorption times. The two most frequently used materials in the current generation of BRS are poly-L-lactic acid (PLLA) and magnesium.

PLLA

- PLLA is the most commonly used polymer for BRS and strut thickness generally amounts to 150 μm in PLLA-based BRS.
- PLLA is degraded through hydrolysis, with the final conversion of lactates into CO_2 and O_2 in the Krebs cycle. However, PLLA degradation is a complex process, which requires months to years [67].
- The degradation of PLLA-BRS can be modulated by altering the ratio between semicrystalline and amorphous polymer status [68].

Magnesium

- Magnesium is mixed with rare earth metals to increase radial strength and control degradation process. Magnesium degradation requires up to 12 months according to its composition, and magnesium-based BRS are finally converted into soft amorphous hydroxyapatite.
- Of note, magnesium is more electronegative than other materials and antithrombotic properties related to electronegative charges have been described.

Other Materials

- Other materials for BRS include tyrosine polycarbonate which requires 2–3 years for resorption; it is used in REVA BRS and REVA ReZolve (Reva Medical, San Diego, CA, USA).

- The polylactic anhydride which takes approximately 15 months for resorption is used in the Ideal BioStent (Xenogenics Corp, Canton, MA, USA) [69].

CE-Approved Bioresorbable Vascular Scaffolds

- So far, three BRS have received the CE mark of approval for coronary use:
  - The Absorb vascular scaffold (BVS 1.1, Abbott Vascular, Santa Clara, CA, USA)
  - The DESolve scaffold (Elixir Medical Corporation, Sunnyvale, CA, USA)
  - The Magmaris scaffold (Biotronik AG, Bülach, Switzerland)
- Moreover, the Absorb BVS has been approved by the FDA in 2016. However, most clinical data are available for the BVS 1.1, which currently represents the only BRS to have been investigated in randomized trials.

Absorb BVS

- The BVS is an everolimus-eluting, balloon-expandable BRS consisting of a PLLA matrix (150 μm) coated with a 1:1 mixture of poly-D,L-lactide and everolimus (8.2 μg/mm).
- Preclinical and imaging-based studies have shown favorable healing characteristics, with restoration of vasomotor function of the treated segment and a positive vessel remodeling after resorption [70].
- Currently, six randomized trials have compared BVS 1.1 with new-generation DES, mainly Xience EES:
  - ABSORB China (n = 480)
  - ABSORB II (n = 501)
  - ABSORB III (n = 2008)
  - ABSORB Japan (n = 400), EVERBIO II (n = 158)
  - TROFI II (n = 191)
- A study-level meta-analysis of these trials (n = 3738) showed that BVS compared with EES had a similar 12-month risk of target-lesion failure (OR 1.20, 95% CI 0.90–1.60, $p = 0.21$), target-lesion revascularization (OR 0.97, 95% CI 0.66–1.43, $p = 0.87$), myocardial infarction (OR 1.36, 95% CI 0.98–1.89, $p = 0.06$), and death (OR 0.95, 95% CI 0.45–2.00, $p = 0.89$) [71].

- Patients treated with BVS had a higher risk of definite or probable stent thrombosis than those treated with metallic stents (OR 1.99, 95% CI 1.00–3.98, $p = 0.05$), with the highest risk observed between 1 and 30 days after implantation (OR 3.11, 95% CI 1.24–7.82, $p = 0.02$) [71].

- In a patient-level meta-analysis of ABSORB II, ABSORB Japan, ABSORB China, and ABSORB III, BVS compared with EES had a similar 1-year risk of patient-oriented (RR 1.09, 95% CI 0.89–1.34, $p = 0.38$) and device-oriented clinical endpoints (RR 1.22, 95% CI 0.91–1.64, $p = 0.17$).

- Treatment with BVS was associated with a significantly higher risk of target-vessel myocardial infarction (RR 1.45, 95% CI 1.02–2.07, $p = 0.04$) due in part to a numerically higher rate of periprocedural myocardial infarction and stent thrombosis (RR 2.09, 95% CI 0.92–4.75, $p = 0.08$) [72].

- When addressing angiographic efficacy by using the primary endpoint of in-segment late lumen loss, BVS was found to be associated with somewhat greater late lumen loss than metallic DES (0.05 mm; 95% CI 0.01–0.09—data from 4 studies [n = 1131]) [73].

- Data on long-term follow-up of randomized trials have also been reported. In the ABSORB II trial, the co-primary endpoint of angiographic vasomotor reactivity was not significantly improved among patients treated with BVS (superiority hypothesis) and the co-primary endpoint of late luminal was not non-inferior to the EES (non-inferiority hypothesis) at 3-year follow-up [74].

- The minimum lumen diameter was significantly smaller in the BVS compared with EES group (1.86 mm vs. 2.25 mm, $p < 0.001$) and the percentage diameter stenosis was higher (25.8% vs. 15.7%, $p < 0.001$).

- In terms of clinical outcomes, the 3-year rates of myocardial infarction (8% vs. 2%, $p = 0.0295$), device-oriented composite endpoint (10% vs. 5%, $p = 0.0425$), and definite or probable scaffold or stent thrombosis (3% vs. 0%) were significantly higher in the BVS compared with the EES group [74].
- At 2 years, a higher rate of target-lesion failure among patients treated with BVS compared with EES was observed in the ABSORB Japan trial (7.3% vs. 3.8%, $p = 0.018$), in which there were four cases of very late scaffold thrombosis while no very late stent thrombosis event [75].
- It is important to note that these trials were not designed to assess clinical outcomes and thus long-term follow-up from ABSORB III is needed to better evaluate the clinical profile of BVS.
- In the meantime, it is important to improve procedural techniques for BVS implantation, such as more aggressive plaque modification before BRS deployment, routine use of high-pressure, noncompliant balloon post-dilatation to ensure sufficient scaffold expansion, and more frequent use of intravascular imaging [76].

DESolve Scaffold

- The DESolve BRS is made of PLLA and elutes a mixture of novolimus and PLLA. The strut thickness is 150 μm (more recently 100 μm) and >95% of the device is resorbed after approximately 1 year.
- The first-in-man study ($n = 15$) reported a late lumen loss at 6-month angiographic follow-up amounting to 0.19 ± 0.19 mm [77].

Magnesium-Based BRS

- The DREAMS 2G, now called Magmaris, is a balloon-expandable, sirolimus-eluting (1.4 mcg/mm^2) BRS, whose scaffold is made from a magnesium alloy with two permanent X-ray markers made from tantalum at the proximal and distal scaffold ends. Approximately 95% of the magnesium is converted in an amorphous matrix of calcium phosphate at 12 months.

- The BIOSOLVE II (First in Man Study of the DREAMS 2nd Generation Drug Eluting Absorbable Metal Scaffold) trial enrolled 123 patients with up to 2 de novo lesions with a reference vessel diameter between 2.2 and 3.7 mm [78]. At 6-month follow-up angiography, in-segment late lumen loss was 0.27 ± 0.37 mm, with 80% of patients presenting a restoration of vasomotion [78]. At 12 months, a second angiographic follow-up was performed in 42 patients and the mean paired in-segment late lumen loss at 6 and 12 months was 0.20 ± 0.21 mm and 0.25 ± 0.22 mm ($p = 0.12$). The 1-year rate of TVR and TLR was 3.4% and 1.7%, respectively [79].

Conclusions

- Coronary artery stents constitute the most important advance in the field of PCI since the introduction of balloon angioplasty. Stents are used in more than 90% of coronary procedures today and have enabled the technique to become one of the most frequently performed therapeutic interventions in medicine.
- The most important benefit of coronary artery stents has been the effective treatment of abrupt or threatened vessel closure, eliminating the need of emergency bypass surgery required in 5–8% of patients in the balloon angioplasty era.
- In addition, the technique of coronary artery stenting has allowed reproducible results and resulted in a short procedure requiring only minutes in uncomplicated cases. Moreover, the ease and predictable outcome in the context of excellent peri-procedural safety, as well as cost considerations, contribute to the justification for ad hoc procedures as the preferred approach for patient care.
- Controlled release of antiproliferative drugs from polymer coatings immobilized on the stent surface was realized in the form of drug-eluting stents. These devices effectively reduced restenosis and lowered the need of repeat revascularization of the target lesion to below 5%. Of note,

new-generation DES have overcome the limitation of first-generation DES—the problem of very late stent thrombosis—thus combining improved safety while maintaining an excellent efficacy profile.

References

1. Sigwart U, Puel J, Mirkovitch V, Joffre F, Kappenberger L. Intravascular stents to prevent occlusion and restenosis after transluminal angioplasty. N Engl J Med. 1987;316:701–6.
2. Lindsay J, Hong MK, Pinnow EE, Pichard AD. Effects of endoluminal coronary stents on the frequency of coronary artery bypass grafting after unsuccessful percutaneous transluminal coronary vascularization. Am J Cardiol. 1996;77:647–9.
3. Dotter CT. Transluminally-placed coilspring endarterial tube grafts. Long-term patency in canine popliteal artery. Invest Radiol. 1969;4:329–32.
4. Roubin GS, Cannon AD, Agrawal SK, Macander PJ, Dean LS, Baxley WA, Breland J. Intracoronary stenting for acute and threatened closure complicating percutaneous transluminal coronary angioplasty. Circulation. 1992;85:916–27.
5. Serruys PW, De Jaegere P, Kiemeneij F, Macaya C, Rutsch W, Heyndrickx G, Emanuelsson H, Marco J, Legrand V, Materne P, Belardi J, Sigwart U, Colombo A, Goy JJ, Van den Heuvel P, Delcan J, Morel MA. A comparison of balloon-expandable-stent implantation with balloon angioplasty in patients with coronary artery disease. N Engl J Med. 1994;331:489–95.
6. Fischman DL, Leon MB, Baim DS, Schatz RA, Savage MP, Penn I, Detre K, Veltri L, Ricci D, Nobuyoshi M, Cleman M, Heuser R, Almond D, Teirstein PS, Fish RD, Colombo A, Brinker J, Moses J, Shaknovich A, et al. A randomized comparison of coronary-stent placement and balloon angioplasty in the treatment of coronary artery disease. N Engl J Med. 1994;331:496–501.
7. Praz L, Cook S, Meier B. Percutaneous coronary interventions in Europe in 2005. EuroIntervention. 2007;3:442–6.
8. Serruys PW, van Hout B, Bonnier H, Legrand V, Garcia E, Macaya C, Sousa E, van der Giessen W, Colombo A, Seabra-Gomes R, Kiemeneij F, Ruygrok P, Ormiston J, Emanuelsson H, Fajadet J, Haude M, Klugmann S, Morel MA. Randomised comparison of implantation of heparin-coated stents with balloon angioplasty in selected patients with coronary artery disease (Benestent II). Lancet. 1998;352:673–81.
9. Stefanini GG, Taniwaki M, Windecker S. Coronary stents: novel developments. Heart. 2014;100:1051–61.
10. Hwang CW, Wu D, Edelman ER. Physiological transport forces govern drug distribution for stent-based delivery. Circulation. 2001;104:600–5.
11. Daemen J, Serruys PW. Drug-eluting stent update 2007: part I. A survey of current and future generation drug-eluting stents: meaningful advances or more of the same? Circulation. 2007;116:316–28.
12. Tanner FC, Boehm M, Akyurek LM, San H, Yang ZY, Tashiro J, Nabel GJ, Nabel EG. Differential effects of the cyclin-dependent kinase inhibitors p27(Kip1), p21(Cip1), and p16(Ink4) on vascular smooth muscle cell proliferation. Circulation. 2000;101:2022–5.
13. Zohlnhofer D, Klein CA, Richter T, Brandl R, Murr A, Nuhrenberg T, Schomig A, Baeuerle PA, Neumann FJ. Gene expression profiling of human stent-induced neointima by cDNA array analysis of microscopic specimens retrieved by helix cutter atherectomy: detection of FK506-binding protein 12 upregulation. Circulation. 2001;103:1396–402.
14. Koster R, Vieluf D, Kiehn M, Sommerauer M, Kahler J, Baldus S, Meinertz T, Hamm CW. Nickel and molybdenum contact allergies in patients with coronary in-stent restenosis. Lancet. 2000;356:1895–7.
15. Kastrati A, Mehilli J, Dirschinger J, Dotzer F, Schuhlen H, Neumann F-J, Fleckenstein M, Pfafferott C, Seyfarth M, Schomig A. Intracoronary stenting and angiographic results: strut thickness effect on restenosis outcome (ISAR-STEREO) trial. Circulation. 2001;103:2816–21.
16. Pache J, Kastrati A, Mehilli J, Schuhlen H, Dotzer F, Hausleiter J, Fleckenstein M, Neumann FJ, Sattelberger U, Schmitt C, Muller M, Dirschinger J, Schomig A. Intracoronary stenting and angiographic results: strut thickness effect on restenosis outcome (ISAR-STEREO-2) trial. J Am Coll Cardiol. 2003;41:1283–8.
17. Kolandaivelu K, Swaminathan R, Gibson WJ, Kolachalama VB, Nguyen-Ehrenreich KL, Giddings VL, Coleman L, Wong GK, Edelman ER. Stent thrombogenicity early in high-risk interventional settings is driven by stent design and deployment and protected by polymer-drug coatings. Circulation. 2011;123:1400–9.
18. Valgimigli M, Sabate M, Kaiser C, Brugaletta S, de la Torre Hernandez JM, Galatius S, Cequier A, Eberli F, de Belder A, Serruys PW, Ferrante G. Effects of cobalt-chromium everolimus eluting stents or bare metal stent on fatal and non-fatal cardiovascular events: patient level meta-analysis. BMJ. 2014;349:g6427.
19. Palmerini T, Benedetto U, Biondi-Zoccai G, Della Riva D, Bacchi-Reggiani L, Smits PC, Vlachojannis GJ, Jensen LO, Christiansen EH, Berencsi K, Valgimigli M, Orlandi C, Petrou M, Rapezzi C, Stone GW. Long-term safety of drug-eluting and bare-metal stents: evidence from a comprehensive network meta-analysis. J Am Coll Cardiol. 2015;65:2496–507.
20. Kang SH, Park KW, Kang DY, Lim WH, Park KT, Han JK, Kang HJ, Koo BK, Oh BH, Park YB, Kandzari DE, Cohen DJ, Hwang SS, Kim HS. Biodegradable-polymer drug-eluting stents vs. bare metal stents vs. durable-polymer drug-eluting stents: a systematic review and Bayesian approach network meta-analysis. Eur Heart J. 2014;35:1147–58.

21. Sabate M, Brugaletta S, Cequier A, Iniguez A, Serra A, Jimenez-Quevedo P, Mainar V, Campo G, Tespili M, den Heijer P, Bethencourt A, Vazquez N, van Es GA, Backx B, Valgimigli M, Serruys PW. Clinical outcomes in patients with ST-segment elevation myocardial infarction treated with everolimus-eluting stents versus bare-metal stents (EXAMINATION): 5-year results of a randomised trial. Lancet. 2016;387:357–66.

22. Stone GW, Kedhi E, Kereiakes DJ, Parise H, Fahy M, Serruys PW, Smits PC. Differential clinical responses to everolimus-eluting and Paclitaxel-eluting coronary stents in patients with and without diabetes mellitus. Circulation. 2011;124:893–900.

23. Kaul U, Bangalore S, Seth A, Arambam P, Abhaychand RK, Patel TM, Banker D, Abhyankar A, Mullasari AS, Shah S, Jain R, Kumar PR, Bahuleyan CG, Investigators TU-I. Paclitaxel-eluting versus everolimus-eluting coronary stents in diabetes. N Engl J Med. 2015;373:1709–19.

24. Piccolo R, Stefanini GG, Franzone A, Spitzer E, Blochlinger S, Heg D, Juni P, Windecker S. Safety and efficacy of resolute zotarolimus-eluting stents compared with everolimus-eluting stents: a meta-analysis. Circ Cardiovasc Interv. 2015;8:e002223.

25. Serruys PW, Farooq V, Kalesan B, de Vries T, Buszman P, Linke A, Ischinger T, Klauss V, Eberli F, Wijns W, Morice MC, Di Mario C, Corti R, Antoni D, Sohn HY, Eerdmans P, Rademaker-Havinga T, van Es GA, Meier B, Juni P, Windecker S. Improved safety and reduction in stent thrombosis associated with biodegradable polymer-based biolimus-eluting stents versus durable polymer-based sirolimus-eluting stents in patients with coronary artery disease: final 5-year report of the LEADERS (Limus eluted from a durable versus ERodable stent coating) randomized, noninferiority trial. JACC Cardiovasc Interv. 2013;6:777–89.

26. Raber L, Kelbaek H, Baumbach A, Tuller D, Ostojic M, Juni P, Von Birgelen C, Kornowski R, Luscher T, Roffi M, Pedrazzini G, Engstrom T, Vukcevic D, Heg D, Windecker S. Long-term clinical outcomes of biolimus-eluting stents with biodegradable versus bare-metal stents in patients with acute STEMI: 5 Year results of the randomized COMFORTABLE AMI trial. Eur Heart J. 2016;37. (Abstract supplement).

27. Raungaard B, Jensen LO, Tilsted HH, Christiansen EH, Maeng M, Terkelsen CJ, Krusell LR, Kaltoft A, Kristensen SD, Botker HE, Thuesen L, Aaroe J, Jensen SE, Villadsen AB, Thayssen P, Veien KT, Hansen KN, Junker A, Madsen M, Ravkilde J, Lassen JF, Scandinavian Organization for Randomized Trials with Clinical O. Zotarolimus-eluting durable-polymer-coated stent versus a biolimus-eluting biodegradable-polymer-coated stent in unselected patients undergoing percutaneous coronary intervention (SORT OUT VI): a randomised non-inferiority trial. Lancet. 2015;385:1527–35.

28. Christiansen EH, Jensen LO, Thayssen P, Tilsted HH, Krusell LR, Hansen KN, Kaltoft A, Maeng M, Kristensen SD, Botker HE, Terkelsen CJ, Villadsen AB, Ravkilde J, Aaroe J, Madsen M, Thuesen L, Lassen JF. Biolimus-eluting biodegradable polymer-coated stent versus durable polymer-coated sirolimus-eluting stent in unselected patients receiving percutaneous coronary intervention (SORT OUT V): a randomised non-inferiority trial. Lancet. 2013;381:661–9.

29. Smits PC, Hofma S, Togni M, Vazquez N, Valdes M, Voudris V, Slagboom T, Goy JJ, Vuillomenet A, Serra A, Nouche RT, den Heijer P, van der Ent M. Abluminal biodegradable polymer biolimus-eluting stent versus durable polymer everolimus-eluting stent (COMPARE II): a randomised, controlled, non-inferiority trial. Lancet. 2013;381:651–60.

30. Natsuaki M, Kozuma K, Morimoto T, Kadota K, Muramatsu T, Nakagawa Y, Akasaka T, Igarashi K, Tanabe K, Morino Y, Ishikawa T, Nishikawa H, Awata M, Abe M, Okada H, Takatsu Y, Ogata N, Kimura K, Urasawa K, Tarutani Y, Shiode N, Kimura T. Final 3-year outcome of a randomized trial comparing second-generation drug-eluting stents using either biodegradable polymer or durable polymer: NOBORI biolimus-eluting versus XIENCE/PROMUS everolimus-eluting stent trial. Circ Cardiovasc Interv. 2015;8:e002817.

31. Windecker S, Haude M, Neumann FJ, Stangl K, Witzenbichler B, Slagboom T, Sabate M, Goicolea J, Barragan P, Cook S, Piot C, Richardt G, Merkely B, Schneider H, Bilger J, Erne P, Waksman R, Zaugg S, Juni P, Lefevre T. Comparison of a novel biodegradable polymer sirolimus-eluting stent with a durable polymer everolimus-eluting stent: results of the randomized BIOFLOW-II trial. Circ Cardiovasc Interv. 2015;8:e001441.

32. Zbinden R, Piccolo R, Heg D, Roffi M, Kurz DJ, Muller O, Vuillomenet A, Cook S, Weilenmann D, Kaiser C, Jamshidi P, Franzone A, Eberli F, Juni P, Windecker S, Pilgrim T. Ultrathin strut biodegradable polymer sirolimus-eluting stent versus durable-polymer everolimus-eluting stent for percutaneous coronary revascularization: 2-year results of the BIOSCIENCE trial. J Am Heart Assoc. 2016;5:e003255.

33. von Birgelen C, Kok MM, van der Heijden LC, Danse PW, Schotborgh CE, Scholte M, Gin RM, Somi S, van Houwelingen KG, Stoel MG, de Man FH, Louwerenburg JH, Hartmann M, Zocca P, Linssen GC, van der Palen J, Doggen CJ, Lowik MM. Very thin strut biodegradable polymer everolimus-eluting and sirolimus-eluting stents versus durable polymer zotarolimus-eluting stents in allcomers with coronary artery disease (BIO-RESORT): a three-arm, randomised, non-inferiority trial. Lancet. 2016;388:2607–17.

34. Jensen LO, Thayssen P, Maeng M, Ravkilde J, Krusell LR, Raungaard B, Junker A, Terkelsen CJ, Veien KT, Villadsen AB, Kaltoft A, Tilsted HH, Hansen KN, Aaroe J, Kristensen SD, Hansen HS, Jensen SE, Madsen M, Botker HE, Berencsi K, Lassen JF, Christiansen EH. Randomized comparison of a biodegradable polymer ultrathin strut sirolimus-eluting

stent with a biodegradable polymer biolimus-eluting stent in patients treated with percutaneous coronary intervention: the SORT OUT VII trial. Circ Cardiovasc Interv. 2016;9:e003610.

35. Saito S, Valdes-Chavarri M, Richardt G, Moreno R, Iniguez Romo A, Barbato E, Carrie D, Ando K, Merkely B, Kornowski R, Eltchaninoff H, James S, Wijns W, Investigators CI. A randomized, prospective, intercontinental evaluation of a bioresorbable polymer sirolimus-eluting coronary stent system: the CENTURY II (Clinical Evaluation of New Terumo Drug-Eluting Coronary Stent System in the Treatment of Patients with Coronary Artery Disease) trial. Eur Heart J. 2014;35:2021–31.

36. Kereiakes DJ, Meredith IT, Windecker S, Lee Jobe R, Mehta SR, Sarembock IJ, Feldman RL, Stein B, Dubois C, Grady T, Saito S, Kimura T, Christen T, Allocco DJ, Dawkins KD. Efficacy and safety of a novel bioabsorbable polymer-coated, everolimus-eluting coronary stent: the EVOLVE II randomized trial. Circ Cardiovasc Interv. 2015;8:e002372.

37. Wijns W, Suttorp MJ, Zagozdzon L, Morice MC, McClean D, Stella P, Donohoe D, Knape C, Ormiston J. Evaluation of a crystalline sirolimus-eluting coronary stent with a bioabsorbable polymer designed for rapid dissolution: two-year outcomes from the DESSOLVE I and II trials. EuroIntervention. 2016;12:352–5.

38. Han Y, Xu B, Jing Q, Lu S, Yang L, Xu K, Li Y, Li J, Guan C, Kirtane AJ, Yang Y, Investigators IL-I. A randomized comparison of novel biodegradable polymer- and durable polymer-coated cobalt-chromium sirolimus-eluting stents. JACC Cardiovasc Interv. 2014;7:1352–60.

39. Haude M, Lee SW, Worthley SG, Silber S, Verheye S, Erbs S, Rosli MA, Botelho R, Meredith I, Sim KH, Stella PR, Tan HC, Whitbourn R, Thambar S, Abizaid A, Koh TH, Den Heijer P, Parise H, Cristea E, Maehara A, Mehran R. The REMEDEE trial: a randomized comparison of a combination sirolimus-eluting endothelial progenitor cell capture stent with a paclitaxel-eluting stent. JACC Cardiovasc Interv. 2013;6:334–43.

40. Cassese S, Desch S, Kastrati A, Byrne RA, King L, Tada T, Lauer B, Schomig A, Thiele H, Pache J. Polymer-free sirolimus-eluting versus polymer-based paclitaxel-eluting stents: an individual patient data analysis of randomized trials. Rev Esp Cardiol (Engl Ed). 2013;66:435–42.

41. Urban P, Meredith IT, Abizaid A, Pocock SJ, Carrie D, Naber C, Lipiecki J, Richardt G, Iniguez A, Brunel P, Valdes-Chavarri M, Garot P, Talwar S, Berland J, Abdellaoui M, Eberli F, Oldroyd K, Zambahari R, Gregson J, Greene S, Stoll HP, Morice MC, Investigators LF. Polymer-free drug-coated coronary stents in patients at high bleeding risk. N Engl J Med. 2015;373:2038–47.

42. Garot P, Morice MC, Tresukosol D, Pocock SJ, Meredith IT, Abizaid A, Carrie D, Naber C, Iniguez A, Talwar S, Menown IB, Christiansen EH, Gregson J, Copt S, Hovasse T, Lurz P, Maillard L, Krackhardt F, Ong P, Byrne J, Redwood S, Windhovel U, Greene S, Stoll HP, Urban P, Investigators LF. Two-year outcomes of high bleeding risk patients after polymer-free drug-coated stents. J Am Coll Cardiol. 2017;69(2):162–71.

43. Carrie D, Berland J, Verheye S, Hauptmann KE, Vrolix M, Violini R, Dibie A, Berti S, Maupas E, Antoniucci D, Schofer J. A multicenter randomized trial comparing amphilimus- with paclitaxel-eluting stents in de novo native coronary artery lesions. J Am Coll Cardiol. 2012;59:1371–6.

44. Romaguera R, Gomez-Hospital JA, Gomez-Lara J, Brugaletta S, Pinar E, Jimenez-Quevedo P, Gracida M, Roura G, Ferreiro JL, Teruel L, Montanya E, Fernandez-Ortiz A, Alfonso F, Valgimigli M, Sabate M, Cequier A. A randomized comparison of reservoir-based polymer-free amphilimus-eluting stents versus everolimus-eluting stents with durable polymer in patients with diabetes mellitus: the RESERVOIR clinical trial. JACC Cardiovasc Interv. 2016;9:42–50.

45. Worthley S, Abizaid A, Kirtane A, Simon D, Windecker S, Stone GW. Stent strut coverage and apposition at 1 and 3 months after implantation of a novel drug-filled coronary stent: first report from the RevElution study. J Am Coll Cardiol. 2016;67:422.

46. Windecker S, Kolh P, Alfonso F, Collet JP, Cremer J, Falk V, Filippatos G, Hamm C, Head SJ, Juni P, Kappetein AP, Kastrati A, Knuuti J, Landmesser U, Laufer G, Neumann FJ, Richter DJ, Schauerte P, Sousa Uva M, Stefanini GG, Taggart DP, Torracca L, Valgimigli M, Wijns W, Witkowski A. 2014 ESC/EACTS Guidelines on myocardial revascularization: The Task Force on Myocardial Revascularization of the European Society of Cardiology (ESC) and the European Association for Cardio-Thoracic Surgery (EACTS) Developed with the special contribution of the European Association of Percutaneous Cardiovascular Interventions (EAPCI). Eur Heart J. 2014;35:2541–619.

47. Byrne RA, Serruys PW, Baumbach A, Escaned J, Fajadet J, James S, Joner M, Oktay S, Juni P, Kastrati A, Sianos G, Stefanini GG, Wijns W, Windecker S. Report of a European Society of Cardiology-European Association of Percutaneous Cardiovascular Interventions task force on the evaluation of coronary stents in Europe: executive summary. Eur Heart J. 2015;36:2608–20.

48. Windecker S, Stortecky S, Stefanini GG, da Costa BR, Rutjes AW, Di Nisio M, Silletta MG, Maione A, Alfonso F, Clemmensen PM, Collet JP, Cremer J, Falk V, Filippatos G, Hamm C, Head S, Kappetein AP, Kastrati A, Knuuti J, Landmesser U, Laufer G, Neumann FJ, Richter D, Schauerte P, Sousa Uva M, Taggart DP, Torracca L, Valgimigli M, Wijns W, Witkowski A, Kolh P, Juni P. Revascularisation versus medical treatment in patients with stable coronary artery disease: network meta-analysis. BMJ. 2014;348:g3859.

49. Roffi M, Patrono C, Collet JP, Mueller C, Valgimigli M, Andreotti F, Bax JJ, Borger MA, Brotons C, Chew

DP, Gencer B, Hasenfuss G, Kjeldsen K, Lancellotti P, Landmesser U, Mehilli J, Mukherjee D, Storey RF, Windecker S, Baumgartner H, Gaemperli O, Achenbach S, Agewall S, Badimon L, Baigent C, Bueno H, Bugiardini R, Carerj S, Casselman F, Cuisset T, Erol C, Fitzsimons D, Halle M, Hamm C, Hildick-Smith D, Huber K, Iliodromitis E, James S, Lewis BS, Lip GY, Piepoli MF, Richter D, Rosemann T, Sechtem U, Steg PG, Vrints C, Luis Zamorano J. 2015 ESC Guidelines for the management of acute coronary syndromes in patients presenting without persistent ST-segment elevation: Task Force for the Management of Acute Coronary Syndromes in Patients Presenting without Persistent ST-Segment Elevation of the European Society of Cardiology (ESC). Eur Heart J. 2016;37:267–315.

50. Kalesan B, Pilgrim T, Heinimann K, Raber L, Stefanini GG, Valgimigli M, da Costa BR, Mach F, Luscher TF, Meier B, Windecker S, Juni P. Comparison of drug-eluting stents with bare metal stents in patients with ST-segment elevation myocardial infarction. Eur Heart J. 2012;33:977–87.

51. Piccolo R, Cassese S, Galasso G, Niglio T, De Rosa R, De Biase C, Piscione F. Long-term clinical outcomes following sirolimus-eluting stent implantation in patients with acute myocardial infarction. A meta-analysis of randomized trials. Clin Res Cardiol. 2012;101:885–93.

52. Piccolo R, Cassese S, Galasso G, De Rosa R, D'Anna C, Piscione F. Long-term safety and efficacy of drug-eluting stents in patients with acute myocardial infarction: a meta-analysis of randomized trials. Atherosclerosis. 2011;217:149–57.

53. Raber L, Kelbaek H, Ostojic M, Baumbach A, Heg D, Tuller D, von Birgelen C, Roffi M, Moschovitis A, Khattab AA, Wenaweser P, Bonvini R, Pedrazzini G, Kornowski R, Weber K, Trelle S, Luscher TF, Taniwaki M, Matter CM, Meier B, Juni P, Windecker S. Effect of biolimus-eluting stents with biodegradable polymer vs. bare-metal stents on cardiovascular events among patients with acute myocardial infarction: the COMFORTABLE AMI randomized trial. JAMA. 2012;308:777–87.

54. Sabate M, Cequier A, Iniguez A, Serra A, Hernandez-Antolin R, Mainar V, Valgimigli M, Tespili M, den Heijer P, Bethencourt A, Vazquez N, Gomez-Hospital JA, Baz JA, Martin-Yuste V, van Geuns RJ, Alfonso F, Bordes P, Tebaldi M, Masotti M, Silvestro A, Backx B, Brugaletta S, van Es GA, Serruys PW. Everolimus-eluting stent versus bare-metal stent in ST-segment elevation myocardial infarction (EXAMINATION): 1 year results of a randomised controlled trial. Lancet. 2012;380:1482–90.

55. Sabate M, Raber L, Heg D, Brugaletta S, Kelbaek H, Cequier A, Ostojic M, Iniguez A, Tuller D, Serra A, Baumbach A, von Birgelen C, Hernandez-Antolin R, Roffi M, Mainar V, Valgimigli M, Serruys PW, Juni P, Windecker S. Comparison of newer-generation drug-eluting with bare-metal stents in patients with acute ST-segment elevation myocardial infarc-

tion: a pooled analysis of the EXAMINATION (Clinical Evaluation of the Xience-V stent in Acute Myocardial INfArcTION) and COMFORTABLE-AMI (Comparison of Biolimus Eluted From an Erodible Stent Coating With Bare Metal Stents in Acute ST-Elevation Myocardial Infarction) trials. JACC Cardiovasc Interv. 2014;7:55–63.

56. Bangalore S, Kumar S, Fusaro M, Amoroso N, Kirtane AJ, Byrne RA, Williams DO, Slater J, Cutlip DE, Feit F. Outcomes with various drug eluting or bare metal stents in patients with diabetes mellitus: mixed treatment comparison analysis of 22,844 patient years of follow-up from randomised trials. BMJ. 2012;345:e5170.

57. Siontis GC, Stefanini GG, Mavridis D, Siontis KC, Alfonso F, Perez-Vizcayno MJ, Byrne RA, Kastrati A, Meier B, Salanti G, Juni P, Windecker S. Percutaneous coronary interventional strategies for treatment of in-stent restenosis: a network meta-analysis. Lancet. 2015;386:655–64.

58. Piccolo R, Pilgrim T, Heg D, Franzone A, Rat-Wirtzler J, Raber L, Silber S, Serruys PW, Juni P, Windecker S. Comparative effectiveness and safety of new-generation versus early-generation drug-eluting stents according to complexity of coronary artery disease: a patient-level pooled analysis of 6,081 patients. JACC Cardiovasc Interv. 2015;8:1657–66.

59. Mehilli J, Richardt G, Valgimigli M, Schulz S, Singh A, Abdel-Wahab M, Tiroch K, Pache J, Hausleiter J, Byrne RA, Ott I, Ibrahim T, Fusaro M, Seyfarth M, Laugwitz KL, Massberg S, Kastrati A, Investigators I-L-MS. Zotarolimus- versus everolimus-eluting stents for unprotected left main coronary artery disease. J Am Coll Cardiol. 2013;62:2075–82.

60. Stone GW, Sabik JF, Serruys PW, Simonton CA, Genereux P, Puskas J, Kandzari DE, Morice MC, Lembo N, Brown WM 3rd, Taggart DP, Banning A, Merkely B, Horkay F, Boonstra PW, van Boven AJ, Ungi I, Bogats G, Mansour S, Noiseux N, Sabate M, Pomar J, Hickey M, Gershlick A, Buszman P, Bochenek A, Schampaert E, Page P, Dressler O, Kosmidou I, Mehran R, Pocock SJ, Kappetein AP, Investigators ET. Everolimus-eluting stents or bypass surgery for left main coronary artery disease. N Engl J Med. 2016;375:2223–35.

61. Makikallio T, Holm NR, Lindsay M, Spence MS, Erglis A, Menown IB, Trovik T, Eskola M, Romppanen H, Kellerth T, Ravkilde J, Jensen LO, Kalinauskas G, Linder RB, Pentikainen M, Hervold A, Banning A, Zaman A, Cotton J, Eriksen E, Margus S, Sorensen HT, Nielsen PH, Niemela M, Kervinen K, Lassen JF, Maeng M, Oldroyd K, Berg G, Walsh SJ, Hanratty CG, Kumsars I, Stradins P, Steigen TK, Frobert O, Graham AN, Endresen PC, Corbascio M, Kajander O, Trivedi U, Hartikainen J, Anttila V, Hildick-Smith D, Thuesen L, Christiansen EH, NOBLE study investigators. Percutaneous coronary angioplasty versus coronary artery bypass grafting in treatment of unprotected left main stenosis (NOBLE): a prospective, ran-

domised, open-label, non-inferiority trial. Lancet. 2016;388:2743–52.

62. Lanka V, Patel VG, Saeed B, Kotsia A, Christopoulos G, Rangan BV, Mohammad A, Luna M, Garcia S, Abdullah SM, Grodin J, Hastings JL, Banerjee S, Brilakis ES. Outcomes with first- versus second-generation drug-eluting stents in coronary chronic total occlusions (CTOs): a systematic review and meta-analysis. J Invasive Cardiol. 2014;26:304–10.

63. Mehilli J, Pache J, Abdel-Wahab M, Schulz S, Byrne RA, Tiroch K, Hausleiter J, Seyfarth M, Ott I, Ibrahim T, Fusaro M, Laugwitz KL, Massberg S, Neumann FJ, Richardt G, Schomig A, Kastrati A. Is Drug-Eluting-Stenting Associated with Improved Results in Coronary Artery Bypass Grafts I. Drug-eluting versus bare-metal stents in saphenous vein graft lesions (ISAR-CABG): a randomised controlled superiority trial. Lancet. 2011;378:1071–8.

64. Aggarwal V, Stanislawski MA, Maddox TM, Nallamothu BK, Grunwald G, Adams JC, Ho PM, Rao SV, Casserly IP, Rumsfeld JS, Brilakis ES, Tsai TT. Safety and effectiveness of drug-eluting versus bare-metal stents in saphenous vein bypass graft percutaneous coronary interventions: insights from the Veterans Affairs CART program. J Am Coll Cardiol. 2014;64:1825–36.

65. Piccolo R, Giustino G, Mehran R, Windecker S. Stable coronary artery disease: revascularisation and invasive strategies. Lancet. 2015;386:702–13.

66. Tamai H, Igaki K, Kyo E, Kosuga K, Kawashima A, Matsui S, Komori H, Tsuji T, Motohara S, Uehata H. Initial and 6-month results of biodegradable poly-l-lactic acid coronary stents in humans. Circulation. 2000;102:399–404.

67. Raber L, Brugaletta S, Yamaji K, O'Sullivan CJ, Otsuki S, Koppara T, Taniwaki M, Onuma Y, Freixa X, Eberli FR, Serruys PW, Joner M, Sabate M, Windecker S. Very late scaffold thrombosis: intracoronary imaging and histopathological and spectroscopic findings. J Am Coll Cardiol. 2015;66:1901–14.

68. Onuma Y, Serruys PW. Bioresorbable scaffold: the advent of a new era in percutaneous coronary and peripheral revascularization? Circulation. 2011;123:779–97.

69. Wiebe J, Nef HM, Hamm CW. Current status of bioresorbable scaffolds in the treatment of coronary artery disease. J Am Coll Cardiol. 2014;64:2541–51.

70. Iqbal J, Onuma Y, Ormiston J, Abizaid A, Waksman R, Serruys P. Bioresorbable scaffolds: rationale, current status, challenges, and future. Eur Heart J. 2014;35:765–76.

71. Cassese S, Byrne RA, Ndrepepa G, Kufner S, Wiebe J, Repp J, Schunkert H, Fusaro M, Kimura T, Kastrati A. Everolimus-eluting bioresorbable vascular scaffolds versus everolimus-eluting metallic stents: a meta-analysis of randomised controlled trials. Lancet. 2016;387:537–44.

72. Stone GW, Gao R, Kimura T, Kereiakes DJ, Ellis SG, Onuma Y, Cheong WF, Jones-McMeans J, Su X, Zhang Z, Serruys PW. 1-year outcomes with the Absorb bioresorbable scaffold in patients with coronary artery disease: a patient-level, pooled meta-analysis. Lancet. 2016;387:1277–89.

73. Windecker S, Koskinas KC, Siontis GC. Bioresorbable scaffolds versus metallic drug-eluting stents: are we getting any closer to a paradigm shift? J Am Coll Cardiol. 2015;66:2310–4.

74. Serruys PW, Chevalier B, Sotomi Y, Cequier A, Carrie D, Piek JJ, Van Boven AJ, Dominici M, Dudek D, McClean D, Helqvist S, Haude M, Reith S, de Sousa Almeida M, Campo G, Iniguez A, Sabate M, Windecker S, Onuma Y. Comparison of an everolimus-eluting bioresorbable scaffold with an everolimus-eluting metallic stent for the treatment of coronary artery stenosis (ABSORB II): a 3 year, randomised, controlled, single-blind, multicentre clinical trial. Lancet. 2016;388:2479–91.

75. Onuma Y, Sotomi Y, Shiomi H, Ozaki Y, Namiki A, Yasuda S, Ueno T, Ando K, Furuya J, Igarashi K, Kozuma K, Tanabe K, Kusano H, Rapoza R, Popma JJ, Stone GW, Simonton C, Serruys PW, Kimura T. Two-year clinical, angiographic, and serial optical coherence tomographic follow-up after implantation of an everolimus-eluting bioresorbable scaffold and an everolimus-eluting metallic stent: insights from the randomised ABSORB Japan trial. EuroIntervention. 2016;12:1090–101.

76. Tamburino C, Latib A, van Geuns RJ, Sabate M, Mehilli J, Gori T, Achenbach S, Alvarez MP, Nef H, Lesiak M, Di Mario C, Colombo A, Naber CK, Caramanno G, Capranzano P, Brugaletta S, Geraci S, Araszkiewicz A, Mattesini A, Pyxaras SA, Rzeszutko L, Depukat R, Diletti R, Boone E, Capodanno D, Dudek D. Contemporary practice and technical aspects in coronary intervention with bioresorbable scaffolds: a European perspective. EuroIntervention. 2015;11:45–52.

77. Verheye S, Ormiston JA, Stewart J, Webster M, Sanidas E, Costa R, Costa JR Jr, Chamie D, Abizaid AS, Pinto I, Morrison L, Toyloy S, Bhat V, Yan J, Abizaid A. A next-generation bioresorbable coronary scaffold system: from bench to first clinical evaluation: 6- and 12-month clinical and multimodality imaging results. JACC Cardiovasc Interv. 2014;7:89–99.

78. Haude M, Ince H, Abizaid A, Toelg R, Lemos PA, von Birgelen C, Christiansen EH, Wijns W, Neumann FJ, Kaiser C, Eeckhout E, Lim ST, Escaned J, Garcia-Garcia HM, Waksman R. Safety and performance of the second-generation drug-eluting absorbable metal scaffold in patients with de-novo coronary artery lesions (BIOSOLVE-II): 6 month results of a prospective, multicentre, non-randomised, first-in-man trial. Lancet. 2016;387:31–9.

79. Haude M, Ince H, Abizaid A, Toelg R, Lemos PA, von Birgelen C, Christiansen EH, Wijns W, Neumann FJ, Kaiser C, Eeckhout E, Lim ST, Escaned J, Onuma Y, Garcia-Garcia HM, Waksman R. Sustained safety and performance of the second-generation drug-eluting absorbable metal scaffold in patients with de novo coronary lesions: 12-month clinical results and angiographic findings of the BIOSOLVE-II first-in-man trial. Eur Heart J. 2016;37:2701–9.

Percutaneous Coronary Intervention: Adjunctive Pharmacology

12

Paul A. Gurbel and Udaya S. Tantry

About Us Inova Heart and Vascular Institute provides the full spectrum of diagnostic, therapeutic, surgical, and interventional cardiac services including a nationally recognized program for treating atrial fibrillation, heart and lung transplantation, innovative minimally invasive surgical techniques, robot-assisted surgery, and implantation of artificial heart devices. Yearly we perform more than 4000 cardiac diagnostic investigations, 5000 cardiac catheterizations, 170 TAVR procedures, and 500 CABG surgeries.

Professor Paul A. Gurbel is an interventional cardiologist at Inova Heart and Vascular Institute. He specializes in the catheter-based treatment of patients with complex cardiovascular disease and he has performed over 15,000 percutaneous cardiac and peripheral procedures. He is currently the Director of the Inova Center for Thrombosis Research and Drug Development, Professor of Medicine at the Johns Hopkins University School of Medicine, and Adjunct Professor of Medicine at Duke University School of Medicine. For over 15 years his research has focused on defining the effects of antiplatelet agents, developing antiplatelet agents, and understanding the relation of

platelet reactivity to ischemic event occurrence in patients undergoing stenting. Dr. Udaya S Tantry is the Director of the Thrombosis Research Laboratory.

Platelet Function in Percutaneous Coronary Intervention

- Percutaneous coronary intervention (PCI) promotes thrombosis by inducing extreme vascular injury. The concomitant presence of dysfunctional endothelium, vulnerable plaque, and endothelial erosion promotes further thrombotic risk.
- Platelet adhesion to newly exposed collagen and von Willebrand factor by specific receptors and binding of thrombin generated by tissue factor to protease-activated receptors (PARs) cause initial platelet activation.
- Following activation, adenosine diphosphate (ADP) is released from dense granules and thromboxane A_2 is generated by cyclooxygenase-1 (COX-1). Although both thromboxane A_2 and ADP amplify platelet activation and aggregation, continuous ADP-$P2Y_{12}$ receptor signaling is essential for sustained activation of the GPIIb/IIIa receptor and stable thrombus generation.
- Simultaneously, platelet activation exposes the phosphatidylserine surface providing binding sites for coagulation factors and the

P. A. Gurbel (✉) · U. S. Tantry
Inova Center for Thrombosis Research and Drug Development, Inova Heart and Vascular Institute, Falls Church, VA, USA
e-mail: Paul.Gurbel@inova.org; udaya.tantry@inova.org

© Springer International Publishing AG, part of Springer Nature 2018
A. Myat et al. (eds.), *The Interventional Cardiology Training Manual*,
https://doi.org/10.1007/978-3-319-71635-0_12

generation of thrombin. Thrombin converts fibrinogen to fibrin and activates factor XIII that cross-links the fibrin network, stabilizes the platelet-fibrin clot at the site of vascular injury, and impairs myocardial blood supply [1, 2].

- Therefore, the rationale for antithrombotic therapy during and following PCI is to prevent thrombus formation within the target lesion

and also in nontarget vessels by attenuating platelet activation and aggregation and arresting coagulation processes. Since clot formation involves multiple pathways including platelet activation and aggregation and coagulation, simultaneous blockade of these pathways is essential to prevent periprocedural and post-PCI ischemic event occurrences (Fig. 12.1).

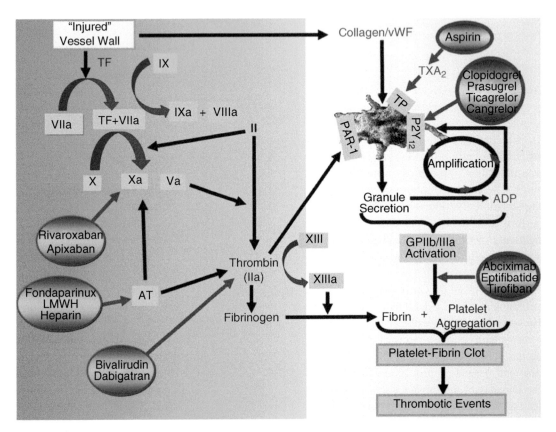

Fig. 12.1 Antiplatelet and antithrombotic agents in percutaneous coronary intervention (PCI). During PCI, at the site of vascular injury, exposure of the subendothelial matrix leads to adhesion and activation of platelets and subsequent release of secondary agonists, TxA$_2$ and ADP. These two locally generated secondary agonists play a critical role in the sustained activation of GPIIb/IIIa receptors and stable platelet aggregation. Simultaneously, platelet activation exposes the phosphatidylserine surface providing binding sites for coagulation factors and the generation of large amounts of thrombin. Thrombin converts fibrinogen to fibrin and activates factor XIII which cross-links the fibrin network, and stabilizes the platelet-fibrin clot at the site of vascular injury. Since clot formation involves multiple pathways including platelet activation, aggregation, and coagulation, simultaneous blockade of these pathways is essential to prevent periprocedural and post-PCI ischemic events. Antiplatelet strategies include (**a**) inhibition of platelet cyclooxygenase-1 enzyme by aspirin; (**b**) inhibition of the P2Y$_{12}$ receptor by clopidogrel, prasugrel, ticagrelor, or cangrelor; and (**c**) inhibition of activated GPIIb/IIIa receptors by abciximab, eptifibatide, and tirofiban. Major antithrombotic agents include (**a**) indirect thrombin inhibitors such as heparin, and low-molecular-weight heparins; (**b**) direct thrombin inhibitors such as bivalirudin and dabigatran; and (**c**) direct Xa inhibitors such as rivaroxaban and apixaban. Key: *AT* antithrombin, *ADP* adenosine diphosphate, *TxA$_2$* thromboxane-A$_2$, *vWF* von Willebrand factor, *TF* tissue factor, *TP* thromboxane A$_2$ receptor, *PAR-1* protease-activated receptor-1, *GP* glycoprotein, *Factor II* prothrombin, *Factor IIa* thrombin. Adapted from Gurbel PA et al. *JACC Heart Fail.* 2014;2:1–14 [2]

- Optimal inhibition of these pathways is essential for maximizing antithrombotic effects and minimizing bleeding risk and is critically dependent on individual patient risk.

Antiplatelet Agents

Aspirin

- Aspirin remains the bedrock of antiplatelet treatment strategies in patients undergoing PCI. The antithrombotic property of aspirin is primarily attributed to irreversible acetylation of the platelet COX-1 enzyme. Subsequently, the generation of TxA_2- and TxA_2-induced platelet aggregation is inhibited.
- The optimal aspirin dose remains controversial. In the Clopidogrel Optimal Loading Dose Usage to Reduce Recurrent Events– Organization to Assess Strategies in Ischemic Syndromes (CURRENT OASIS-7) trial, aspirin 300–325 mg daily as compared to aspirin 75–100 mg daily was

associated with increased 30-day gastrointestinal bleeding, but there was no significant differences in the outcome of cardiovascular death, MI, or stroke and no differences in major bleeding observed between groups (Fig. 12.2) [3].
- Current revascularization guidelines recommend immediate treatment with an initial loading dose of non-enteric-coated aspirin 150–300 mg (or 80–150 mg IV) followed by a lifelong maintenance dose of 75–100 mg per day [4–6] (Table 12.1).
- The most common side effect of aspirin treatment is gastrointestinal intolerance.

P2Y$_{12}$ Receptor Blockers

The most widely used oral $P2Y_{12}$ receptor blockers are the thienopyridines (clopidogrel and prasugrel), and ticagrelor (Fig. 12.3). The European Commission issued marketing authorization for cangrelor, an intravenous $P2Y_{12}$ receptor blocker, in March 2015.

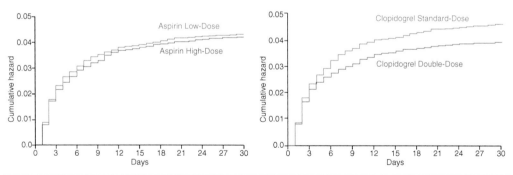

Cardiovascular Death, myocardial infraction or stroke

	Aspirin Low Dose	Aspirin High Dose	HR (95% CI, p value)	Clopidogrel Standard	Clopidogrel Double	HR (95% CI, p value)
CV Death/MI/Stroke (%)						
Overall (n=25,086)	4.4	4.2	0.97 (0.86-1.09), p=0.61	4.4	4.2	0.94 (0.83-1.06), p=0.30
PCI Cohort (n=17,263)	4.2	4.1	0.98 (0.84-1.13), p=0.73	4.5	3.9	0.86 (0.74-0.99), p=0.039
Myocardial Infraction (%)	2.4	2.3	0.97 (0.80-1.19), p=0.80	2.6	2.0	0.79 (0.64-0.96), p=0.018
CURENT Major Bleeding (%)	1.3	1.5	1.18 (0.92-1.53), p=0.20	1.1	1.6	1.41 (1.09-1.83), p=0.009

Fig. 12.2 Primary outcome in CURRENT OASIS 7 trial: invasive cohort. Adapted from Mehta et al. *Lancet.* 2010;376:1233–43 [3]

Table 12.1 European Society of Cardiology Guidelines for Myocardial Revascularization [4–6]

European Society of Cardiology Guidelines	Class of recommendation Level of evidence		
	SCAD	NSTEMI	STEMI
Pretreatment with antiplatelet therapy			
600 mg Clopidogrel in elective PCI patients once anatomy is known and decision to proceed with PCI preferably 2 h or more before the procedure	I A		
It is recommended to give P2Y12 inhibitors at the time of first medical contact			
Pretreatment with clopidogrel may be considered in patients with high probability for significant coronary artery disease	IIb C		
P2Y12 inhibitors at the time of first medical contact			
Pretreatment with prasugrel in patients whom coronary anatomy is not known is not recommended		III B	
Pretreatment with GP IIb/IIIa inhibitor in patients whom coronary anatomy is not known is not recommended		III A	
Upstream use of a GP IIb/IIIa inhibitor (vs. in-lab use) may be considered in high-risk patients undergoing transfer for primary PCI			
In patients on a maintenance dose of 75 mg clopidogrel, a new loading dose of 600 mg or more may be considered once the indication for PCI is confirmed	IIb C		
Clopidogrel 75 mg daily is indicated as an alternative in case of aspirin intolerance	I B		
Antiplatelet therapy during PCI			
ASA before elective stenting	I B		
ASA oral loading dose 150–300 mg (or 80–150 mg IV) if not pretreated	I C		
ASA is recommended for all patients without contraindications at an initial oral loading dose of 150–300 mg (or 80–150 mg IV) and a maintenance dose of 75–100 mg daily long-term regardless of treatment strategy		I A	I B
Clopidogrel (600 mg loading dose or more, 75 mg daily maintenance dose) for elective stenting	I A		
Cangrelor may be considered in $P2Y_{12}$ inhibitor-naive patients undergoing PCI		IIb A	IIb A
GP IIb/IIIa antagonists only for bailout or a thrombotic complication	IIa C	IIa C	IIa C
It is not recommended to administer GP IIb/IIIa inhibitors in patients in whom coronary anatomy is not known		III A	
Antiplatelet therapy after stenting			
$P2Y_{12}$ inhibitor administration in addition to aspirin beyond 1 year may be considered after careful assessment of the ischemic and bleeding risks of the patient		IIb A	
DAPT for at least 1 month after BMS implantation	I A		
DAPT for 6 months after DES implantation	I B		
Shorter DAPT duration (<6 months) may be considered after DES implantation in patients at high bleeding risk	IIb A		
Lifelong single-antiplatelet therapy, usually ASA	I A		

Table 12.1 (continued)

European Society of Cardiology Guidelines	Class of recommendation / Level of evidence		
	SCAD	NSTEMI	STEMI
Instruction of patients about the importance of complying with antiplatelet therapy	I C		
DAPT may be used for more than 6 months in patients at high ischemic risk and low bleeding risk	IIb C		
A P2Y$_{12}$ inhibitor is recommended in addition to ASA and maintained over 12 months unless there are contraindications such as excessive risk of bleeding. Options are:		I A	
• Prasugrel (60 mg loading dose, 10 mg daily dose) if no contraindication		I B	I A
• Ticagrelor (180 mg loading dose, 90 mg twice daily) if no contraindication		I B	I A
• Clopidogrel (600 mg loading dose, 75 mg daily dose), only when prasugrel or ticagrelor is not available or is contraindicated		I B	I A
GP IIb/IIIa antagonists should be considered for bailout situation or thrombotic complications		IIa C	
GP IIb/IIIa inhibitors should be considered for bailout or evidence of no-reflow or a thrombotic complication			IIa C
Upstream use of a GP IIb/IIIa inhibitor (vs. in-lab use) may be considered in high-risk patients undergoing transfer for primary PCI			
Anticoagulant therapy			
Unfractionated heparin 70–100 U/kg	I B		I C
Bivalirudin (0.75 mg/kg IV bolus followed by IV infusion of 1.75 mg/kg/h for up to 4 h after the procedure) in case of heparin-induced thrombocytopenia	I C		I C
Bivalirudin 0.75 mg/kg IV bolus followed by IV infusion of 1.75 mg/kg/h during the procedure in patients at high bleeding risk	IIa A		
Enoxaparin IV 0.5 mg/kg	IIa B		
Anticoagulation is recommended for all patients in addition to antiplatelet therapy during PCI		I A	I C
The anticoagulation is selected according to both ischemic and bleeding risks, and according to the efficacy–safety profile of the chosen agent		I C	
Bivalirudin (0.75 mg/kg IV bolus followed by IV infusion of 1.75 mg/kg/h for up to 4 h after the procedure) as alternative to UFH plus GP IIb/IIIa during PCI		I A	
UFH if patients cannot receive bivalirudin		I C	
UFH 70–100 IU/kg IV (50–70 IU/kg if concomitant with GPIIb/IIIa inhibitors) is recommended in patients undergoing PCI who did not receive any anticoagulant		I B	
In patients on fondaparinux (2.5 mg daily S.C.), a single-IV-bolus UFH (70–85 IU/kg, or 50–60 IU/kg) in the case of concomitant use of GP IIb/IIIa inhibitor during PCI		I B	
Enoxaparin should be considered as anticoagulant for PCI in patients pretreated with subcutaneous enoxaparin		IIa B	

(continued)

Table 12.1 (continued)

European Society of Cardiology Guidelines	Class of recommendation Level of evidence		
	SCAD	NSTEMI	STEMI
Discontinuation of anticoagulation should be considered after an invasive procedure unless otherwise indicated		IIa C	
Crossover of UFH and LMWH is not recommended		III B	
Unfractionated heparin: 70–100 U/kg IV bolus when no GP IIb/IIIa inhibitor is planned; 50–70 U/kg IV bolus with GP IIb/IIIa inhibitor			
Routine use of enoxaparin IV should be considered			IIa A
Routine use of bivalirudin should be considered			IIa A
Fondaparinux is not recommended for primary PCI			III B
Antithrombotic treatment in patients undergoing PCI who require oral anticoagulation			
Dual therapy of new oral anticoagulant and clopidogrel 75 mg/day may be considered as an alternative to initial triple therapy in selected patients	IIb B		
The use of ticagrelor and prasugrel as part of initial triple therapy is not recommended	III C		
In selected patients who receive ASA and clopidogrel, low-dose rivaroxaban (2.5 mg twice daily) may be considered in the setting of PCI for ACS if the patient is at low bleeding risk	IIb B		
It is recommended to use additional parenteral anticoagulation, regardless of the timing of the last dose of new oral anticoagulant	I C		
Periprocedural parenteral anticoagulants (bivalirudin, enoxaparin, or UFH) should be discontinued immediately after primary PCI	IIa C		
Platelet function testing or genetic testing may be considered in specific high-risk situations (e.g., history of stent thrombosis; compliance issue; suspicion of resistance; high bleeding risk)	IIb C		
Routine platelet function testing or genetic testing (clopidogrel and ASA) to adjust antiplatelet therapy before or after elective stenting is not recommended	III A		
It is recommended not to interrupt antiplatelet therapy within the recommended duration of treatment	I C		

Key: *SCAD* stable coronary artery disease, *NSTEMI* non-ST-segment-elevation myocardial infarction, *STEMI* ST-segment-elevation myocardial infarction, *PCI* percutaneous coronary intervention, *GP* glycoprotein, *ASA* acetylsalicylic acid, *DAPT* dual-antiplatelet therapy, *BMS* bare-metal stent, *DES* drug-eluting stent, *UFH* unfractionated heparin, *LMWH* low-molecular-weight heparin

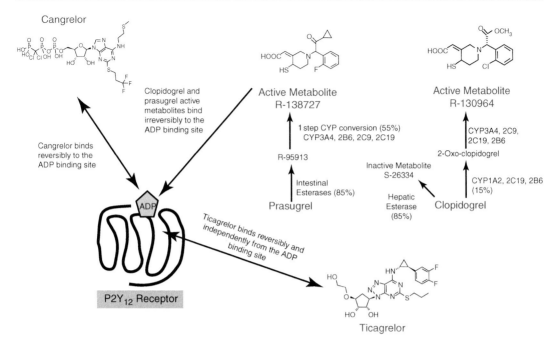

Fig. 12.3 Metabolism and mechanism of action of $P2Y_{12}$ inhibitors

Clopidogrel

- Clopidogrel, a second-generation thienopyridine, remains the most widely prescribed oral $P2Y_{12}$ receptor blocker. Following absorption, nearly ~85% of clopidogrel is hydrolyzed to an inactive carboxylic metabolite and the remaining 15% is rapidly and extensively metabolized by CYP450-dependent two-step process in liver to a highly unstable active metabolite R-130964. Plasma concentrations of the parent compound are below the detection limit beyond 2 h post-dosing. The active metabolite binds specifically and irreversibly to the platelet $P2Y_{12}$ receptor during passage through the hepatic circulation and inhibits the $P2Y_{12}$ receptor for the life span of platelets.

- Results of the earlier landmark trials strongly influenced the widely implemented strategy of dual-antiplatelet therapy for the PCI patient as the standard of care. In the CURRENT OASIS-7 trial a strategy of double-dose clopidogrel (600 mg on day 1, 150 mg on days 2–7, then 75 mg daily) was compared to standard-dose clopidogrel (300 mg on day 1, then 75 mg daily) in patients with ACS. In an analysis of 78% of patients who underwent PCI, double-dose clopidogrel therapy was associated with a 14% reduction in the rate of the primary outcome, 46% reduction in the secondary outcome of definite stent thrombosis, and 41% more CURRENT defined major bleeding (Fig. 12.2) [3].

- The presence of single-nucleotide polymorphisms (SNPs) of the gene encoding CYP450 2C19, particularly the loss-of-function (*LoF*) allele (*CYP2C19*2, *3, *4, and *5*), has been shown to be independently associated with reduced clopidogrel active metabolite generation, reduced inhibition of ADP-induced platelet aggregation, and increased post-PCI ischemic events. Measurements of ex vivo platelet function indicative of $P2Y_{12}$ receptor activity demonstrated a slow onset of action, wide response variability, and an absence of inhibition (resistance) in ~30% of patients undergoing PCI treated with a 300 mg clopidogrel added to aspirin therapy [5].

- In multiple studies of patients undergoing PCI, high on-treatment platelet reactivity during clopidogrel therapy was associated with an increased risk of ischemic event occurrence.

- Currently available evidence supports the concept of a threshold for on-treatment platelet reactivity to ADP in patients treated with dual-antiplatelet therapy that may be used to stratify patient risk for ischemic/thrombotic events following PCI, including stent thrombosis.
- Pharmacodynamic studies have demonstrated that therapy with potent $P2Y_{12}$ receptor blockers such as prasugrel or ticagrelor is an optimal strategy to overcome high on-treatment platelet reactivity and genetic polymorphisms [7].
- Selective, but not routine, platelet function testing or genetic testing may be considered in determining an antiplatelet strategy in patients with a history of stent thrombosis and in patients prior to undergoing high-risk PCI.

Prasugrel

- Prasugrel, a third-generation thienopyridine, is rapidly absorbed after oral administration with modest intra- and inter-recipient variability.
- Prasugrel is extensively hydrolyzed by intestinal and plasma esterases to an inactive short-lived thiolactone metabolite that is further metabolized to the pharmacologically active metabolite, R-138727, mainly by hepatic CYP3A4 and CYP2B6 in a one-step oxidation process (Fig. 12.3).
- Prasugrel is associated with a more rapid onset of action and greater active metabolite generation resulting in less response variability, a lower prevalence of non-responsiveness, and greater inhibition of ADP-induced platelet aggregation compared with clopidogrel.
- In the TRITON-TIMI 38 trial, in ACS patients undergoing planned PCI, prasugrel (60 mg load/10 mg daily maintenance) plus aspirin treatment (75–162 mg/day) was associated with a 19% reduction in the primary composite endpoint of cardiovascular death, nonfatal MI, and nonfatal stroke at a median 14.5-month

follow-up compared with clopidogrel (300 mg load/75 mg daily maintenance) plus aspirin treatment.

- However, these benefits were associated with significantly increased key safety end points of TIMI major bleeding, including life-threatening and fatal bleeding in patients treated with prasugrel as compared to clopidogrel (2.4% vs. 1.8%; $p < 0.03$) (Fig. 12.4) [8].
- Prasugrel is not recommended in patients with active pathological bleeding or a history of TIA or stroke.
- In patients ≥ 75 years of age, prasugrel is generally not recommended because of increased risk of fatal and intracranial bleeding and uncertain benefit.
- It is recommended not to start prasugrel therapy in patients likely to undergo urgent CABG. When possible, prasugrel should be discontinued at least 7 days before any surgery [4].
- In the Comparison of Prasugrel at the Time of Percutaneous Coronary Intervention or as Pretreatment at the Time of Diagnosis in Patients with Non-ST Elevation Myocardial Infarction (ACCOAST) trial, NSTE-ACS patients with positive troponin levels, scheduled to undergo coronary angiography within 2–48 h after randomization, were treated with either prasugrel 30 mg loading dose pre-angiography and 30 mg at PCI (pretreatment group) or 60 mg at PCI. The rate of the primary efficacy composite endpoint of cardiovascular death, MI, stroke, urgent revascularization, or glycoprotein IIb/IIIa bailout through day 7 did not differ between the treatment groups (HR, 95% CI = 1.02, 0.84–1.25; $p = 0.81$), but the key safety endpoint of TIMI major bleeding (CABG or non-CABG) was increased in pretreated patients (HR, 95% CI = 1.90, 1.19–3.02; $p = 0.006$). These results suggest that pretreatment with prasugrel in NSTE ACS patients is not beneficial in reducing ischemic risk but is associated with elevated bleeding risk [9].

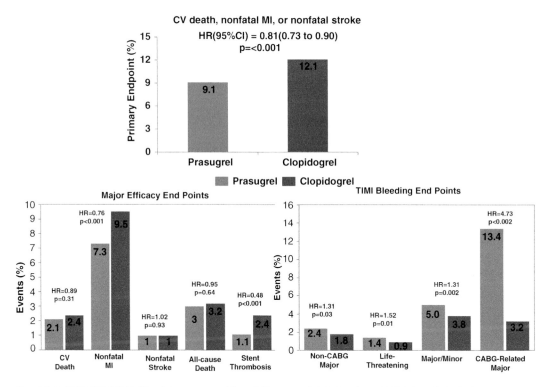

Fig. 12.4 TRITON TIMI 38 trial outcomes (Key: *MI* myocardial infarction, *TIMI* Thrombolysis in Myocardial Infarction, *HR* hazard ratio, *CI* confidence interval, *CV* cardiovascular, *CABG* coronary artery bypass graft) [8]

Ticagrelor

- Ticagrelor (AZD6140), a cyclopentyltriazo-lopyrimidine derivative, is an oral, reversibly binding, direct-acting $P2Y_{12}$ inhibitor.
- In stable coronary artery disease (CAD) patients, ticagrelor therapy was associated with a rapid onset of action, a greater level of inhibition that persisted during maintenance therapy, and a more rapid offset of pharmacodynamic action compared with clopidogrel [10].
- In a prespecified analysis of PLATO trial involving ACS patients in whom an invasive strategy was planned (72% of total patients), ticagrelor (180 mg loading/90 mg bid) versus clopidogrel (300–600 mg loading dose/75 mg per day) was associated with a significant reduction in the primary efficacy endpoint of CV death, MI, or stroke (event rate at 360 days = 9.0% vs. 10.7%, HR = 0·84, 95% CI = 0·75–0·94; p = 0·0025). Similarly, there

were significant reductions in the secondary key endpoints of all-cause death plus MI plus stroke (9.4% vs. 11.2%; p = 0.0016), all-cause death (3.9% vs. 5.0%; p = 0.013), and MI (5.3% vs. 6.6%; p = 0.0023) in favor of ticagrelor therapy (Fig. 12.5) [11].
- There were no differences in TIMI major bleeding (7.9% vs. 7.9%, p = 1.00), or TIMI non-CABG-related major bleeding (2.8% vs. 2.2%, p = 0.08) in patients treated with ticagrelor vs. clopidogrel.
- The ticagrelor benefit remained significant (vs. clopidogrel) whether or not patients were given standard or higher loading doses of clopidogrel, and in those already on clopidogrel at the start of the study.
- The PLATO trial demonstrated a significant reduction in mortality associated with ticagrelor therapy. An absence of clinical benefit associated was, however, noted among the

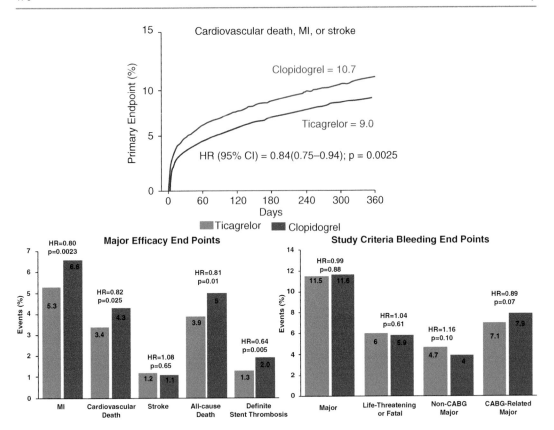

Fig. 12.5 PLATO trial outcomes: invasive cohort. Adapted from Cannon et al. *Lancet.* 2010;375:283–93 [11]. (Key: *MI* myocardial infarction, *HR* hazard ratio, *CI* confidence interval, *CABG* coronary artery bypass graft)

North American patient population enrolled in the PLATO trial. This has been attributed to the concomitant use of high-dose aspirin (aspirin >100 mg/day). Therefore, 75–81 mg per day aspirin is recommended in all patients treated with ticagrelor.

- Ticagrelor therapy is associated with side effects including dyspnea, which is rarely severe enough to cause discontinuation of treatment, and bradycardia.
- When possible, ticagrelor should be discontinued at least 5 days before surgery [4].
- In the ATLANTIC study, prehospital treatment with ticagrelor in STEMI patients was associated with a similar proportion of patients without ≥70% resolution of ST-segment elevation before PCI or the proportion of patients without TIMI flow grade 3 at initial angiography in the infarct-related artery as compared to in-hospital treatment. Similarly no differences in 30-day major adverse car-

diovascular events or bleeding events were also observed [12].

- The TWILIGHT (Ticagrelor With Aspirin or Alone in High-risk Patients After Coronary Intervention; ClinicalTrials.gov NCT02270242) study will determine the benefit of ticagrelor monotherapy alone versus ticagrelor plus low-dose aspirin for 12 months in reducing bleeding among high-risk patients undergoing PCI who have completed a 3-month course of aspirin plus ticagrelor.

Cangrelor

- Cangrelor is a parenterally administered adenosine triphosphate (ATP) analog with a short half-life (3–6 min), with rapid onset/offset of action, and dose-dependent and predictable pharmacodynamic effects.
- Cangrelor directly, reversibly, and competitively inhibits binding of ADP to the $P2Y_{12}$ receptor.

- In patients with stable CAD or ACS undergoing PCI in the CHAMPION-PHOENIX trial, a bolus and infusion of cangrelor therapy versus a loading dose of 600 mg or 300 mg of clopidogrel was associated with a significantly reduced primary endpoint of death, MI, ischemia-driven revascularization, or stent thrombosis at 48 h [4.7% vs. 5.9%, odds ratio (95% CI) = 0.78 (0.66–0.93), p = 0.005]. The primary safety endpoint of severe bleeding at 48 h was similar between the treatment groups [0.16% vs. 0.11% odds ratio (95% CI) = 1.50 (0.53–4.22), p = 0.44]. The rate of stent thrombosis was lower in the cangrelor group compared with clopidogrel group [0.8% vs. 1.4%, odds ratio (95%CI) = 0.62 (0.43–0.90), p = 0.01]. Furthermore, the benefits associated with cangrelor were consistent across the subgroups of stable angina (n = 1991), NSTEMI (n = 2810), and STEMI (n = 6138) (interaction, p = 0.98), and whether the patient received clopidogrel 300 mg LD or 600 mg LD (interaction, p = 0.61). GUSTO severe bleeding was similar between groups [13].
- Cangrelor has been recommended in Europe to be co-administered with aspirin, for the reduction of thrombotic cardiovascular events in adult patients with coronary artery disease undergoing PCI who have not received an oral $P2Y_{12}$ inhibitor prior to the PCI procedure and in whom oral therapy with $P2Y_{12}$ inhibitors is not feasible or desirable.

Glycoprotein (GP) IIb/IIIa Inhibitors

- The GPIIb/IIIa receptor, a member of the integrin family of receptors, is the most abundant platelet glycoprotein receptor (~80,000 per platelet).
- Platelet activation by various agonists and stimuli induces a conformational change in GPIIb/IIIa that markedly enhances its affinity for fibrinogen. The pharmacological agents that directly block the binding of fibrinogen to the GPIIb/IIIa receptor are more effective in inhibiting platelet aggregation than any oral antiplatelet strategy.

- In addition to inhibition of platelet aggregation, GPIIb/IIIa inhibitors also induce platelet disaggregation and may attenuate microembolization, and release of vasoconstrictors [14].
- All of the GPIIb/IIIa inhibitors have been associated with an increase in bleeding as compared to treatment with heparin alone. However, GPIIb/IIIa inhibitors are frequently incorrectly dosed, and overdosing has been associated with increased bleeding. Moreover, in current practice the activated clotting time target during the time of GPIIb/IIIa inhibitor use for PCI is lower than in earlier studies.
- Efficacy and increased safety have been reported with use of GPIIb/IIIa inhibitors in conjunction with heparin at activating clotting time (ACT) levels of 200–250 s [15].
- Most of the clinical trials demonstrating a favorable net clinical efficacy of GP IIb/IIIa inhibitor therapy predated the era of early invasive therapy, PCI with uniform or near-uniform stenting, and thienopyridine pretreatment. These older studies supported the upstream use of a GP IIb/IIIa inhibitor in combination with aspirin and an anticoagulant in high-risk patients.
- The efficacy of glycoprotein (GP) IIb/IIIa inhibitor therapy has been established particularly among high-risk patients undergoing PCI with elevated cardiac biomarkers, and diabetes. Most often, in the current era of PCI, GPIs are used for "bailout" when visible thrombus is present in the target vessel.
- According to guidelines, upstream use of GPI (vs. in-lab use) can be considered only in high-risk patients undergoing transfer for primary PCI and routine upstream use of GP IIb/IIIa inhibitor in NASTE-ACS patients undergoing angiography is not recommended.
- Following the development of fast-acting, potent oral $P2Y_{12}$ receptor blockers, such as prasugrel and ticagrelor, the use of GPIs in high-risk patients waned and now is more limited in current interventional practice as compared to two decades ago.
- Moreover, cangrelor, an intravenous $P2Y_{12}$ receptor antagonist with very fast onset and offset of action, represents a new strategy of

modulating peri-PCI platelet reactivity. The characteristics and recommended dosing of three commercially available GP IIb/IIIa inhibitors, abciximab, eptifibatide, and tirofiban, are given in Table 12.2.

Duration of Dual-Antiplatelet Therapy

- The optimal duration of DAPT after stenting is not yet clearly defined. The risk for recurrent thrombotic event occurrences following stenting is high during the first 3 months and thrombotic events continue to increase for at least 3 years.
- Complete stent endothelialization, the most desired outcome, has been observed within a month with bare-metal stent (BMS) implantation, whereas drug-eluting stent (DES) implantation has been associated with highly suppressed early healing and poor endothelial cell coverage that may persist for years.
- In addition, recent randomized clinical trials (RCT's) of longer duration DAPT suggested a continued reduction of thrombotic events at about 3 years in patients treated with prolonged DAPT and this event reduction was mostly observed in non-culprit lesion vessels. In this line, the duration of DAPT appears dependent on stent type (BMS vs. earlier generation DES vs. newer generation DES vs. biodegradable stents), presence or absence of prior MI, balance between ischemic and bleeding risk, and cost versus benefit.
- There are numerous trials that have investigated the duration of DAPT in patients treated with bare-metal stents and drug-eluting stents including newer generation stents. Since none of these trials are powered for ischemic endpoints; all were open label and the time for stenting to randomization varied among these trials.

Table 12.2 GPIIb/IIIa inhibitors: properties and administration

	Abciximab	Eptifibatide	Tirofiban
Type	Antibody fab fragment	Synthetic cyclic heptapeptide	Nonpeptide mimetic
Molecular weight	Large molecule (47.6 KDa)	Small molecule (832 Da)	Small molecule (495 Da)
Receptor specificity	Nonspecific (GPIIb/IIIa, vitronectin, Mac-1)	Specific for GPIIb/IIIa	Specific for GPIIb/IIIa
Mechanism of receptor inhibition	Irreversible; steric hindrance and conformational change	Reversible: Competitive inhibition (KGD recognition sequence)	Reversible: Competitive inhibition (RGD recognition sequence)
Receptor binding	Long acting, high affinity	Short acting, low affinity	Short acting, low affinity
Plasma half-life	10–30 min	~2.5 h	~2 h
Platelet function recovery	~48 h	4–8 h	4–8 h
Elimination route	Senescent platelets (spleen)	Renal (50%)	Renal (65%)
Administration: Normal renal function	Bolus 0.25 mg/kg IV Infusion 0.125 µg/kg/min (max.10 µg/min) for 12 h	Double bolus 180 µg/kg IV (at 20-min interval) Infusion 2 µg/kg/min for 18 h	25 ug/kg within 3 min and then 0.15 ug/kg/min for 18 h
Renal insufficiency	No specific recommendations Careful consideration of bleeding risk	**GFR < 50 mL/min/1.73 m²** No adjustment of bolus, reduce infusion rate to 1 µg/kg/min	**GFR ≤ 60 mL/min/1.73 m²** 25 ug/kg within 5 min and then 0.075 ug/kg/min
Severe renal insufficiency (GFR < 30 mL/min/1.73 m²)		Contraindicated in severe renal insufficiency	

- Numerous meta-analyses have also addressed the duration of DAPT. Based on the available evidence, it is recommended that DAPT be administered for at least 1 month after BMS implantation in stable CAD, for 6 months after new-generation DES implantation in stable CAD, and for up to 1 year in patients after ACS, irrespective of revascularization strategy [4].
- In the DAPT study, 9961 patients treated with standard thienopyridine therapy (clopidogrel or prasugrel) and aspirin for 12 months and who were without any ischemic or bleeding events were randomly assigned to receive DAPT or aspirin alone for another 18 months. The prolonged DAPT therapy was associated with a 71% relative (1% absolute) reduction in stent thrombosis ($p < 0.001$), a 53% relative (2.0% absolute) reduction in MI ($p < 0.001$), a 29% relative (1.6% absolute) reduction in

major adverse cardiovascular and cerebrovascular events ($p < 0.001$), and a 1.0% absolute increase in GUSTO moderate or severe bleeding ($p = 0.001$) (Fig. 12.6) [16].
- Trials of prolonged or extended DAPT suggest that the benefit/risk ratio of prolonged DAPT may be more favorable for those with prior MI, with an absolute decrease in ischemic events of ≈1% to 2% at the cost of an absolute increase in bleeding events of ≈1% over the course of several years of prolonged or extended therapy (median durations of therapy: 18–33 months) [17].
- A new risk score (the "DAPT score"), derived from the DAPT study, may be useful for decisions about whether to continue (prolong or extend) in patients treated with coronary stent implantation (Table 12.3) [18].
- The PEGASUS-TIMI 54 study provided some evidence regarding the long-term efficacy of

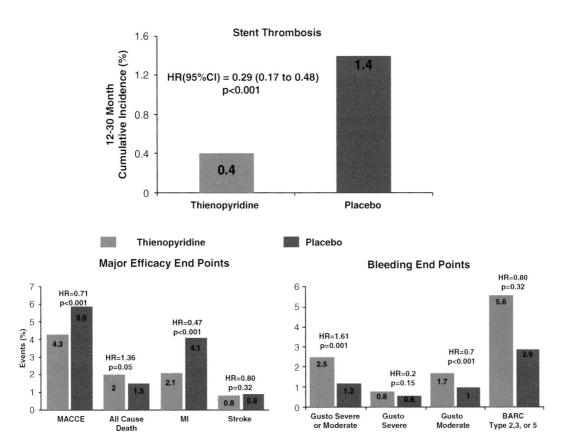

Fig. 12.6 DAPT trial outcomes [16]. (Key: *HR* hazard ratio, *MACCE* major adverse cardiovascular and cerebrovascular events, *MI* myocardial infarction, *BARC* bleeding academic research consortium)

Table 12.3 Factors used to calculate a "DAPT score"

Variable	Points
Age ≥75 years	-2
Age 65 to <75 years	-1
Age <65 years	0
Current cigarette smoker	1
Diabetes mellitus	1
Myocardial infarction at presentation	1
Prior percutaneous coronary intervention or prior myocardial infarction	1
Stent diameter <3 mm	1
Paclitaxel-eluting stent	1
Congestive heart failure or left ventricular ejection fraction <30%	2
Saphenous vein graft percutaneous coronary intervention	2

A score of ≥2 is associated with a favorable benefit/risk ratio for prolonged DAPT while a score of <2 is associated with an unfavorable benefit/risk ratio

Adapted from Levine et al. *J Am Coll Cardiol.* 2016;68:1082–115 [17]

ticagrelor therapy in the setting of post-MI and post-PCI. Here 21,162 patients (83% underwent PCI), 1–3 years post-MI, were treated with 90 mg bid ticagrelor, 60 mg bid ticagrelor, or placebo in addition to low-dose aspirin for a median duration of 33 months. Prolonged ticagrelor therapy was associated with 14–15% reduction in the primary efficacy endpoint of CV death, MI, or stroke, but 2.3–2.7-fold increased risk for clinically significant bleeding. However, the 60 mg dose was associated with a better safety and tolerability profile with numerically lower rates of bleeding and other side effects such as dyspnea. In light of this, the European Medicines Agency in October 2016 recommended a 60 mg twice-daily dose when an extended treatment (for up to 3 years) is required for patients with a history of MI of at least 1 year earlier and a high risk of an atherothrombotic event [19].

Antithrombotics

Indirect Thrombin Inhibitors

- Unfractionated heparin (UFH) is a heterogeneous mixture of polysaccharide molecules. The pentasaccharide sequence of UFH binds to antithrombin and enhances the inhibition of thrombin and also factor Xa.
- UFH binds plasma proteins strongly, leading to unpredictable levels of free heparin in the circulation. UFH therefore exhibits significant variability in antithrombotic effect and requires close monitoring.
- Most of the benefits of UFH are short term. Its other disadvantages include the need for continuous intravenous administration and the infrequent but serious complication of immunogenic heparin-induced thrombocytopenia. Despite this, UFH is the standard of care for prevention of thrombus generation in the setting of PCI in all patients.
- Low-molecular-weight heparins (LMWHs) were developed with the goal of providing improved anticoagulation over that of UFH.
- LMWHs have less direct effect on thrombin, less plasma binding, better bioavailability, less platelet activation, and more effect on factor Xa, and a lower risk of immune-mediated thrombocytopenia than UFH.
- LMWH therapy can be administered subcutaneously on a weight basis and does not require dose adjustments or monitoring. Patients with renal insufficiency require lower dosing of LMWHs, since LMWH is mainly cleared by the kidneys.
- In the STEEPLE trial, the primary endpoint of 48-h non-CABG-related bleeding was lower with low-dose enoxaparin (0.5 mg/kg) but not with the higher dose (0.75 mg/kg) as compared to UFH, whereas major bleeding was decreased with similar efficacy with both doses as compared to UFH in stable CAD patients undergoing PCI.
- The enoxaparin low-dose therapy was stopped prematurely because of a nonsignificant trend towards excess mortality not related to ischemic events and not confirmed at 1 year of follow-up [20].
- In recent studies, enoxaparin therapy did not demonstrate increased benefit over UFH when pre-randomization anticoagulation was not consistent with the study treatment or when there was a post-randomization crossover.
- In the ATOLL trial, enoxaparin (0.5 mg/kg) did not significantly reduce the primary composite endpoint of death, MI, procedure

failure, or major bleeding as compared to UFH ($p = 0.069$) and there was no indication for higher incidence of bleeding with enoxaparin versus UFH in patients undergoing primary PCI.

- In the per-protocol analysis of the ATOLL trial, that included 87% of patients, enoxaparin was superior to UFH in reducing the primary endpoint (relative risk 0.76, $p = 0.012$), mortality (RR = 0.46, $p = 0.05$), and major bleeding (RR = 0.46, $p = 0.0002$) [21].
- Based on these favorable results, enoxaparin with or without GPI should be considered as an alternative to UFH for primary PCI according to European guidelines [4].

Fondaparinux

- Fondaparinux, an indirect factor Xa inhibitor, is a synthetic pentasaccharide that binds (reversibly with high affinity) to antithrombin III, thereby catalyzing the antithrombin III-mediated inhibition of factor Xa.
- Fondaparinux is not preferred during PCI due to the risk of catheter thrombosis [4].
- In NSTE-ACS patients undergoing PCI in the OASIS 5 trial (6239 out of 22,078 patients), fondaparinux 2.5 mg subcutaneous once-daily dose as compared to enoxaparin was associated with significantly lower major bleeding (including access-site complications) at 9 days (2.3% vs. 5.1%, HR = 0.45, $p < 0.001$). Catheter thrombus formation, however, was observed more frequently with fondaparinux (0.9% vs. 0.4%) and was abolished by injection of an empirically determined bolus of UFH at the time of PCI.
- Therefore, a single-bolus UFH (85 IU/kg, or 60 IU/kg in the case of concomitant use of GP IIb/IIIa receptor inhibitors) is indicated during PCI in patients with NSTEMI treated with fondaparinux.

Direct Thrombin Inhibitors

- Direct thrombin inhibitors are small molecules that bind to thrombin (both fluid phase and fibrin bound) and block thrombin-induced conversion of fibrinogen to fibrin and activation of FV, FVII, and FIX. They have limited interaction with plasma proteins and cells, making dosing and bioavailability much more predictable.
- The major direct thrombin inhibitors available are dabigatran, argatroban, and bivalirudin of which bivalirudin is widely used during coronary intervention.
- In the ISAR-REACT-3 trial, among stable CAD patients undergoing PCI and pretreated with clopidogrel, bivalirudin (bolus 0.75 mg/kg; infusion 1.75 mg/kg/h) showed similar net clinical outcomes as compared with UFH, but higher-than-recommended dosage of UFH (140 IU/kg) was attributed to excess major bleeding [22]. A lower dose of UFH (100 IU/kg) was associated with similar major bleeding as compared to bivalirudin and a trend towards less ischemic events in the UFH arm [23].
- Therefore, UFH is the standard anticoagulant treatment for elective PCI and bivalirudin should be considered in patients at high risk of bleeding.
- In the ACUITY trial, moderate- to high-risk patients ($n = 13,819$) with NSTE-ACS managed with contemporary pharmacotherapy and undergoing an early invasive strategy were randomized to UFH or enoxaparin plus planned GPI, bivalirudin plus planned GPI, or bivalirudin monotherapy.
- Bivalirudin monotherapy met non-inferiority criteria with respect to the 30-day primary ischemic endpoint (death, MI, or unplanned revascularization), with a significantly lower risk of major bleeding [24]. Among patients who underwent PCI ($n = 7789$) (57% received PCI through femoral access), there was no difference in the primary ischemic endpoint or stent thrombosis, but bivalirudin monotherapy was associated with a significant reduction in major bleeding, minor bleeding, and transfusion requirements (Fig. 12.7) [25].
- In the ISAR-REACT 4 trial, the safety and efficacy of bivalirudin monotherapy versus UFH plus GPI in NSTE-ACS patients undergoing PCI through femoral access and pretreated with clopidogrel were assessed. This

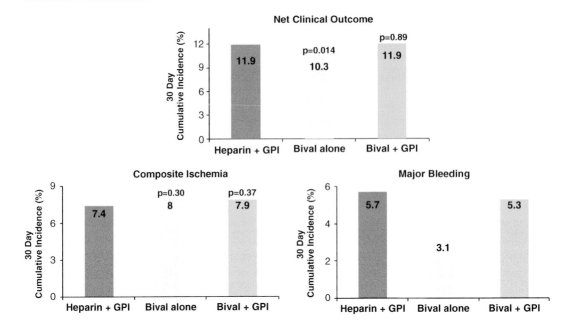

Fig. 12.7 ACUITY trial outcomes [24]. (1) Composite ischemia endpoint = death from any cause, myocardial infarction, or unplanned revascularization for ischemia. (2) Major bleeding = not related to CABG. (3) Net clinical outcome endpoint = the composite ischemia endpoint or major bleeding. (Key: *Bival* bivalirudin, *GPI* glycoprotein inhibitor)

trial provided further evidence in favor of bivalirudin with similar primary ischemic endpoint and significantly lower major bleeding that was attributed to lower access-site bleeding [26]. It should be noted that most of the evidence in support of bivalirudin was derived from trials where it was compared to UFH plus GPI, a combination which is no longer routinely implemented in the current practice.

- In the HORIZON-AMI trial, among patients with STEMI undergoing primary PCI through femoral access (93%), bivalirudin plus provisional GPI was found to be superior to UFH plus routine GPIs with respect to 30-day major bleeding (4.9% vs. 8.3%, RR = 0.60, $p = 0.001$) and 30-day net adverse clinical events including all-cause death, reinfarction, repeat revascularization, definite stent thrombosis, stroke, or major bleeding (9.2% vs. 121.1%, RR = 0.76, $p = 0.005$). The clinical benefit of bivalirudin therapy persisted for 3 years. However, a higher incidence of stent thrombosis was observed during the first 24 h in the bivalirudin arm (1.3% vs. 0.3%,

$p < 0.001$), but no difference was observed at 30 days. Pre-randomization use of UFH and 600 mg loading dose of clopidogrel were independent predictors of lower risk of acute and subacute stent thrombosis [27].

- The recent EUROMAX trial compared a strategy of prehospital bivalirudin therapy with UFH or LMWH with optional use of GPIs (69%) in 2218 STEMI patients, with frequent use of radial access (47%) and pretreatment with $P2Y_{12}$ inhibitors (98%). Prehospital use of bivalirudin was associated with significantly lower 30-day primary endpoint of death or non-CABG major bleeding as compared to UFH group (5.1% vs. 8.5%, RR = 0.60, $p < 0.001$) that was driven by a significant reduction in major bleeding (2.6% vs. 6.0%, RR = 0.43, $p < 0.001$). Similar to HORIZON-AMI, 30-day stent thrombosis was more frequent in the bivalirudin group (1.6 vs. 0.5%, RR = 2.89, $p = 0.002$) that was solely driven by a difference during the first 24 h and was paralleled by a trend towards a higher rate of re-infarction (1.7% vs. 0.9%, RR = 1.93, $p = 0.08$) despite the use of prasugrel and ticagrelor in more than half of patients. Again, the mortality benefit observed in the HORIZON-AMI trial was not demonstrated in the EUROMAX trial [28].

- The HEAT-PPCI trial compared bivalirudin ($n = 905$) with UFH alone ($n = 907$) in STEMI patients who were planned to undergo primary PCI. In this trial, GPI use was allowed only for bailout (15%), and prasugrel or ticagrelor, and radial access was frequently used (89% and 80% of patients, respectively). Bivalirudin therapy was associated with higher rates of the 30-day primary composite endpoint of all-cause death, cerebrovascular accidents, recurrent infarction, and urgent target-vessel revascularization (8.7% vs. 5.7%, HR = 1.52, $p = 0.01$), and stent thrombosis (3.4% vs. 0.9%, RR = 3.91, $p = 0.001$). Bivalirudin had a similar primary safety endpoint of major BARC 3–5 bleeding (3.5% vs. 3.1%, $p = 0.59$) and similar mortality rate (5.1% vs. 4.3%) as compared to UFH therapy.

- Finally, the results of these trials further reinforced the higher risk of stent thrombosis associated with bivalirudin therapy as compared to UFH without systematic use of GPIs while there were small differences in major bleeding [29]. These concerns were reflected in the recent European guidelines that downgraded the recommendation for the use of bivalirudin in primary PCI from Class I A to Class IIa A [4].

Non-vitamin K Oral Anticoagulants

Factor Xa Inhibitors

- Direct factor Xa inhibitors apixaban, rivaroxaban, darexaban, and otamixaban have been, or, are currently being, investigated in patients with ACS, either in the acute phase during intervention or in the secondary prevention after the acute event.

- In the preplanned interim analysis of the TAO trial, otamixaban did not reduce the rate of ischemic events relative to unfractionated heparin plus eptifibatide but did increase bleeding in patients with NSTE-ACS undergoing planned early PCI [30].

- In the landmark ATLAS-ACS 2 TIMI 51 trial that enrolled patients with recent ACS, low-dose rivaroxaban (2.5 mg bid, 25% of the total dose used for atrial fibrillation), added to aspirin and clopidogrel, reduced major cardiovascular adverse events (9.1% vs. 10.7%, $p = 0.02$), and cardiovascular death (2.7% vs. 4.1%, $p = 0.002$) and all-cause death (2.9% vs. 4.5%, $p = 0.002$), but with an increased risk of non-CABG major bleeding (1.8% vs. 0.6%, $p < 0.001$) and intracranial hemorrhage (0.4% vs. 0.2%, $p = 0.04$) but not the risk of fatal bleeding. In this study, time from index event to randomization was 4.7 days and ~60% of patients underwent PCI or CABG for the index event [31].

- The APPRAISE trial (a phase III trial) that compared 5 mg bid apixaban (full dose) added to DAPT vs. DAPT alone in high-risk ACS patients was prematurely stopped due to excess bleeding risk in the absence of benefit with respect to ischemic outcomes [32].

- In the WOEST trial, 573 patients undergoing PCI were randomized to receive clopidogrel plus oral anticoagulant (double therapy) or clopidogrel plus aspirin plus oral anticoagulant (triple therapy) for 30 days after BMS placement (35%) and 1 year for DES placement (65%). The primary endpoint of any TIMI bleeding was significantly lower in the dual-therapy arm (19.5% vs. 44.9%, HR = 0.49, $p < 0.001$). Furthermore, dual therapy was associated with similar rates of MI, stroke, target-vessel revascularization, or stent thrombosis but lower all-cause death [33].

- In the PIONEER AF-PCI trial, in patients with atrial fibrillation undergoing PCI with stenting, the administration of either 15 mg once daily rivaroxaban plus a $P2Y_{12}$ inhibitor or 2.5 mg twice-daily rivaroxaban was associated with a lower rate of clinically significant bleeding than was standard therapy with a vitamin K antagonist plus DAPT and a similar rate of the efficacy endpoint of CV death, MI, or stroke [34].

- Based on encouraging results from above trials, the safety of 2.5 mg bid rivaroxaban was compared to 100 mg daily aspirin on top of clopidogrel or ticagrelor in patients with MI in the GEMINI-ACS trial and >84% of patients were stented. Randomized therapy was started a median of 5.5 days after the index event and continued a median of 291 days. The primary endpoint of TIMI non-CABG clinically significant bleeding and the composite exploratory ischemic endpoint (cardiovascular death, MI, stroke, or definite stent thrombosis) were similar between groups. In a *post hoc* analysis, rivaroxaban was associated with numerically higher occurrence of the primary and ischemic composite endpoints in the first 30 days, but thereafter safety and efficacy appeared the same. There was numerically more ISTH and BARC 3 bleeding with rivaroxaban [35]. GEMINI-ACS was not powered for ischemic outcomes, and conclusions about the comparative efficacy of aspirin versus low-dose rivaroxaban cannot be made, but there was no signal of an antithrombotic benefit of rivaroxaban over aspirin [36].

- In summary, evidence supports the benefit of addition of low-dose Xa inhibitor in high-risk ACS patients treated with aspirin and clopidogrel who were stabilized after an index event. Far more robust evidence is required to support the addition of a low-dose oral Xa inhibitor on top of DAPT with ticagrelor or prasugrel or to replace aspirin with a Xa inhibitor in high-risk ACS patients undergoing PCI or stabilized after PCI.

Summary of Current Evidence

- Ischemic events during and following PCI are strongly influenced by platelet function and coagulation; simultaneous blockade of these pathways is essential to reduce ischemic events. Optimal inhibition of these pathways is needed for maximizing total antithrombotic effects. Minimizing bleeding risk is also a critical goal in the treatment of the PCI patient.
- Aspirin remains the bedrock oral antiplatelet agent. The totality of evidence supports dual-antiplatelet therapy with aspirin plus a $P2Y_{12}$ receptor blocker as the standard of care during and following PCI.

- Both of the newer oral $P2Y_{12}$ inhibitors, prasugrel and ticagrelor, are associated with a faster onset of action, greater platelet inhibition, and lower on-treatment platelet reactivity than clopidogrel. These superior pharmacodynamic properties have translated into lower ischemic outcomes as compared to clopidogrel in the treatment of the ACS/PCI patient. However, greater non-CABG-related major bleeding was associated with prasugrel and ticagrelor therapy.
- The new intravenous $P2Y_{12}$ receptor blocker, cangrelor, is associated with a faster onset and offset of effect and represents a new strategy of modulating peri-PCI platelet reactivity. It has been associated with lower ischemic event rates than clopidogrel loading at the time of PCI. The clinical efficacy of cangrelor has never been evaluated in patients treated with prasugrel or ticagrelor.
- The pharmacological agents that directly block the binding of fibrinogen to the GPIIb/IIIa receptor (GPIIb/IIIa inhibitors) are highly effective and more potent in inhibiting platelet aggregation than cangrelor. The increased use of the $P2Y_{12}$ inhibitors with a rapid onset of potent pharmacodynamic effects (prasugrel, ticagrelor, or cangrelor) may challenge the role of GPIIb/IIIa inhibitors in the treatment of the PCI patient. There have been no head-to-head clinical studies of cangrelor versus GPIs.
- The optimal duration of DAPT in patients treated with PCI remains controversial. Based on the available evidence, it is recommended that DAPT be administered for at least 1 month after BMS implantation in stable CAD, for 6 months after new-generation DES implantation in stable CAD, and for up to 1 year in patients after ACS.
- Recent randomized trials in patients treated with new-generation coronary artery stents have suggested shorter duration DAPT. However these trials were underpowered.
- The DAPT and PEGASUS trials compared the efficacy of long-term (>12 months) $P2Y_{12}$ inhibitor therapy on top of aspirin. Both trials demonstrated enhanced efficacy of long-term DAPT at the expense of greater bleeding.

- In addition to antiplatelet therapy, anticoagulation is recommended in ACS patients undergoing PCI. Current choices are heparin, UFH, and bivalirudin.
- Evidence supports the benefit of adding low-dose Xa inhibitor in high-risk ACS patients who are stabilized after the index event and treated with aspirin and clopidogrel.
- Stronger evidence is required to support the addition of a low-dose oral Xa inhibitor on top of DAPT with ticagrelor or prasugrel or to replace aspirin with a low-dose Xa inhibitor in high-risk ACS patients undergoing PCI.

References

1. Tantry US, Etherington A, Bliden KP, Gurbel PA. Antiplatelet therapy: current strategies and future trends. Future Cardiol. 2006;2:343–66.
2. Gurbel PA, Tantry US. Antiplatelet and anticoagulant agents in heart failure: current status and future perspectives. JACC Heart Fail. 2014;2:1–14.
3. Mehta SR, Tanguay JF, Eikelboom JW, et al. CURRENT-OASIS 7 trial investigators. Double-dose versus standard-dose clopidogrel and high-dose versus low-dose aspirin in individuals undergoing percutaneous coronary intervention for acute coronary syndromes (CURRENT-OASIS 7): a randomised factorial trial. Lancet. 2010;376:1233–43.
4. Windecker S, Kolh P, Alfonso F, et al. 2014 ESC/EACTS Guidelines on myocardial revascularization: The Task Force on Myocardial Revascularization of the European Society of Cardiology (ESC) and the European Association for Cardio-Thoracic Surgery (EACTS)Developed with the special contribution of the European Association of Percutaneous Cardiovascular Interventions (EAPCI). Eur Heart J. 2014;35:2541–619.
5. Roffi M, Patrono C, Collet JP, et al. Management of Acute Coronary Syndromes in Patients Presenting without Persistent ST-Segment Elevation of the European Society of Cardiology. 2015 ESC Guidelines for the management of acute coronary syndromes in patients presenting without persistent ST-segment elevation: Task Force for the Management of Acute Coronary Syndromes in Patients Presenting without Persistent ST-Segment Elevation of the European Society of Cardiology (ESC). Eur Heart J. 2016;37:267–315.
6. Steg PG, James SK, Atar D, et al. ESC Guidelines for the management of acute myocardial infarction in patients presenting with ST-segment elevation. Eur Heart J. 2012;33:2569–619.
7. Tantry US, Bonello L, Aradi D, et al. Working Group on On-Treatment Platelet Reactivity. Consensus and update on the definition of on-treatment platelet reactivity to adenosine diphosphate associated with ischemia and bleeding. J Am Coll Cardiol. 2013;62:2261–73.
8. Wiviott SD, Braunwald E, McCabe CH, et al. TRITON-TIMI 38 Investigators. Prasugrel versus clopidogrel in patients with acute coronary syndromes. N Engl J Med. 2007;357:2001–15.
9. Montalescot G, Bolognese L, Dudek D, et al. ACCOAST Investigators. Pretreatment with prasugrel in non-ST-segment elevation acute coronary syndromes. N Engl J Med. 2013;369:999–1010.
10. Gurbel PA, Bliden KP, Butler K, et al. Randomized double-blind assessment of the ONSET and OFFSET of the antiplatelet effects of ticagrelor versus clopidogrel in patients with stable coronary artery disease: the ONSET/OFFSET study. Circulation. 2009;120:2577–85.
11. Cannon CP, Harrington RA, James S, et al. PLATelet Inhibition and Patient Outcomes Investigators. Comparison of ticagrelor with clopidogrel in patients with a planned invasive strategy for acute coronary syndromes (PLATO): a randomised double-blind study. Lancet. 2010;375:283–93.
12. Montalescot G, van 't Hof AW, Lapostolle F, et al. ATLANTIC Investigators. Prehospital ticagrelor in ST-segment elevation myocardial infarction. N Engl J Med. 2014;371:1016–27.
13. Bhatt DL, Stone GW, Mahaffey KW, et al. CHAMPION PHOENIX Investigators. Effect of platelet inhibition with cangrelor during PCI on ischemic events. N Engl J Med. 2013;368:1303–13.
14. Lefkovits J, Plow EF, Topol EJ. Platelet glycoprotein IIb/IIIa receptors in cardiovascular medicine. N Engl J Med. 1995;332:1553–9.
15. Hanna EB, Rao SV, Manoukian SV, Saucedo JF. The evolving role of glycoprotein IIb/IIIa inhibitors in the setting of percutaneous coronary intervention strategies to minimize bleeding risk and optimize outcomes. JACC Cardiovasc Interv. 2010;3:1209–19.
16. Mauri L, Kereiakes DJ, Yeh RW, et al. DAPT study Investigators. Twelve or 30 months of dual antiplatelet therapy after drug-eluting stents. N Engl J Med. 2014;371:2155–66.
17. Levine GN, Bates ER, Bittl JA, et al. 2016 ACC/AHA Guideline Focused Update on Duration of Dual Antiplatelet Therapy in Patients With Coronary Artery Disease: A Report of the American College of Cardiology/American Heart Association Task Force on Clinical Practice Guidelines. J Am Coll Cardiol. 2016;68:1082–115.
18. Yeh RW, Secemsky EA, Kereiakes DJ, et al. DAPT Study Investigators. Development and validation of a prediction rule for benefit and harm of dual antiplatelet therapy beyond 1 year after percutaneous coronary intervention. JAMA. 2016;315:1735–49.
19. Bonaca MP, Bhatt DL, Cohen M, et al. PEGASUS-TIMI 54 Steering Committee and Investigators. Long-term use of ticagrelor in patients with prior myocardial infarction. N Engl J Med. 2015;372:1791–800.

20. Montalescot G, White HD, Gallo R, et al. Enoxaparin vs. unfractionated heparin in elective percutaneous coronary intervention. N Engl J Med. 2006;355:1006–17.

21. Collet J-P, Huber K, Cohen M, et al. A direct comparison of intravenous enoxaparin with unfractionated heparin in primary percutaneous coronary intervention (from the ATOLL trial). Am J Cardiol. 2013;112:1367–72.

22. Kastrati A, Neumann FJ, Mehilli J, et al. Bivalirudin vs. unfractionated heparin during percutaneous coronary intervention. N Engl J Med. 2008;359:688–96.

23. Schulz S, Mehilli J, Neumann FJ, et al. Intracoronary Stenting and Antithrombotic Regimen: Rapid Early Action for Coronary Treatment (ISAR-REACT) 3A Trial Investigators. ISAR-REACT 3A: a study of reduced dose of unfractionated heparin in biomarker negative patients undergoing percutaneous coronary intervention. Eur Heart J. 2010;31:2482–91.

24. Stone GW, McLaurin BT, Cox DA, et al. Bivalirudin for patients with acute coronary syndromes. N Engl J Med. 2006;355:2203–16.

25. Stone GW, White HD, Ohman EM, et al. Acute Catheterization and Urgent Intervention Triage strategy (ACUITY) Trial Investigators. Bivalirudin in patients with acute coronary syndromes undergoing percutaneous coronary intervention: a subgroup analysis from the Acute Catheterization and Urgent Intervention Triage strategy (ACUITY) trial. Lancet. 2007;369:907–19.

26. Kastrati A, Neumann F-J, Schulz S, et al. Abciximab and heparin vs. bivalirudin for non-ST-elevation myocardial infarction. N Engl J Med. 2011;365:1980–9.

27. Stone GW, Witzenbichler B, Guagliumi G, et al. HORIZONS-AMI Trial Investigators. Bivalirudin during primary PCI in acute myocardial infarction. N Engl J Med. 2008;358:2218–30.

28. Steg PG, van 't Hof AW, Hamm CW, et al. Bivalirudin started during emergency transport for primary PCI. N Engl J Med. 2013;369:2207–17.

29. Shahzad A, Kemp I, Mars C, et al. for the HEAT-PPCI trial investigators. Unfractionated heparin versus bivalirudin in primary percutaneous coronary intervention (HEAT-PPCI): an open-label, single centre, randomized controlled trial. Lancet. 2014;384:1848.

30. Steg PG, Mehta SR, Pollack CV Jr, Investigators TAO. Anticoagulation with otamixaban and ischemic events in non-ST-segment elevation acute coronary syndromes: the TAO randomized clinical trial. JAMA. 2013;310:1145–55.

31. Mega JL, Braunwald E, Wiviott SD, et al., the AACSTIRivaroxaban in patients with a recent acute coronary syndrome. N Engl J Med. 2012;366:9–19.

32. Alexander JH, Lopes RD, James S, et al. Apixaban with antiplatelet therapy after acute coronary syndrome. N Engl J Med. 2011;365:699–708.

33. Dewilde WJ, Oirbans T, Verheugt FW, et al. Use of clopidogrel with or without aspirin in patients taking oral anticoagulant therapy and undergoing percutaneous coronary intervention: an open label, randomised, controlled trial. Lancet. 2013;381:1107–15.

34. Gibson CM, Mehran R, Bode C, et al. Prevention of bleeding in patients with atrial fibrillation undergoing PCI. N Engl J Med. 2016;375:2423–34.

35. Ohman EM, Roe MT, Steg PG, et al. Clinically significant bleeding with low-dose rivaroxaban versus aspirin, in addition to P2Y12 inhibition, in acute coronary syndromes (GEMINI-ACS-1): a double-blind, multicentre, randomised trial. Lancet. 2017;389:1799–808.

36. Gurbel PA, Tantry US. GEMINI-ACS-1: toward unearthing the antithrombotic therapy cornerstone for acute coronary syndromes. Lancet. 2017;89:1773–5.

Adjunctive Technologies (Rotablation, Excimer Laser, Aspiration Thrombectomy, Distal Embolic Protection)

13

Michael S. Lee and Jeremy Kong

About Us The UCLA Medical Center team of physicians, nurses, and health professionals provide comprehensive cardiovascular care and offer the most advanced treatments available, ranging from catheter-based coronary and structural heart interventions and heart transplantations. Most recently, UCLA Medical Center is the world's leader in the research of coronary orbital atherectomy. In addition to being one of the nation's largest heart and lung transplant programs, UCLA provides state-of-the-art interventional and surgical treatment of cardiac arrhythmias. The center also offers cutting-edge heart surgery, including minimally invasive robotic heart valve surgery, and utilizes a world-class circulatory assist device program. As with other leading academic programs, UCLA also integrates education and innovative cardiovascular research into its practice, emphasizing the importance of evidence-based medicine as a crucial instrument in improving overall quality of care. Both single- and multicenter observational studies are conducted on a regular basis to continually advance our clinical practices.

Key Points

Rotational Atherectomy

- Rotational atherectomy improves the procedural success rate of percutaneous coronary intervention (PCI) in heavily calcified lesions, but does not decrease restenosis. Late lumen loss was higher in patients treated with rotational atherectomy followed by drug-eluting stenting compared with patients without rotational atherectomy.
- Pericardiocentesis kits and covered stents should be readily available given the risk of coronary perforation.

Excimer Laser

- Excimer laser coronary atherectomy improves procedural success but does not decrease restenosis in moderately calcified lesions.
- Excimer laser coronary atherectomy can be used in situations that are difficult to treat including in-stent restenosis, suboptimal stent expansion, and subtotally occluded lesions uncrossable by exchange catheters.

M. S. Lee (✉) · J. Kong
Division of Cardiology, UCLA Medical Center,
Los Angeles, CA, USA
e-mail: MSLee@mednet.ucla.edu;
JKong@mednet.ucla.edu

© Springer International Publishing AG, part of Springer Nature 2018
A. Myat et al. (eds.), *The Interventional Cardiology Training Manual*,
https://doi.org/10.1007/978-3-319-71635-0_13

Aspiration Thrombectomy

- Routine use of thrombectomy for acute myocardial infarction (AMI) is not recommended.
- The benefits of up-front manual aspiration thrombectomy in AMI remain questionable, but the procedure may become necessary in bailout situations.

Embolic Protection Devices

- Embolic protection devices can capture liberated debris during saphenous vein graft (SVG) intervention to decrease the risk of distal embolization and periprocedural MI.
- Embolic protection devices do not appear to protect against no-reflow or improve clinical outcomes in PCI of native coronary vessels.
- Embolic protection devices provide clinical benefit in SVG intervention but remain underutilized.

Rotational Atherectomy

Synopsis

- Coronary artery calcification (CAC) increases the complexity of PCI. Severe CAC can create undilatable lesions, limit

stent expansion, predispose vessels to dissection during high-pressure balloon inflations, and increase the risk of major adverse cardiac events (MACE).
- Rotational atherectomy (RA) (Boston Scientific, Maple Grove, MN, USA) is an invaluable tool for modifying severely calcified lesions.

Techniques to Quantify Degree of Coronary Artery Calcification

- Quantifying the degree of CAC is important, as appropriate patient selection is vital to RA success.
- Patients with moderate-to-severe CAC are appropriate candidates. Various imaging modalities are used to identify the presence of moderate-to-severe CAC (Table 13.1).

Fluoroscopy and Angiography
- Fluoroscopy and angiography are limited in their ability to identify and quantify CAC. Hazy angiographic images make distinguishing between thrombus, dissection, distorted lumen, and irregular plaque morphology difficult [1–3].
- Fluoroscopy cannot differentiate between medial calcification, superficial calcification, and calcification narrowing the lumen diameter [4]. Angiography cannot clearly visualize vascular wall components.

Table 13.1 Summary of coronary diagnostic techniques

	Angioscopy	Coronary arteriography	Intravascular ultrasound	Optical coherence tomography
Picture expression	3-dimension	2-dimension	2-dimension	2-dimension and 3-dimension
Color tone	Color	Black and white	Black and white	False color (e.g., sepia) or black and white
Quantification	–	++	++	++
High resolution	++	+	+	+++
General picture	–	–	++	++
Tissue characterization				
Plaque characterization	++	+	++	++
Intraluminal	++	+	+	++
Intramural	–	–	++	+
Calcification	–	+	++	+++
Thrombus	++	+	–	+++

++: excellent; +: good; –: poor
Adapted from Regar E, Weissman NJ, Muhlestein JB. Intravascular ultrasound, optical coherence tomography, and angioscopy of coronary circulation. In: UpToDate, Post TW (ed), UptoDate, Waltham, MA. (Accessed on November 2, 2016)

- These techniques alone are inadequate to determine whether lesions require plaque modification.

Intravascular Ultrasound (See Also Chap. 14)

- Intravascular ultrasound (IVUS) is superior to angiography alone in evaluating CAC [5]. IVUS can distinguish between discrete stenosis, dissection, plaque morphologies, and lumen irregularities [6].
- It provides a tomographic view of vessels with high resolution that improves delineation of the extent, composition, morphology, and distribution of arterial plaque [7, 8].
- The normal coronary anatomy produces a "three-layer appearance." The denser intima and adventitia produce a bright hyper-echoic appearance bordering the darker hypo-echoic middle media layer. Dense calcium also appears hyper-echoic on IVUS.
- Although IVUS cannot penetrate calcium itself, it helps quantify the arc and length of CAC. Atherectomy should be considered if the arc of calcium is ≥270°.
- Limitations include increased cost and duration of the procedure compared to angiography alone. Periprocedural risks, including vessel spasm and dissection, are uncommon.

Tips and Tricks

- Intracoronary administration of nitroglycerin can decrease the risk of coronary vasospasm.
- Vigorously flushing with normal saline can remove air from the catheter prior to insertion into the guiding catheter.
- The IVUS catheter should not be flushed due to the risk of air embolism once in the guiding catheter.

Optical Coherence Tomography (See Also Chap. 14)

- Optical coherence tomography (OCT) is analogous to pulse-echo imaging, but uses infrared light instead of sound [9].
- Its fiber-optic technology accurately characterizes the extent and morphology of CAC, limits artifacts, and produces a tenfold higher image resolution than IVUS [10–12].

- Two types of OCT include time-domain (TD-OCT) and Fourier-domain optical coherence tomography (FD-OCT). TD-OCT is the first-generation OCT, but has limited use given relatively slow data acquisition. FD-OCT has higher rates of wavelength scanning, faster image acquisition, and greater penetration depth.
- Typically, OCT penetrates 1–2 mm compared to 4–8 mm with IVUS [13]. Although OCT is inferior to IVUS in delineating reference vessel diameter given its limited range of visualization, it characterizes the structure of coronary artery disease in greater detail. Its ability to visualize calcification without blooming artifact prevents overestimation of CAC extent. Furthermore, it is superior in identifying neointimal hyperplasia, a surrogate marker for stent thrombosis [14].
- Limitations are similar to those of IVUS, increasing PCI cost and time. TD-OCT requires removal of blood during image acquisition to prevent red blood cell light scattering. Balloon occlusion of the vessel with subsequent saline irrigation can prevent this [12].
- The newer FD-OCT improves scanning times and pullback speeds, obviating the need for balloon occlusion [13]. Complication rates are similar to IVUS in head-to-head comparisons [15–17].

Tips and Tricks

- The catheter should be introduced distally into the coronary artery after administration of intracoronary nitroglycerin to minimize vasospasm.
- Some clinicians continue dual-antiplatelet therapy for 14 days to 1 month after OCT imaging due to endothelial damage observed in animal studies.

Indications for Rotational Atherectomy

- RA is reserved for selected patients with moderate-to-severe CAC. The decision to perform RA is based on clinical judgment and should be considered when there is a low likelihood of successful stent delivery and expansion without plaque modification.
- RA utilization is also determined by the degree of coronary calcium, as benefits are diminished

Fig. 13.1 Treatment algorithm for atherectomy (Plate A) and components of the rotablation system (Plate B = range of burrs available, also available in 2.15, 2.25, 2.38, and 2.50 mm; Plate C = system components). Adapted from Lee MS, Shah N. J Invasive Cardiol 2015

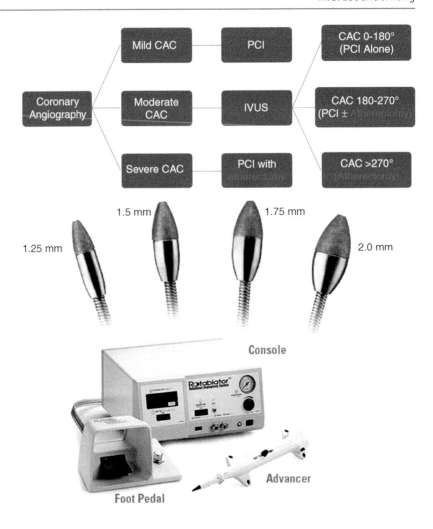

with minimal calcium (Fig. 13.1). The ACCF/AHA/SCAI guidelines for PCI provide a class IIa recommendation for utilizing RA for fibrotic or heavily calcified lesions that cannot be traversed by balloon catheters or adequately dilated before stent implantation [18].

- It should not be performed routinely for de novo lesions or in-stent restenosis (ISR) (class III recommendation) [18].

Tips and Tricks
- IVUS and OCT help determine CAC severity. Atherectomy should be used if the calcium arc is ≥270°.
- If coronary atherectomy for a calcified lesion is not the initial strategy, balloon inflation at nominal pressure should be performed to

determine if the balloon fully expands without dissecting the vessel.
- If the balloon doesn't fully expand, coronary atherectomy can still be performed as long as a dissection has not occurred.

Contraindications for Rotational Atherectomy

- Absolute contraindications to RA include:
  - Presence of thrombus
  - Saphenous vein graft (SVG) lesions
  - Coronary dissection
- Relative contraindications in general include:
  - The lack of cardiothoracic surgery availability

- Severe three-vessel or unprotected left main disease
- Severe left ventricular dysfunction
- Lesions >25 mm
- Lesion angulation >45° [19]

Rotational Atherectomy Technique

- A rapidly rotating olive-shaped burr coated with 2000–3000 microscopic diamond chips modifies calcified plaque to facilitate stent delivery and expansion [20].
- The burr, which is bonded to the drive shaft, has a size range of 1.25 mm to 2.5 mm and is advanced over a 0.009 in. RotaWire (Boston Scientific). The other components include the console and turbine that is activated via foot pedal (Fig. 13.1).
- The mechanism of action is differential cutting, whereby the burr ablates inelastic tissue (calcium, fibrous tissue) and spares healthy tissue due to its elastic properties that deflect diamond microchip edges [20]. The differential cutting and longitudinal friction via changes in circumferential direction aid burr advancement through lesions. The typical burr-to-artery ratio is 0.5, as the purpose of RA is plaque modification rather than debulking.

Tips and Tricks

- A workhorse wire can traverse the lesion by swapping out the RotaWire through an over-the-wire balloon or any other exchange catheter, as the RotaWire is often difficult to advance across the lesion.
- Once the burr is advanced proximal to the lesion, the following maneuvers can be performed prior to ablation to reduce slack from the system and prevent the burr from jumping forward when activated: (1) gently pulling back the drive shaft and removing stored tension from the advancing shaft; (2) loosening the advancer knob and moving it back and forth; and (3) briefly activating dynaglide.
- Avoid adding vasodilators in the rota-flush solution to decrease the risk of periprocedural hypotension [21].

- A "single-operator" technique can be used to advance the drive shaft when a skilled assistant is not available to hold the RotaWire [22].
- If the RotaWire is inadvertently pulled back with the drive shaft on it, the RotaWire can be readvanced forward while activating dynaglide.
- Briefly tapping on dynaglide can facilitate the delivery of the burr that is difficult to advance.
- Constant normal saline flushes during each pass decrease heat generation.
- The burr should be advanced with a slow (1 mm/s) pecking technique.
- Each pass should be kept to a short duration (<15–20 s) to minimize excessive friction that can injure vessels, activate platelets, or release large debris [19].
- Burr deceleration of >5000 rpm indicates that it should be advanced more slowly or pulled back.
- Prophylactic placement of a temporary pacemaker should be considered if the patient has baseline bradycardia, a long diffuse lesion in the right coronary artery, or a dominant left circumflex artery [23].
- If a temporary pacemaker is not placed, nurses should have atropine readily available if heart block is induced.
- Nurses should have phenylephrine readily available if severe hypotension develops.
- Patients with left ventricular systolic dysfunction should be evaluated for a hemodynamic support device [24].

Clinical Data

- The ERBAC trial demonstrated that RA had the best initial procedural success rate compared to excimer laser and balloon angioplasty (89% vs. 77% vs. 80%, $p = 0.009$) [25].
- The COBRA trial reported that RA provided higher procedural success rates compared to balloon angioplasty (85% vs. 78%, $p < 0.05$) with no difference in rates of restenosis, target lesion revascularization, or symptomatic outcome at 6 months [26].

• The ROTAXUS trial showed that RA had a higher overall strategy success rate in patients with severe CAC lesions compared to PCI alone (92.5% vs. 83.3%, $p = 0.03$) [27]. The rates of in-stent restenosis, target-lesion revascularization, and MACE were similar between both groups at 9 months. There were also no differences in MACE rates at 2 years [28].

Complications/Troubleshooting

Vascular Complications

• The risk of coronary vasospasm can be reduced with prophylactic intracoronary nitroglycerin.
• A smaller burr-to-artery ratio (<0.7) may reduce angiographic complications compared to aggressive burr sizing (>0.7) [29, 30]. A smaller burr-to-artery ratio can additionally decrease the risk of coronary perforation.
• Coronary dissection is also concerning given its association with greater residual stenosis and greater need for surgical revascularization. Predictors of dissection include vessel tortuosity and angulation. Meticulous technique, slow burr movement, and avoiding atherectomy altogether in tortuous and angulated vessels will minimize both perforation and dissection risks.
• Larger catheters and frequent catheter exchanges increase the risk of cerebrovascular events possibly due to calcified arterial debris embolizing to the cerebral vasculature [31]. Careful advancement to minimize drop in speed, lower rotational speeds (150,000 rather than 180,000 rpm), and intermittent lesion contact may allow perfusion to better clear debris.

Slow/No-Reflow

• Reduced coronary flow (TIMI grade 2), or slow flow, is secondary to atherosclerotic debris showering followed by subsequent thrombotic phenomena, neurohormonal mediator release, and platelet activation in the absence of stenosis, thrombus, or dissection. No-reflow is TIMI grade 0–1 in the coronary

Table 13.2 Prevention and treatment strategies for slow or no reflow during rotational atherectomy

Mechanism of slow/no-reflow	Therapeutic options
Atheromatous debris embolus	Avoidance of significant deceleration Short duration of ablation Small burr sizing
Intraprocedural hypotension	Vasopressor: • Phenylephrine for immediate response • Dopamine or norepinephrine if sustained Intra-aortic balloon pump
Neurohormonal reflex bradycardia	Atropine
Microcirculatory vasospasm	Vasodilatory agents: • Nitroprusside • Nicardipine • Adenosine
Platelet activation, aggregation	Bailout glycoprotein IIb/IIIa inhibitor Optimal antiplatelet therapy

Adapted from Tomey M, Kini A, Sharma S. Current status of rotational atherectomy. JACC: Cardiovascular Interventions 2014;4:345–353

vasculature without obvious secondary cause. The interplay of both local features at the level of the coronary artery and systemic pathophysiologic factors may cause these disturbances in coronary flow [32].
• To minimize the risk of slow/no-reflow, strategies such as prophylactic intracoronary administration of vasodilatory agents, appropriate device sizing, and slow and short-duration passes are recommended (Table 13.2).
• Treatment of slow/no-reflow includes intracoronary nitroprusside, adenosine, or calcium-channel blockade [33].

Burr Entrapment

• Burr entrapment is a rare phenomenon. The burr only ablates during advancement since only the distal half has diamond chips. The proximal portion of the burr can become entrapped in an incompletely ablated calcified lesion due to its inability to perform retrograde ablation.
• Various techniques can remove the entrapped burr, including deep intubation with the

guiding catheter or balloon angioplasty at the location of burr entrapment [34].

- Strategies to decrease the risk of burr entrapment include using smaller burrs with higher mobility and short-duration passes with intermittent advancement ("pecking" motion) to help avoid burr deceleration and stalling [19]. High-speed (>170,000 rpm) atherectomy may allow the burr to cross calcified lesions easier.
- Utilizing tactile, auditory, and visual senses can help minimize complications. Signs of impending entrapment include excessive vibration from the burr encountering extra resistance, changes in the pitch related to burr resistance, and poor burr advancement on fluoroscopy.

Summary

- RA is an invaluable tool to modify complex and heavily calcified coronary lesions.
- Intravascular imaging is a vital tool to identify the presence and degree of CAC and assist the operator in determining the need for atherectomy.
- Operator training, appropriate device selection, and experience are imperative to improving clinical outcomes in patients with complex coronary lesions.

Excimer Laser

Synopsis

Various coronary atherectomy methods are used to modify calcified lesions and reduce rates of PCI complications. One such technique is excimer laser coronary atherectomy (ELCA), a form of laser angioplasty (LA), which can improve successful stenting in lesions with CAC.

Techniques to Quantify Degree of Coronary Artery Calcification

Invasive imaging modalities like IVUS and OCT are used to quantify CAC and assist the operator

in determining whether patients require adjunctive treatment with coronary atherectomy. These are covered in detail in the rotational atherectomy section previously (see also Chap. 14).

Indications for Excimer Laser Coronary Atherectomy

- The ACCF/AHA/SCAI guidelines for PCI provide a class IIb recommendation for utilizing LA in fibrotic or moderately calcified lesions that cannot be crossed or dilated with conventional balloon angioplasty [16].
- LA should not be used routinely during PCI (class III recommendation) [16].
- Procedural success using ELCA for crossing and debulking calcified chronic total occlusions and balloon-resistant lesions was high (>90%) with no perforation or no-reflow in the LEONARDO study and the study by Bilodeau et al. [35, 36].
- ELCA can also be used synergistically with RA in heavily calcified subtotally occluded lesions. If a standard 0.014 in. wire traverses the subtotally occluded lesion but an exchange catheter cannot cross, ELCA can modify the lesion to create a channel through which the RotaWire can subsequently be delivered distally through an exchange catheter [37]. This ELCA and RA combination is termed the RASER technique and is particularly effective for calcified stenosis during PCI [38–40].
- Suboptimal stent expansion can be treated with ELCA as it modifies the underlying resistant atheroma by delivering energy to the outer stent surface without disrupting stent architecture [41, 42]. This weakens plaque resistance behind the stent to facilitate further stent expansion.
- ELCA is effective in treating in-stent restenosis (see also Chap. 31). In a study of 107 restenotic lesions in 98 patients, lesions treated with ELCA had greater IVUS cross-sectional area and luminal gain compared to balloon angioplasty alone [43]. ELCA resulted in more ablation of intimal hyperplasia and a trend toward lower rates of 6-month

target-vessel revascularization (21% vs. 38%; $p = 0.083$). Data also support long-term efficacy of ELCA with balloon angioplasty in treating ISR, showing less frequent need for repeat target-vessel revascularization [44].

Tips and Tricks

- If the rate of advancement of the catheter distal tip does not correspond directly to the rate of proximal shaft advancement on fluoroscopy, reassess lesion morphology.
- The laser catheter tip should never pass the guide-wire tip.
- Avoid withdrawing the guide wire inside the laser catheter.

Table 13.3 Indications for excimer laser coronary atherectomy (ELCA) and the preferred laser catheter

ELCA indication	Preferred laser catheter (mm)
Acute myocardial infarct, intracoronary thrombus	0.9–1.4
Uncrossable lesions	0.9 × 80
Chronic total occlusions	0.9 × 80
Under-expanded stent	0.9 × 80
In-stent restenosis	0.9–2.0 (concentric or eccentric)
Saphenous vein grafts	0.9–2.0

Adapted from Rawlins J, Din J, Talwar S, O'Kane P. Coronary Intervention With The Excimer Laser: Review Of The Technology And Outcome Data. Interventional Cardiology Review 2016;11 (1):27–32

Contraindications for Excimer Laser Coronary Atherectomy

- An absolute contraindication to ELCA is the presence of coronary dissection.
- Relative contraindications to atherectomy are similar to rotational atherectomy.
- ELCA has minimal ablative effects on calcium and relies on ablation of more pliable lesion tissue, suggesting that severely calcified vessels may have less luminal gain following ELCA [45, 46]. Sequential IVUS analysis following ELCA has failed to demonstrate quantitative (measurable decrease in calcium arc or superficial calcium) or qualitative (visual evidence of reduced shadowing and increased ultrasound penetration) calcium ablation [46].

Excimer Laser Coronary Atherectomy Technique

- ELCA utilizes fiber-optic technology to produce monochromatic light energy to ablate plaque without directly affecting the surrounding healthy tissue [20]. Ultraviolet pulses debulk moderately calcified plaque, fibrous tissue, atheroma, and thrombus.
- Continuous versus pulsed laser waves affect the degree to which coronary plaque is affected. One of ELCA's initial limitations was the constant power output inducing significant thermal damage [47–49]. The current ELCA model delivers high energy in a pulsatile fashion, breaking chemical bonds in tissue without damaging surrounding material or causing heat damage [50]. ELCA can also vaporize concomitant thrombi, decreasing the risk of platelet aggregation [51].
- Coronary catheters are available in 0.9, 1.4, 1.7, and 2.0 mm diameters. Laser catheter size is primarily based on:
  - Lesion severity
  - Reference vessel diameter
  - Target-material consistency [37]
- The 0.9 mm X80 catheter is selected in most balloon failure cases because it provides the widest range of power and repetition (Table 13.3).
- The ELCA catheter is advanced on a short monorail segment, compatible with any standard 0.014 in. guide wire [37]. This is a major advantage over alternative coronary atherectomy techniques that require dedicated guide wires.

Tips and Tricks

- Operators control two factors during usage: wave frequency administered and amount of energy (fluence) [50]. There is a fine balance between the pulse repetition rate and fluence

Fig. 13.2 Workflow for successful laser atherectomy. Adapted from: Rawlins J, Din J, Talwar S, O'Kane P. Coronary Intervention With The Excimer Laser: Review Of The Technology And Outcome Data. Interventional Cardiology Review 2016;11 (1):27–32

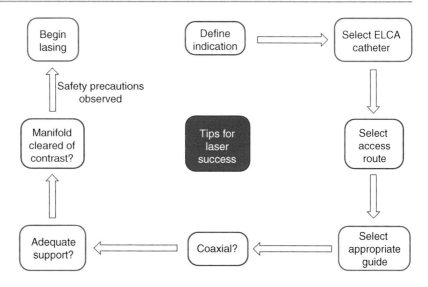

administered to minimize thermal effects during the procedure [52].

- A frequency/fluency of 40/40 is typically the initial setting. Settings can be increased after several passes.
- Effective plaque removal via slow advancement of the catheter (1 mm/s) creates a smoother, larger vessel diameter.
- ELCA should not be performed while injecting contrast media because contrast and blood have high absorption of emission light, increasing the risk of dissection and perforation [53, 54].
- Constant saline flushing during catheter advancement can decrease the risk of complications.
- A systematic approach improves the workflow for successful ELCA (Fig. 13.2).

Complications/Troubleshooting

Vascular Complications

- Coronary vasospasm occurred in 6.1% of cases in one multicenter analysis [36] but can be reduced with prophylactic intracoronary nitroglycerin. Coronary perforation and dissection are more troublesome complications.
- A 16-trial analysis reported high rates of dissection (22.0%) and perforation (2.4%) with LA [55]. Logistic regression analysis revealed a correlation between dissections and utilization of larger catheter sizes ($p = 0.0005$), lesion length > 10 mm ($p = 0.001$), and high energy per pulse levels ($p = 0.0001$ for native vessels) [55].

Slow/No-Reflow

Slow/no-reflow phenomena increase periprocedural complications due to induced ischemia and MIs. Their pathophysiology, prophylaxis, and treatment are covered in the rotational atherectomy section.

Summary

ELCA is used to modify complex and moderately calcified coronary lesions. Although its role is not as widely accepted as that of RA, it provides another option for treating undilatable lesions. Its versatility also allows operators to address difficult-to-treat lesions, including in-stent restenosis.

Aspiration Thrombectomy

Synopsis

- PCI is the preferred method of reestablishing coronary perfusion after thrombotic coronary occlusion in acute ST-elevation myocardial infarction (STEMI). However, PCI risks distal thrombus embolization.

Fig. 13.3 Angiojet™ mechanical thrombectomy system. High-pressure saline jets create a vacuum effect that induces fragmentation and aspiration of large-volume thrombus (image courtesy of Boston Scientific, Inc.)

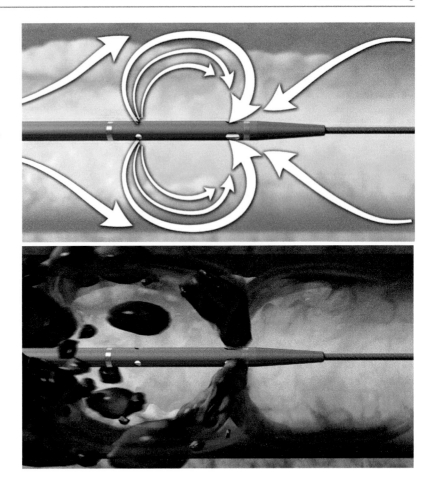

- Thrombectomy procedures have been studied in acute myocardial infarction (AMI), which includes completely occlusive STEMI or partially occlusive unstable angina and non-ST-elevation MI (NSTEMI).
- The goal of thrombectomy is to debulk intraluminal thrombus to improve flow and reduce distal embolization (Fig. 13.3). Early trials demonstrated mortality benefit with up-front routine thrombectomy in STEMI patients. However, subsequent trials have contradicted these findings.

No-Reflow Phenomenon

- No-reflow is a profound reduction in coronary blood flow (TIMI grade flow $\leq$ 2) in the absence of stenosis, thrombus, dissection, or spasm [56–58]. Thrombectomy may provide protective benefit against this phenomenon.
- A study of 260 patients undergoing primary PCI reported that no-reflow was most common in patients with large thrombus burden without thrombectomy, followed by those who underwent thrombectomy [59].
- A retrospective study of 116 AMI patients treated with conventional angioplasty and 89 AMI patients treated with angioplasty plus manual aspiration thrombectomy reported that no-reflow phenomenon was significantly lower in the thrombectomy group (8 vs. 18%, $p < 0.05$) [60]. Although this suggests that thrombectomy may decrease the risk of no-reflow, the reduction of adverse clinical events is not well

established since many higher risk patients did not benefit from the procedure, or were excluded from studies.

Thrombectomy

Large thrombus burden is associated with a higher rate of stent thrombosis and worse clinical outcomes [61]. Two types of thrombectomy have been studied in AMI patients: manual aspiration and mechanical thrombectomy.

Manual Aspiration Thrombectomy

- In aspiration thrombectomy, a dual-lumen catheter replaces a traditional balloon catheter. The catheters are deployed in rapid exchange or over-the-wire format with a second port connected to a vacuum syringe. The operator aspirates thrombus upon reaching the target lesion by turning the vacuum syringe stopcock.
- The 2015 ACC/AHA/SCAI primary PCI for STEMI patients' focused update does not recommend routine use of aspiration thrombectomy [62, 63]. Three large randomized studies provide the bulk of evidence for aspiration thrombectomy utilization (Table 13.4).
- The TAPAS trial, which randomized 1071 STEMI patients, reported that the primary endpoint of myocardial blush grade 0 or 1 occurred less frequently in patients treated with aspiration thrombectomy with the 6F Export catheter (Medtronic, Minneapolis, MN) compared with PCI alone (17.1% vs. 26.3%, $p < 0.001$) [64]. Although 30-day MACE rates were similar (6.8% vs. 9.4%;

$p = 0.12$), MACE and overall mortality were significantly lower in those who achieved better myocardial blush. This benefit persisted at 1-year follow-up [65].

- The TASTE trial randomized 7244 STEMI patients to aspiration thrombectomy or PCI alone [66]. The primary endpoint of death from any cause at 30 days was similar in both groups (2.8% vs. 3.0%, $p = 0.63$), as were rates of 30-day MACE and 1-year mortality (5.3% vs. 5.6%, $p = 0.57$) [67].
- The TOTAL study, designed to clarify the mixed findings in the TAPAS and TASTE trials, randomized 10,732 STEMI patients to up-front manual aspiration thrombectomy with the Export catheter (Medtronic) versus PCI alone [68]. The primary outcome of the composite of cardiovascular death, recurrent MI, cardiogenic shock, or New York Heart Association class IV heart failure within 180 days occurred with similar frequency in both groups (6.9% vs. 7.0%, $p = 0.86$). Stroke within 30 days occurred more frequently with aspiration thrombectomy (0.7 vs. 0.3%, $p = 0.02$), as did stroke at 180 days (1.0 vs. 0.5%, $p = 0.002$). Outcomes at 1 year also showed a potential increase in stroke and no reduction in longer term clinical outcomes [69].
- Although aspiration thrombectomy showed promising clinical benefits in the TAPAS trial, the TASTE and TOTAL trials curbed early enthusiasm. Taking the cumulative data of these trials, the routine use of aspiration thrombectomy has been downgraded to bailout in cases of heavy thrombus burden and poor flow.

Table 13.4 Major RCTs of manual aspiration thrombectomy (MAT)

Trial	Publication date	Size	Device	30-day MACE MAT arm (%)	30-day MACE control arm (%)	1-year MACE MAT arm (%)	1-year MACE control arm (%)
TAPAS	2008	1071	Export	6.8	9.4	5.6[a]	9.9[a]
TASTE	2013	7244	Multiple	3.3[a]	3.9[a]	8.0	8.5
TOTAL	2015	10,732	Export	6.9	7.0	8.0	8.0

MAT Manual aspiration thrombectomy, *TAPAS* the Thrombus Aspiration during Percutaneous Coronary Intervention in Acute Myocardial Infarction Study, *TASTE* the Thrombus Aspiration in ST-Elevation Myocardial Infarction in Scandinavia trial, *TOTAL* the Trial of Routine Aspiration Thrombectomy with PCI versus PCI Alone in Patients with STEMI
[a]Mortality or myocardial infarction

Mechanical Thrombectomy

- Mechanical thrombectomy utilizes moving, machine-driven parts to macerate and aspirate thrombus. One such device is the Angiojet (Boston Scientific, Marlborough, MA), which uses rheolytic thrombectomy (RT). The 6F compatible system shoots high-pressure, high-velocity saline jets from its catheter tip to form a low-pressure zone, creating a vacuum that dissociates and aspirates thrombi via the Venturi-Bernoulli effect (Fig. 13.3). However, the AiMI and JETSTENT trials raised safety concerns.
- The AiMI trial randomized 480 patients presenting within 12 h of a STEMI to PCI alone versus RT [70]. The primary endpoint of infarct size was larger in the RT group (12.5% vs. 9.8%, $p < 0.02$). The RT group also had higher rates of 30-day MACE (6.7% vs. 1.7%; $p = 0.01$) and mortality (4.6% vs. 0.8%; $p = 0.02$) [70].
- The JETSTENT trial randomized 501 patients with STEMI in vessels >2.5 mm and visible thrombus to RT versus direct stenting [71]. The protocol required the device be activated prior to crossing the lesion. Although the rates of 6-month MACE (11.2% vs. 19.4%; $p = 0.009$) and 12-month event-free survival (85.2% vs. 75%; $p = 0.009$) were improved with Angiojet, the primary endpoint of infarct size was similar in both groups.
- A meta-analysis that included seven trials comparing mechanical thrombectomy to conventional PCI reported no significant difference in the incidence of MACE or death [72]. However, there was a trend toward a higher rate of all strokes with mechanical thrombectomy (1.3% vs. 0.4%, $p = 0.07$) [73].
- The manual devices in general are more user friendly with shorter learning curves. Despite effective thrombus removal, mechanical thrombectomy used during primary PCI does not appear to reduce infarct size or improve TMPG, TIMI flow grade, ST-segment resolution, or 30-day MACE [74].

Summary

- Thrombectomy during primary PCI does not provide benefit across most large randomized trials. The ACC/AHA/SCAI guidelines relegated routine aspiration thrombectomy utilization from class IIa to class III in 2015.
- However, its utility should be individually tailored for each case when flow cannot be restored with balloon inflation alone.
- Mechanical thrombectomy has yet to show equivalent benefits to manual aspiration. Thus, interventionalists must be familiar with aspiration thrombectomy techniques in complex reperfusion cases that may require adjunctive PCI treatment.

Distal Embolic Protection

Synopsis

- Reestablishing coronary perfusion after STEMI is crucial to improve patient outcomes. However, manipulation of culprit lesions with wires and catheters risks distal embolization of atheromatous material and thrombus.
- Embolic protection devices (EPDs) were designed for adjunctive use during PCI to address this issue. Early randomized trials analyzing EPD efficacy in native coronary vessels did not show additional benefit when used with primary or rescue PCI.
- Patients with SVG lesions have different risk factors and rates of vascular complications. Subsequent trials investigating EPD efficacy in SVG intervention demonstrated clinical benefits not seen in the native circulation.

Types of Distal Embolic Protection Devices (See Also Chap. 30)

EPDs capture and retrieve friable, lipid-rich plaque particles dislodged during PCI. EPDs can

Table 13.5 Embolic protection device type based on mechanism of action: strengths and limitations

	Proximal occlusion	Distal occlusion	Distal filter
Embolization on wiring/predilatation/device crossing	−	+	+
Failure to capture debris <100 μm	−	−	+
Failure to capture soluble mediators	−	−	+
Ischemia during balloon occlusion	+	+	−
Limited contrast opacification	+	+	−
Unlimited debris capture	+	+	−
Shunting of debris into proximal side branches	−	+	−
Graft lesion location			
Ostial (<12 mm)	−	+	+
Middle	+	+	+
Distal (<20 mm)	+	−	−

Adapted from Bangalore S, Bhatt DL. Embolic protection devices. Circulation 2014 Apr 29;129 (17):e470–6

be separated into three categories based on their mechanism of operation: proximal occlusion aspiration devices, distal occlusion aspiration devices, and distal embolic filters (Table 13.5).

Proximal Occlusion Aspiration
- A proximal occlusion aspiration device utilizes a guiding catheter with an inflatable balloon tip deployed proximal to the lesion. This occludes antegrade flow, creating a column of stagnant blood containing debris that is later aspirated through the guiding catheter.
- The Proxis (7F; St. Jude Medical, Minneapolis, MN), which is no longer commercially available, provides protection prior to crossing the lesion, potentially recovering all particles and vasoreactive substances, and can be used in lesions without a distal landing zone. The type of guide wire can also be tailored to procedural requirements.
- Disadvantages include limited contrast opacification and ischemia during balloon occlusion.

Distal Occlusion Aspiration
- A distal occlusion aspiration device contains an inflatable occlusion balloon attached to a hypotube (small tube acting as an interventional guide wire for balloon angioplasty or stenting).

- The occlusion balloon is inflated several centimeters distal to the lesion, obstructing antegrade flow and trapping plaque debris. Debris is subsequently removed via an aspiration catheter (Export or FlushCath).
- The PercuSurge GuardWire (6F; Medtronic, Minneapolis, MN) and TriActiv system (7F or 8F; Kensey Nash Corp, Exton, PA) are examples of such devices. These EPDs capture particles <100 μm and soluble vasoactive mediators with unlimited debris capture, but risk embolization during the wiring and device-crossing phase.
- Other disadvantages include ischemia during balloon occlusion, limited contrast opacification, and risk of shunting debris into proximal side branches. Operators also cannot tailor the guide wire type to procedural requirements.

Distal Embolic Filter
- A distal embolic filter has a filter bag attached to the distal portion of a 0.014 in. guide wire with a delivery sheath (3.2F). The filter bag has 100–110 μm pore sizes to filter particles >100–110 μm. The filter bag with debris is later retrieved with a retrieval catheter (4.2F–4.9F).
- Devices that work with this principle include the FilterWire (Boston Scientific, Natick, Mass.), Interceptor Plus Coronary Filter System (Medtronic Vascular, Santa Rosa, CA), and the Spider (Medtronic, Minneapolis, MN).

- Advantages include the ability to maintain perfusion and contrast opacification during the procedure.
- Disadvantages include the potential risk of distal embolization during the wiring and device-crossing phases, inability to filter soluble vasoactive substances, large-diameter delivery sheath requirement, and embolization of debris during filter retrieval.

Clinical Data in Native Coronary Circulation

- Data on EPD efficacy in STEMI patients have failed to consistently demonstrate significant benefit on clinical outcomes or myocardial reperfusion (Table 13.6) [75].
- The EMERALD trial analyzed EPD efficacy in 501 STEMI patients who underwent

Table 13.6 Major trials of embolic protection devices for ST-segment-elevation myocardial infarction involving the native coronary arteries

Trial	Device	Patients (n)	Primary endpoint	Result (%)	P-value
Proximal occlusion device					
PREPARE	Proxis vs. conventional PCI	284	Complete ST-segment resolution at 60 min	80 vs. 72	0.14
Distal occlusion device					
EMERALD	GuardWire Plus vs. conventional guide wire	501	ST-segment resolution at 30 min Infarct size	63.3 vs. 61.9 12.0 vs. 9.5	0.78 0.34
ASPARAGUS	GuardWire Plus vs. conventional guide wire	329	TIMI grade 3 flow TMP grade 3	77 vs. 78 25.2 vs. 20.3	0.73 0.26
MICADO	GuardWire Plus vs. conventional guide wire	167	No-reflow TIMI grade 3 flow TMP grade 3	4 vs. 3 80 vs. 76 58 vs. 44	0.73 0.182 0.054
Ohala et al.	GuardWire Plus vs. abciximab	120	TIMI grade 3 flow	89 vs. 89	>0.05
Tahk et al[a]	GuardWire Plus vs. conventional guide wire	116	TIMI grade 3 flow TMP grade 3 Hyperemic average peak velocity	96 vs. 81 65 vs. 38 39.2 ± 16.7 vs. 30.6 ± 10.8 cm/s	0.016 0.001 0.014
Distal filter device					
DEDICATION	FilterWire vs. conventional PCI	626	ST-segment resolution at 90 min	72 vs. 76	0.29
PROMISE	FilterWire EX vs. conventional guide wire	200	Maximum adenosine-induced flow velocity	34 ± 17 vs. 36 ± 20 cm/s	0.46
PREMIAR	SpiderRX vs. conventional PCI	140	ST-segment resolution at 60 min	60 vs. 60	0.99
UpFlow MI	FilterWire EX vs. conventional guide wire	100	TIMI grade 3 flow TMP grade 3 ST-segment resolution at 60 min	88.2 vs. 93.9 68.1 vs. 66 9.4 vs. 10.7	>0.05 > 0.05 > 0.05

ASPARAGUS Aspiration of Liberated Debris in Acute Myocardial Infarction With GuardWire Plus System, *DEDICATION* Drug Elution and Distal Protection During Percutaneous Coronary Intervention in ST Elevation Myocardial Infarction trial, *EMERALD* Enhanced Myocardial Efficacy and Removal by Aspiration of Liberated Debris, *MICADO* Multicenter Investigation of Coronary Artery Protection With a Distal Occlusion Device in Acute Myocardial Infarction, *PREPARE* Proximal Embolic Protection in Acute Myocardial Infarction and Resolution of ST-Elevation, *PREMIAR* Protection of Distal Embolization in High-Risk Patients with Acute ST-Segment Elevation Myocardial Infarction, *PROMISE* Protection Devices in PCI Treatment of Myocardial Infarction for Salvage of Endangered Myocardium, TIMI Thrombolysis in Myocardial Infarction, *TMP* Thrombolysis in Myocardial Infarction myocardial perfusion, *UpFlow MI* Use of Protective FilterWire to Improve Flow in Acute Myocardial Infarction study
Adapted from Bangalore S, Bhatt DL. Embolic protection devices. Circulation 2014 Apr 29;129 (17):e470–6
[a]No difference in major adverse cardiac events at 6 months

primary PCI or rescue intervention after failed fibrinolysis [76]. There was no significant difference in the co-primary endpoint of infarct size between patients randomized to PCI with a GuardWire and those randomized to primary PCI alone (median, 12.0% vs. 9.5%, $p = 0.15$). The secondary endpoint of MACE at 6 months was also comparable in the two groups (10.0% vs. 11.0%, $p = 0.66$).

- The PROMISE and DEDICATION trials were of similar design to the EMERALD trial, but used the FilterWire rather than the GuardWire [77, 78]. The two groups (PCI with and without EPDs) were equivalent in infarct size, maximal adenosine-induced flow velocity, and 30-day mortality in the PROMISE trial. Likewise, complete ($\geq 70\%$) ST-segment resolution was similar between the two study arms in the DEDICATION trial. In fact, 15-month follow-up results of the DEDICTATION trial suggest an increased incidence of stent thrombosis and target-vessel revascularization with routine EPD use [79].
- It is hypothesized that the native coronary circulation may have smaller embolic burdens than SVG, accounting for the apparent lack of benefit with EPD utilization. There is no role for EPD use during PCI of native coronary vessels in STEMI.

Clinical Data in Saphenous Vein Grafts

- The ACCF/AHA/SCAI guidelines provide a class I indication to the use of EPDs during SVG intervention when technically feasible [18]. EPDs may have a greater impact on SVG lesions given their potentially higher embolic burden compared to native vessels.
- Degenerated vein grafts have more friable lipid-rich plaque, more diffuse lesions with thinner fibrous caps, and thus a greater propensity to embolize distally [80, 81]. In fact, MACE rates double in SVG intervention compared to those in native coronary vessels [82].
- The SAFER trial randomized 801 patients with SVG stenosis to stent placement over the shaft of a GuardWire device or a conventional angioplasty guide wire [83]. EPD utilization significantly reduced the frequency of no-reflow (3% vs. 9%, $p = 0.02$) and MI (8.6% vs. 14.7%, $p = 0.008$).

- The FIRE trial compared the PercuSurge GuardWire against the FilterWire Ex in 651 patients who received SVG stenting [82]. Equivalent results were recorded for the 30-day composite endpoint of death, MI, or target-vessel revascularization (11.6 vs. 9.9%, $p = 0.53$).
- The PRIDE trial compared the TriActiv System to both the PercuSurge GuardWire and the FilterWire Ex system [84]. The TriActiv System was not inferior to the other devices in terms of MACE, but may be associated with more bleeding complications.
- In-stent restenosis of SVG lesions consists primarily of neointimal proliferation and may have lower embolic potential, potentially negating the need for distal embolic protection. A study of 54 patients undergoing PCI for SVG in-stent restenosis without EPDs showed no procedure-related MI or no-reflow episodes during the procedure [85]. More data are needed to clarify the role of EPD in the treatment of SVG in-stent restenosis.
- The PROXIMAL trial evaluated the use of the Proxis device in 594 patients undergoing stenting in 639 SVGs [86]. Patients were randomized to either current care (distal EPD whenever possible, no EPD when not) or a test arm (proximal protection device whenever possible, distal embolic protection when proximal protection not feasible). The test arm was noninferior to the current care in the primary composite endpoint of death, MI, or target-vessel revascularization at 30 days (10.0% vs. 9.2%, $p = 0.0061$).
- Overall, the trials above demonstrate the efficacy of all three EPD classes in minimizing adverse outcomes in PCI for SVG stenosis (see also Chap. 30). Other studies comparing newer devices against the GuardWire reference standard have also been found to be noninferior in efficacy (Table 13.7). Although these devices have become part of a more common standard of care, they are currently underutilized in SVG intervention [87].

Table 13.7 Major trials of embolic protection devices for saphenous vein graft intervention

Trial	Device	Patients (n)	30-day MACE (%)	P-value	Design
Proximal occlusion device					
PROXIMAL	Proxis vs. FilterWire or GuardWire	594	9.2 vs. 10	0.006	Noninferiority
Distal occlusion device					
SAFER	GuardWire vs. conventional guide wire	801	9.6 vs. 16.5	0.004	Superiority
PRIDE	TriActiv vs. GuardWire	631	11.2 vs. 10.1	0.02	Noninferiority
Distal filter device					
AMEthyst	Interceptor PLUS vs. FilterWire or GuardWire	797	8.0 vs. 7.3	0.025	Noninferiority
SPIDER	SPIDER vs. FilterWire or GuardWire	732	9.1 vs. 8.4	0.012	Noninferiority
CAPTIVE	CardioShield vs. GuardWire	652	11.4 vs. 9.1	>0.05	Noninferiority
FIRE	FilterWire vs. GuardWire	651	9.9 vs. 11.6	0.0008	Noninferiority
TRAP	TRAP vs. conventional guide wire	358	12.7 vs. 17.3	0.24	Superiority

AMEthyst Assessment of the Medtronic Ave Interceptor Saphenous Vein Graft Filter System trial, *CAPTIVE* CardioShield Application Protects During Transluminal Intervention of Vein Grafts by Reducing Emboli trial, *FIRE* FilterWire EX Randomized Evaluation trial, *MACE* major adverse cardiac event, *PRIDE* Protection During Saphenous Vein Graft Intervention to Prevent Distal Embolization trial, *PROXIMAL* Proximal Protection During Saphenous Vein Graft Intervention trial, *SAFER* Saphenous Vein Graft Angioplasty Free of Emboli Randomized trial, *SPIDER* Saphenous Vein Graft in a Distal Embolic Protection Randomized trial, *TRAP* Trap Vascular Filtration System to Reduce Embolic Complications During Stenting of Diseased Saphenous Vein Grafts trial
Adapted from Bangalore S, Bhatt DL. Embolic protection devices. Circulation 2014 Apr 29;129 (17):e470–6

Summary

Routine EPD use as an adjunctive therapy to primary PCI in patients with acute STEMI in the native circulation is not recommended. However, evidence supports the routine use of EPDs in the setting of PCI for SVG lesions.

Disclosure Statement No conflicts of interest to report.

References

1. Higgins CL, Marvel SA, Morrisett JD. Quantification of calcification in atherosclerotic lesions. Arterioscler Thromb Biol. 2005;25:1567–76.
2. Bezerra H, Guagliumi G, Valescchi O, et al. Unraveling the lack of neointimal hyperplasia detected by intravascular ultrasound using optical coherence tomography: lack of spatial resolution or a true biological effect? J Am Coll Cardiol. 2009;53(Suppl A):90A.
3. Witzenbichler B, Maehara A, Weisz G, et al. Relationship between intravascular ultrasound guidance and clinical outcomes after drug-eluting stents: the ADAPT-DES Study. American Heart Association Scientific Sessions. Dallas, TX. 2013.
4. Tuzcu EM, Berkalp B, De Franco A, et al. The dilemma of diagnosing coronary calcification: angiography versus intravascular ultrasound. J Am Coll Cardiol. 1996;27:832–8.
5. Mintz G, Popma J, Pichard A, et al. Patterns of calcification in coronary artery disease. A statistical analysis of intravascular ultrasound and coronary angiography in 1155 lesions. Circulation. 1995;91:1959–65.
6. Ziada KM, Tuzcu EM, De Franco AC, et al. Intravascular ultrasound assessment of the prevalence and causes of angiographic "haziness" following high-pressure coronary stenting. Am J Cardiol. 1997;80:116.
7. Yock P, Fitzgerald P, Popp R. Intravascular ultrasound. Sci Am Sci Med. 1995;2:68.
8. Fitzgerald PJ, St Goar FG, Connolly AJ, et al. Intravascular ultrasound imaging of coronary arteries. Is three layers the norm? Circulation. 1992;86:154–8.
9. Huang D, Swanson EA, Lin CP, et al. Optical coherence tomography. Science. 1991;254:1178.
10. Mintz GS, Nissen SE, Anderson WD, et al. American College of Cardiology clinical expert consensus document on standards for acquisition, measurement and reporting of intravascular ultrasound studies (IVUS). A report of the American College of Cardiology task force on clinical expert consensus documents. J Am Coll Cardiol. 2001;37:1478–92.
11. Prati F, Regar E, Mintz GS, et al. Expert review document on methodology, terminology, and clinical applications of optical coherence tomography: physical principles, methodology of image acquisition, and clinical application for assessment of coronary arteries and atherosclerosis. Eur Heart J. 2010;31(4):401.

12. Terashima M, Kaneda H, Suzuki T. The role of optical coherence tomography in coronary intervention. Korean J Intern Med. 2012;1-12(53):27.

13. Bezerra HG, Costa MA, Guagliumi G, et al. Intracoronary optical coherence tomography: a comprehensive review. J Am Coll Cardiol Interv. 2009;2(11):1035–46.

14. Bouma BE, Tearney GJ, Yabushita H, et al. Evaluation of intracoronary stenting by intravascular optical coherence tomography. Heart. 2003;89:317.

15. Serruys PW, Ormiston JA, Onuma Y, et al. A bioabsorbable everolimus-eluting coronary stent system (ABSORB): 2-year outcomes and results from multiple imaging methods. Lancet. 2009;373:897–910.

16. Kubo T, Imanishi T, Kitabata H, et al. Comparison of vascular response after sirolimus-eluting stent implantation between patients with unstable and stable angina pectoris: a serial optical coherence tomography study. J Am Coll Cardiol Imaging. 2008;1:475–84.

17. Yamaguchi T, Terashima M, Akasaka T, et al. Safety and feasibility of an intravascular optical coherence tomography image wire system in the clinical setting. Am J Cardiol. 2008;101:562–7.

18. Levine GN, Bates ER, Blankenship JC, et al. 2011 ACCF/AHA/SCAI Guideline for Percutaneous Coronary Intervention. A report of the American College of Cardiology Foundation/American Heart Association Task Force on Practice Guidelines and the Society for Cardiovascular Angiography and Interventions. J Am Coll Cardiol. 2011;58:e44–122.

19. Tomey M, Kini A, Sharma S. Current status of rotational atherectomy. J Am Coll Cardiol Intv. 2014;7(4):345–53.

20. Akkus NI, Abdulbaki A, Jimenez E, et al. Atherectomy devices: technology update. Med Devices. 2015;8:1–10.

21. Lee MS, Kim MH, Rha SW. Alternative rota-flush solution for patients with severe coronary artery calcification who undergo rotational atherectomy. J Invasive Cardiol. 2017;29:25–8.

22. Lee MS, Weisner P, Rha SW. Novel technique of advancing the rotational atherectomy device: "single-operator" technique. J Invasive Cardiol. 2016;28(5):183–6.

23. Baim DS. Coronary angioplasty. In: Baim DS, Grossman W, editors. Cardiac catheterization, angiography and intervention. Baltimore, MD: Williams & Wilkins; 1996. p. 551.

24. O'Neill WW, Kleiman NS, Moses J, et al. A prospective, randomized clinical trial of hemodynamic support with Impella 2.5 versus intra-aortic balloon pump in patients undergoing high-risk percutaneous coronary intervention: the PROTECT II study. Circulation. 2012;126:1717–27.

25. Reifart N, Vandormael M, Krajcar M, et al. Randomized comparisons of angioplasty of complex coronary lesions at a single center. Excimer laser, rotational atherectomy, and balloon angioplasty comparison (ERBAC) study. Circulation. 1997;96:91–8.

26. Dill T, Dietz U, Hamm CW, et al. A randomized comparison of balloon angioplasty versus rotational atherectomy in complex coronary lesions (COBRA study). Eur Heart J. 2000;21:1759–66.

27. Abdel-Wahab M, Richardt G, Joachim Buttner H, et al. High-speed rotational atherectomy before paclitaxel-eluting stent implantation in complex calcified coronary lesions: the randomized ROTAXUS (Rotational Atherectomy Prior to Taxus Stent Treatment for Complex Native Coronary Artery Disease) trial. J Am Coll Cardiol Intv. 2013;6:10–9.

28. de Waha S, Allali A, Buttner HJ, Toelg R, Geist V, Neumann FJ, Khattab AA, Richardt G, Abdel-Wahab M. Rotational atherectomy before paclitaxel-eluting stent implantation in complex calcified coronary lesions: two-year clinical outcome of the randomized ROTAXUS trial. Catheter Cardiovasc Interv. 2016;87(4):691–700.

29. Whitlow PL, Bass TA, Kipperman M, et al. Results of the study to determine rotablator and transluminal angioplasty strategy (STRATAS). Am J Cardiol. 2001;87:699–705.

30. Clavijo LC, Steinberg DH, Torguson R, et al. Sirolimus-eluting stents and calcified coronary lesions: clinical outcomes of patients treated with and without rotational atherectomy. Catheter Cardiovasc Interv. 2006;68:873–8.

31. Eggebrecht H, Oldenburg O, Dirsch O, et al. Potential embolization by atherosclerotic debris dislodged from aortic wall during cardiac catheterization: histological and clinical findings in 7,621 patients. Catheter Cardiovasc Interv. 2000;49:389–94.

32. Wang X, Nie SP. The coronary slow flow phenomenon: characteristics, mechanisms and implications. Cardiovasc Diagn Ther. 2011;1(1):37–43.

33. Walton AS, Pomerantsev EV, Oesterle SN, et al. Outcome of narrowing related side branches after high-speed rotational atherectomy. Am J Cardiol. 1996;77:370.

34. Sulimov DS, Abdel-Wahab M, Toelg R, et al. Stuck rotablator: the nightmare of rotational atherectomy. Euro Interv. 2013;9:251–8.

35. Ambrosini V, Sorropago G, Laurenzano E, Golino L, Casafina A, Schiano V, Gabrielli G, Ettori F, Chizzola G, Bernardi G, Spedicato L, Armigliato P, Spampanato C, Furegato M. Early outcome of high energy laser (Excimer) facilitated coronary angioplasty ON hARD and complex calcified and balloon-resistant coronary lesions: LEONARDO study. Cardiovasc Revasc Med. 2015;16:141–6.

36. Bilodeau L, Fretz EB, Taeymans Y, Koolen J, Taylor K, Hilton DJ. Novel use of a high-energy laser catheter for calcified and complex coronary artery lesions. Catheter Cardiovasc Interv. 2004;62:155–61.

37. Topaz O, Safian RD. Eximer laser coronary angioplasty. In: Safian RD, Freed MS, editors. Manual of interventional cardiology. 3rd ed. Royal Oaks, MI: Physicians Press; 2001. p. 681–91.

38. Fernandez JP, Hobson AR, McKenzie D, et al. Beyond the balloon: excimer coronary laser atherectomy

used alone or in combination with rotational atherectomy in the treatment of chronic total occlusions, non-crossable and nonexpansible coronary lesions. EuroIntervention. 2013;9:243–50.

39. McKenzie DB, Talwar S, Jokhi PP, et al. How should I treat severe coronary artery calcification when it is not possible to inflate a balloon or deliver a RotaWire? EuroIntervention. 2011;6:779–83.

40. Fernandez JP, Hobson AR, McKenzie D, et al. Treatment of calcific coronary stenosis with the use of excimer laser coronary atherectomy and rotational atherectomy. Int J Cardiol. 2010;2:801–6.

41. Papaioannou T, Yadegar D, Vari S, et al. Excimer laser (308 nm) recanalization of in-stent restenosis: thermal considerations. Lasers Med Sci. 2001;16:90–100.

42. Burris N, Lippincott RA, Elfe A, et al. Effects of 308 nanometer excimer laser energy on 316 L stainless-steel stents: implications for laser atherectomy of in-stent restenosis. J Invasive Cardiol. 2000;12:555–9.

43. Mehran R, Mintz GS, Satler LF, et al. Treatment of in-stent restenosis with excimer laser coronary angioplasty: mechanisms and results compared with PTCA alone. Circulation. 1997;96:2183–9.

44. Rawlins J, Sambu N, O'Kane P. Strategies for the management of massive intra-coronary thrombus in acute myocardial infarction. Heart. 2013;99:510.

45. Bittl JA. Clinical results with excimer laser coronary angioplasty. Semin Interv Cardiol. 1996;1:129–34.

46. Mintz GS, Kovach JA, Javier SP, et al. Mechanisms of lumen enlargement after excimer laser coronary angioplasty. An intravascular ultrasound study. Circulation. 1995;92:3408–14.

47. Abela GS, Crea F, Smith W, et al. In vitro effects of argon laser radiation on blood: quantitative and morphologic analysis. J Am Coll Cardiol. 1985;5:231–7.

48. Grundfest WS, Litvack F, Forrester JS, et al. Laser ablation of human atherosclerotic plaque without adjacent tissue injury. J Am Coll Cardiol. 1985;5:929–33.

49. Geschwind HJ, Boussignac G, Teisseire B, et al. Conditions for effective Nd-YAG laser angioplasty. Br Heart J. 1984;52:484–9.

50. Biamino G. The excimer laser: science fiction fantasy or practical tool? J Endovasc Ther. 2004;11(Suppl 2):II207–22.

51. Topaz O, Ebersole D, et al. Excimer laser in myocardial infarction: a comparison between STEMI patients with established Q-wave versus patients with non-SEMI (non-Q). Lasers Med Sci. 2008;23(1):1–10.

52. Taylor K, Reiser C. Next generation catheters for excimer laser coronary angioplasty. Lasers Med Sci. 2001;16:133–40.

53. Isner JM, Pickerin JG, Mosseri M. Laser-induced dissections: pathogenesis and implications for therap. J Am Coll Cardiol. 1992;19:1619–21.

54. Van Leeuwen TG, Meertens JH, Velema E, et al. Intraluminal vapor bubble induced by excimer laser pulse causes microsecond arterial dilation and invagination leading to extensive wall damage in the rabbit. Circulation. 1993;87:1258–63.

55. Baumbach A, Bittl JA, Fleck E, Geschwind HJ, Sanborn TA, Tcheng JK, Karch KR. Acute complications of excimer laser coronary angioplasty: a detailed analysis of multicenter results. Coinvestigators of the U.S. and European Percutaenous Excimer Laser Coronary Angioplasty (PELCA) Registries. J Am Coll Cardiol. 1994;23(6):1305–13.

56. Rezkalla SH, Kloner RA. Coronary no-reflow phenomenon. Curr Treat Options Cardiovasc Med. 2005;7:75.

57. Eeckhout E, Kern MJ. The coronary no-reflow phenomenon: a review of mechanisms and therapies. Eur Heart J. 2001;22:729.

58. Henriques JP, Zijlstra F, Ottervanger JP, et al. Incidence and clinical significance of distal embolization during primary angioplasty for acute myocardial infarction. Eur Heart J. 2002;23:1112.

59. Ahn SG, Choi HH, Lee JK, Lee JW, Youn YJ, Yoo SY, Cho BR, Lee SH, Yoon J. The impact of initial and residual thrombus burden on the no-reflow phenomenon in patients with ST-segment elevation myocardial infarction. Coron Artery Dis. 2015;26(3):245–53.

60. Kishi T, Yamada A, Okamatsu S, Sunagawa K. Percutaneous coronary arterial thrombectomy for acute myocardial infarction reduces no-reflow phenomenon and protects against left ventricular remodeling related to the proximal left anterior descending and right coronary artery. Int Heart J. 2007;48(3):287–302.

61. Sianos G, Papafaklis MI, Daemen J, et al. Angiographic stent thrombosis after routine use of drug-eluting stents in ST-segment elevation myocardial infarction: the importance of thrombus burden. J Am Coll Cardiol. 2007;50(7):573–83.

62. Levine GN, Bates ER, Blankenship JC, et al. 2015 ACC/AHA/SCAI Focused Update on Primary Percutaneous Coronary Intervention for Patients With ST-Elevation Myocardial Infarction: An Update of the 2011 ACCF/AHA/SCAI Guideline for Percutaneous Coronary Intervention and the 2013 ACCF/AHA Guideline for the Management of ST-Elevation Myocardial Infarction. J Am Coll Cardiol. 2016;67:1235.

63. Levine GN. 2015 ACC/AHA/SCAI focused update on primary percutaneous coronary intervention. J Am Coll Cardiol. 2016;67:12135.

64. Svilaas T, Vlaar PJ, van der Horst IC, et al. Thrombus aspiration during primary percutaneous coronary intervention. N Engl J Med. 2008;358:557.

65. Vlaar PJ, Svilaas T, van der Horst IC, et al. Cardiac death and reinfarction after 1 year in the Thrombus Aspiration during Percutaneous coronary intervention in Acute myocardial infarction Study (TAPAS): a 1-year follow-up study. Lancet. 2008;371(9628):1915–20.

66. Frobert O, Lagerqvist B, Olivecrona GK, et al. Thrombus aspiration during ST-segment elevation myocardial infarction. N Engl J Med. 2013;369:1587.

67. Lagerqvist B, Frobert O, Olivecrona GK, et al. Outcomes 1 year after thrombus aspiration for myocardial infarction. N Engl J Med. 2014;371:1111.

68. Jolly SS, Cairns JA, Yusuf S, et al. Randomized trial of primary PCI with or without routine manual thrombectomy. N Engl J Med. 2015;372:1389.

69. Jolly SS, Cairns JA, et al. Outcomes after thrombus aspiration for ST elevation myocardial infarction: 1-year follow-up of the prospective randomized TOTAL trial. Lancet. 2016 Jan 9;387(10014):127–35.

70. Ali A, Cox D, Dib N, et al. Rheolytic thrombectomy with percutaneous coronary intervention for infarct size reduction in acute myocardial infarction: 30-day results from a multicenter randomized study. J Am Coll Cardiol. 2006;48(2):244–52.

71. Migliorini A, Stabile A, Rodriguez AE, et al. Comparison of AngioJet rheolytic thrombectomy before direct infarct artery stenting with direct stenting alone in patients with acute myocardial infarction. The JETSTENT trial. J Am Coll Cardiol. 2010;56(16):1298–306.

72. Gibson CM, Cannon CP, Murphy SA, Ryan KA, Mesley R, Marble SJ, et al. Relationship of TIMI myocardial perfusion grade to mortality after administration of thrombolytic drugs. Circulation. 2000;101(2):125–30.

73. Kumbhani DJ, Bavry AA, Desai MY, et al. Role of aspiration and mechanical thrombectomy in patients with acute myocardial infarction undergoing primary angioplasty: an updated meta-analysis of randomized trials. J Am Coll Cardiol. 2014;62:1409.

74. Ali A, Cox D, Dib N, et al. Rheolytic thrombectomy with percutaneous coronary intervention for infarct size redution in acute myocardial infarction: 30-day results from a multicenter randomized study. J Am Coll Cardiol. 2006;48:244.

75. Bavry AA, Kumbhani DJ, Bhatt DL. Role of adjunctive thrombectomy and embolic protection devices in acute myocardial infarction: a comprehensive meta-analysis of randomized trials. Eur Heart J. 2008;29:2989–3001.

76. Stone GW, Webb J, Cox DA, et al. Distal microcirculatory protection during percutaneous coronary intervention in acute ST-segment elevation myocardial infarction: a randomized controlled trial. JAMA. 2005;293:1063.

77. Gick M, Jander N, Bestehorn HP, et al. Randomized evaluation of the effects of filter-based distal protection on myocardial perfusion and infarct size after primary percutaneous catheter intervention in myocardial infarction with and without ST-segment elevation. Circulation. 2005;112:1462.

78. Kelbaek H, Terkelsen CJ, Helqvist S, et al. Randomized comparison of distal protection versus conventional treatment in primary percutaneous coronary intervention: the drug elution and distal protection in ST-elevation myocardial infarction (DEDICATION) trial. J Am Coll Cardiol. 2008;51:899.

79. Kaltoft A, Kelbaek H, Kløvgaard L, Terkelsen CJ, Clemmensen P, Helqvist S, Lassen JF, Thuesen L. Increased rate of stent thrombosis and target lesion revascularization after filter protection in primary percutaneous coronary intervention for ST-segment elevation myocardial infarction: 15-month follow-up of the DEDICATION (Drug Elution and Distal Protection in ST Elevation Myocardial Infarction) trial. J Am Coll Cardiol. 2010;55:867–71.

80. White CJ, Ramee SR, Collins TJ, Mesa JE, Jain A. Percutaneous angioscopy of saphenous vein coronary bypass grafts. J Am Coll Cardiol. 1993;21:1181–5.

81. Silva JA, White CJ, Collins TJ, Ramee SR. Morphologic comparison of atherosclerotic lesions in native coronary arteries and saphenous vein graphs with intracoronary angioscopy in patients with unstable angina. Am Heart J. 1998;136:156–63.

82. Stone GW, Rogers C, Hermiller J, et al. Randomized comparison of distal protection with a filter-based catheter and a balloon occlusion and aspiration system during percutaneous intervention of diseased saphenous vein aorto-coronary bypass grafts. Circulation. 2003;108:548–53.

83. Baim DS, Wahr D, George B, et al. Randomized trial of a distal embolic protection device during percutaneous intervention of saphenous vein aorto-coronary bypass grafts. Circulation. 2002;105:1285.

84. Carrozza JP Jr, Mumma M, Breall JA, et al. Randomized evaluation of the TriActiv balloon-protection flush and extraction system for the treatment of saphenous vein graft disease. J Am Coll Cardiol. 2005;46:1677.

85. Ashby DT, Dangas G, Aymong EA, et al. Effect of percutaneous coronary interventions for in-stent restenosis in degenerated saphenous vein grafts without distal embolic protection. J Am Coll Cardiol. 2003;41:749.

86. Mauri L, Cox D, Hermiller J, et al. The PROXIMAL trial: proximal protection during saphenous vein graft intervention using the proxis embolic protection system: a randomized, prospective, multicenter clinical trial. J Am Coll Cardiol. 2007;50:1442.

87. Mauri L, Rogers C, Baim DS. Devices for distal protection during percutaneous coronary revascularization. Circulation. 2006;113:2651–6.

Intracoronary Imaging

14

Takashi Kubo and Takashi Akasaka

About us Wakayama Medical University is located in the southwestern part of Japan. Areas of our expertise are intracoronary imaging (OCT, IVUS, NIRS, CT, and MRI) and coronary physiology (CFR and FFR). We have participated in a number of international clinical trials and worked as an imaging core laboratory. We will continue our efforts to elucidate the mechanisms of coronary atherosclerosis and establish the clinical significance of imaging- and physiology-oriented percutaneous coronary intervention.

Introduction

Intravascular imaging provides a valuable opportunity to assess coronary atherosclerosis in living people and to guide percutaneous coronary intervention (PCI). Several catheter-based, invasive, intravascular imaging methods are currently available for research and clinical purposes. Intravascular ultrasound (IVUS) and optical coherence tomography (OCT) are commonly used intravascular imaging methods in our daily clinical practice.

T. Kubo (✉) · T. Akasaka
Department of Cardiovascular Medicine, Wakayama Medical University, Wakayama, Japan
e-mail: takakubo@wakayama-med.ac.jp;
akasat@wakayama-med.ac.jp

IVUS

Grayscale IVUS

- IVUS uses high-frequency (20–60 MHz) sound waves and produces cross-sectional, monochrome images of a coronary vessel with a resolution of 100–200 μm. IVUS enables visualization of not only the lumen of the coronary arteries but also the atherosclerotic plaque within the vessel wall, which cannot be seen by angiography.
- In the IVUS image, the coronary artery wall is visualized as three layers. Moving outward from the lumen, the first layer includes a complex of intima, plaque, and internal elastic membrane. The second layer includes the media with external elastic membrane (EEM), which is usually less echogenic than the intima. The third and outer layer includes the adventitia and periadventitial tissues.
- The plaque is classified into high, iso, or low echo-reflectance type. The high echoic plaque is usually regarded as "hard" or "calcified"; the iso echoic plaques as "fibrotic"; and the low echoic plaques as "soft" or "lipid rich."
- The low or iso echoic plaque with ultrasound attenuation behind the plaque, in the absence of calcification, is described as "attenuated plaque." This is considered to be atheroma with a lipid-rich necrotic core. However,

diagnostic accuracy of grayscale IVUS for plaque tissue characterization is modest.

- For guiding PCI, IVUS is useful to assess angiographically ambiguous lesions including intermediate lesions of uncertain stenotic severity, aneurysmal lesions, ostial stenoses, tortuous vessels, diffuse disease, left main lesions, bifurcation stenosis, sites with plaque rupture, stent edge dissection, intraluminal filling defects, angiographically hazy lesions, and angiographically foreshortened vessels.

- In addition, IVUS is capable of measuring lumen and vessel diameter, plaque and stent area, and plaque eccentricity and vascular remodeling index, which are helpful information to determine balloon and stent size (Figs. 14.1 and 14.2).

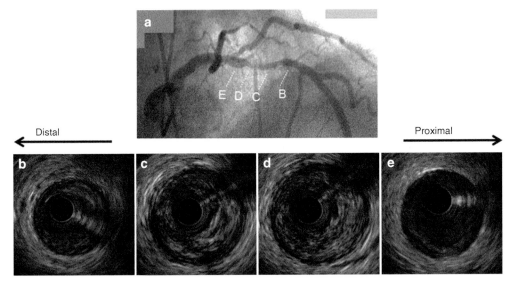

Fig. 14.1 Positive vessel remodeling. Coronary angiography shows an intermediate lesion in the proximal left anterior descending coronary artery (**a**). Grayscale IVUS demonstrates that the lesion EEM area (**c** and **d**) is greater than the reference EEM area (**b** and **e**)

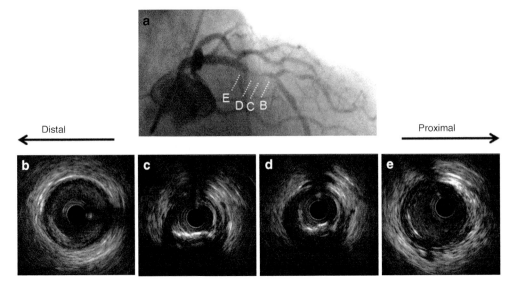

Fig. 14.2 Negative vessel remodeling. Coronary angiography shows a severe stenosis lesion in the proximal left anterior descending coronary artery (**a**). Grayscale IVUS demonstrates that the lesion EEM area (**c** and **d**) is smaller than the reference EEM area (**b** and **e**). The plaque in the lesion (**c** and **d**) is usually regarded as "calcified"

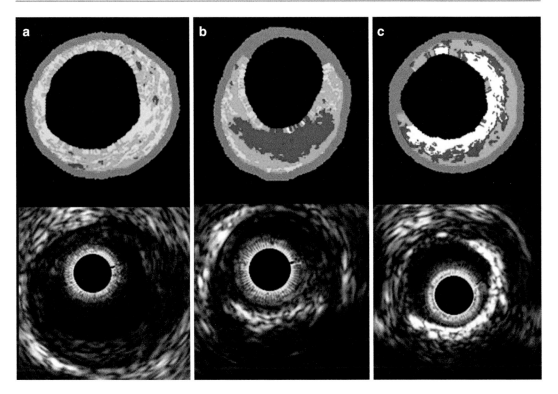

Fig. 14.3 Plaque type classification by VH-IVUS. VH-IVUS shows pathological intimal thickening (**a**), thin-capped fibroatheroma (**b**), and fibrocalcific plaque (**c**)

Virtual Histology (VH)-IVUS

- Based on the radiofrequency analysis of ultrasound backscattered signals, VH-IVUS allows automatic assessment of plaque tissue composition.
- VH-IVUS identifies four different tissue types and produces a color-coded map of the plaque (fibrous = green, fibro-fatty = yellow green, dense calcium = white, and necrotic core = red).
- In the VH-IVUS image, the plaque is classified into pathological intimal thickening, thin-capped fibroatheroma (TCFA), thick-capped fibroatheroma, fibrotic plaque, or fibrocalcific plaque (Fig. 14.3).
- Pathological intimal thickening consists of mainly a mixture of fibrous and fibro-fatty tissue with <10% confluent necrotic core and <10% confluent dense calcium.
- VH-derived TCFA is defined as a fibroatheroma (>10% confluent necrotic core) without evidence of a fibrous cap (necrotic core abutting the lumen >30°) because the resolution of IVUS is

insufficient for detecting the thin fibrous cap of <65 μm determined by pathology.
- Thick-capped fibroatheroma is defined as a fibroatheroma with a definable fibrous cap. Fibrotic plaque consists of mainly fibrous tissue with <10% confluent necrotic core, <15% fibro-fatty tissue, and <10% confluent dense calcium.
- Fibrocalcific plaque is composed of nearly all fibrous tissue and dense calcium with <10% confluent necrotic core.
- In the stent-treated lesion, stent struts exhibit a VH-IVUS appearance of white surrounded by a red "halo" and neointima within the stent is indicated predominantly by a mixture of fibrous and fibro-fatty tissue.

OCT

- OCT is an optical analog of IVUS using near-infrared light (wavelength: 1250–1350 nm). OCT provides an extraordinarily high-resolution (10–20 μm) image.

- However, the visible range of OCT is limited in the vessel surface because the depth of penetration of near-infrared light is shallow (<2 mm, depended on the tissue type).
- OCT enables visualization of the intima (high-signal-intensity inner layer), media (low-signal-intensity middle layer), and adventitia (high-signal-intensity outer layer) in the coronary artery wall.
- OCT is capable of differentiating three types of coronary plaque: fibrous, calcified, and lipidic.
- The OCT images of fibrous plaque are characterized by a homogeneous, signal-rich region; fibrocalcific plaque by a well-delineated, signal-poor region with sharp border; and lipid-rich plaque by a signal-poor region with diffuse border.
- OCT delineates unstable plaque features including plaque rupture, erosion, and calcified nodule(s) in the culprit lesion of an acute coronary syndrome.
- Plaque rupture is characterized by the presence of fibrous-cap discontinuity with a clear cavity formed inside the plaque (Fig. 14.4); OCT-derived erosion by the presence of attached thrombus overlying an intact plaque (Fig. 14.5); and OCT-derived calcified nodule by the fibrous-cap disruption over a calcified plaque with protruding calcification, superficial calcium, and substantive calcium proximal and/or distal to the lesion (Fig. 14.6).
- Furthermore, OCT has the potential to detect key features of vulnerable plaque such as TCFA, macrophage accumulation, cholesterol crystals, and the vasa vasorum. The high resolution of OCT can directly identify the thin fibrous cap of <65 μm overlying a lipid-rich necrotic core.
- OCT-derived macrophage accumulation is characterized by signal-rich, distinct, or confluent punctuate regions with shadowing; cholesterol crystal by a thin, linear region of high signal intensity within the lipid plaque; and vasa vasorum by a signal-poor, well-delineated void within plaque. Microchannels in chronic total occlusions give a "lotus root" appearance on OCT (Fig. 14.7).
- The high resolution of OCT is beneficial for guidance of PCI. The clear image of OCT permits automated quantitative analyses, which provides accurate and highly reproducible measurements of lumen.

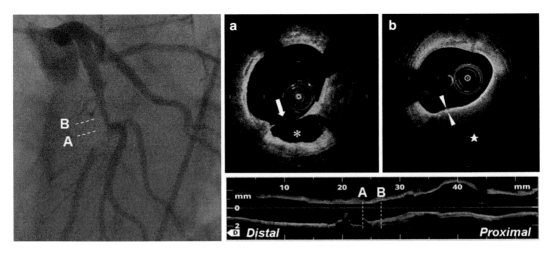

Fig. 14.4 Plaque rupture. Images were obtained from a 72-year-old female with ST-segment-elevation myocardial infarction. Coronary angiography showed an occlusion in the proximal left anterior descending coronary artery. OCT after aspiration thrombectomy demonstrated fibrous-cap disruption (arrow) and core cavity (star) (**a**), and thin-capped fibroatheroma (fibrous cap = arrowheads, and lipid core = asterisk) (**b**)

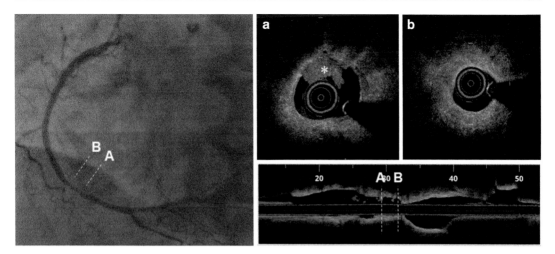

Fig. 14.5 Erosion. Images were obtained from a 63-year-old female with ST-segment-elevation myocardial infarction. Coronary angiography showed a lesion with haziness and a filling defect in mid-right coronary artery. OCT demonstrated a probable erosion which was characterized by intracoronary thrombosis (**a**, asterisk) overlying a fibrous plaque (**b**)

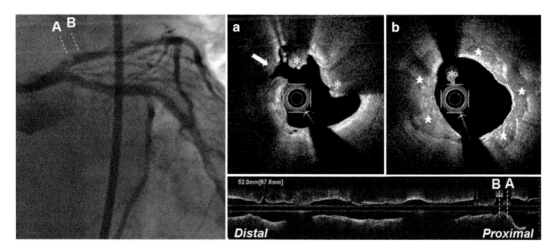

Fig. 14.6 Calcified nodule. Images were obtained from a 78-year-old male with non-ST-segment-elevation myocardial infarction. Coronary angiogram showed a filling defect and haziness in the ostial left anterior descending coronary artery. OCT demonstrated a calcified nodule, which was characterized by thrombus (**a**, asterisks) and rupture (**a**, arrow) of calcified plaque (**b**, stars) without lipid (courtesy of Dr. Kadotani. Kakogawa Central City Hospital, Kakogawa, Japan)

- OCT identifies stent malapposition, tissue protrusion, and stent-edge dissection immediately after PCI and detects thin neointima over drug-eluting stents and neoatherosclerosis (defined as a development of atherosclerosis in the neointima) at late follow-up. Furthermore, in the case of bioresorbable scaffolds, OCT provides information regarding the time course of scaffold dissolution.

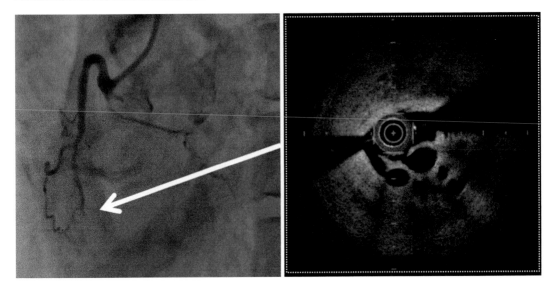

Fig. 14.7 Lotus root appearance in chronic total occlusion. Coronary angiography shows an occlusion in the mid-right coronary artery. OCT after pre-dilatation with a small balloon demonstrates multiple channels within the lesion

IVUS Versus OCT

- Each method has advantages and disadvantages in technology.
- Advantages of IVUS are deeper signal penetration that allows visualization of the whole vessel wall and longer pullback distance that permits assessment from distal coronary artery to aorto-ostial junction. However, IVUS has had no fundamental advances in the technology in more than a decade.
- Advantages of OCT are higher resolution image that is easy to interpret and faster pullback speed that enables 3-dimensional reconstruction of coronary arteries.
- However, for reliable image acquisition, OCT requires injection of contrast media to displace blood from the vessel lumen because the OCT signal is attenuated by the presence of red blood cells. Therefore, OCT is not suited for assessing coronary artery ostia and totally or subtotally occluded lesions.

Indications for Use

- Both IVUS and OCT are powerful tools for research. These methods increase our knowledge of the nature of atherosclerosis, pathophysiology of vulnerable plaques, and mechanism of restenosis and thrombosis following PCI.
- In addition, IVUS and OCT are widely used in daily clinical practice. These methods provide valuable information that has a great influence on the procedural strategy for lesion preparation and stent optimization especially in PCI to complex lesions.
- However, routine use of intravascular imaging in PCI may be limited by the cost of the imaging catheter and the extra time for imaging procedures in addition to angiography guidance alone.

Evidence Base

IVUS

- A plaque burden of at least 70%, a minimal luminal area of 4.0 mm^2 or less, and the presence of VH-derived TCFA were independent risk factors of subsequent major adverse cardiovascular events [1].
- Increase of plaque volume is associated with increased risk of future cardiac event. Decrease of plaque volume is observed during intensive statin treatment.

- IVUS is useful for the assessment of angiographically intermediate left main stenosis: IVUS-measured minimum lumen area of <4.8 mm^2 is reported to be the cutoff for predicting myocardial ischemia [2].
- Stent under-expansion is associated with stent restenosis and stent thrombosis: IVUS-measured minimum stent area of <5.3–5.5 mm^2 is reported to be the cutoff for predicting late restenosis in second-generation drug-eluting stents [3].
- Optimal stent-edge landing zone is a segment with less plaque: IVUS-measured residual plaque burden of >55% in the stent-edge segment is reported to be the cutoff for predicting stent-edge restenosis [4].
- Attenuated plaque and VH-derived fibro-fatty tissue are associated with angiographic slow flow during PCI and periprocedural myocardial infarction (MI).
- Late-acquired stent malapposition is often observed in very late drug-eluting stent thrombosis. IVUS is helpful for guidance of coronary stent implantation, particularly in cases with long stenting (stent length >28 mm) [5] or left main coronary artery stenting [6]. Several studies have demonstrated that IVUS-guided PCI reduced major adverse cardiac events including stent thrombosis, MI, and target-lesion revascularization after drug-eluting stent implantation compared with angiography-guided PCI [7].

OCT

- OCT-derived TCFA and vasa vasorum are potential predictors of subsequent plaque progression and lumen narrowing.
- Increase of fibrous-cap thickness and decrease of lipid arc and macrophage density are observed during lipid-lowering therapy with statin and/or eicosapentaenoic acid.
- OCT-derived TCFA and lipid-rich plaque (lipid arc >180°) are associated with angiographic slow flow during PCI and periprocedural MI [8].
- A registry study reported that OCT-derived irregular tissue protrusions as well as small minimal stent area were associated with target-lesion revascularization within 1 year after PCI (Fig. 14.8) [9].
- Optimal stent-edge landing zone is a segment with less lipidic plaque: OCT-measured lipid arc of >180° in the stent-edge segment is reported to be the cutoff for predicting stent-edge restenosis [10].

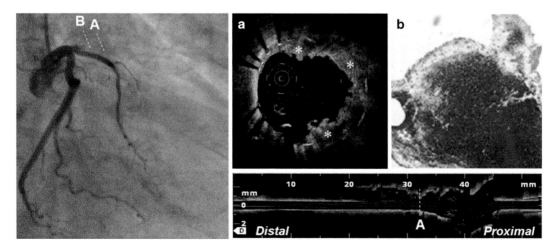

Fig. 14.8 Early stent thrombosis. Images were obtained from a 63-year-old male with stent thrombosis 13 days after second-generation drug-eluting stent implantation. Coronary angiography showed an occlusion in the previously stented segment in the proximal left anterior descending coronary artery. OCT demonstrated in-stent thrombus (**a**, asterisks). After OCT imaging, red thrombi, which consisted mainly of red blood cells, were obtained from the infarct-related lesion by aspiration thrombectomy (**b**)

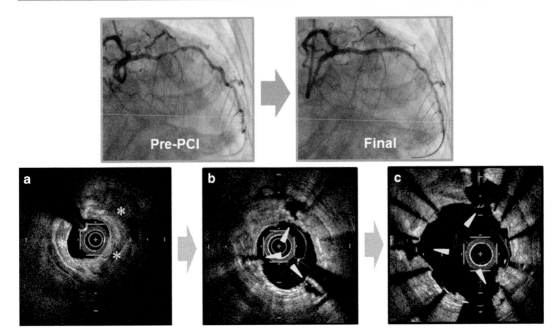

Fig. 14.9 Calcium fracture. Coronary angiography showed a significant stenosis in the proximal left anterior descending coronary artery. OCT before PCI demonstrated circumferential calcium in the lesion (**a**, asterisks). We used a cutting balloon for lesion preparation and successfully induced calcium fracture (**b**, arrowheads). We then implanted a stent and achieved adequate lumen expansion (**c**)

- In bifurcation PCI, OCT-measured small side-branch angle (<50°) and long carina-tip length (>1.7 mm) are predictors of side-branch occlusion after main-vessel stenting [11]. The guidance with 3-dimensional OCT imaging is helpful in bifurcation PCI for guide wire recrossing into the jailed side branch after main-vessel stenting.
- In circumferentially calcified lesions, if the calcium is thin (OCT-measured minimum calcium thickness <500 μm), high-pressure ballooning or cutting balloon angioplasty before stenting is effective for inducing calcium fracture which is associated with adequate stent expansion and favorable late outcomes (Fig. 14.9); and if it is thick (>500 μm), use of rotablator is recommended [12].
- In small-vessel stenting (≤2.5 mm), OCT-measured minimum stent area of <3.5 mm² is reported to be the cutoff for predicting late restenosis in second-generation drug-eluting stents [13].
- There is no evidence demonstrating direct relationship between OCT-identified stent strut without neointimal coverage and very late stent thrombosis.
- In in-stent restenosis with OCT-derived homogenous signal-rich neointima, drug-coated balloon therapy is reported to be effective for preventing repeat revascularization [14].
- Late-acquired stent malapposition and OCT-derived neoatherosclerosis are often observed in very late drug-eluting stent thrombosis (Fig. 14.10). Only one registry study demonstrated that OCT-guided PCI reduced cardiac death and MI compared with angiography-guided PCI [15].

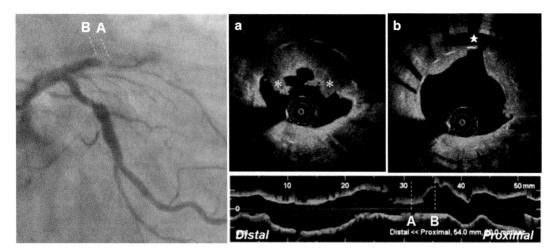

Fig. 14.10 Very late stent thrombosis. Images were obtained from a 71-year-old male with stent thrombosis 5 years after first-generation drug-eluting stent implantation. Coronary angiography showed an occlusion in the previously stented segment in the proximal left anterior descending coronary artery. OCT demonstrated in-stent thrombus (**a**, asterisks) and late-acquired stent malapposition (**b**, star)

Conclusion

IVUS and OCT are useful in assessing coronary atherosclerosis, guiding and optimizing PCI, and determining mechanisms of stent failure. Use of intravascular imaging in addition to angiography has a potential to improve clinical outcomes in patients undergoing PCI.

References

1. Stone GW, Maehara A, Lansky AJ, de Bruyne B, Cristea E, Mintz GS, Mehran R, McPherson J, Farhat N, Marso SP, Parise H, Templin B, White R, Zhang Z, Serruys PW, PROSPECT Investigators. A prospective natural-history study of coronary atherosclerosis. N Engl J Med. 2011;364:226–35.

2. Kang SJ, Lee JY, Ahn JM, Song HG, Kim WJ, Park DW, Yun SC, Lee SW, Kim YH, Mintz GS, Lee CW, Park SW, Park SJ. Intravascular ultrasound-derived predictors for fractional flow reserve in intermediate left main disease. JACC Cardiovasc Interv. 2011;4:1168–74.

3. Song HG, Kang SJ, Ahn JM, Kim WJ, Lee JY, Park DW, Lee SW, Kim YH, Lee CW, Park SW, Park SJ. Intravascular ultrasound assessment of optimal stent area to prevent in-stent restenosis after zotarolimus-, everolimus-, and sirolimus-eluting stent implantation. Catheter Cardiovasc Interv. 2014;83:873–8.

4. Kang SJ, Cho YR, Park GM, Ahn JM, Kim WJ, Lee JY, Park DW, Lee SW, Kim YH, Lee CW, Mintz GS, Park SW, Park SJ. Intravascular ultrasound predictors for edge restenosis after newer generation drug-eluting stent implantation. Am J Cardiol. 2013;111:1408–14.

5. Hong SJ, Kim BK, Shin DH, Nam CM, Kim JS, Ko YG, Choi D, Kang TS, Kang WC, Her AY, Kim YH, Hur SH, Hong BK, Kwon H, Jang Y, Hong MK, IVUS-XPL Investigators. Effect of intravascular ultrasound-guided vs. angiography-guided everolimus-eluting stent implantation: the IVUS-XPL randomized clinical trial. JAMA. 2015;314:2155–63.

6. Park SJ, Kim YH, Park DW, Lee SW, Kim WJ, Suh J, Yun SC, Lee CW, Hong MK, Lee JH, Park SW, MAIN-COMPARE Investigators. Impact of intravascular ultrasound guidance on long-term mortality in stenting for unprotected left main coronary artery stenosis. Circ Cardiovasc Interv. 2009;2:167–77.

7. Witzenbichler B, Maehara A, Weisz G, Neumann FJ, Rinaldi MJ, Metzger DC, Henry TD, Cox DA, Duffy PL, Brodie BR, Stuckey TD, Mazzaferri EL Jr, Xu K, Parise H, Mehran R, Mintz GS, Stone GW. Relationship between intravascular ultrasound guidance and clinical outcomes after drug-eluting stents: the assessment of dual antiplatelet therapy with

drug-eluting stents (ADAPT-DES) study. Circulation. 2014;129:463–70.

8. Tanaka A, Imanishi T, Kitabata H, Kubo T, Takarada S, Tanimoto T, Kuroi A, Tsujioka H, Ikejima H, Komukai K, Kataiwa H, Okouchi K, Kashiwaghi M, Ishibashi K, Matsumoto H, Takemoto K, Nakamura N, Hirata K, Mizukoshi M, Akasaka T. Lipid-rich plaque and myocardial perfusion after successful stenting in patients with non-ST-segment elevation acute coronary syndrome: an optical coherence tomography study. Eur Heart J. 2009;30:1348–55.

9. Soeda T, Uemura S, Park SJ, Jang Y, Lee S, Cho JM, Kim SJ, Vergallo R, Minami Y, Ong DS, Gao L, Lee H, Zhang S, Yu B, Saito Y, Jang IK. Incidence and clinical significance of poststent optical coherence tomography findings: one-year follow-up study from a multicenter registry. Circulation. 2015;132:1020–9.

10. Ino Y, Kubo T, Matsuo Y, Yamaguchi T, Shiono Y, Shimamura K, Katayama Y, Nakamura T, Aoki H, Taruya A, Nishiguchi T, Satogami K, Yamano T, Kameyama T, Orii M, Oota S, Kuroi A, Kitabata H, Tanaka A, Hozumi T, Akasaka T. Optical coherence tomography predictors for edge restenosis after everolimus-eluting stent implantation. Circ Cardiovasc Interv. 2016;9:e004231.

11. Watanabe M, Uemura S, Sugawara Y, Ueda T, Soeda T, Takeda Y, Kawata H, Kawakami R, Saito Y. Side branch complication after a single-stent crossover technique: prediction with frequency domain optical coherence tomography. Coron Artery Dis. 2014;25:321–9.

12. Kubo T, Shimamura K, Ino Y, Yamaguchi T, Matsuo Y, Shiono Y, Taruya A, Nishiguchi T, Shimokado A, Teraguchi I, Orii M, Yamano T, Tanimoto T, Kitabata H, Hirata K, Tanaka A, Akasaka T. Superficial calcium fracture after PCI as assessed by OCT. JACC Cardiovasc Imaging. 2015;8:1228–9.

13. Matsuo Y, Kubo T, Aoki H, Satogami K, Ino Y, Kitabata H, Taruya A, Nishiguchi T, Teraguchi I, Shimamura K, Shiono Y, Orii M, Yamano T, Tanimoto T, Yamaguchi T, Hirata K, Tanaka A, Akasaka T. Optimal threshold of postintervention minimum stent area to predict in-stent restenosis in small coronary arteries: an optical coherence tomography analysis. Catheter Cardiovasc Interv. 2016;87:E9–E14.

14. Tada T, Kadota K, Hosogi S, Miyake K, Amano H, Nakamura M, Izawa Y, Kubo S, Ichinohe T, Hyoudou Y, Eguchi H, Hayakawa Y, Otsuru S, Hasegawa D, Shigemoto Y, Habara S, Tanaka H, Fuku Y, Kato H, Goto T, Mitsudo K. Association between tissue characteristics evaluated with optical coherence tomography and mid-term results after paclitaxel-coated balloon dilatation for in-stent restenosis lesions: a comparison with plain old balloon angioplasty. Eur Heart J Cardiovasc Imaging. 2014;15:307–15.

15. Prati F, Di Vito L, Biondi-Zoccai G, Occhipinti M, et al. Angiography alone versus angiography plus optical coherence tomography to guide decision-making during percutaneous coronary intervention: the Centro per la Lotta contro l'Infarto-Optimisation of Percutaneous Coronary Intervention (CLI-OPCI) study. EuroIntervention. 2012;8:823–9.

Physiologic Lesion Assessment: Fractional Flow Reserve

Mohammad Sahebjalal and Nicholas Curzen

About Us University Hospital Southampton is a large teaching hospital in the south of England. It is a regional center for complex cardiac intervention as well as TAVI. Professor Curzen was Chief Investigator of the RIPCORD, FFRCT RIPCORD, COMET studies and is CI of the ongoing multicenter randomized RIPCORD II and FORECAST trials, both of which study the effect of physiology in addition to coronary anatomy.

Introduction

- Patient outcome following percutaneous coronary intervention (PCI) is predominantly determined by three factors: clinical presentation, comorbidities, and the decision-making process before, during, and after the PCI procedure.
- In order to justify *any intervention*, there needs to be reason to think that this will result in either (a) an improvement of symptoms or (b) an improvement in prognosis or (c) both.

M. Sahebjalal
Coronary Research Group, University Hospital Southampton NHS Foundation Trust, Southampton, UK

N. Curzen (✉)
Coronary Research Group, University Hospital Southampton NHS Foundation Trust, Southampton, UK

Faculty of Medicine, University of Southampton, Southampton, UK
e-mail: nick.curzen@uhs.nhs.uk

- For the interventionalist, the skillful application of modern diagnostic tools and reference to the appropriate evidence base can facilitate delivery of optimal patient care.
- Coronary angiography has been used as a diagnostic tool for more than half a century; however it is now well established that coronary angiography alone has important flaws and, in particular, can correlate poorly with the functional importance of a stenosis within the epicardial arteries.
- Further, the evidence base increasingly points to lesion-level ischemia as our target for revascularization. The availability of invasive physiological lesion assessment has revolutionized our ability to define with precision the presence or absence of lesion-level ischemia [1].
- The aim of this chapter is to review the evidence for and the expanding role of physiological lesion assessment in our everyday interventional practice.
  NOTE: Since this chapter was originally written, 2 large randomised trials (DEFINE FLAIR & SWEDEHEART) have demonstrated the equivalent clinical utility of iFR to direct management strategy compared to FFR. Specifically, *in these trials an iFR-guided revascularisation strategy was non-inferior to an FFR-guided strategy with respect to MACE*. Although outside the remit of this chapter, the authors support the use of either FFR or iFR for the purpose of improving the diagnostic accuracy and personalised

© Springer International Publishing AG, part of Springer Nature 2018
A. Myat et al. (eds.), *The Interventional Cardiology Training Manual*,
https://doi.org/10.1007/978-3-319-71635-0_15

management of patients. The message is: USE FFR or IFR MORE in routine practice... don't waste energy on arguing which modality is best because they are both now well validated.

Coronary Physiology

Structure of Coronary Arteries

- Normal coronary arteries have a trilaminar structure consisting of the intima, media, and adventitia.
- The endothelial cells of the tunica intima, although once thought of as inert, play an important and dynamic role in regulation of hemostasis and vascular tone. They have a synthetic and metabolic capability to respond to any changes in hemodynamic forces, and it is this balance which maintains vascular homeostasis [2].
- Any disturbance in this balance, however, will predispose the vasculature to vasoconstriction and therefore disturbance of coronary blood flow. The complex interaction between chronic vascular inflammation and endothelial dysfunction is a precursor to the development of atheroma and its subsequent natural history.

Coronary Arteries and Perfusion

- The function of the coronary vasculature has been traditionally, and artificially, divided into three groups:
  - The epicardial vessels which are visible on angiography and offer little resistance to blood flow
  - The small arteries and arterioles (>400 µm)
  - The capillary system and arterioles (<400 µm), also known as restrictive vessels, which primarily control the myocardial distal flow [3–6]
- During increased oxygen demand, the resistance of the microvascular segment decreases, thus allowing for an increase in blood flow.
- The same can apply when there is an increase in resistance to blood flow in epicardial arteries due to a stenosis. The resistance in microvascular structure consequently reduces,

thereby maintaining total resistance and in turn preserving the resting coronary flow.
- Once the epicardial artery stenosis increases further, the total upstream resistance increases and results in decreased myocardial flow regardless of the small vessel bed. This consequently leads to myocardial ischemia and angina [2, 7].

Coronary Blood Flow

- The myocardium has the highest oxygen demand per tissue mass. The resting coronary blood flow is about 250 mL/min.
- Vascular tone plays an important role in regulating coronary blood flow and is determined by four main factors: perfusion pressure, myocardial compression, myocardial metabolism, and neurohormonal control [8].

Perfusion Pressure
- Coronary blood flow occurs mainly during diastole and, under normal conditions, coronary pressures are equal to the central aortic pressure throughout the epicardial vessel.
- It is this unique property of coronary perfusion, which has allowed interventionists the use of an unequivocal reference value during physiological assessment of a lesion (i.e., the central aortic pressure, Pa).

Myocardial Metabolism
- Coronary vascular resistance is primarily under metabolite control and even if neurohormonal controls are cut off the myocardium has the ability to match blood flow to its metabolic requirement [8].
- The exact nature of this is unclear; however, adenosine and adenosine triphosphate (ATP)-sensitive potassium channels have received considerable attention as effectors of coronary vascular tone.
- Adenosine is a potent coronary vasodilator and a metabolite of cardiac myocytes. It is believed that myocytes release adenosine as myocardial PO_2 falls resulting in increased coronary blood flow. Chilian et al. used dipyridamole, a nucleoside transport inhibitor, to promote release of endogenous adenosine and examine its effect on coronary

resistance. They discovered that during controlled conditions, the microvascular resistance fell to 27% indicating that adenosine exerts its greatest vasodilatory effect on microvasculature.

- ATP is another metabolic agent, which is believed to effect coronary vascular resistance. ATP-sensitive potassium channels are usually inhibited by intracellular ATP; thus, during hypoxia which results in decreased intracellular ATP, these channels are activated resulting in relaxation of smooth muscles, and therefore vasodilation.

Neurohormonal Controls

- Branches of the parasympathetic and sympathetic division of the autonomic nervous system supply the coronary vasculature. Both fibers are located within the vascular wall of large arteries with denser innervation being present in resistance arterioles and capillary tree.
- The stellate ganglion is the major source of cardiac sympathetic innervation and the vagus nerve supplies the efferent cholinergic nerves [8].
- Sympathetic control is mediated via α-adrenergic and β-adrenergic receptors within the microvascular structure. The response of the coronary microcirculation to α-adrenergic activation is vasoconstriction whereas activation of β-adrenergic receptors of the coronary vasculature produces vasodilation.

The Flaws of Angiographic Lesion Assessment

- Since its advent, the use of the angiogram to determine the presence and extent of coronary artery disease (CAD) has become a standard platform for patient diagnosis and management.
- It is clear, however, *that even very experienced operators cannot accurately define whether a specific angiographic stenosis is "significant" in a proportion of lesions, perhaps around 30%, if the currency of significance in this context is lesion-specific ischemia.*
- Observational reports derived from a variety of trials and studies have reinforced this discrepancy between the angiographic and physiological significance of stenosis. Thus, as shown in Fig. 15.1, there are mild-to-moderate lesions that do cause ischemia and severe-looking lesions that do not.
- As the evidence increases that ischemia should be the target for revascularization, it becomes increasingly obvious that making an accurate diagnosis regarding lesion-specific ischemia is critical to accurate, bespoke management of patients [9].

Physiological Indices of the Coronary Circulation

Several indicators for measuring cardiac physiology have been proposed to guide clinical decision-making. These include coronary flow reserve (CFR), index of microvascular resistance (IMR), instantaneous wave-free ratio (iFR), and fractional flow reserve (FFR).

Coronary Flow Reserve

- Myocardial blood flow represents approximately 5% of cardiac flow. Due to the nature of myocardial activity there is a high oxygen demand, even at rest, and as a result the oxygen extraction is much higher compared to other organs.
- Coronary blood flow is able to supply oxygen effectively for any given myocardial demand and normally increases substantially in response to the increase in myocardial oxygen demand. This increase from baseline to maximal flow is termed the coronary flow reserve (CFR).
- CFR can be defined as the ratio of hyperemic blood flow to resting myocardial flow with a normal value of 4–6, indicating that the microvascular resistance can reduce by a factor of 4–6 [7].
- CFR measurement, however, is of limited value for clinical decision-making during PCI as it is a combined measurement of resistance in epicardial vessels as well as the microvasculature [2].

Index of Microvascular Resistance

- IMR is a relatively novel specific index of microvascular function, which, unlike CFR, is

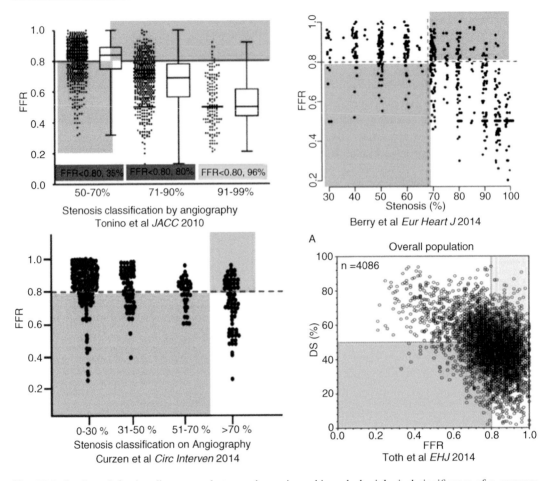

Fig. 15.1 Studies reinforcing discrepancy between the angiographic and physiological significance of a coronary artery stenosis [9]

independent of epicardial vascular disease and hemodynamic influences [7].

- Fearon and colleagues introduced the concept of Index of microvascular resistance with a notion that the mean transient time during hyperemia is inversely proportional to flow and therefore suggested that IMR can be calculated during maximum hyperemia using the following formula [1, 7]:

$$IMR = \text{distal coronary pressure}(Pd) \\ \times \text{mean transient time}$$

- They validated this using a coronary thermo-dilution concept, which involved using a regular pressure wire with a microsensor mounted 3 cm from the tip of the wire to enable simul-taneous pressure and temperature measurement after injecting 3 mL of saline at room temperature. From this they could measure the mean transit time [9].

- IMR has been well validated in animal studies and was recently used as an independent prognostic factor in patients with ST-segment-elevation myocardial infarction (STEMI). This study, in which 253 patients underwent IMR assessment immediately after having primary PCI, concluded that IMR measurement at the time of primary PCI for STEMI is an independent predictor for long-term clinical outcome, including death [10].

- IMR may be a useful method for predicting clinical outcome in acute MI patients in the future, although larger studies are required.

Fractional Flow Reserve

- Flow, pressure, and resistance are the important parameters in circulatory function, in an analogous manner to electrical circuits (Ohm's: law V=IR). Absolute flow and resistance are very difficult to calculate as they are both dependent on myocardial mass and therefore no unequivocal normal value exists, making their impact on clinical decision-making modest [2, 7].
- Myocardial perfusion pressures, on the other hand, equal the central aortic pressure and therefore, across a normal coronary artery, the pressure is transmitted completely without any pressure loss to the most distal region.
- This is the basis for the concept that, *if downstream resistance can be assumed to be negligible* (i.e., the microcirculatory resistance is minimal), the pressure drop across an epicardial stenosis is proportional to flow, and the flow measured can therefore be expressed as a fraction of what the flow would have been if no epicardial stenosis was present. Negligible

distal resistance is achieved by inducing maximal hyperemia in the microcirculation using agents including adenosine, papaverine, and regadenoson.
- *Fractional flow reserve (FFR) is thus the ratio of maximal blood flow in a stenotic artery distal to the stenosis in relation to the maximum blood flow in that artery if no stenosis was present.*
- This physiological parameter has been painstakingly correlated with noninvasive parameters of ischemia in order to produce an artificial, but highly reproducible, binary cutoff for the labelling of ischemic or non-ischemic stenosis around the FFR value of 0.8. This is important as the extent and presence of ischemia in CAD are the most relevant factors to patient outcome [2].
- Out of all the available indices of coronary physiology (Fig. 15.2), FFR is the best validated index aiding the interventionist in their clinical decision-making, although iFR data (see below) have accumulated quickly indicating the value of this parameter.

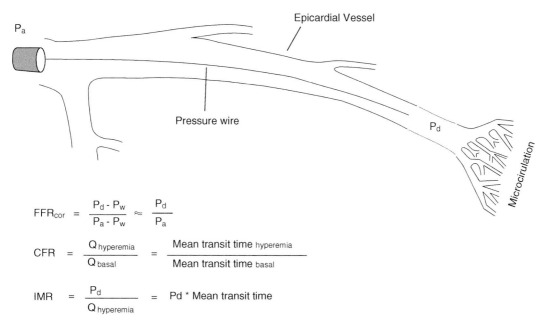

$$FFR_{cor} = \frac{P_d - P_w}{P_a - P_w} \approx \frac{P_d}{P_a}$$

$$CFR = \frac{Q_{hyperemia}}{Q_{basal}} = \frac{Mean\ transit\ time_{hyperemia}}{Mean\ transit\ time_{basal}}$$

$$IMR = \frac{P_d}{Q_{hyperemia}} = P_d * Mean\ transit\ time$$

Fig. 15.2 Established measures of coronary physiology. The fractional flow reserve (FFR) is an index of epicardial coronary physiology and is measured during maximal hyperemia. The coronary flow reserve (CR) is a measure of both the epicardial and microvascular physiology and is expressed as the ratio of hyperemic to basal flow, simpli-fied to the ratio of basal to hyperemic mean transit time. The index of microcirculatory resistance (IMR) is a specific index of the microcirculation and is expressed as the product of Pd and mean transit time. Pw here indicates the coronary wedge pressure. Reproduced with permission from Haddad et al. *Circ Heart Fail* 2012;5:759–768

FFR Studies: The Evidence Base

The DEFER Study [11]

- DEFER is one of the three most important original trials which have set the benchmark for clinical use of FFR to determine best practice with prognostic benefit (Table 15.1).
- This multicenter randomized controlled trial was carried out in 12 hospitals across Europe and 2 hospitals in Asia between 1997 and 1998, recruiting 325 patients.

Key Finding
Note that NOT stenting coronary lesions that are FFR negative, regardless of the visual angiographic severity, is associated with an excellent clinical outcome on optimal medical therapy alone.

Table 15.1 Summary of the DEFER trial

Study components	Description
Design	Multicenter, prospective randomized controlled trial
Settings/method	Patients who had PCI planned were randomized to PCI or deferral of PCI. All patients then had FFR measurement. In both arms patients with FFR <0.75 received PCI and formed the control group In the PCI group, patients with FFR ≥0.75 received PCI and formed the PERFORM group. In the deferral of PCI group these patients did not receive PCI and were labelled the DEFER group
Type of stent	Bare-metal stents
Inclusion criteria	Elective PCI of a single angiographically significant stenosis (>50%) in a native coronary artery
Primary endpoint	Freedom from major adverse cardiac events (MACE) at 2-year follow-up
Results	89% vs. 83% (DEFER vs. PERFORM) of patients reached the primary endpoint ($p = 0.27$). Event-free survival at 5 years was 79% vs. 71% (DEFER vs. PERFORM)
Conclusion	In patients with stable angina and FFR of ≥0.75 or above, stenting does not improve their outcome
Clinical impact	Currently patients with stable angina and FFR ≥0.75 are treated with optimal medical therapy

Fractional Flow Reserve Versus Angiography for Guiding PCI in Patients with Multivessel Coronary Artery Disease (FAME) Study [12]

- FAME is one of the most important trials for determining clinical interventional practice since the advent of drug-eluting stents. It recruited patients who had already been committed to multivessel PCI by their supervising cardiologist.
- It set out to test the hypothesis that an FFR-guided strategy would be superior to an angiogram-guided strategy for these patients.
- This was a multicenter, randomized controlled trial across 5 centers in the USA and 15 in Europe between 2006 and 2007, recruiting a total of 1005 patients (Table 15.2).

Key Finding
Patients with multivessel disease considered to require PCI, an FFR-guided approach is associated with fewer vessels being stented, less stenting overall, as well as less contrast and radiation, but with a superior clinical outcome than an angiographically guided approach.

Table 15.2 Summary of the FAME trial

Study components	Description
Design	Multicenter, randomized controlled trial
Settings/method	Patients were assessed for PCI by angiogram, then randomized to FFR- or angiogram-guided therapy. In the FFR group, cardiologists only stented lesions with FFR ≤0.8
Type of stent	Drug-eluting stents (96.9%)
Inclusion criteria	Multivessel coronary disease with ≥50% stenosis in ≥2 epicardial vessels
Primary endpoint	Composite of death, MI, and repeat revascularization at 1 year
Main results	The primary outcome occurred in 18.3% vs. 12.2% (angio vs. FFR; $p = 0.02$), despite fewer vessels being treated with less stents, and using less contrast and flouroscopy, in the FFR group. MACE at 2 years occurred in 22.4% vs. 17.9% (angio vs. FFR)
Conclusion	MACE was significantly lower in FFR-guided PCI at 1 year
Clinical impact	Increase in the use of FFR-guided coronary intervention in patients with multivessel disease

FAME II Study [13]

- FAME II was designed in response to the findings of the COURAGE trial, which controversially demonstrated that there was no clinical outcome advantage, over and above OMT, in PCI for patients with stable angina (Table 15.3).
- FAME II compared clinical outcome in patients with stable angina, and in whom there was at least one FFR-positive lesion, randomised to either OMT alone or OMT plus PCI.
- FAME II was conducted in 28 sites in Europe and North America, enrolling 1220 patients between 2010 and January 2012, at which point the trial was stopped early due to a significant difference in the primary endpoint between the two groups.
- Although FAME II suggests that there was a significant benefit in terms of a lower rate of the combined clinical endpoint, this was driven by a difference in urgent revascularization. There was no difference in the rate of death or MI. Nevertheless, it does demonstrate a superior clinical outcome in such patients for an OMT plus PCI strategy.

Key Finding

In patients with FFR-positive lesions, OMT alone is associated with a worse clinical outcome than stenting plus OMT.

Does Routine Pressure Wire Assessment Influence Management Strategy at Coronary Angiography for Diagnosis of Chest Pain? (RIPCORD) Study [14]

- RIPCORD recruited 200 patients with stable chest pain who were listed for a diagnostic angiogram across 10 centers in the UK between 2008 and 2012 (Table 15.4).

Table 15.4 Summary of the RIPCORD trial

Study components	Description
Design	Multicenter, open label
Settings/method	Patients with cardiac sounding chest pain underwent a coronary angiogram (CA), the supervising cardiologist (SC) made a management plan based on CA Patients then had FFR assessment of all vessels of stentable/graftable diameter with results disclosed to the SC to make a second management plan. Management options were: OMT alone; PCI; CABG; more information required
Inclusion criteria	Patients awaiting elective angiogram for investigation of chest pain
Primary outcome	Effect on management of knowing FFR data + angiographic data compared to only knowing angiographic data
Results	Overall, management plan after disclosure of FFR data changed in 26% of patients and localization of functionally significant stenoses changed in 32%
Conclusion	There was a change in management strategy in just over a quarter of patients when FFR data was known compared to angiography assessment alone
Clinical impact	If FFR was measured routinely in all stentable/graftable vessels at the diagnostic angiogram stage, management of patients would be different in around one quarter of patients. This generates the hypothesis and provides the power calculation for the RIPCORD2 randomised trial

Table 15.3 Summary of the FAME II trial

Study components	Description
Design	Multicenter, randomized controlled trial
Settings/method	All patients underwent FFR assessment. Where FFR ≤0.8, patients were randomized to PCI + OMT or OMT alone. If FFR was >0.8, patients were included in a registry and 166 were randomly selected for follow-up
Type of stent	Drug-eluting stents
Inclusion criteria	Stable angina or documented ischemia on noninvasive testing with ≥50% stenosis in a major epicardial vessel
Primary outcome	Composite of all-cause mortality, MI, and urgent revascularization at 2 years
Main results	For the primary endpoint, there was a significant difference between the PCI + OMT (4.3%) vs. OMT only (12.7%); $p < 0.001$
Conclusion	Outcomes were better in patients with stable coronary artery disease and FFR ≤0.8 if they had FFR-guided PCI
Clinical impact	Lesions with FFR ≤0.8 in patients with stable CAD are treated with PCI + OMT as a result of this study

- It asked the question: What difference to an angiogram-derived management plan would having FFR data of all stentable vessels make?

> **Key Finding**
> That having FFR data of all coronary vessels of stentable/graftable size, regardless of the severity of angiographic disease, routinely on patients undergoing diagnostic angiography changes the management in 26% of the population, because in 32% of lesions the angiogram does not predict significance as determined by FFR assessment of lesion-specific ischemia.

A Prospective Natural History Study of Coronary Atherosclerosis Using Fractional Flow Reserve [15]

This study by the FAME investigators reported the 2-year clinical outcomes of 607 patients in whom FFR had been measured.

> **Key Finding**
> In patients with stable CAD, stenosis severity as assessed by FFR is a major and independent predictor of lesion-related outcome. *In other words, the lower the FFR, the worse the outcome for that lesion.* This probably reflects the amount of myocardium at risk.

Key Points for Fractional Flow Reserve [1, 2, 7]

1. Universal normal value
   Fractional flow reserve (FFR) has a universal "NORMAL" value of 1.
2. Immune from changes in hemodynamics
   FFR measurement is not influenced by changes in systemic hemodynamics.
3. *Reproducible:* FFR is a reproducible and reliable measurement and it has been shown to be independent of any cardiac risk factors.
4. *Size matters*: The larger the myocardial mass supplied by an epicardial artery, the greater the flow, resulting in a larger gradient across a lesion and therefore lower FFR. This also

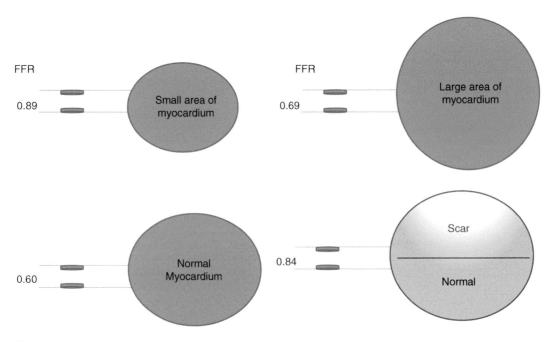

Fig. 15.3 Relationship between FFR and degree of myocardial mass

applies to FFR measurements after MI, where some of the muscle may have been replaced by scar tissue (Fig. 15.3).

Clinical Applications

Equipment [2, 7, 16]

Catheters

- It is our opinion that guide catheters should be used as default when pressure wire studies are being conducted.
- This not only provides better support than diagnostic catheters, but also gives the operator the option of proceeding using the pressure wire as the coronary angioplasty wire in rare cases of complication, or when PCI is the obvious appropriate treatment.
- **Catheter size**: We recommend using 6F catheters, although FFR measurements are frequently done using 5, 7, and 8F catheters. In the case of using large catheters, care should be taken to disengage the catheter from the coronary ostium when measurements are taken if there is any sign of pressure damping.
- **Side holes or no side holes**: Using a catheter with side holes can introduce error into FFR measurements. For example, a pressure gradient may exist between the side holes and the tip of the catheter, which can be more pronounced during maximal hyperemia causing inaccurate FFR readings. We therefore recommend using a guide catheter with no side holes to avoid incorrect FFR measurements.

Hyperemia

- The induction of maximum hyperemia is crucial to the principle of FFR measurement, as stated above, in order to ensure that the microvascular resistance is minimal and constant.
- Maximum hyperemia is achieved pharmacologically, with adenosine being the drug of choice.
- There has been controversy regarding use of intravenous (IV) versus intracoronary (IC) adenosine. This was addressed by Jeremias et al. who examined this in 52 patients and concluded that intracoronary adenosine is equivalent to intravenous infusion in achieving maximum hyperemia [17]. Furthermore, contemporary data help to define the optimal intracoronary doses to be used.

- In our center we use intracoronary adenosine for most of our FFR measurements *except when there is an aorto-ostial lesion*, or if a pullback is desired, in which case an IV adenosine infusion is employed.
- Likewise it is important to make sure that epicardial vessels are also free of any unwanted spasm; *thus it is important to administer 200–300 mcg of intracoronary nitrates* to prevent and treat any unwanted spasm due to wire manipulation, prior to giving adenosine and taking FFR measurements [17].

Anticoagulation

- As soon as the decision is made to instrument the coronary tree, the use of the same anticoagulation regime as PCI is recommended.
- Patients should receive weight-adjusted unfractionated heparin (70–100 u/kg), achieving an activated clotting time (ACT) of ≥250 s [18].

Pressure Wire

- There are several pressure wires currently available for clinical use such as PrimeWire PRESTIGE (Volcano), PressureWire Aeris (St. Jude Medical), and COMET (Boston Scientific). Pressure sensors are either piezoelectric or optical.
- The pressure wire is a 0.014 in. wire with a 3 cm radio-opaque tip at the distal point on which the transducer is mounted (Fig. 15.4).
- Pressure wires have a tip load of 0.6–1.6 g (depending on the manufacturer) (Fig. 15.5) and are generally more challenging to handle compared to workhorse coronary wires, although this is improving with each new device and iteration.

Fig. 15.4 Pressure wire structure

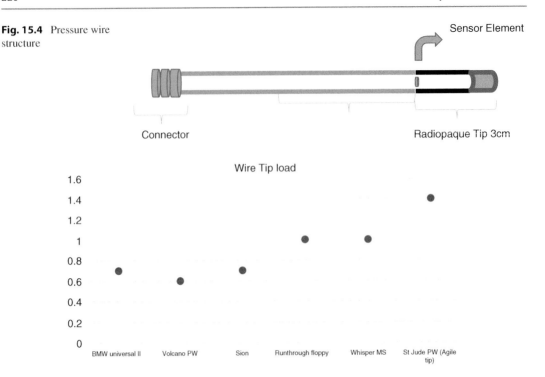

Fig. 15.5 Pressure wire tip loads. Comparison of pressure wire (PW) tip load to standard coronary wires

FFR Assessment of a Single Epicardial Lesion

How to Perform a Pressure Wire Study?

- The main indication for FFR measurement is to assess the functional/physiological relevance of a stenosis within an epicardial vessel [7, 19].
- A pressure wire study is an interventional skill and the wire needs to be handled with care and precision to minimize any complications.
- To be valid, FFR measurements should be undertaken with meticulous attention to detail. The following steps should be followed in order to successfully perform a pressure wire study of a non-ostial lesion.

- Step 1: Choose an appropriate guide catheter and engage the coronary artery, monitoring for any pressure damping.
- Step 2: Prepare the wire. Using the port at the end of the pressure wire holder, flush the pres-

sure wire using a 20 mL syringe, then while resting the holder on a flat surface connect the pressure wire to the console, and zero the pressures. The pressure wire is now ready to be used.
- Step 3: Prior to advancing the wire, anticoagulation should be considered in the form of 70–100u/Kg of unfractionated heparin.
- Step 4: To avoid any epicardial vessel spasm, administer 200–300 mcg of intracoronary nitrates.
- Step 5: Once the pressure wire is ready, shape the tip of the wire to the desired angle to aid maneuverability of the wire.
- Step 6: Using the introducer needle, advance the wire through the Y-connector and up the catheter until the pressure sensor is just within the tip of the guide catheter.
- Step 7: Once happy with the position of the sensor and if there is no pressure damping evident, the pressure wire should be equalized, after which the Pd/Pa reading should be 1.0 (Fig. 15.6). Note that if an introducer needle was used, this needs to be removed and the Y-connector shut, *before equalization*.

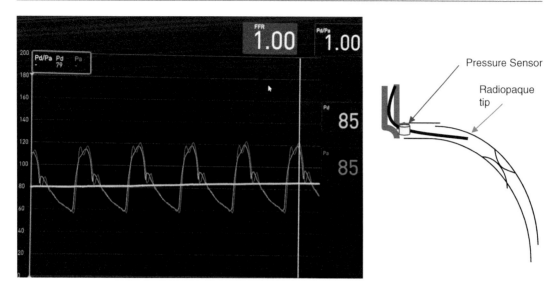

Fig. 15.6 Pressure wire equalization. The transducer is placed at the tip of the guide catheter before equalization is performed. The FFR value should be 1 before proceeding to assessing coronary lesions

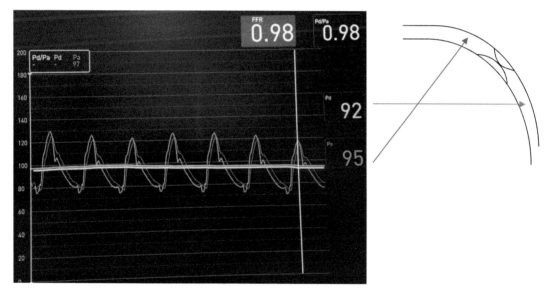

Fig. 15.7 Standard FFR readout. The pressure before the lesion is represented by the red line (Pa) and the pressure after the lesion is presented by blue line (Pd). The FFR result here is 0.98

- Step 8: Advance the wire distally until the pressure sensor is at least 2–3 cm beyond the lesion of interest. It is well established that there is turbulence within 1–2 cm distal to a stenosis and this turbulence can negate an accurate FFR reading, so the pressure transducer needs to be beyond this area. Remove

your introducer needle and make sure that the Y-connector is closed.
- Step 9: To ensure maximum hyperemia and no epicardial vasoconstriction, administer 200–300 mcg of intracoronary nitrates.
- Step 10: When the pressure reading is stable, take the reading as the baseline Pd/Pa (Fig. 15.7).

- Step 11: Once happy with the resting FFR and position of the sensor, start adenosine infusion/administer IC adenosine, warning the patient of possible side effects. If IC adenosine is used, ensure that the guide catheter is well engaged and there is no pressure damping. It's a good idea to record a short test shot to document the position of the wire and catheter.
- Step 12: When the pressure tracing has stabilized at the lowest reading, this can be taken as FFR at maximum hyperemia. After IC adenosine this will occur within 10–15 s, but with IV adenosine a steady-state FFR often takes between 1 and 2 min.
- Step 13: If satisfied with the FFR measurement, the pressure wire should be pulled back so that the pressure sensor is once again within the guide catheter. This is to check for any drift, which can render the FFR measurement invalid (Fig. 15.8). The FFR at this point should be 1.0.
- Step 14: A check angiogram should be performed to make sure that there is no damage to the vessel.
- Note: The term "FFR" is only valid for measurements taken at maximal hyperemia. At all other times the reading is Pd/Pa, not FFR.

Tips and Tricks

- Be careful that you know where the pressure transducer is on the wire you are using. Generally, the transducer sits at the junction of the radiopaque tip, which is between 3 and 3.5 cm from the leading tip depending upon the manufacturer.
- Choose the appropriate guide for the vessel size to avoid any pressure damping or ventricularization of the pressure trace. Until such pressure distortion is resolved, FFR readings will not be valid.
- If an introducer needle is used, make sure that this is fully outside and the Y-connector closed before equalizing or taking any measurements.
- The transducer needs to be mid-chest (5 cm below the sternum) for equalization and measurement.
- Drift of the pressure can occur, especially after a long procedure, and this can affect the accuracy of the measurements. This can be identified from the waveform as both curves will be identical in shape with a dicrotic notch clearly visible. If suspected, you should check for drift by bringing the pressure wire back so that the sensor is at the tip of the guide. If there

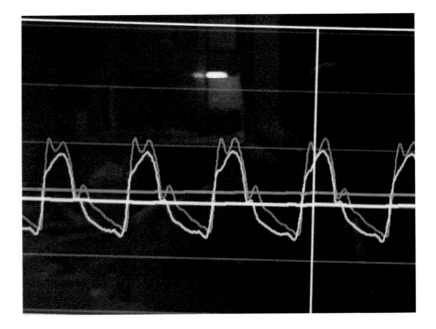

Fig. 15.8 Example of pressure wire drift. Red (Pa) and green (Pd) waveforms are identical with the dicrotic notch visible

were drift or any doubt about the FFR measurement, it is safer to re-equalize and take the FFR measurement again (i.e., if the measurement just doesn't seem to make sense then start again!) (Fig. 15.8).

- If the decision is made to treat a lesion, the pressure wire can be disconnected from the transducer to allow PCI treatment to be carried out. On reconnecting the wire, however, care needs to be taken to ensure that the electrodes at the end of the wire are clean and dry before inserting this back into the transducer.

- There is actually quite good evidence that rechecking the FFR distal to the stented segment can predict outcome after the PCI, and so this can be used to check the physiological outcome of the intervention. The lower the post-stent FFR, the higher the MACE rate at follow-up [20].

FFR Assessment in Multiple Epicardial Lesions

Assessment of Diffusely Diseased Vessels

- Given that atherosclerosis can be diffuse and affect long segments of the epicardial coronary artery it is therefore possible for the FFR to be positive in vessels in which there is no obvious discrete coronary lesion.

- This is a relatively common reason for a vessel being labelled as angiographically not being significant but is FFR positive [1, 7, 16, 19].

Serial Stenoses

- When there are several lesions along the course of an artery, FFR taken distal to all the lesions is still perfectly valid to assess whether the vessel is ischemic. However, this will not identify the relative contributions of the stenoses that have been included. It simply assesses the overall drop in pressure along the measured length of the vessel. Increasingly, a pull-back FFR measurement is recommended for this situation.

- The principle of pullback is that, *during continuous maximal hyperemia induced by adenosine infusion*, the wire is slowly pulled back from distal to proximal within the vessel, paying particular attention to points at which the FFR steps up sharply, thus indicating a more important stenosis inducing hemodynamic alteration. This can be an extremely effective technique, if done very carefully, with which to identify the most important lesion.

- However, it introduces extensive potential for misinterpretation of the result. *If the most distal lesion is the most hemodynamically significant in a series of two or more then the FFR reading proximal to that lesion will underestimate all upstream lesions until the distal lesion is treated.*

- As a result, the hemodynamically significant distal lesion tends to falsely reduce the pressure gradient across the proximal lesion, resulting in overestimation of the FFR [1, 16].

FFR Assessment of an Ostial Lesion

Pressure wire assessment of an ostial lesion requires precision and care especially when it is the left main stem (LMS).

Left Main Stem Assessment

- The presence of significant disease in the LMS is prognostically important and requires treatment. By contrast, there is good evidence that revascularization of hemodynamically insignificant LMS lesions is not beneficial.

- The use of FFR assessment for LMS lesions, as long as the basic rules of data acquisition in relation to avoiding damping and ventricularization of the trace are followed, has a good evidence base [1, 7, 16].

- It is also essential to bear in mind that in the presence of other epicardial vessel lesions, the serial stenosis principle is highly relevant when assessing LMS lesions. Specifically, downstream lesions in the left anterior descending (LAD) and circumflex (LCx) arteries can have a major influence on the interpretation of the result.
- This was looked at by Fearon and De Bruyne in 2012, by using a previously validated *in vitro* model of coronary circulation to create a fixed intermediate stenosis of the LMS and variable downstream LAD and LCx stenoses, and concluded that in the presence of proximal or mid-LAD or LCx disease LM SFFR can be reliably measured if the pressure wire is placed in the uninvolved epicardial artery [21].
- The implication of this study from a clinical standpoint is that if FFR of a LMS lesion taken in a relatively disease-free branch is ≤0.8, this indicates that the LMS is hemodynamically significant, regardless of disease in the other main branch.
- Only rarely could the FFR in the disease-free branch be >0.8 when assessing a LM lesion, and be underestimating the FFR because of a tight proximal lesion in the other branch.

Tips and Tricks of Performing a Pressure Wire Study of an Ostial Lesion

- All the steps previously explained on how to conduct a pressure wire study still apply and the following additional steps need to be taken into account when performing an ostial lesion pressure wire study:
  - Guide catheter needs to be disengaged slightly. *This therefore mandates IV adenosine infusion use to induce maximal hyperemia.*
  - Guide with side holes should not be used.
  - The pressure wire needs to be equalized in the aorta with the guide slightly disengaged.

FFR in Acute Coronary Syndromes

FFR in ST-Elevation Myocardial Infarction

- During STEMI, the aim of primary PCI is to restore TIMI 3 flow.
- FFR measurement of the culprit vessel is unreliable because of high microvascular resistance in the distal bed resulting from vessel spasm, thrombus embolization, and edema. By contrast, there is no contraindication to measurement of FFR in non-culprit vessels in STEMI patients [22].
- In DANAMI3-PRIMULTI, patients presenting with STEMI who had other clinically significant coronary stenoses in addition to the lesion in the infarct-related artery (IRA) were randomized to FFR-guided intervention versus no intervention of the non-culprit lesions after successful intervention of the IRA [23].
- The authors concluded that not only use of FFR is safe in functional assessment of non-culprit lesions in STEMI patients but also complete revascularization guided by FFR measurements significantly reduced the risk of repeat revascularization [22].
- The safety of guidewire-based measurement of coronary physiology using IV adenosine was also assessed by Berry et al. in a prospective study where the FFR was measured at the end of primary PCI. They found that invasive FFR measurement in STEMI patients is feasible and can be performed safely using IV adenosine [24].

FFR in Non-ST-Elevation Myocardial Infarction

- It is believed that microvascular resistance in the infarcted territory is inversely proportional to the amount of viable myocardium rendering the FFR measurement of an epicardial vessel lesion valid [1, 20].
- The concept of FFR-guided management of patients with non-ST-elevation myocardial infarction (NSTEMI) was examined in the

FAMOUS-NSTEMI trial. This prospective, multicenter, randomized controlled trial enrolled 350 NSTEMI patients with ≥1 coronary stenoses of at least 30% as assessed on angiography.

- FFR was measured in both groups, but the results were only disclosed to the operator in the FFR-guided group [25].
- The study showed that the number of patients treated with OMT (without revascularization) was significantly higher in the FFR-guided group compared to the angio-guided group (22.7% vs. 13.2%; $p = 0.02$).
- Berry et al. also confirmed the safety and feasibility of using FFR measurement in 350 NSTEMI patients [24].

FFR After Coronary Intervention

- FFR measurement after PCI can also be used as a prognostic tool. Specifically, an FFR value of 0.9 has been associated with better long-term outcome and a reduction in revascularization.
- Pijls et al. examined 750 patients with postprocedural FFR measurement and related this to MACE at 6 months.
- The authors found that in patients with a postprocedural FFR of 0.9–0.95 the event rate at 6 months was 6% compared to 32% of patients with postprocedural FFR of less than 0.9. They therefore concluded that FFR after stenting is a strong predictor of outcome at 6 months [18, 19].
- One recent meta-analysis of 8 relevant studies (including a total of 1337 patients) concluded that persistently low FFR following PCI is associated with an adverse clinical outcome [20].

Low FFR Despite a Good Angiographic Result

- Despite achieving an apparently good angiographic result after stenting, a repeat FFR measurement distal to the stented segment may still be suboptimal [1, 7, 16]. This can be due to several causes.
- Most commonly it is due to either suboptimal stent size or inadequate expansion of the stented segment, or due to geographical miss of the hemodynamically significant lesion.
- This scenario is a cast-iron indication for intracoronary imaging assessment.

Conclusion

- The clinical applicability of pressure wire assessment of CAD is the product of many years of meticulous validation. The clinical trial data have provided us with clear evidence that FFR-guided PCI practice is associated with better clinical outcomes at lower overall cost than purely angiographic guidance.
- The next important challenge is to apply the increasing persuasive evidence that FFR guidance is useful at the stage of the diagnostic angiogram in order to optimize patient management.
- RIPCORD showed that patient management plans were affected in 26% of cases when FFR measurements were revealed to the operator, because the angiogram did not predict whether a lesion was ischemic or not in 32% of vessels [14].
- A large number of studies have now confirmed the same discrepancy between the assessment of angiographic lesion severity and FFR assessment of ischemia.
- This has occurred consistently in around 30% of lesions and this leads to a management change in between 22 and 48% of cases [25–31].
- It is clear that there are angiographically tight lesions that are FFR negative and mild-looking lesions that are FFR positive. The consequence of this is that it is NOT logical to target FFR only at "intermediate" lesions.
- The appropriate use of FFR requires meticulous attention to detail and a thorough understanding of the technique.

References

1. Blows LJ, Redwood SR. The pressure wire in practice. Heart. 2007;93(4):419–22.
2. Redwood S, Curzen N, Banning A. Oxford textbook of interventional cardiology. Oxford: Oxford University Press; 2010.
3. Kern MJ, Lerman A, Bech JW, De Bruyne B, Eeckhout E, Fearon WF, et al. Physiological assessment of coronary artery disease in the cardiac catheterization laboratory: a scientific statement from the American Heart Association Committee on Diagnostic and Interventional Cardiac Catheterization, Council on Clinical Cardiology. Circulation. 2006;114(12):1321–41.
4. Hoffman JI, Spaan JA. Pressure-flow relations in coronary circulation. Physiol Rev. 1990;70(2):331–90.
5. Jones CJ, Kuo L, Davis MJ, Chilian WM. Distribution and control of coronary microvascular resistance. Adv Exp Med Biol. 1993;346:181–8.
6. Spaan JA, Cornelissen AJ, Chan C, Dankelman J, Yin FC. Dynamics of flow, resistance, and intramural vascular volume in canine coronary circulation. Am J Physiol Heart Circ Physiol. 2000;278(2):H383–403.
7. De Bruyne B, Hersbach F, Pijls NH, Bartunek J, Bech JW, Heyndrickx GR, et al. Abnormal epicardial coronary resistance in patients with diffuse atherosclerosis but "normal" coronary angiography. Circulation. 2001;104(20):2401–6.
8. Kaplan JA. Essentials of cardiac anesthesia. Philadelphia, PA: Saunders/Elsevier; 2008. http://www.sciencedirect.com/science/book/9781416037866
9. Longman K, Curzen N. Should ischemia be the main target in selecting a percutaneous coronary intervention strategy? Expert Rev Cardiovasc Ther. 2013;11(8):1051–9.
10. Fearon WF, Shah M, Ng M, Brinton T, Wilson A, Tremmel JA, et al. Predictive value of the index of microcirculatory resistance in patients with ST-segment elevation myocardial infarction. J Am Coll Cardiol. 2008;51(5):560–5.
11. Pijls NH, van Schaardenburgh P, Manoharan G, Boersma E, Bech JW, van't Veer M, et al. Percutaneous coronary intervention of functionally nonsignificant stenosis: 5-year follow-up of the DEFER study. J Am Coll Cardiol. 2007;49(21):2105–11.
12. Tonino PA, De Bruyne B, Pijls NH, Siebert U, Ikeno F, van' t Veer M, et al. Fractional flow reserve versus angiography for guiding percutaneous coronary intervention. N Engl J Med 2009;360(3):213-224.
13. De Bruyne B, Pijls NH, Kalesan B, Barbato E, Tonino PA, Piroth Z, et al. Fractional flow reserve-guided PCI versus medical therapy in stable coronary disease. N Engl J Med. 2012;367(11):991–1001.
14. Curzen N, Rana O, Nicholas Z, Golledge P, Zaman A, Oldroyd K, et al. Does routine pressure wire assessment influence management strategy at coronary angiography for diagnosis of chest pain?: the RIPCORD study. Circ Cardiovasc Interv. 2014;7(2):248–55.
15. Barbato E, Toth G, Johnson N, et al. A prospective natural history study of coronary atherosclerosis using fractional flow reserve. J Am Coll Cardiol. 2016;68:2247–55.
16. Redwood S, Curzen N, Thomas MR, editors. Coronary physiology in clinical practice. Chapter 9. In: Oxford Textbook Of Interventional Cardiology. Oxford: Oxford University Press.
17. Jeremias A, Filardo SD, Whitbourn RJ, Kernoff RS, Yeung AC, Fitzgerald PJ, et al. Effects of intravenous and intracoronary adenosine 5′-triphosphate as compared with adenosine on coronary flow and pressure dynamics. Circulation. 2000;101(3):318–23.
18. Niccoli G, Banning AP. Heparin dose during percutaneous coronary intervention: how low dare we go? Heart. 2002;88(4):331–4.
19. Pijls NH, De Bruyne B, Peels K, Van Der Voort PH, Bonnier HJ, Bartunek JKJJ, et al. Measurement of fractional flow reserve to assess the functional severity of coronary-artery stenoses. N Engl J Med. 1996;334(26):1703–8.
20. Wolfrum M, Fahrni G, de Maria GL, Knapp G, Curzen N, Kharbanda RK, et al. Impact of impaired fractional flow reserve after coronary interventions on outcomes: a systematic review and meta-analysis. BMC Cardiovasc Disord. 2016;16(1):177.
21. Daniels DV, van't Veer M, Pijls NH, van der Horst A, Yong AS, De Bruyne B, et al. The impact of downstream coronary stenoses on fractional flow reserve assessment of intermediate left main disease. JACC Cardiovasc Interv. 2012;5(10):1021–5.
22. Ntalianis A, Sels J, Davidavicius G, et al. Fractional flow reserve for the assessment of nonculprit coronary artery Stenoses in patients with acute myocardial infarction. J Am Coll Cardiol Interv. 2010;3:1274–81.
23. Engstrom T, Kelbaek H, Helqvist S, Hofsten DE, Klovgaard L, Holmvang L, et al. Complete revascularisation versus treatment of the culprit lesion only in patients with ST-segment elevation myocardial infarction and multivessel disease (DANAMI-3-PRIMULTI): an open-label, randomised controlled trial. Lancet. 2015;386(9994):665–71.
24. Ahmed N, Layland J, Carrick D, Petrie MC, McEntegart M, Eteiba H, et al. Safety of guidewire-based measurement of fractional flow reserve and the index of microvascular resistance using intravenous adenosine in patients with acute or recent myocardial infarction. Int J Cardiol. 2016;202:305–10.
25. Layland J, Oldroyd KG, Curzen N, Sood A, Balachandran K, Das R, et al. Fractional flow reserve vs. angiography in guiding management to optimize outcomes in non-ST-segment elevation myocardial infarction: the British Heart Foundation FAMOUS-NSTEMI randomized trial. Eur Heart J. 2015;36(2):100–11.
26. Sant'Anna FM, Silva EE, Batista LA, Ventura FM, Barrozo CA, Pijls NH. Influence of routine assessment of fractional flow reserve on decision making during coronary interventions. Am J Cardiol. 2007;99(4):504–8.

27. Baptista SB, Raposo L, Santos L, et al. Impact of routine fractional flow reserve evaluation during coronary angiography on management strategy and clinical outcome: one-year results of the POST-IT. Circ Cardiovasc Interv. 2016;9(7):e003288.

28. Nakamura M, Yamagishi M, Ueno T, et al. Modification of treatment strategy after FFR measurement: CVIT-DEFER registry. Cardiovasc Interv Ther. 2015;30(1):12–21.

29. Van Belle E, Rioufol G, Pouillot C, et al. Outcome impact of coronary revascularization strategy reclassification with fractional flow reserve at time of diagnostic angiography: insights from a large French multicenter fractional flow reserve registry. Circulation. 2014;129(2):173–85.

30. Tonino PA, Fearon WF, De Bruyne B, et al. Angiographic versus functional severity of coronary artery stenoses in the FAME study fractional flow reserve versus angiography in multivessel evaluation. J Am Coll Cardiol. 2010;55(25):2816–21.

31. Toth G, Hamilos M, Pyxaras S, et al. Evolving concepts of angiogram: fractional flow reserve discordances in 4000 coronary stenoses. Eur Heart J. 2014;35(40):2831–8.

Primary Percutaneous Coronary Intervention for ST-Elevation Myocardial Infarction

16

Lene Holmvang and Francis R. Joshi

Abbreviations

ACT	Activated clotting time
AHA	American Heart Association
CT	Computed tomography
ESC	European Society of Cardiology
FFR	Fractional flow reserve
LAD	Left anterior descending coronary artery
LCX	Left circumflex artery
PET	Positron emission tomography
PPCI	Primary percutaneous coronary intervention
RCA	Right coronary artery
RCT	Randomized controlled trial
STEMI	ST-elevation myocardial infarction

About Us Rigshospitalet, Copenhagen University Hospital, is Denmark's most highly specialized hospital, providing treatment for people in Denmark, the Faroe Islands, and Greenland. Rigshospitalet is a part of the Danish public healthcare system, which is financed through general taxation.

The Heart Center covers a population of 2.6 million people for primary percutaneous coronary intervention (PPCI), cardiac surgery, cardiac transplantation, and percutaneous structural interventions. It serves one million people for elective PCI and electrophysiology.

The typical annual workload for coronary disease includes 5000 coronary angiographies, 1000 primary PCI procedures, and 1500 elective and subacute cases. Four catheter laboratories are dedicated to PCI procedures with pressure wire and intracoronary imaging readily at hand. We have a structured chronic total occlusion (CTO) program including prior advanced noninvasive assessment with positron emission tomography (PET) and CT. Our center also specializes in the treatment of cardiogenic shock and out-of-hospital cardiac arrest for which hemodynamic support with Impella and/or extracorporeal membrane oxygenation (ECMO) is available. Complex cases are discussed on a daily basis in a Heart Team conference with cardiothoracic surgical colleagues.

The staff consists of 7–8 interventional cardiologists, 1–2 Danish interventional fellows, and 1 international fellow.

The Heart Center has 20–30 PhD students and an equal number of full-time study nurses. Our research is centered on reperfusion therapy, medical as well as device treatment of heart failure, stem cell research, and treatment after cardiac arrest. Research output is approximately 250 peer-reviewed papers annually.

L. Holmvang · F. R. Joshi (✉)
The Heart Center, Rigshospitalet, Copenhagen, Denmark
e-mail: lene.holmvang@regionh.dk

© Springer International Publishing AG, part of Springer Nature 2018
A. Myat et al. (eds.), *The Interventional Cardiology Training Manual*,
https://doi.org/10.1007/978-3-319-71635-0_16

Assessment of the STEMI Patient at the Rigshospitalet

- About 80–90% of our patients with suspected STEMI are triaged directly from the ambulance to the catheterization lab, bypassing both more local hospitals and our own emergency room. Diagnosis and triage are confirmed by telemedicine.
- During transportation, the patients are accompanied by paramedics or anesthesiologists working in the prehospital setting. On arrival, a medical history and bedside echocardiography are obtained while the patient is prepared for angiography. This strategy enables a mean door-to-balloon time of 26 min.
- Direct triage means that the lab functions as an emergency room, and inevitably there are some false activations of PPCI teams.

Preferred to missing genuine STEMI cases, an ideal false-activation rate has not been well defined. Though most studies suggest that this is around 20%, the prognosis of patients with final diagnoses other than STEMI is not always benign; some will have life-threatening alternative diagnoses such as aortic dissection (Fig. 16.1), pulmonary embolism (Fig. 16.2), tako-tsubo cardiomyopathy (Fig. 16.3), or sepsis.

- Deserving special mention are those patients presenting with chest pain and a (presumed) new left bundle branch block (LBBB)—considered a STEMI equivalent. It has been shown that LBBB activations for primary PCI are likely to involve older patients, with a greater prevalence of cardiogenic shock and poorer survival. Although ECG criteria (such as those

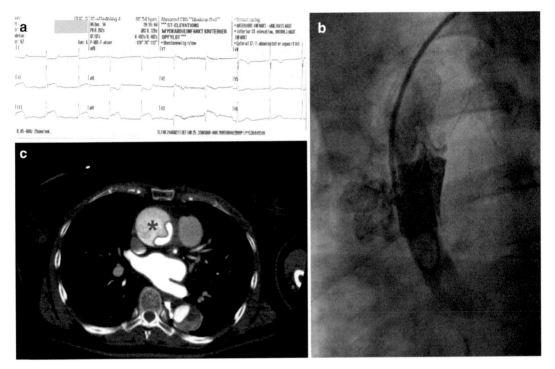

Fig. 16.1 Mimics of STEMI: acute aortic syndrome. Female patient presenting with acute chest pain. She received prehospital aspirin, ticagrelor, and intravenous heparin. (**a**) Prehospital ECG with evident inferior ST elevation. (**b**) It was not possible to advance a catheter to the aortic root. Aortography demonstrated that the catheter was in the false lumen of a type A aortic dissection. (**c**) CT angiography confirming extensive dissection. The right coronary artery is perfused via the false lumen (*asterisk*)

Fig. 16.2 Mimics of STEMI: submassive pulmonary embolism. A 28-year-old male presenting with acute chest pain and dyspnea. (**a**) ECG with suspicion of anterior ST elevation. Note, however, the deep S-wave in lead I, with a Q-wave and T-wave inversion in lead III, indicative of right-heart strain. (**b**) After bedside echocardiography, CT pulmonary angiography revealed bilateral pulmonary emboli (*yellow arrows*)

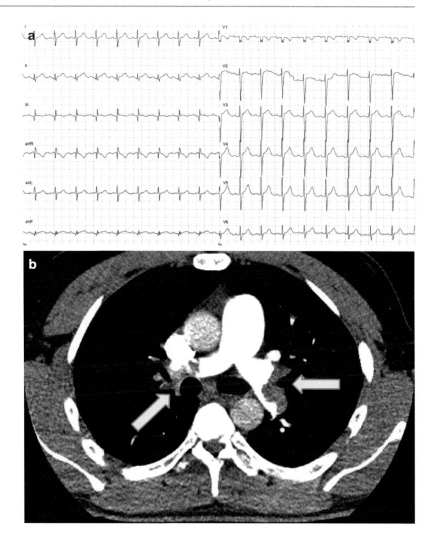

defined by Sgarbossa) exist, none have yet been shown to demonstrate adequate discriminative value for the identification of culprit coronary occlusions.

- Electronic medical records, such as the Sundhedsplatform that exists in East Denmark, allow clinicians to rapidly check old records. Where previous ECGs do not exist, and in the absence of a readily apparent alternative diagnosis in the field, there is a low threshold for accepting patients for clinical evaluation and diagnostic coronary angiography.

- Of note the new ESC STEMI guidelines published in 2017 suggest the following criteria which can be used to improve the diagnostic accuracy of STEMI in LBBB:
  - Concordant ST-segment elevation ≥1 mm in leads with a positive QRS complex
  - Concordant ST-segment depression ≥1 mm in V1–V3
  - Discordant ST-segment elevation ≥5 mm in leads with a negative QRS complex
  - The presence of RBBB may confound the diagnosis of STEMI

Adjunctive Pharmacotherapy for PPCI at the Rigshospitalet

Patients triaged to PPCI are pretreated with 300 mg of aspirin and 10,000 units of intravenous heparin. In line with data from the ATLANTIC study, only those with expected transfer times >30 min receive loading doses of ticagrelor in the field, subject to individual bleeding risks and/or concerns about the possibility of mechanical complications of STEMI or acute aortic syndrome.

Unfractionated heparin is used as an anticoagulant; an activated clotting time (ACT) is checked on arrival, after vascular access is obtained. Further doses of intravenous heparin are given as necessary to a target of >250 s, with repeat measurement of the ACT every 30 min. Bivalirudin is no longer used, in view of its cost and in light of the HEAT-PPCI study data. Eptifibatide is used as bailout for no-reflow or for a large intracoronary thrombus burden. Generally, infusions are continued for 18 h, though may be given for up to 48 h in selected cases.

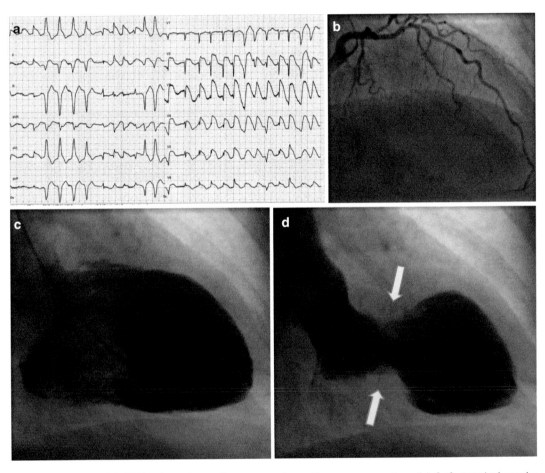

Fig. 16.3 Mimics of STEMI: tako-tsubo cardiomyopathy. A 90-year-old female presenting with chest pain, dyspnea, and pre-shock. (**a**) ECG with evident anterolateral ST elevation and non-sustained ventricular tachycardia. (**b**) Angiography with good flow in the left anterior descending coronary artery. (**c**) Left ventriculography (end-diastolic frame). (**d**) Left ventriculography (end-systolic frame) showing basal hyperkinesis (*yellow arrows*) and ballooning of the apex

Guideline-Mandated Timelines for Reperfusion Therapy in STEMI

- PPCI is a swift and effective method to ensure reperfusion of the occluded coronary artery in patients with STEMI. Compared with systemic fibrinolysis, the obvious advantage is the avoidance of side effects related to fibrinolytic therapy such as bleeding, but rapid clinical assessment (including urgent bedside echocardiography) and diagnostic coronary angiography are also advantageous in the 15–20% of field-triaged patients with diagnoses other than STEMI.
- The initial trials documenting a mortality benefit from PPCI compared with fibrinolysis were performed prior to the era of prehospital diagnosis of STEMI. Time from symptom onset to reperfusion (either fibrinolysis or PPCI) is important with regard to mortality and morbidity; healthcare systems have thus evolved to provide the earliest possible initiation of reperfusion therapy.
- When initiated as part of coordinated systems, it is accepted that PPCI is superior to fibrinolysis. However, some patients are not offered reperfusion by PPCI either because of long transportation times, because of a lack of suitable PPCI centers, or because the healthcare system has failed to establish a successful prehospital diagnostic program with field triage of patients directly to PCI centers.

- Previous focus on door-to-balloon (DTB) times has been important to further streamline in-hospital care, but before the patient even reaches the hospital several factors should be in focus in order to reduce delays. Door-to-balloon time alone is a poor parameter to evaluate the efficacy of a healthcare system offering PPCI (Fig. 16.4).
- In the ESC STEMI guidelines from 2012, PPCI is the recommended reperfusion therapy over fibrinolysis if performed by an experienced team within 120 min of first medical contact whereas the AHA/ACCF guidelines from 2013 recommend fibrinolysis if PPCI cannot be performed within 90 min of first medical contact. The European time standard has not changed in the new ESC STEMI guidelines published in 2017.
- A thorough meta-analysis in the 2013 British NICE guidelines on the acute management of myocardial infarction with ST-segment elevation concluded that acute coronary angiography, with follow-on PPCI if indicated, should be the preferred coronary reperfusion strategy if PPCI can be delivered within 120 min of the time when fibrinolysis could have been given.
- Because of the initial confusion regarding the exact definition of several of the performance measures described in the above-mentioned guidelines, the 2014 ESC/EACTS revascularization guidelines have attempted to further

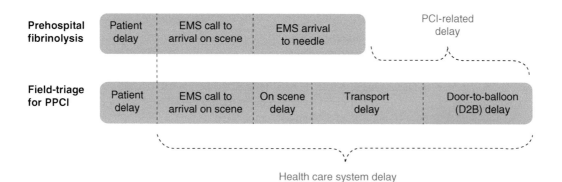

Fig. 16.4 Delays when treating STEMI patients with fibrinolysis or primary PPCI. "Healthcare system delay" is the total delay from emergency medical service (EMS) call to PPCI. "PCI-related delay" is the extra delay that one may use to perform PPCI while still achieving comparable outcomes to fibrinolysis. Adapted with permission from Terkelsen, C. Herz 2014;39:672–676

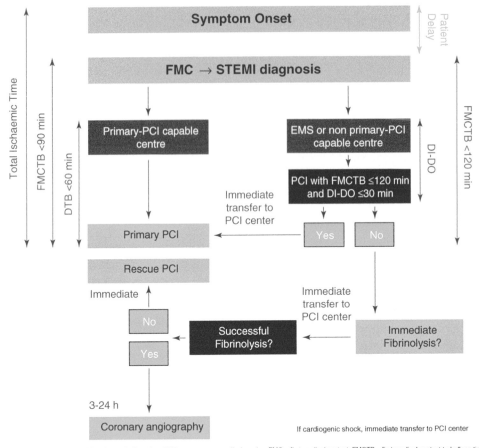

Fig. 16.5 Transportation and reperfusion strategies for patients presenting with ST-elevation myocardial infarction. Reproduced with permission from Oxford University Press on behalf of the European Society of Cardiology guidelines on myocardial revascularization. Windecker S, et al. Eur Heart J 2014;35:2541–2619

define when to choose between fibrinolysis and PPCI (Fig. 16.5). In these guidelines first medical contact is defined as the time when the STEMI diagnosis is established either by the emergency medical system in the field or in hospital.

- Fibrinolysis is limited to patients with symptom onset within 12 h but whether PPCI is effective in patients presenting even later is not well documented. Revascularization is recommended for patients with cardiogenic shock up to 36 h after symptom debut and should also be considered in "late pre-

senters" with ongoing ischemia or if hemodynamically unstable.

The Role of Fibrinolysis in the Era of Primary PCI

- The initial studies comparing fibrinolysis with conventional therapy for myocardial infarction focused on those patients already in hospital; few studies have compared prehospital fibrinolysis with PPCI. The CAPTIM study was terminated early because of a lack of funding but demonstrated equipoise (and even a trend for reduced mortality) for those patients given fibrinolysis within 2 h of the onset of symptoms [1].

- Thus, very early prehospital fibrinolysis would appear to be as effective as PPCI, where the latter is not readily available. This should be followed by systematic angiography as this has been shown to be superior to a more conservative approach.
- Even in the CAPTIM trial, however, 26% of patients required so-called rescue PCI for failed thrombolysis (ongoing pain or unresolved ST elevation), and this is not without some risk.
- The STREAM trial explored prehospital fibrinolysis with tenecteplase for patients within 3 h of the onset of symptoms, yet unable to undergo PPCI within 1 h, with transfer to a PPCI center, versus direct transfer. 36% of patients in the fibrinolysis arm required emergent (or rescue) angiography. There was no difference in the primary outcome of death, shock, heart failure, or re-infarction at 30 days, though the fibrinolysis arm was associated with a significantly increased risk of intracranial hemorrhage [2].
- These data should be put into context with those obtained from studies of facilitated PPCI with fibrinolytic therapy. The ASSENT-4 study comparing PPCI versus PPCI with prior full-dose tenecteplase showed that facilitated therapy was associated with greater mortality, re-infarction, and stroke [3].
- Similarly, the FINESSE study showed no improvement in clinical outcomes with facilitated PPCI with combinations of reteplase plus abciximab, or abciximab alone [4]. There is no role for facilitated approaches in contemporary PPCI.
- Taken together, these data suggest that in stable patients given successful fibrinolysis, angiography should be deferred, unless there is evidence of re-infarction or hemodynamic instability.

> **Reperfusion Therapy for Patients Presenting with STEMI on Denmark's Offshore Islands**
>
> While excellent outcomes have been obtained for patients transferred by helicopter from the Baltic island of Bornholm (distance 160 km, flight time 45 min), patients presenting with STEMI on the Faroe Islands and Greenland are given fibrinolysis. If there is successful reperfusion, and the patient remains stable, angiography is generally deferred for 24 h

Thrombectomy in Primary PCI

- PPCI effectively restores epicardial coronary blood flow but restoration of microvascular perfusion remains a challenge. Distal embolization of macroscopic thrombus occurs in 10–15% of cases, and is associated with poorer long-term outcomes. Impaired microvascular perfusion is evident in up to a third of patients; an absent myocardial blush (Grade 0 or 1) is associated with a significantly poorer 1-year survival than cases with normal (Grade 3) perfusion.
- Thrombectomy therefore appears as an attractive means of reducing thrombus burden at the culprit lesion, and reducing distal embolization (see also Chap. 13). The first large supportive evidence using a simple aspiration device was the TAPAS trial, a single-center study demonstrating significant reduction in absent myocardial blush (Grade 0 or 1), 17.1% in the aspiration thrombectomy arm compared to 26.3% in the standard arm ($p < 0.001$). Though underpowered for this outcome, thrombectomy was also associated with a significant reduction in mortality at 1 year [5]. Meta-analyses subsequently confirmed that manual thrombectomy was associated with a significant improvement in surrogate markers of microvascular perfusion including blush grade, ST-segment resolution, and distal embolization. This led to significant enthusiasm for this simple adjunct to PPCI.

- More recently, however, appropriately powered multicenter clinical studies have since cast doubt on the efficacy of routine thrombectomy in PPCI. The TASTE (Thrombus Aspiration in ST-Elevation Myocardial Infarction in Scandinavia) study randomized 7244 patients to thrombus aspiration and PCI or PCI alone, with outcomes determined from extensive registry data. There was no difference in all-cause mortality at 30 days (2.8% thrombectomy vs. 3.0% PCI alone, $p = 0.63$) or at 1-year follow-up [6].

- The larger ($n = 10,732$) multicenter prospective TOTAL trial randomized patients to routine manual thrombectomy versus PCI alone with bailout thrombectomy (TIMI 0-1 flow after pre-dilatation or persistent large thrombus after stenting). Bailout thrombectomy occurred in 7.0% in the PCI-alone group. The primary outcome was a composite of death from cardiovascular causes, recurrent myocardial infarction, cardiogenic shock, or NYHA class IV heart failure within 180 days. This was not different between the two study arms (6.9% in the aspiration thrombectomy group vs. 7.0% in the PCI-alone group; $p = 0.86$) [7].

- The main safety concern with manual thrombectomy remains the risk of dragging thrombus back into the aorta when the catheter is retracted. In the TOTAL trial, the incidence of stroke was 0.7% in the aspiration thrombectomy arm compared to 0.3% in the PCI-alone group ($p = 0.02$)—though the strokes seen accumulated over 30 days. It is difficult to explain these data mechanistically; they would seem inconsistent with dragging thrombus back into the aorta during PPCI. It seems probable that these are chance findings.

- The evidence thus does not support routine use of thrombectomy with the aim of improving outcomes, but some interventionalists continue to use it to assist their procedures. Identifying specific subgroups of patients who may benefit prognostically has not been possible; neither TASTE nor TOTAL showed a benefit for the primary outcome in patients with high thrombus burden. Nevertheless there will likely continue to be individual cases where the operator feels that thrombectomy is likely to be of some benefit.

- Interestingly, an OCT sub-study of TOTAL suggested that even though we can collect thrombus from the artery, and see angiographic improvement, aspiration dose not reduce the mean absolute thrombus volume (pre-stenting) at the culprit lesion. This suggests that angiography is an insensitive means of assessing thrombus burden, and that simple aspiration catheters are not as effective as we might hope.

- Beyond these therefore, though less widely available, rheolytic catheters which use saline jets to disrupt organized thrombus before aspiration are also available, and allow more effective clearance of large thrombi. Locally, we have experience of the ClearLumen System (Walk Vascular, Irvine, CA, USA), and have found this useful in selected cases (Fig. 16.6).

- It is also possible to perform thrombus aspiration using a Guideliner (Vascular Solutions, Inc., Minneapolis, MN, USA) or even the guide catheter—this may be especially useful as bailout in the setting of a critically unstable patient with a large thrombus burden in the left main coronary artery.

Manual Thrombectomy During Primary PCI: Hints and Tips

Do:
    Consider it but think again about routine use.

Don't:
    Expect to improve clinical outcomes in all cases.
    Forget that there may be individual cases where it may be helpful.

Safety tips:
    Maintain suction as the aspiration catheter is removed from the coronary artery.
    Ensure that the guide catheter is well engaged in the coronary ostium.
    Open the O-ring and allow the guide catheter to bleed back and/or aspirate from the guide to ensure that the system is free of thrombus.

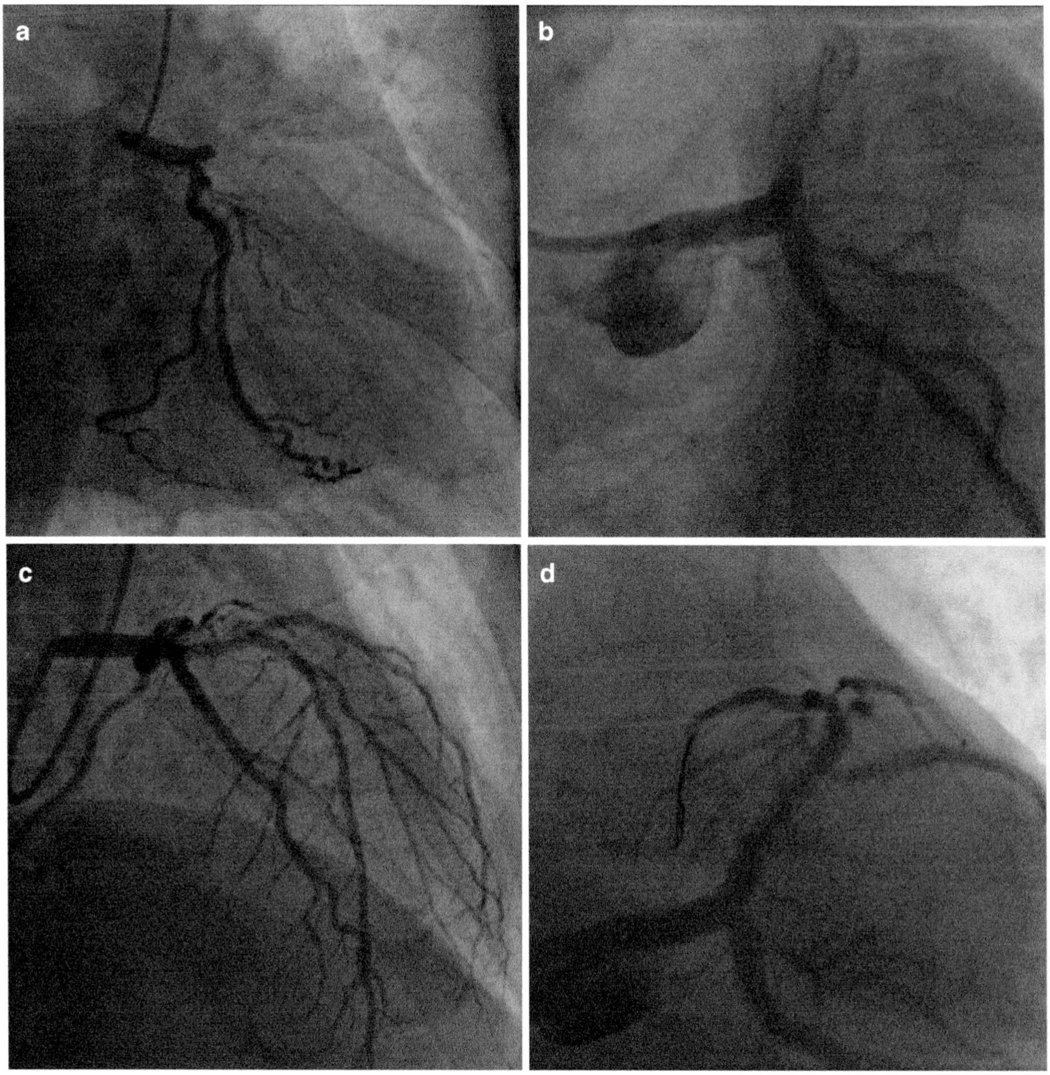

Fig. 16.6 Thrombectomy using the ClearLumen system. A 76-year-old man with prior stent thrombosis stopped dual-antiplatelet therapy 3 days before a brain biopsy for suspected malignancy. He presented with an anterior STEMI secondary to acute stent thrombosis 2 days later. (a) Proximal occlusion of the LAD (RAO caudal projection). TIMI 0 flow. (b) LAO caudal projection. (c) After thrombectomy with ClearLumen system (RAO cranial) with TIMI 3 flow. (d) LAO caudal projection

Embolic Protection Devices in Primary PCI

- Though crossing the culprit lesion with a wire itself leads to distal embolization, it is appreciated that further manipulation of the culprit lesion may lead to more distal embolization and/or increase the risk of no-reflow.

- Protection devices have been used in the percutaneous treatment of bypass graft stenoses (see also Chaps. 13 and 30) and may be characterized as those providing distal balloon occlusion, distal filtering, or proximal balloon occlusion.
- Though it is feasible to use filter-based protection devices such as the FilterWire-EZ (Boston Scientific, Santa Clara, CA, USA; Fig. 16.7)

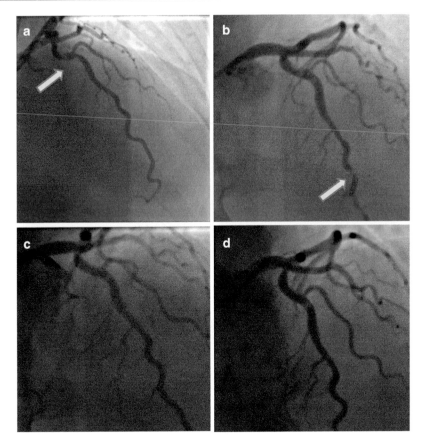

Fig. 16.7 Use of a FilterWire distal protection device in native coronary arteries. (**a**) Presentation with acute stent thrombosis (*yellow arrow*) and TIMI 2 flow. (**b**) After delivery of FilterWire. The basket is open, and there is adjacent coronary spasm. (**c**) After intracoronary nitrates. (**d**) Result after thrombectomy and restoration of TIMI 3 flow. The patient was given an eptifibatide infusion for 18 h thereafter, before further evaluation 2 days later. No thrombus material was observed in the filter. While delivery of such protection devices is feasible, evidence does not support their routine use

or distal balloon occlusion devices such as the GuardWire Plus (Medtronic Vascular, US) in native coronary arteries, studies, including the DEDICATION study conducted here in Denmark, have consistently shown that routine use does not lead to better microvascular perfusion, reduced infarct size, or improved outcomes at 1 month.

- Indeed, longer term follow-up data from the DEDICATION study suggest that the routine use of distal protection in STEMI increases the risk of stent thrombosis and clinically driven target-vessel revascularization, perhaps because of spasm leading to undersizing of the implanted stent or vessel injury during deployment.

- A more recent study of the Proxis proximal occlusion system (St. Jude Medical, Minneapolis, MN, USA) which entirely occludes antegrade coronary flow during PPCI suggests that it does not lead to more complete ST-segment resolution at 60 min after PPCI.

- These negative results likely relate to the oft-required pre-dilatation to facilitate delivery of bulky devices (that themselves may then cause embolization during deployment), unprotected side branches, and incomplete capture of embolized debris. Routine use of distal protection devices in PPCI cannot be recommended.

STEMI and Cardiogenic Shock

- These patients continue to have a poor prognosis, with only 40–50% of patients surviving to hospital discharge. Professional guidance continues to recommend complete, multivessel revascularization in such patients (Fig. 16.8), though this is derived from now-historical SHOCK trial data, with patients presenting relatively late after STEMI. The CULPRIT-SHOCK (clinicaltrials.gov identifier NCT01927549) trial, in contrast, demonstrated a reduction in the 30-day risk of a composite of death or severe renal failure in those who initially underwent culprit-vessel PPCI compared to those receiving immediate multivessel PCI in the context of acute MI complicated by cardiogenic shock.

- Beyond revascularization, mechanical hemodynamic support devices exist and are used variably around the world (see also Chap. 23). The IABP-SHOCK II study has shown that

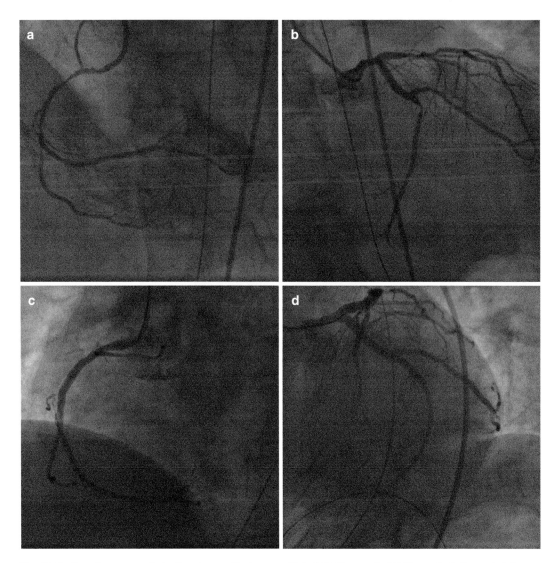

Fig. 16.8 Complete revascularization in a patient presenting with inferior STEMI, multivessel disease, and shock. An Impella mechanical circulatory support device was placed after PCI but the patient died 24 h later. (**a**) Culprit RCA stenosis. (**b**) Non-culprit disease in left coronary artery. (**c**) After primary PCI of RCA. (**d**) After PCI of LAD and LCX

Fig. 16.9 Complete revascularization in a patient presenting with inferior STEMI, shock, and dual-acute stent thromboses. (**a**) Culprit RCA occlusion secondary to stent thrombosis. (**b**) Acute stent thrombosis of previously placed LAD stent. (**c**) After primary PCI of RCA (thrombectomy and balloon angioplasty). (**d**) PCI of LAD (thrombectomy and balloon angioplasty). (**e**) An Impella mechanical circulatory support device was placed after PCI. The patient survived to discharge

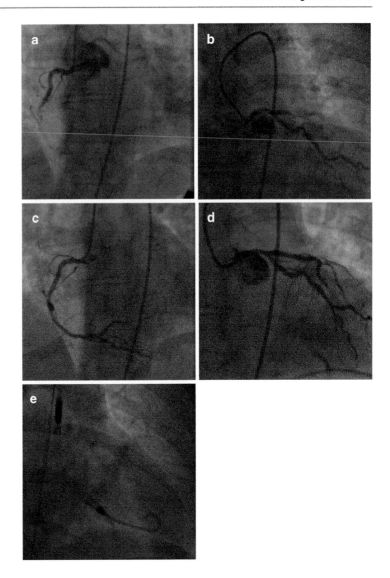

routine use of intra-aortic balloon pumps in such cases is not associated with improved outcomes, though most of these were implanted after PPCI.

- Local practice is to consider short-term support using a percutaneous catheter-based Impella axial pump (Abiomed, Inc., Danvers, MA, USA; Fig. 16.9). The ongoing DAN-SHOCK trial (clinicaltrials.gov identifier NCT01633502) aims to outline the role for the Impella CP (flow up to 3.75 L/min) in such patients—randomized to either conventional therapy with inotropic support or percutaneous insertion of an Impella CP during PPCI. The study aims to enroll 360 patients—

though in keeping with other studies in this area, recruitment has been slow and perhaps limited by notional lack of equipoise among interventionalists.

Complete Versus Culprit Revascularization in Multivessel Disease STEMI Without Shock

- Approximately 40% of patients with STEMI have multivessel disease and treatment options for these patients may include:
  - *Culprit artery-only PPCI*, with PCI of non-culprit arteries only for spontaneous

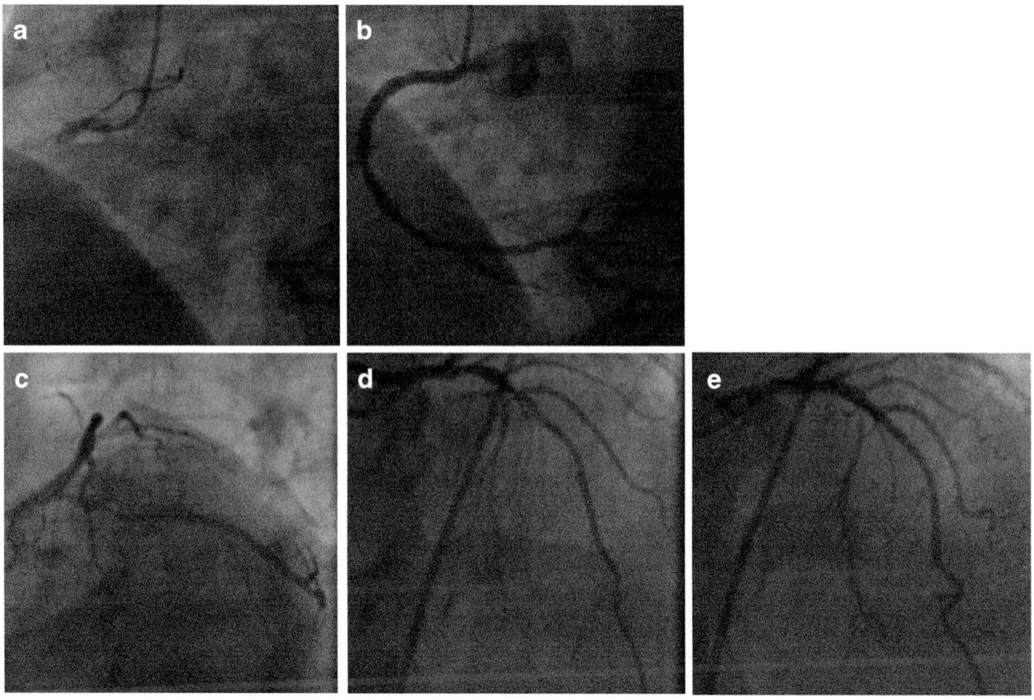

Fig. 16.10 Complete revascularization with staged PCI after presentation with inferior STEMI. (**a**) Occluded RCA. (**b**) After primary PCI of RCA. (**c**) Staged, FFR-guided, PCI 2 days later. FFR LCx 0.97. (**d**) Proximal LAD stenosis with FFR 0.61. (**e**) After PCI of the proximal LAD

ischemia or intermediate- or high-risk findings on pre-discharge noninvasive testing
– *Multivessel PCI* at the time of PPCI
– *Culprit artery-only PPCI* followed by *staged PCI* (or in certain cases CABG; Figs. 16.10 and 16.11) of non-culprit lesions
• Professional guidelines have previously recommended against PCI of non-culprit stenoses at the time of PPCI in hemodynamically stable patients with STEMI. However, the strategy of routine, staged PCI of such lesions was not addressed in these previous guidelines, and considered only in the limited context of spontaneous ischemia or high-risk findings on pre-discharge noninvasive testing. The earlier recommendations were primarily based on the findings from many observational studies and meta-analyses that showed trends toward or statistically significant worse outcomes in those who underwent multivessel primary PCI.
• After publication of the 2014 ESC/EACTS guidelines on myocardial revascularization,

four RCTs have since suggested that a strategy of multivessel PCI, either at the time of PPCI or as a planned, staged procedure, may be beneficial and safe in selected patients with STEMI. The four studies were different regarding treatment strategies, sample size, and inclusion rates, but all showed either a definite benefit with regard to the composite primary endpoint (PRAMI [8], CVLPRIT [9], DANAMI 3-PRIMULTI [10]) or no between-group difference (PRAGUE-13).
• The larger of the studies, DANAMI 3-PRIMULTI ($n = 627$) as well as CVLPRIT ($n = 296$), found the benefit primarily related to a reduction in unplanned revascularizations whereas PRAMI ($n = 465$) also found a mortality benefit of complete revascularization.
• The ongoing COMPLETE study is currently enrolling patients and will be the largest randomized study to date to address the question of complete versus culprit-only revascularization in STEMI. Results are expected in 2018.

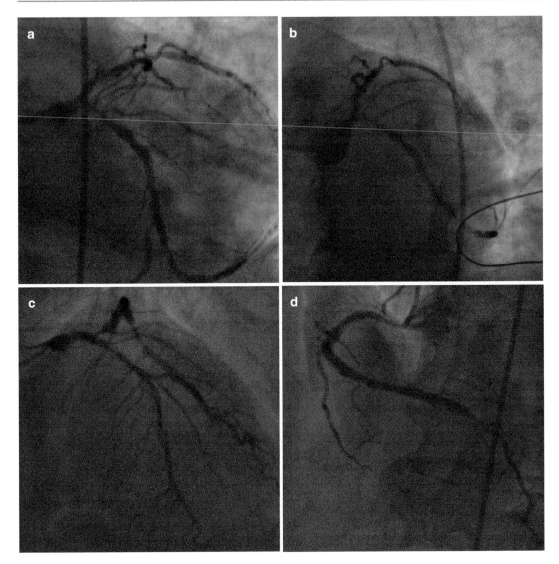

Fig. 16.11 Complete revascularization by coronary artery bypass grafting 3 days after presentation with inferior STEMI. (**a–c**) Angiography of left coronary artery. Significant stenoses are seen in the proximal LAD and LCx. (**d**) Angiography of likely culprit PDA stenosis, with TIMI 3 flow. The patient was pain free on arrival in the cath lab. He underwent bypass surgery 3 days after presentation with a left internal mammary artery graft to the LAD and sequential vein graft to the obtuse marginal and PDA

Multivessel Disease in STEMI Patients Without Shock: Local Practice at Rigshospitalet

After the completion of the DANAMI-3-PRIMULTI trial, all patients with STEMI and multivessel disease are revascularized in full with a staged, FFR-guided procedure 1–2 days after the index procedure. However, in patients with relative contraindications to an early second procedure (i.e., heart failure, reduced kidney function, infection) we find it safe to postpone the second procedure, since the positive effect in DANAMI-3-PRIMULTI was mainly driven by a reduction in unplanned revascularization, rather than harder endpoints.

Conclusions

- PPCI is a swift and effective method to ensure reperfusion of the occluded coronary artery in patients with STEMI. Compared with systemic fibrinolysis, the obvious advantage is the avoidance of side effects related to fibrinolytic therapy such as bleeding, but rapid clinical assessment (including urgent bedside echocardiography) and diagnostic coronary angiography are also advantageous in the 15–20% of field-triaged patients with diagnoses other than STEMI. Time from symptom onset to reperfusion (either fibrinolysis or PPCI) is important with regard to mortality and morbidity; healthcare systems have thus evolved to provide the earliest possible initiation of reperfusion therapy.

- In most cases, PPCI with wiring of the culprit vessel, pre-dilation, and stenting is highly effective and this is well practiced around the world. The routine use of adjunctive fibrinolysis, thrombectomy, or distal protection devices is not associated with benefits in hard endpoints. Several questions remain, however, including the optimal management of hemodynamically stable patients with multivessel coronary artery disease, as well as optimizing outcomes for patients presenting with STEMI and shock. A schematic of what is new in the 2017 European STEMI guidelines can be seen in Fig. 16.12.

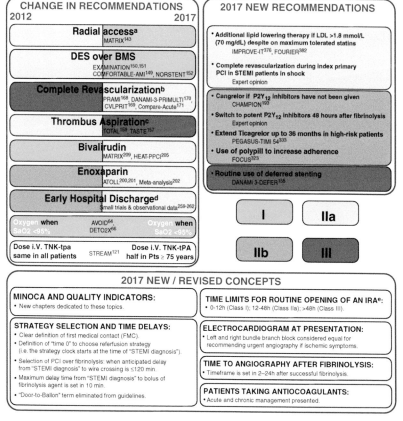

Fig. 16.12 European Society of Cardiology STEMI Guidelines 2017. What is new in the 2017 ESC STEMI Guidelines compared with 2012. In left and mid panels, below each recommendation, the most representative trial (acronym) driving the indication is mentioned. Reproduced with permission from Oxford University Press on behalf of the European Society of Cardiology. Ibanez et al. Eur Heart J 2017;00:1–66 doi:https://doi.org/10.1093/eurheartj/ehx393. Key: *BMS* bare-metal stent, *DES* drug-eluting stent, *IRA* infarct-related artery, *i.v.* intravenous, *LDL* low-density lipoprotein, *PCI* percutaneous coronary intervention, *SaO2* arterial oxygen saturation, *STEMI* ST-elevation myocardial infarction, *TNK-tPA* tenecteplase tissue plasminogen activator. ᵃOnly for experienced radial operators. ᵇBefore hospital discharge (either immediate or staged). ᶜRoutine thrombus aspiration (bailout in certain cases may be considered). ᵈIn 2012 early discharge was considered after 72 h, in 2017 early discharge is 48–72 h. ᵉIf symptoms or hemodynamic instability IRA should be opened regardless of the time from symptom onset

References

1. Bonnefoy E, Lapostolle F, Leizorovicz A, et al. Primary angioplasty versus prehospital fibrinolysis in acute myocardial infarction: a randomised study. Lancet. 2002;360:825–9.
2. Armstrong PW, Gershlick AH, Goldstein P, et al. Fibrinolysis or primary PCI in ST-segment elevation myocardial infarction. N Engl J Med. 2013;368:1379–87.
3. Assessment of the Safety and Efficacy of a New Treatment Strategy with Percutaneous Coronary Intervention (ASSENT-4 PCI) investigators. Primary versus tenecteplase-facilitated percutaneous coronary intervention in patients with ST-segment elevation acute myocardial infarction (ASSENT-4 PCI): randomised trial. Lancet. 2006;367:569–78.
4. Ellis SG, Tendera M, de Belder MA, et al. Facilitated PCI in patients with ST-elevation myocardial infarction. N Engl J Med. 2008;358:2205–17.
5. Svilaas T, Vlaar PJ, van der Horst IC, et al. Thrombus aspiration during primary percutaneous coronary intervention. N Engl J Med. 2008;358:557–67.
6. Fröbert O, Lagerqvist B, Olivecrona GK, et al. Thrombus aspiration during ST-segment elevation myocardial infarction. N Engl J Med. 2013;369:1587–97.
7. Jolly SS, Cairns JA, Yusuf S, et al. Randomized trial of primary PCI with or without routine manual thrombectomy. N Engl J Med. 2015;372:1389–98.
8. Wald DS, Morris JK, Wald NJ, et al. Randomized trial of preventive angioplasty in myocardial infarction. N Engl J Med. 2013;369:1115–23.
9. Gershlick AH, Khan JN, Kelly DJ, et al. Randomized trial of complete versus lesion-only revascularization in patients undergoing primary percutaneous coronary intervention for STEMI and multivessel disease: the CvLPRIT trial. J Am Coll Cardiol. 2015;65:963–72.
10. Engstrøm T, Kelbæk H, Helqvist S, et al. Complete revascularisation versus treatment of the culprit lesion only in patients with ST-segment elevation myocardial infarction and multivessel disease (DANAMI-3—PRIMULTI): an open-label, randomised controlled trial. Lancet. 2015;386:665–71.

Percutaneous Coronary Interventions for NSTEMI and Unstable Angina

17

Stéphane Noble and Marco Roffi

About Us The University Hospital of Geneva is a tertiary center with 1000 beds, 2 cardiac catheterization laboratories, and 4 full staff interventional cardiologists sharing, in addition to the entire spectrum of structural heart interventions as well as peripheral and carotid interventions, around 800 percutaneous coronary interventions (PCI) per year with an 80% rate of radial approach for PCI. The city of Geneva and its catchment area count approximately 500,000 inhabitants and the transportation time by ambulance is generally less than 30 min. Of note, we have a helicopter with an anesthesiologist on board and two car ambulances with a paramedic as well as an emergency medicine doctor who can be called in support of the paramedic teams in the field for emergencies including STEMI and NSTEMI with hemodynamic instability. Since 2007, we rely upon a STEMI alarm system, which is initiated by the emergency specialist doctor in the field and leads to automatic activation of the cardiac catheterization laboratory team [1]. In the last few years we have been treating STEMI and NSTEMI patients referred by a regional hospital located 28 km away. While STEMI patients per protocol receive a loading dose of prasugrel when not contraindicated, patients with suspected

NSTEMI are not pretreated with a P1Y$_{12}$ inhibitor. Our protocol for antiplatelet therapy is shown in Fig. 17.1. Periprocedural anticoagulation is achieved with unfractionated heparin. Our clinical and research interests are multiple and varied: acute coronary syndromes; antiplatelet therapy; stent devices; progression/regression of atherosclerosis; structural, peripheral, as well as carotid interventions; and pulmonary hypertension.

Definitions and Biomarkers

- Acute coronary syndromes (ACS) have been traditionally divided into unstable angina (UA), non-ST-elevation myocardial infarction (NSTEMI), and ST-elevation myocardial infarction (STEMI). This book chapter focuses on the first two presentations.
- Table 17.1 summarizes the conditions that increase the likelihood of non-ST-segment elevation acute coronary syndromes (NSTE-ACS).
- Unstable angina is defined by the presence of ischemic symptoms at rest, or at minimal effort in the absence of myocardial injury (i.e., absence of elevation of high-sensitivity cardiac troponins). These patients are at low risk of life-threatening arrhythmias, myocardial infarction (MI), or death. In the absence of recurrent symptoms, continuous rhythm monitoring is not mandatory. Moreover, in UA

S. Noble · M. Roffi (✉)
Cardiology Division, University Hospital of Geneva, Geneva, Switzerland
e-mail: Stephane.Noble@unige.ch; Marco.Roffi@hcuge.ch

© Springer International Publishing AG, part of Springer Nature 2018
A. Myat et al. (eds.), *The Interventional Cardiology Training Manual*,
https://doi.org/10.1007/978-3-319-71635-0_17

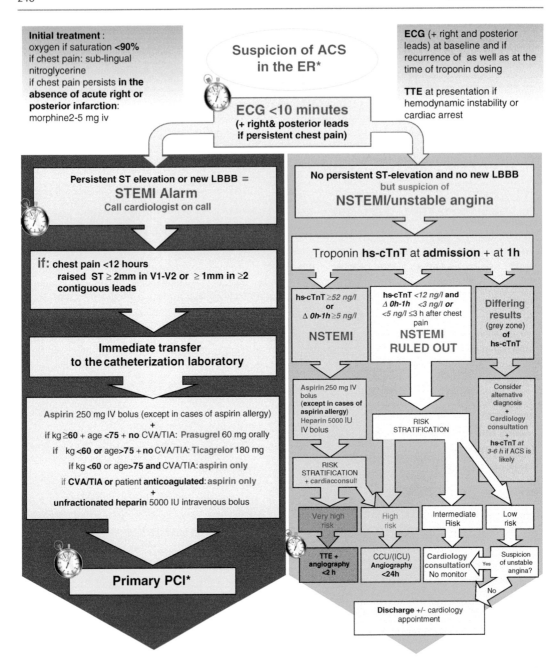

Fig. 17.1 Management algorithm for patients with suspected acute coronary syndromes at the University Hospital of Geneva, Switzerland. Key: *ACS* acute coronary syndrome, *CCU* coronary care unit, *CVA* cerebrovascular accident, *ER* emergency room, *ICU* intensive care unit, *LBBB* left bundle branch block, *PCI* percutaneous coronary interventions, *TIA* transient ischemic attack, *TTE* transthoracic echocardiography. *In cases of out of hospital (e.g., in the ambulance) suspicion of acute myocardial infarction → 12-lead ECG → if ST elevation → STEMI ALARM → direct transfer to the cardiac catheterization laboratory for primary PCI

patients, the benefit of intensive antiplatelet therapy and early revascularization is modest.

• By definition, NSTEMI is characterized by myocardial injury which translates into an increased risk of life-threatening arrhythmias and death. These patients derive a benefit from intensive antiplatelet therapy and revascularization.

• The universal definition of MI requires the presence of typical ischemic symptoms or

Table 17.1 Conditions increasing the likelihood of NSTE-ACS [16]

Older age
Male gender
Family history of coronary artery disease
Diabetes
Hyperlipidemia
Hypertension
Renal insufficiency
Previous manifestation of coronary artery disease
Other evidence of systemic atherosclerosis such as peripheral or carotid artery disease

Table 17.2 Diagnostic Criteria for Myocardial Infarction with Non-Obstructive Coronary Artery (MINOCA) [3]

The diagnosis of MINOCA is made in the presence of all of the following criteria:
1. Acute myocardial infarction criteria
(a) Positive cardiac biomarker (preferably cardiac troponin) defined as a rise and/or fall in serial levels, with at least one value above the 99th percentile upper reference limit
and
(b) Corroborative clinical evidence of infarction evidenced by at least one of the following:
I. Symptoms of ischemia
II. New or presumed new significant ST-T changes or new left bundle branch block
III. Development of pathological Q-waves
IV. Imaging evidence of new loss of viable myocardium or new regional wall motion abnormality
V. Intracoronary thrombus evident on angiography or at autopsy
2. Nonobstructive coronary arteries on angiography:
Defined as the absence of obstructive coronary artery disease on angiography (i.e., no coronary artery stenosis $\geq 50\%$), in any potential infarct-related artery. This includes both patients with:
• Normal coronary arteries (no stenosis >30%)
• Mild coronary atheroma (stenosis >30% but <50%)
3. No clinically overt specific cause for the acute presentation:
At the time of angiography, the underlying cause of the clinical presentation and myocardial injury is not apparent
→ As soon as the working diagnosis of MINOCA is made, evaluate the patient for the underlying cause of the MINOCA presentation

ischemic ECG changes in addition to a troponin level above the 99th percentile of healthy individuals, with a rise and/or fall of the biomarker [2]. While there are five different types of MI, we focus on type 1 and 2, which are defined below. Type 3 corresponds to MI resulting in death and with no biomarkers available. Type 4 and 5 are MI post-PCI and coronary artery bypass graft (CABG), respectively.

- Type 1 MI corresponds to plaque rupture, ulceration, fissuring, or erosion in the coronary artery, whereas type 2 MI is related to extra-coronary conditions which contribute to an imbalance between demand and myocardial oxygen supply, such as tachy/bradyarrhythmias, anemia, hypotension, severe hypertension, respiratory failure, severe aortic stenosis, or atrial fibrillation with poorly controlled ventricular response. Two coronary conditions not associated with plaque instability may also be the underlying mechanism of type 2 MI, namely coronary spasm and coronary embolism.
- Up to 20% of patients with NSTE-ACS have either no coronary artery disease (CAD) or nonobstructive lesions of epicardial coronary arteries, a condition recently described as MINOCA (myocardial infarction with nonobstructive coronary artery) [3]. In this population, acute MI is present (as defined by the universal definition of MI previously described) but in the absence of obstructed coronary arteries on the angiogram (arbitrarily defined as <50%) and without any overt clinical cause (e.g., pulmonary embolism, myocarditis) for the acute presentation at the time of the coronary angiogram.

- The MINOCA syndrome is heterogeneous with no common pathophysiological mechanism. This working diagnosis should initiate an in-depth search for the cause of underlying myocardial injury. The MINOCA diagnostic criteria are summarized in Table 17.2.
- Creatine kinase (CK) and its MB fraction (CK-MB) were the traditional markers of cardiomyocyte damage, but are less sensitive and specific than cardiac troponin. Serial CK levels may help quantify the extent and/or timing of MI, but cardiac troponins (and preferably high-sensitivity cardiac troponins) are the preferred biomarker to diagnose or rule out acute MI and to quantify cardiomyocyte injury.
- Co-peptin is a quantitative marker of endogenous stress and nearly universally elevated in

Table 17.3 Etiologies of high-sensitivity cardiac troponin elevations in patients with suspected acute coronary syndromes [16]

• Mild troponin elevation associated with:
– Tachy- or bradyarrhythmias
– Heart failure
– Hypertensive emergencies
– Critical illnesses
– Perimyocarditis
– Aortic stenosis
– Aortic dissection
– Pulmonary embolism
• Substantial troponin elevation (>10 times the 99th percentile) associated with:
– Non-ST-elevation myocardial infarction
– Takotsubo cardiomyopathy
– Myocarditis

the first hours of MI. It has a very small, if any, added value when used in combination with high-sensitivity cardiac troponin.

- The replacement of conventional cardiac troponin assays by the introduction of high-sensitivity troponin assays results in earlier detection of MI, and provides an approximately 20% relative increase (4% absolute increase) in the detection of type 1 MI, with a corresponding decrease in the diagnosis of unstable angina. It also favors a marked increase in type 2 MI (100%) [4]. Table 17.3 summarizes the association of the level of troponin elevation and causes.

- To confirm NSTEMI, high-sensitivity troponin should be assessed at presentation as well as after 1 or 3 h, depending on the assay and algorithms used. The greatest advantage from the higher sensitivity and diagnostic accuracy of the high-sensitivity cardiac troponin assays is observed in patients presenting early after chest pain onset as well as in patients with a small MI.

- As a general rule, the higher the troponin level, the greater the likelihood of MI; in addition, rising and/or falling of troponin differentiate acute from chronic cardiomyocyte damage (the more pronounced the change, the higher the likelihood of MI).

- The positive predictive value for MI in patients classified as rule in by the high-sensitivity car-

diac troponin at baseline at 0 and 1 h (0 h/1 h protocol) using tested essays (Elecsys or Architect) is 70–80%, while the negative predictive value (i.e., the ability to rule out MI) exceeds 98% [4]. In association with clinical presentation and 12-lead ECG, the 0 h/1 h protocol allows an early detection of candidates for early coronary angiography.

- Finally cardiac troponin remains elevated for several days and thus is of limited value to detect early re-infarction in acute MI. Therefore, CK-MB levels can be helpful in diagnosing subacute MI as well as to detect re-infarction since they fall much more rapidly after MI than troponin.

Timing of Intervention

- The timing of coronary intervention varies according to the clinical presentation, presence or absence of 12-lead ECG modification, and troponin results. Additional ischemic risk stratification can be easily and accurately performed using the Global Registry of Acute Coronary Events (GRACE) 2.0 risk calculator [4].

- According to guidelines, all NSTEMI patients require an early invasive strategy (i.e., coronary angiography within 24 h).

- Importantly, the occlusion of vessels supplying blood to the lateral or posterolateral myocardium may not cause ST-segment elevation on a standard 12-lead ECG. Indeed approximately 50% of acute circumflex coronary artery occlusions may not cause ST-segment elevation on the 12-lead ECG [5]. In patients with persistent symptoms suggestive of ongoing myocardial ischemia and a nondiagnostic 12-lead ECG, additional leads should be examined (i.e., posterior, right ventricular) and thereafter immediate coronary angiography may be required.

- Almost a quarter of NSTEMI patients have an acutely occluded coronary artery and in two-thirds of the cases collateralization of this artery is seen at coronary angiography [5].

- In NSTEMI cases with obstructive CAD, 40–80% of patients have multivessel disease and multiple ruptured plaques may coexist as shown by pathological and intracoronary imaging studies. Furthermore, the identification of the culprit lesion based on the angiography may sometimes be difficult especially when the coronary flow is normal in the presumptive infarct-related artery (approximately 50% of the cases).

- In patients presenting with hemodynamic instability, acute heart failure related to ACS, shock, or cardiac arrest, the ESC guidelines recommend transthoracic echocardiography prior to immediate coronary angiography to assess left ventricular function and exclude mechanical complications (wall perforation, ventricular septal defect, severe mitral regurgitation) and noncoronary conditions such as massive pulmonary embolism or aortic stenosis [4].

Early Invasive Approach

- An early invasive approach is defined by the performance of coronary angiography within 24 h of the first medical contact.
- Patients with simple lesion(s) or requiring immediate revascularization in the context of ongoing or recurrent ischemia, hemodynamic instability, acute heart failure, recurrent ventricular arrhythmias, or total occlusion of the culprit vessel should benefit from ad hoc PCI.
- In patients with complex multivessel CAD, stable hemodynamic conditions, and TIMI III grade flow in the culprit vessel in the absence of ongoing ischemia, heart team discussions should be favored to guide management (PCI vs. CABG).
- Whenever possible, complete revascularization should be pursued, as it is associated with better prognosis than incomplete revascularization in NSTE-ACS.

An Early Invasive Strategy According to Risk

- The recommended maximal time delay between hospital admission and coronary angiography varies according to patient risk.

- Patients at **very high risk** (i.e., hemodynamic instability, recurrent or ongoing chest pain refractory to medical therapy, mechanical complication of MI, acute heart failure related to ACS, life-threatening arrhythmias or cardiac arrest, recurrent dynamic ST-T wave changes, particularly with intermittent ST elevation) should undergo immediate coronary angiography, meaning in less than 2 h. For patients admitted in a center without PCI facilities, transfer to PCI center should be immediate.
- Patients at **high risk** (i.e., rise or fall of troponin compatible with MI, symptomatic or silent dynamic ST- or T-wave changes, or GRACE score >140) should undergo a coronary angiography with a maximum delay of 24 h.
- For the **intermediate risk** patients (i.e., diabetes mellitus, renal GFR <60 mL/min/1.73 m^2, LVEF <40% or congestive heart failure, early post-infarction angina, prior PCI, prior CABG, GRACE risk score >109 but <140) the coronary angiography should be performed within 72 h of admission.
- Finally for **low-risk patients** (i.e., none of the above-mentioned characteristics) a noninvasive test may be performed before or shortly after hospital discharge and coronary angiography planned according to the presence or extent of ischemia.

Vascular Access, Stent Type, and Antiplatelet Therapy

- In patients with invasively treated ACS, transradial approach (TRA) should be the default access [4, 6, 7] and centers with cardiac catheterization laboratories treating ACS patients using a transfemoral approach should implement a transition to TRA.
- In patients on a vitamin K antagonist (VKA), radial approach should more than ever be favored. Of note, if the INR is >2.5, limited data suggest that there is no benefit to adding parenteral anticoagulation during PCI in order to prevent periprocedural ischemic events and catheter thrombosis, whereas when the INR is

<2.5 parenteral anticoagulation (commonly unfractionated heparin) is administered for the procedure [8].

- When TRA is not feasible and the patient is at intermediate risk, VKA may be stopped and transfemoral coronary angiography may be postponed until the INR is <2 [8]. In patients on non-vitamin K oral anticoagulants, additional parenteral anticoagulation for PCI is recommended independently of the timing of the last dose of drugs.

- With respect to stent choice, the use of new-generation drug-eluting stents rather than bare-metal stents is recommended (Class I, level of evidence A) and should be considered (Class IIa, level of evidence B) even in those requiring chronic anticoagulation therapy [4].

- Dual-antiplatelet therapy (DAPT), defined as the combination of aspirin and a $P2Y_{12}$ inhibitor, is recommended for 12 months in NSTE-ACS patients independently of the revascularization strategy. However, shorter or longer DAPT durations may be considered based on individual bleeding and ischemic risks of the patients. Among the $P2Y_{12}$ inhibitors, ticagrelor and prasugrel are superior to clopidogrel, but they are contraindicated in patients on oral anticoagulation (e.g., with atrial fibrillation, mechanical valve, pulmonary embolism). In these patients undergoing stenting, triple therapy (i.e., aspirin, clopidogrel, and one anticoagulant) may be given for a period of time ranging from 1 (with the BIOFREEDOM stent) [9, 10] to 6 months based on the estimated bleeding risk. Thereafter the combination with one antiplatelet and one anticoagulant (either vitamin K antagonist or non-vitamin K antagonist oral anticoagulant) should be continued up to 1 year. In the absence of high-risk features (e.g., diffuse multivessel disease, left main or multiple stenting, recurrent ischemic symptoms) after 1-year anticoagulation may be continued alone.

- When non-vitamin K oral anticoagulants are used in combination with DAPT, the lowest tested for the prevention of stroke dose should be used (i.e., dabigatran 110 mg twice a day, rivaroxaban 15 mg daily, apixaban 2.5 mg twice a day).

- Pretreatment with $P2Y_{12}$ inhibitors in patients scheduled for coronary angiography has been a source of debate and remains controversial. The only randomized, controlled trial assessing $P2Y_{12}$ pretreatment in NSTEMI patients is the ACCOAST (Comparison of Prasugrel at the Time of Percutaneous Coronary Intervention or as Pretreatment at the Time of Diagnosis in Patients with Non-ST Elevation Myocardial Infarction) trial [11]. The conclusions of this trial of 4033 patients (6% were treated with surgery, 69% underwent PCI, and the remaining 25% were treated conservatively) were that up to day 7 TIMI major bleeding episodes related or not related to CABG increased in the pretreatment group (TIMI major and life-threatening bleeding not related to CABG were increased by three- and sixfold, respectively) and the rate of the primary outcomes (i.e., composite of death from cardiovascular cause, MI, stroke, urgent revascularization, or glycoprotein inhibitor rescue therapy) was not decreased by the pretreatment strategy with prasugrel. All the results were confirmed at 30 days.

- In a subgroup analysis of the 2770 patients who underwent PCI, the ACCOAST-PCI study, pretreatment with prasugrel was still not associated with a decrease in any ischemic events and there was no impact on the presence of thrombus before PCI or on stent thrombosis post-PCI while the bleeding complications significantly increased [12].

- Therefore, in the ESC guidelines pretreatment with prasugrel is not recommended in patients for whom the coronary anatomy is not known (Class III, evidence C).

- With respect to other $P2Y_{12}$ inhibitors (i.e., ticagrelor and clopidogrel), the timing of administration has not been adequately investigated and no recommendations were formulated for or against pretreatment in the ESC guidelines.

- Importantly, morphine delays the biological effect of oral $P2Y_{12}$ inhibitors by slowing intestinal absorption. In PCI bailout situations or thrombotic complications glycoprotein (GP) IIb/IIIa inhibitors should be considered (ESC Class IIa, level of evidence C). When GPIIb/IIIa inhibitors are used, platelet count should be followed during the first 24 h and perfusion discontinued if platelet count falls to <100,000 μL or drops by >50% from baseline. To avoid a low platelet count due to platelet aggregate on ethylenediaminetetraacetic acid (EDTA) tubes, platelet count should be performed on a sodium citrate tube.

Conservative Strategy

- In very elderly or frail patients or in the presence of comorbidities (e.g., severe chronic renal insufficiency, cancer at high risk of bleeding or dementia), conservative treatment may be favored. Although there is no upper age limit for 1-year DAPT treatment in these patients, the bleeding risk should be assessed carefully.
- In the setting of medically managed patients, DAPT using ticagrelor is superior to clopidogrel—according to the PLATO study [13]—whereas prasugrel was not superior to clopidogrel—according to the TRILOGY ACS trial [14]—in terms of ischemic event reduction, but both medications caused more bleeding complications than clopidogrel.
- The ESC guidelines recommend in NSTE-ACS patients with a planned conservative treatment to introduce $P2Y_{12}$ inhibitor (preferably ticagrelor) in the absence of contraindication when the diagnosis is confirmed.
- Clopidogrel is recommended only for patients who cannot receive ticagrelor or in those who require chronic oral anticoagulation, which is a clear contraindication for the more potent $P2Y_{12}$ inhibitors.
- In NSTEMI patients allergic to aspirin, there are no prospective data available to guide their management. There are aspirin desensitization protocols consisting of the administration of increasing doses of aspirin (e.g., 5 mg, 10 mg, 20 mg, 40 mg every 30 min followed

by 100 mg the day after), which are well tolerated in the vast majority of patients [8]. In the presence of a true major allergy refractory to desensitization, monotherapy with a potent $P2Y_{12}$ (prasugrel or ticagrelor) may be considered.

PCI Versus CABG

- In the absence of trials performed in the ACS setting, we have to rely on PCI versus CABG comparative studies enrolling stable CAD patients.
- In order to choose between the two revascularization modalities, several factors should be taken into account, including the clinical presentation (e.g., cardiogenic shock/hemodynamic instability, STEMI, NSTEMI, UA), surgical risk, coronary anatomy and lesion complexity, ventricular function, comorbidities, frailty, and life expectancy.
- As previously mentioned, patients with simple lesion(s) or requiring immediate revascularization in the context of ongoing or recurrent ischemia, hemodynamic instability, acute heart failure related to ACS, recurrent ventricular arrhythmias, or total occlusion of the culprit vessel should benefit from ad hoc PCI. In patients with complex multivessel CAD, stable hemodynamic conditions, and TIMI III grade flow in the culprit vessel, in the absence of ongoing ischemia, heart team discussions should be favored to choose between PCI and CABG.
- The ESC guidelines recommend that CABG should be considered (Class IIa, level of evidence B) in the setting of multiple-vessel disease and an acceptable surgical risk profile with a life expectancy of >1 year.
- CABG surgery performed on DAPT is associated with a twofold increase in major bleeding and in reoperation due to bleeding. In the hemodynamically stable patient, surgery should be delayed by 5 days post-ticagrelor and clopidogrel cessation and by 7 days if the patients were on prasugrel.

Secondary Prevention

- Independent of the revascularization strategy, high-dose statin therapy is essential. The latest European guidelines recommend for patients at very high cardiovascular risk (i.e., all patients with ACS) to decrease LDL cholesterol to <1.8 mmol/L or at least by 50% [15].
- Cardiac rehabilitation and lifestyle changes, in addition to cardiovascular risk factor modification, are also crucially important steps to improve the long-term prognosis of ACS patients.

Conclusion

- While early coronary angiography and, if appropriate, revascularization are superior to medical management in NSTEMI patients, patients with suspected unstable angina are at lower risk and may initially undergo a noninvasive assessment first.
- In the absence of dedicated data, the decision between PCI and CABG should be based on clinical presentation, lesion(s) complexity, and comorbidities.
- Independently of the revascularization strategy, DAPT is recommended for 12 months, although shorter or longer durations based on the ischemic and bleeding risk profiles of the individual patient may be applied.
- Timing of ticagrelor administration in patients undergoing an early invasive strategy (pretreatment) is uncertain.
- All patients benefit from cardiovascular risk factor control including high-dose statins, lifestyle changes, and cardiac rehabilitation.

References

1. Grosgurin O, Plojoux J, Keller PF, Niquille M, N'koulou R, Mach F, Sarasin FP, Rutschmann OT. Prehospital emergency physician activation of interventional cardiology team reduces door-to-balloon time in ST-elevation myocardial infarction. Swiss Med Wkly. 2010;140(15–16):228–32.

2. Thygesen K, Alpert JS, Jaffe AS, Simoons ML, Chaitman BR, White HD, Writing Group on the Joint ESC/ACCF/AHA/WHF Task Force for the Universal Definition of Myocardial Infarction, Thygesen K, Alpert JS, White HD, Jaffe AS, Katus HA, Apple FS, Lindahl B, Morrow DA, Chaitman BA, Clemmensen PM, Johanson P, Hod H, Underwood R, Bax JJ, Bonow RO, Pinto F, Gibbons RJ, Fox KA, Atar D, Newby LK, Galvani M, Hamm CW, Uretsky BF, Steg PG, Wijns W, Bassand JP, Menasché P, Ravkilde J, Ohman EM, Antman EM, Wallentin LC, Armstrong PW, Simoons ML, Januzzi JL, Nieminen MS, Gheorghiade M, Filippatos G, Luepker RV, Fortmann SP, Rosamond WD, Levy D, Wood D, Smith SC, Hu D, Lopez-Sendon JL, Robertson RM, Weaver D, Tendera M, Bove AA, Parkhomenko AN, Vasilieva EJ, Mendis S; ESC Committee for Practice Guidelines (CPG). Third universal definition of myocardial infarction. Eur Heart J. 2012;33(20):2551–67.

3. Agewall S, Beltrame JF, Reynolds HR, Niessner A, Rosano G, Caforio AL, et al. ESC working group position paper on myocardial infarction with non-obstructive coronary arteries. Eur Heart J. 2016;38(3):143–53. https://doi.org/10.1093/eurheartj/ehw149.

4. Roffi M, Patrono C, Collet JP, Mueller C, Valgimigli M, Andreotti F, et al. 2015 ESC Guidelines for the management of acute coronary syndromes in patients presenting without persistent ST-segment elevation: Task Force for the Management of Acute Coronary Syndromes in Patients Presenting without Persistent ST-Segment Elevation of the European Society of Cardiology (ESC). Eur Heart J. 2016;37(3):267–315. https://doi.org/10.1093/eurheartj/ehv320.

5. Valgimigli M, Patrono C, Collet JP, Mueller C, Roffi M. Questions and answers on coronary revascularization: a companion document of the 2015 ESC Guidelines for the management of acute coronary syndromes in patients presenting without persistent ST-segment elevation. Eur Heart J. 2015;37(3):e8–e14. https://doi.org/10.1093/eurheartj/ehv408.

6. Noble S. Radial access in patients invasively treated for acute coronary syndromes: a lifesaving approach. JACC Cardiovasc Interv. 2016;9(7):671–3. https://doi.org/10.1016/j.jcin.2016.02.008.

7. Andò GCD. Radial access reduces mortality in patients with acute coronary syndromes: results from an updated trial sequential analysis of randomized trials. JACC Cardiovasc Interv. 2016;9(7):660–70.

8. Collet JP, Roffi M, Mueller C, Valgimigli M, Patrono C, Baumgartner H, et al. Questions and answers on antithrombotic therapy: a companion document of the 2015 ESC Guidelines for the management of acute coronary syndromes in patients presenting without persistent ST-segment elevationdagger. Eur Heart J. 2015. https://doi.org/10.1093/eurheartj/ehv407.

9. Garot PMM, Tresukosol D, Pocock SJ, Meredith IT, Abizaid A, Carrié D, Naber C, Iñiguez A, Talwar S, Menown IB, Christiansen EH, Gregson J, Copt S, Hovasse T, Lurz P, Maillard L,

Krackhardt F, Ong P, Byrne J, Redwood S, Windhövel U, Greene S, Stoll HP, Urban P, LEADERS FREE Investigators. Two-year outcomes of high bleeding risk patients after polymer-free drug-coated stents. J Am Coll Cardiol. 2017;69(2):162–71. https://doi.org/10.1016/j.jacc.2016.10.009.

10. Urban PMI, Abizaid A, Pocock SJ, Carrié D, Naber C, Lipiecki J, Richardt G, Iñiguez A, Brunel P, Valdes-Chavarri M, Garot P, Talwar S, Berland J, Abdellaoui M, Eberli F, Oldroyd K, Zambahari R, Gregson J, Greene S, Stoll HP, Morice MC, LEADERS FREE Investigators. Polymer-free drug-coated coronary stents in patients at high bleeding risk. N Engl J Med. 2015;373(21):2038–47. https://doi.org/10.1056/NEJMoa1503943.

11. Montalescot G, Bolognese L, Dudek D, Goldstein P, Hamm C, Tanguay JF, et al. Pretreatment with prasugrel in non-ST-segment elevation acute coronary syndromes. N Engl J Med. 2013;369(11):999–1010. https://doi.org/10.1056/NEJMoa1308075.

12. Montalescot G, Collet JP, Ecollan P, Bolognese L, Ten Berg J, Dudek D, et al. Effect of prasugrel pretreatment strategy in patients undergoing percutaneous coronary intervention for NSTEMI: the ACCOAST-PCI study. J Am Coll Cardiol. 2014;64(24):2563–71. https://doi.org/10.1016/j.jacc.2014.08.053.

13. Wallentin LBR, Budaj A, Cannon CP, Emanuelsson H, Held C, Horrow J, Husted S, James S, Katus H, Mahaffey KW, Scirica BM, Skene A, Steg PG, Storey RF, Harrington RA, Investigators PLATO, Freij A, Thorsén M. Ticagrelor versus clopidogrel in patients with acute coronary syndromes. N Engl J Med. 2009;361(11):1045–57.

14. Roe MT, Armstrong PW, Fox KA, White HD, Prabhakaran D, Goodman SG, et al. Prasugrel versus clopidogrel for acute coronary syndromes without revascularization. N Engl J Med. 2012;367(14):1297–309. https://doi.org/10.1056/NEJMoa1205512.

15. Catapano AL, Graham I, De Backer G, Wiklund O, Chapman MJ, Drexel H, et al. 2016 ESC/EAS Guidelines for the Management of Dyslipidaemias: The Task Force for the Management of Dyslipidaemias of the European Society of Cardiology (ESC) and European Atherosclerosis Society (EAS)Developed with the special contribution of the European Assocciation for Cardiovascular Prevention & Rehabilitation (EACPR). Eur Heart J. 2016;37:2999–3058. https://doi.org/10.1093/eurheartj/ehw272.

16. Mueller CPC, Valgimigli M, Collet JP, Roffi M. Questions and answers on diagnosis and risk assessment: a companion document of the 2015 ESC Guidelines for the management of acute coronary syndromes in patients presenting without persistent ST-segment elevation. Eur Heart J. 2015. https://doi.org/10.1093/eurheartj/ehv409.

Percutaneous Coronary Intervention for Stable Ischemic Heart Disease

18

William S. Weintraub, Sandra Weiss,
and Abdul Latif Bikak

About Us Christiana Care Health System located in Delaware is a two-campus multispecialty hospital system. The Center for Heart and Vascular Health is part of the Christiana campus with a 900-bed hospital.

The heart and vascular center provides patient-centered cardiology solutions ranging from complex coronary interventions to structural heart procedures including but not limited to left atrial appendage occluders and percutaneous aortic valve implants. We also have a robust acute myocardial infraction response program which is in line with all the metrics set by ACC/AHA, including door to balloon time. The center provides patients with services related to cardiothoracic surgery as well. Our invasive volume is quite robust, with over 4700 diagnostic cases and nearly 1600 interventional coronary cases performed in the fiscal year 2015.

Multidisciplinary heart teams which comprise invasive cardiology, noninvasive cardiology, cardiac surgery, and advance heart failure specialists help make the complex patient- centered decisions ranging from valvular heart disease, advanced heart failure and transplantation and ischemic heart disease.

When it pertains to stable ischemic heart disease (SIHD), we ensure patients are on multiple antianginal medications prior to considering angiography or surgical bypass with strict adherence to appropriate use criteria (AUC) with additional annual internal review of cases with the heart team to verify compliance with those criteria. We also go through the SCAI AUC tool intra-procedurally to chart appropriateness of those cases before percutaneous coronary intervention (PCI) is undertaken.

Introduction

- Coronary angiography and revascularization began in the 1960s and has evolved dramatically into a robust platform for not only diagnosis of coronary disease but also complex percutaneous intervention.
- The phenomenal number of procedures, over a million by the mid-2000s in the United States alone [1], has helped improve operator expertise. This coupled with advances in equipment, specifically in stent technology, has made percutaneous intervention an increasingly preferred modality in various clinical scenarios.
- With this, the world saw ever-increasing revascularization of coronary stenoses in patients ranging from those with asymptomatic lesions to those suffering an acute

W. S. Weintraub (✉) · S. Weiss · A. L. Bikak
The Center for Heart and Vascular Health,
Christiana Care Health System, Newark, DE, USA
e-mail: William.s.Weintraub@medstar.net;
sweiss@christianacare.org;
abdul.l.bikak@christianacare.org

© Springer International Publishing AG, part of Springer Nature 2018
A. Myat et al. (eds.), *The Interventional Cardiology Training Manual*,
https://doi.org/10.1007/978-3-319-71635-0_18

myocardial infarction (MI). However, even though coronary intervention through both PCI and coronary artery bypass grafting (CABG) have greatly improved outcomes in the setting of acute coronary syndrome (ACS), the same has not been systematically true for stable ischemic heart disease (SIHD) [2].

The Early Experience: CABG Versus Medical Therapy

- The first studies that looked at revascularization of SIHD as opposed to medical therapy were the initial CABG trials, including the VA study, CASS trial, and ECSS in Europe [3, 4]. They showed relief from angina symptoms, falling by 50% over 10 years [5]. Nonetheless, the outcomes were suboptimal, highlighting several limitations:
  - First, much of the short-lived benefit was secondary to graft occlusion as internal mammary artery (IMA) grafts were not used as frequently as in contemporary practice [6].
  - Second, medical therapy in both arms was markedly distinct from modern recommendations with a lack of robust lipid lowering, blood pressure control, antianginal medications, antiplatelet medications, and lifestyle modifications—all mainstays of current treatment.
- What these studies were pivotal in highlighting, however, were patient characteristics associated with poorer survival. These included:
  - Low left ventricular ejection fraction (LVEF).
  - Three-vessel coronary disease (>70% stenosis).
  - >50% left main disease.
  - Two- to three-vessel disease which included the proximal left anterior descending (LAD) artery [7].
- Interestingly, what these trials failed to show was a mortality benefit or freedom from subsequent myocardial ischemia for low risk patients. In the CABG Surgery Trialists

Collaboration meta-analysis, even though the high-risk patients showed a benefit with CABG, the lowest risk category trended toward increased mortality with CABG and postsurgical complications [8].

- Although these trials are now more of historical interest, they certainly helped us define three crucial clinical considerations that impact outcomes in the SIHD population:
  - The anatomical complexity and burden of coronary artery disease.
  - Severity of left ventricular dysfunction.
  - Degree and extent of comorbid conditions.

Moving Ahead: Percutaneous Coronary Intervention for SIHD

- With the advent of PCI, trials started looking at this modality in SIHD and how it compared to both medical therapy and traditional bypass graft surgery. The initial trials compared balloon angioplasty to medical therapy. Most notable of these trials was RITA 2 [9]. This trial showed no mortality benefit of PCI in SIHD, something that was reinforced in a subsequent meta-analysis looking at optimal medical therapy (OMT) against balloon angioplasty. Furthermore, while balloon angioplasty was initially better at controlling anginal symptoms, this proved at the expense of more frequent repeat revascularizations and periprocedural MIs.
- Many of these early-experience PCI events were related to the high rate of restenosis and acute vessel closure with balloon angioplasty alone. The advent of coronary stents, and in particular drug eluting stents (DES), significantly reduced the incidence of these complications and the transition into our modern practice [10]. With this, the notion that medical therapy was better at preventing adverse outcomes to intervention was challenged once again.
- Nonetheless, in the years preceding the Clinical Outcomes of Utilizing Revascularization and Aggressive Drug Evaluation (COURAGE) trial, a routine invasive strategy for SIHD was the default. This was despite guideline

recommendations for a strategy of OMT with intensive antianginal medication utilization, lifestyle modifications, and risk factor reduction [2].

- In 2004, >1 million stent procedures were performed in the US with data showing that 85% of PCIs were performed in patients with SIHD [11]. It was assumed that revascularization of a symptomatic coronary stenosis would lead not only to improvement in angina but also a reduction in hard cardiovascular (CV) endpoints.

- Yet, Katritsis and colleagues published a meta-analysis in 2005 including 11 randomized trials and 2950 patients that failed to demonstrate a significant reduction in death, MI, or need for subsequent revascularization with PCI in this population [12]. What was clearly lacking was a single, large randomized study that compared modern PCI techniques to OMT in the treatment of SIHD.

The Modern Era

- The COURAGE Trial aimed to answer this question [13]. The study randomized 2287 patients with SIHD to a strategy of OMT vs. PCI with OMT and evaluated all-cause mortality and nonfatal MI with a median follow-up of 4.6 years.

- Eighty-five percent of the participants had undergone a stress evaluation with 2/3 of the nuclear studies demonstrating multiple perfusion abnormalities. Nearly 70% of participants had multivessel disease on angiography with >30% having involvement of the proximal LAD. Surprisingly, the study revealed no significant difference in the primary outcome.

- Furthermore, even though the PCI arm had a lower incidence of repeat revascularization in the short-term, over 70% of participants in both arms were free of angina by end-of-study.

- Although it has been said the compliance to OMT in COURAGE would be difficult to replicate in the real world, the overall importance of OMT was highlighted and the role of PCI in

SIHD was shown to confer limited long-term symptom benefit with no survival advantage. Indeed, OMT was mandated in both arms of the COURAGE trial and remains the standard of care today, whether revascularization is performed or not.

- Following this, the BARI-2D trial shed further light on the topic. The original BARI trial evaluated CABG vs. PCI and showed no mortality difference in the overall population, but in a subgroup analysis of patients with diabetes, CABG conferred a survival benefit over angioplasty [14].

- The more contemporary BARI-2D trial considered once again a high-risk population with diabetes, and again compared medical therapy alone against prompt revascularization with either CABG or PCI, with OMT in both arms [15]. The trial failed to show a mortality benefit at 5 years with intervention. Of note, when the results were stratified by intended treatment, the CABG arm had significant improvement in major cardiovascular outcomes compared to medical therapy, primarily driven by a nearly 50% reduction in the rate of nonfatal MI (14.6% vs. 7.4%), something that was not seen with PCI.

- The subsequent FREEDOM and BEST trials further supported these findings [16, 17]. These studies compared revascularization with CABG vs. DES-PCI in patients with DM and multivessel CAD. While not specifically comparing revascularization strategies to OMT, these studies showed CABG to be superior to DES-PCI by way of reduction in major adverse cardiovascular events at the expense of an increased rate of stroke.

- The importance of these studies was the use of DES, which in theory would optimize results of PCI revascularization. Of the 1149 patients randomized to PCI in COURAGE, 14% received balloon angioplasty alone, 86% received angioplasty with stent implantation, and 97% of the stents implanted were bare metal stents (BMS); DES, where used, were first generation.

- Yet, despite the widespread use and availability of the best-performing everolimus family of stents used exclusively in the BEST trial, the dramatic decrease in the need for additional procedures with modern DES PCI still failed to match revascularization achieved by CABG.

Why Does PCI Fail?

Degree of Revascularization

- Perhaps some of the unique benefit seen specifically with CABG over medical therapy was tied to the degree of ischemic reduction. In general, complete revascularization confers a long-term survival benefit when compared to incomplete revascularization, especially in those with a large burden of disease. For example, analyses of the SYNTAX trial (a study which evaluated PCI versus CABG in patients using a quantified anatomy-based risk score) allowed for calculation of a residual SYNTAX score [18, 19]. This score defined the degree of remaining disease burden after PCI. A score of >8 after PCI was associated with higher mortality (35.3% mortality with a score > 8 versus 8.7% with score 0–4 and 11.4% with score 4–8, $p < 0.001$) as reviewed in the post hoc analysis of the ACUITY trial and then validated by the SYNTAX trial at 5-year follow-up [18].
- Second, a meta-analysis of 35 trials with almost 90,000 patients demonstrated that complete revascularization resulted in a lower rate of death and MI in long-term follow-up and was more likely achieved when CABG was the treatment modality [20].
- These data point to the fact that in patients with a greater burden of disease, lowering the degree of ischemia was beneficial and CABG appeared best able to accomplish this. However, this remains true for PCI in SIHD as well.
- In an aging population with significant comorbidities, the rate of surgical turndown cannot be discounted. Therefore, the degree of pre and post ischemia burden after PCI may be an important marker for meaningful success [21].

- The forthcoming ISCHEMIA (clinicaltrials. gov NCT01471522) and SYNTAX II (clinicaltrials.gov NCT02015832) trials will hopefully expand on this subject [22]. The ongoing ISCHEMIA trial is enrolling patients with moderate ischemic burden as seen on noninvasive testing with randomization to OMT vs. revascularization plus OMT. As randomization will take place before an invasive ischemic evaluation, it plans to expand our understanding of even the most complex of ischemic disease including left main stenosis.

Effects of Comorbidities

- It has become clear through studies such as BARI-2D that comorbid conditions such as diabetes and left ventricular dysfunction can significantly modify risk. Furthermore, end-organ manifestations of those comorbidities are predictive of a poor long-term prognosis, with degree of severity conferring differential risk.
- It is with this in mind that risk scores such as ACEF, which incorporates, age, serum creatinine, and LVEF have been created and validated in predicting inpatient mortality after CABG. A step further is the incorporation of the anatomical SYNTAX score with components of ACEF to formulate the SYNTAX II score [22]. This score incorporates both anatomical and clinical variables and will attempt to enhance our choice of medical therapy versus revascularization and selection of revascularization modalities where appropriate.
- As an example, a patient with low comorbid complexity and a low anatomical SYNTAX score will have a low SYNTAX II score and will presumably be preferred for medical therapy alone or possibly with PCI, while a patient with significant comorbidities and high anatomical complexity will have a higher SYNTAX II score and may benefit from revascularization, specifically with CABG. The ongoing SYNTAX II trial plans to validate this concept.

Ischemic Burden as a Predictor of Outcomes

- The fact that SIHD patient with diabetes and multivessel CAD garnered benefit from surgical revascularization points to a high burden of anatomical disease, and by extension, degree of ischemia, as a predictor of incremental benefit from revascularization over medical therapy. As this was not consistent with the findings of COURAGE, this begs the question as to whether assessment of degree of jeopardized myocardium should play a role in patient assessment.

- As such, evidence mounts toward classifying patients with SIHD more objectively using both anatomy and ischemic burden. The nuclear sub-study of the COURAGE trial evaluated outcomes based on the degree of ischemic reduction as measured by rest/stress SPECT myocardial perfusion imaging [23]. Significant ischemia reduction was seen more in the PCI and OMT arm as opposed to OMT alone. Although degree of ischemic reduction did not predict outcomes in the overall population, patients with a moderate to severe ischemia burden to start with AND a decrease of >5% ischemia burden showed a significant trend toward event free survival.

- To better quantify this, trials utilizing fractional flow reserve (FFR) were undertaken. The FAME trial showed that limited intervention to lesions with FFR ≤0.8 was effective and safe (see also Chap. 15) [24]. In fact, at 1-year follow-up the primary endpoint of MI, death, or repeat revascularization was significantly reduced in the FFR arm.

- The subsequent FAME 2 trial sought to build upon the findings of FAME and reconcile them with COURAGE by determining if *FFR-guided* PCI with OMT compared to OMT alone could improve outcomes in patients with SIHD [25]. This trial was terminated early given the significant difference in the primary endpoint. At 1 year, the composite endpoint of death, MI, or urgent revascularization was significantly reduced by FFR-guided PCI with OMT versus OMT alone, primarily driven by an eightfold reduction in urgent revascularization for ACS.

- Of those requiring urgent revascularization, just under half presented with significant evidence of ischemia: 21.5% with troponin positivity and 26.8% with unstable angina and ischemic ECG changes. Of note, inclusion of urgent revascularization as an endpoint has been met with some criticism given the overall rate of MI was unchanged by FFR-guided therapy. It therefore remains questionable, given the weight of evidence, whether revascularization with PCI, even with functional assessment of lesion-specific ischemic impact, results in benefit that warrants procedural risks over proven OMT. Further study is necessary.

Conclusion

- Trials looking at OMT versus intervention such as BARI-2D and COURAGE have reinforced our understanding that SIHD can be treated effectively with medical therapy. Intervention has not been shown to offer a survival benefit, and even symptom relief is transient.

- However, we have also come to realize there is a subset of patients who benefit from revascularization, specifically surgical revascularization, highlighting the need for better tools to stratify patients into categories that would confer this benefit, whether anatomical, ischemia-driven, or both.

- How best to incorporate such tools and to improve patient outcomes awaits further study. Since writing this chapter there has been a huge amount of focus and significant discussion on the results of the ORBITA trial [26]. Although beyond the scope of this manuscript to dissect the trial results further, we would strongly recommend the reader to read further on the topic, including an excellent Editorial on a substudy of ORBITA [27, 28].

References

1. Rosamond W, Flegal K, Friday G, et al. Heart disease and stroke statistics-2007 update. Circulation. 2007;115:e69–e171.
2. ACC/AHA/SCAI 2005 guideline update for percutaneous coronary intervention—summary article. A report of the American College of Cardiology/American Heart Association Task Force on practice guidelines (ACC/AHA/SCAI writing committee to update the 2001 guidelines for percutaneous coronary intervention). Circulation. 2006;113:156–75.
3. Varnauskas E. Twelve-year follow-up of survival in the randomized European Coronary Surgery Study. N Engl J Med. 1988;319(6):332–7.
4. Veterans Administration Coronary Artery Bypass Surgery Cooperative Study Group. Eleven-year survival in the veterans administration randomized trial of coronary bypass surgery for stable angina. N Engl J Med. 1984;311(21):1333–9.
5. The VA Coronary Artery Bypass Surgery Cooperative Study Group. Eighteen-year survival in the veterans affairs cooperative study of coronary artery bypasss surgery for stable angina. Circulation. 1992;86(1):121–30.
6. Loop FD, Lytle BW, Cosgrove DM, et al. Influence of the internal-mammary-artery graft on 10-year survival and other cardiac events. N Engl J Med. 1986;314(1):1–6.
7. Coronary artery surgery study (CASS): a randomized trial of coronary artery bypass surgery. Comparability of entry characteristics and survival in randomized patients and nonrandomized patients meeting randomization criteria. J Am Coll Cardiol. 1984;3(1):114–28.
8. Yusuf S, Zucker D, Passamani E, et al. Effect of coronary artery bypass graft surgery on survival: overview of 10-year results from randomised trials by the Coronary Artery Bypass Graft Surgery Trialists Collaboration. Lancet. 1994;344:563–70.
9. Coronary angioplasty versus medical therapy for angina: the second Randomised Intervention Treatment of Angina (RITA-2) trial. RITA-2 trial participants. Lancet. 1997;350(9076):461–8.
10. Pocock SJ, Henderson RA, Rickards AF, Hampton JR, et al. Meta-analysis of randomised trials comparing coronary angioplasty with bypass surgery. Lancet. 1995;346(8984):1184–9.
11. Roger VL, Go AS, Lloyd-Jones DM, et al. Executive summary: heart diseaseand stroke statistics-2011 update: a report from the American Heart Association. Circulation. 2011;123(4):459–63.
12. Katritsis DG, Ioannidis JP. Percutaneous coronary intervention versus conservativetherapy in nonacute coronary artery disease: a meta analysis. Circulation. 2005;111:2906–12.
13. Boden WE, et al. Optimal medical therapy with or without PCI for stable coronary disease. N Engl J Med. 2007;356(15):1503–16.
14. Chaitman BR, Rosen AD, Williams DO, et al. Myocardial infarction and cardiac mortality in the Bypass Angioplasty Revascularization Investigation (BARI) randomized trial. Circulation. 1997;96(7):2162–70.
15. Sobel BE, Frye R, Detre KM, et al. Burgeoning dilemmas in the management of diabetes and cardiovascular disease: rationale for the bypass angioplasty revascularization investigation 2 diabetes (BARI 2D) trial. Circulation. 2003;107(4):636–42.
16. Farkouh ME, Domanski M, Sleeper LA, et al. Strategies for multivessel revascularization in patients with diabetes. N Engl J Med. 2012;367:2375–84.
17. Park SJ, Ahn JM, Kim YH, et al. Trial of everolimus-eluting stents or bypass surgery for coronary disease. N Engl J Med. 2015;372:1204–12.
18. Farooq V, et al. Quantification of incomplete revascularization and its association with five year mortality in the synergy between percutaneous cornary intervention with taxus and cardiac surgery (SYNTAX) trial validation of residual SYNTAX score. Circulation. 2013;128:141–51.
19. Xu B, Yang YJ, Han YL, et al. Validation of residual SYNTAX score with second-generation drug-eluting stents: one-year results from the prospective multicentre SEEDS study. EuroIntervention. 2014;10(1):65–73.
20. Garcia S, et al. Outcomse after complete versus incomplete revascularization of patients with multivessel coronary artery disease: a meta-analysis of 89, 883 patients enrolled in randomized clinical trials and obervational studies. J Am Coll Cardiol. 2013;62:1421–31.
21. Aggarwal V, et al. Clinical outcomes based on completeness of revascularisation in patients undergoing percutaneous coronary intervention: a meta-analysis of multivessel coronary artery disease studies. EuroIntervention. 2012;7:1095–102.
22. Escaned J, Banning A, Farooq V, et al. Rationale and design of the SYNTAX II trial evaluating the short to long-term outcomes of state-of-the-art percutaneous coronary revascularisation in patients with de novo three-vessel disease. EuroIntervention. 2016;12(2):e224–34.
23. Shaw LJ, Berman DS, Maron DJ, et al. Optimal medical therapy with or without percutaneous coronary intervention to reduce ischemic burden: results from the Clinical Outcomes Utilizing Revascularization and Aggressive Drug Evaluation (COURAGE) trial nuclear substudy. Circulation. 2008;117(10):1283–91.
24. Tonino PA, De Bruyne B, Pijls NH, et al. Fractional flow reserve versus angiography for guiding percutaneous coronary intervention. N Engl J Med. 2009;360(3):213–24.

25. Sechtem U. Is FAME 2 a breakthrough for PCI in stable coronary disease? Clin Res Cardiol. 2015;104(4):283–7.
26. Al-Lamee R, Thompson D, Dehbi H-M, et al. Percutaneous coronary intervention in stable angina (ORBITA): a double-blind, randomised controlled trial. Lancet. 2018;391:31–40.
27. Al-Lamee R, Howard J, Shun-Shin M, et al. Fractional flow reserve and instantaneous wave-free ratio as predictors of the placebo-controlled response to percutaneous coronary intervention in stable single vessel coronary artery disease: the physiology-stratified analysis of ORBITA. Circulation. 2018. doi:https://doi.org/10.1161/CIRCULATIONAHA.118.033801 [Epub ahead of print].
28. Kirtane AJ. ORBITA: bringing some oxygen back to pci in stable ischemic heart disease? Circulation. CIRCULATIONAHA.118.035331.

Percutaneous Coronary Intervention for Left Ventricular Systolic Dysfunction

Sophie Zhaotao Gu, Amr Gamal,
Christopher Eggett, Hani Ali, Azfar Zaman,
Richard Edwards, and Vijay Kunadian

About Us The Freeman Hospital is a tertiary teaching hospital, part of the Newcastle Upon Tyne Hospitals NHS Foundation Trust, based in Newcastle upon Tyne in the north east of England. The Cardiothoracic Centre was established in a purpose built facility in 1977 and has expanded extensively to become one of the leading units of its kind in the country. The center is equipped to deliver a highly specialized transplant service, and has performed over 1200 heart, lung, and heart and lung transplants since the late 1980s. Freeman Hospital is the largest volume interventional center in the UK with approximately 3000 angioplasty procedures performed annually. The cardiology team at the Freeman Hospital is led by 20 adult cardiology consultants and 5 consultants specializing in pediatric cardiology and adult congenital heart diseases. We work closely with

the cardiothoracic surgery team consisting of 6 cardiothoracic surgeons and 2 pediatric cardiothoracic surgeons [1]. The department is equipped with a comprehensive range of facilities to include a Coronary Care Unit, 6 catheter laboratories, a screening room, a day-case unit for elective diagnostic procedures, pacemaker and rehabilitation services, in addition to inpatient wards and outpatient clinics. We apply the latest advanced technology to deliver the best care to support high-risk patients. These include invasive haemodynamic support ranging from intra-aortic balloon pump, Impella, extracorporeal membrane oxygenation (ECMO), and left ventricular assist devices as bridge therapy for patients awaiting heart transplant. Our unit is committed to teaching, training, and academic research activities. We have strong ties with Newcastle University. We are actively engaged in training the next generation of cardiologists through our fellowship programs in intervention, electrophysiology, imaging, and congenital heart disease. We also support postgraduate training programs (masters and doctoral programs) in cardiovascular medicine and surgery. We are engaged in several collaborative research projects with the Newcastle Clinical Trials Unit, National Institute of Health Research Newcastle Clinical Research Facility, and Newcastle Magnetic Resonance Imaging Centre. At the department level, we have a dedicated on-site cardiovascular research team consisting of research nurses, clinical trial man-

S. Z. Gu · H. Ali · A. Zaman · V. Kunadian (✉)
Institute of Cellular Medicine,
Newcastle University,
Newcastle upon Tyne, UK

Cardiothoracic Centre, Freeman Hospital,
Newcastle upon Tyne NHS Foundation Trust,
Newcastle upon Tyne, UK
e-mail: azfar.zaman@nuth.nhs.uk;
vijay.kunadian@newcastle.ac.uk;
http://www.ncl.ac.uk/cardio/staff/profile/
vijaykunadian.html#background

A. Gamal · C. Eggett · R. Edwards
Cardiothoracic Centre, Freeman Hospital,
Newcastle upon Tyne NHS Foundation Trust,
Newcastle upon Tyne, UK

agers, and trial coordinators that support the delivery of clinical studies.

This chapter focuses on the diagnosis and management of ischemic cardiomyopathy. We explore the current evidence base to aid clinical decision-making for invasive versus conservative management. Conventional pharmacological therapy for heart failure will not be discussed in detail in this chapter.

Ischaemic Cardiomyopathy

- Heart failure (HF) is a clinical syndrome with symptoms and signs caused by cardiac dysfunction. Its prevalence is estimated at 1–2% in the developed world [2] with an incidence approaching 5–10 per 1000 persons per year. Ischaemic heart disease (IHD) is the most common cause of heart failure in the developed world [3]. Heart failure due to ischaemia is associated with worse mortality compared with a non-ischemic cause. The term ischaemic cardiomyopathy (ICM) has been commonly used to describe impaired left ventricular systolic dysfunction (LVSD—ejection fraction ≤35–40%) resulting from coronary artery disease (CAD).
- Felker and colleagues assessed 1921 patients with symptomatic HF and ejection fraction ≤40%, and found that extensive CAD is independently associated with worse survival outcome whereas patients with single-vessel disease and no prior history of myocardial infarction (MI) or revascularization had similar outcome as those with non-ischemic cardiomyopathy and should be excluded from a diagnosis of ICM for prognostic purposes [4].
- The proposed unified definition for ICM is shown in Table 19.1. Ischemic cardiomyopathy consists of a spectrum of pathophysiological states [5] as summarized in Table 19.2.
- The extent of CAD seen on coronary angiography can provide further information to predict prognosis. Viability assessment by noninvasive

imaging can detect hibernating myocardium, which can potentially improve function once the ischemic burden has been treated.
- Therefore, the diagnostic approach to ICM consists of two steps: the detection of CAD and the detection of viable myocardium.
- Due to the high frequency of IHD as the aetiology of HF, evaluation for CAD by coronary angiography is usually part of the workup of patients with a new diagnosis of HF. The 2013 American College of Cardiology Foundation (ACCF)/American Heart Association (AHA) HF guidelines recommended that coronary angiography is reasonable as an invasive evaluation for HF (Table 19.3) [6].
- Noninvasive tests such as cardiac computed tomography (CT) and cardiac magnetic reso-

Table 19.1 Definition of ischemic cardiomyopathy [4]

Definition of ischaemic cardiomyopathy (ICM)
Left ventricular systolic dysfunction with one or more of:
• A history of prior myocardial infarction or revascularization
• ≥75% stenosis of the left main stem or proximal left anterior descending artery
• ≥75% stenosis of two or more coronary vessels

Table 19.2 Spectrum of pathophysiological states in ischemic cardiomyopathy

	Definition
Myocardial stunning	• Reversible transient hypocontractility that occurs following an episode of acute ischaemia
Hibernation	• Refers to segments of myocardium with chronic, but potentially reversible ischaemic dysfunction • Is a retrospective definition often used interchangeable with the term viable myocardium
Viability	• Is a prospective definition based on imaging findings to predict segments that may recover function following revascularization
Scarring	• Irreversible loss of myocardium due to ischemia, the infarcted tissue cannot recover function after revascularization

nance imaging (CMR) angiography can also be used.

- Several imaging modalities are used to detect viable myocardium, including dobutamine stress echocardiography (DSE), CMR with late gadolinium enhancement (LGE), single-photon-emission CT (SPECT), and positron emission tomography (PET). International guidelines recommend that use of non-invasive imaging to detect myocardial ischaemia and viability is reasonable in HF patients with CAD [2, 6].

Table 19.3 Summary of recommendations for cardiac imaging in patients with heart failure to detect ischemia and viability [2, 6]

Year	Society	Guideline	Recommendations	Class[a]	Level[b]
2013	ACCF/ AHA	Heart failure – Noninvasive cardiac imaging	Noninvasive imaging to detect myocardial ischemia and viability is reasonable in HF and CAD	IIa	C
			Viability assessment is reasonable before revascularization in HF patients with CAD	IIa	B
			MRI is reasonable when assessing myocardial infiltration or scar	IIa	B
2016	ESC	Heart failure – Noninvasive imaging	Noninvasive stress imaging (CMR, stress echocardiography, SPECT, PET) may be considered for the assessment of myocardial ischemia and viability in patients with HF and CAD (considered suitable for coronary revascularization) before the decision on revascularization	IIb	B
			Cardiac CT may be considered in patients with HF and low to intermediate pre-test probability of CAD or those with equivocal noninvasive stress tests in order to rule out coronary artery stenosis	IIb	C
2013	ACCF/ AHA	Heart failure – Invasive evaluation	When ischemia may be contributing to HF, coronary arteriography is reasonable	IIa	C
2016	ESC	Heart failure – Invasive imaging	Invasive coronary angiography is recommended in patients with HF and angina pectoris recalcitrant to pharmacological therapy or symptomatic ventricular arrhythmias or aborted cardiac arrest (who are considered suitable for potential coronary revascularization) in order to establish the diagnosis of CAD and its severity	I	C
			Invasive coronary angiography should be considered in patients with HF and intermediate to high pre-test probability of CAD and the presence of ischaemia in noninvasive stress tests (who are considered suitable for potential coronary revascularization) in order to establish the diagnosis of CAD and its severity	IIa	C

ACCF American College of Cardiology Foundation, *AHA* American Heart Association, *CAD* coronary artery disease, *CMR* cardiac magnetic resonance imaging, *CT* computed tomography, *ESC* European Society of Cardiology, *HF* heart failure, *MRI* magnetic resonance imaging, *PET* positron emission tomography, *SPECT* single-photon emission computed tomography
[a]Class of recommendation
[b]Level of evidence

Viability Testing

Dobutamine Stress Echocardiography (DSE)

- Used to examine the myocardial contractile reserve. Viable myocardium demonstrates improved ejection fraction or regional contractile function (contractile reserve) to inotropic stimulation (Fig. 19.1).
- Viable myocardium is defined as dysfunctional segments at rest that show improved contractility during a low-dose dobutamine (5–10 mcg/kg/min) infusion.
- During higher dose infusion, these viable segments may have deteriorating wall contraction due to inducible ischemia. This biphasic response (Fig. 19.2) has been shown to be highly predictive of viable myocardium that

may recover function following revascularization [7].

Single-Photon Emission Computed Tomography (SPECT)

- Nuclear imaging technique that relies on the demonstration of preserved cellular and metabolic functions in viable myocardium. It utilizes Thallium-201 and Technetium-99 m as tracers.
- Images taken soon after tracer injection indicate delivery of tracer by myocardial blood flow, and images taken 4–24 h later reflect cellular integrity which indicates tissue viability [8].
- SPECT is widely available but has low resolution and higher attenuation artifact. The sensi-

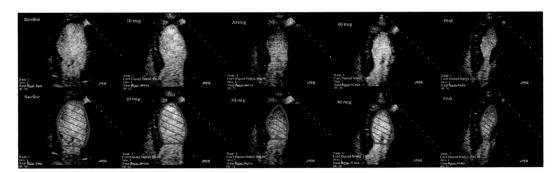

Fig. 19.1 Dobutamine stress echocardiography images demonstrating improved myocardial contraction in response to dobutamine. Images are taken at end systole in apical 4 chamber view. The left ventricular cavity at end systole is outlined in red as shown in the lower row. Contractility (ejection fraction) improves with dobutamine compared to baseline (as end systolic volume reduces), and is at its best at peak dobutamine

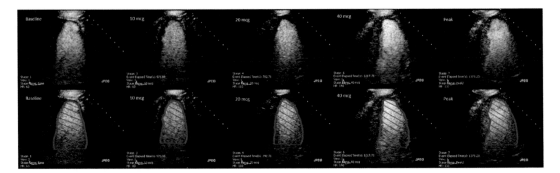

Fig. 19.2 Biphasic response to dobutamine demonstrating inducible ischemia: contractility improves to its best at low-dose 10 mcg/kg/min dobutamine infusion; wall contraction then deteriorates at higher dose infusion

tivity of this investigation is reduced in obese patients and females.

Positron Emission Tomography (PET)

- Nuclear imaging technique that provides comparison of myocardial perfusion to myocardial metabolism. Metabolic tracers such as fluoro-deoxyglucose-18 (FDG), which is a glucose analogue, are used as markers of viability.
- Viable tissue is metabolically active, whereas myocardial scars are metabolically inactive, therefore metabolic activity as reflected by the uptake of glucose by viable tissue is preserved or increased despite reduced perfusion (Table 19.4).
- PET can accurately predict areas of viable myocardium with high possibility of recovering function following revascularization [9]. However, PET is not used in routine clinical practice due to its low availability in many centers and high associated cost.

Cardiac MRI (CMR)

- Provides assessment of global LV function, regional wall motion, thickening, and scarring.
- Gadolinium is a contrast agent that remains in the extracellular/interstitial space. Its washout is decreased in areas of myocardial scar or fibrosis. Late gadolinium enhancement (LGE) can therefore be used as direct scar imaging to assess the amount and spatial location of myocardial scarring.
- Viable tissue can be identified by the use of low-dose dobutamine stress magnetic reso-

nance (LDDSMR), which identifies the presence of contractile reserve. Viable myocardium is defined as [10]:
- Area with contractile dysfunction at rest due to CAD with no myocardial scarring (negative LGE).
- Myocardial scar with less than 50% transmurality shown on LGE and positive LDDSMR test.

Viability and Clinical Outcomes

- Myocardial viability assessment with the use of nuclear imaging, typically SPECT or low-dose DSE and/or CMR is commonly used to predict LV function recovery and numerous studies suggest such methods can predict survival improvement following coronary artery bypass grafting (CABG) [11, 12].
- However, these previous studies are outdated, using retrospective data with uncertainty on the adequacy of baseline variable adjustment, and lack of standardization of optimal medical therapy (OMT).
- The Surgical Treatment for Ischemic Heart Failure (STICH) trial was a prospective randomized study, and its sub-study reported the association between myocardial viability and survival benefit in randomized patients with CAD and LV dysfunction treated with CABG compared to medical therapy alone. However, the trial failed to demonstrate a significant interaction between survival benefit and viable myocardium after baseline variables adjustment [13]. This lack of interaction suggests that viability assessment may not be the sole deciding factor in selecting best therapy for patients with ischemic cardiomyopathy.

Table 19.4 Definition of viability on a PET scan

	Perfusion	Metabolic activity/FDG uptake	
Viable myocardium	↓	↔ or ↑	Perfusion-metabolic mismatch
Nonviable scar tissue	↓	↓or absent	Perfusion-metabolic match

FDG fluorodeoxyglucose

STICH Trial

The STICH trial was the first prospective randomized controlled trial (RCT) to assess the role of CABG compared to standard medical therapy in patients with severe LVSD and CAD. STICH

Table 19.5 Summary of STICHES 10-year outcome, CABG vs. medical therapy [17]

Outcome	CABG group (%)	Medical therapy group (%)	Hazard ratio for CABG vs. medical therapy (95%CI)	P value
Death from any cause	58.9	66.1	0.84 (0.73–0.97)	0.02
Death from cardiovascular causes	40.5	49.3	0.79 (0.66–0.93)	0.006
Death from any cause or hospitalization for cardiovascular causes	76.6	87.0	0.72 (0.64–0.82)	<0.001

enrolled a total of 1212 patients between 2002 and 2007 from 99 sites in 22 countries.

- Patients with EF ≤35% and CAD that was amenable to CABG were recruited for randomization. Of these, 602 patients were randomized to the medical therapy alone group, and 610 patients assigned to medical therapy plus CABG group.
- OMT in the STICH trial included angiotensin-converting enzyme inhibitor (ACE-i) and/or angiotensin receptor blocker (ARB), beta-blocker, aldosterone antagonist, and antiplatelet agents. The use of HMG-CoA reductase inhibitor, diuretic, and digitalis were dependent on specific indications for individual patients. Implantable defibrillators were used in compliance with standard guidelines [14].
- At 5-year follow-up, no significant difference was found between medical therapy alone and medical therapy plus CABG in reaching the primary endpoint of death from any cause (hazard ratio [HR] with CABG 0.86; 95% confidence interval [CI] 0.72–1.04).
- Rates of the secondary outcome of death from cardiovascular causes (HR with CABG 0.81; 95% CI 0.66–1.00) and of death from any cause or hospitalization for cardiovascular causes (HR with CABG 0.74; 95% CI 0.64–0.85) were found to be lower in the CABG group compared to medical therapy alone group [15].
- Further mode-of-death analysis was carried out and found that CABG in addition to medical therapy tended to reduce the most common modes of death: sudden death (HR 0.73; 95% CI 0.54–0.99) and fatal pump failure events (HR 0.64; 95% CI 0.41–1.00) [16].

The risk of death following CABG was 3 times that of the medical therapy group up to 30 days (HR with CABG 3.12; 95% CI 1.33–7.31), and the benefit of CABG only started to outweigh this postoperative risk after 2 years [15].

The STICH Extension Study (STICHES)

- Conducted to follow up ICM patients from the STICH trial for an additional 5 years (at 10 years) to study the long-term effects of CABG.
- Demonstrated a survival benefit for revascularization. At median follow-up of 9.8 years (minimum 3.5 years and maximum 13.4 years), CABG was associated with a more favorable outcome than medical therapy alone across all clinically important long-term outcomes, summarized in Table 19.5.
- Overall, CABG was associated with a median survival benefit of 1.44 years, the number needed to treat to prevent one death was 14, and the number needed to treat to prevent one cardiovascular death was 11 [17].

Optimal Medical Therapy vs. Percutaneous Coronary Intervention vs. Coronary Artery Bypass Graft

- Advances in medical therapy for patients with heart failure has led to current treatment recommendations for use of beta-blockers, ACE inhibitors, ARBs, diuretics, and aldosterone antagonists.
- Device therapy including the use of implantable cardiac defibrillators (ICD) and cardiac resynchronization therapy (CRT) are also recommended for selected patient groups [2].

- International guidelines in general recommend CABG for heart failure patients with more extensive CAD (significant stenosis in the left main [LM] stem or proximal left anterior descending [LAD] artery or triple vessel disease) and/or the presence of severe angina symptoms (see Table 19.6) [2, 6, 18, 19].
- Evidence to support a survival benefit for CABG in patients with impaired LV function with minimal angina symptoms is, however, lacking. On the basis of the STICH trial which

now shows a long-term survival benefit for CABG in addition to OMT compared to OMT alone in patients with severe LV dysfunction and CAD, the current guidelines should be revised to prompt clinicians to evaluate CAD status and consider revascularization for this patient group.

- A meta-analysis of 26 observational studies from our group found that CABG is associated with acceptable operative mortality (on-pump CABG 5.4%; 95% CI 4.5–6.4%; off-pump

Table 19.6 Summary of international guidelines on revascularization in patients with LV systolic dysfunction [2, 6, 18, 19]

Year	Society	Guideline	Recommendations	Class[a]	Level[b]
2011	ACCF/ AHA	CABG	CABG to improve survival is reasonable in patients with mild-moderate LV systolic dysfunction (EF 35% to 50%) and significant (≥70% diameter stenosis) multivessel CAD or proximal LAD coronary artery stenosis, when viable myocardium is present in the region of intended revascularization	IIa	B
			CABG might be considered with the primary or sole intent of improving survival in patients with stable IHD with severe LV systolic dysfunction (EF <35%) whether or not viable myocardium is present	IIb	B
2013	ACCF/ AHA	Heart failure	CABG or percutaneous intervention is indicated for HF patients on guideline-directed medical therapy (GDMT) with angina and suitable coronary anatomy, especially significant left main stenosis or left main equivalent	I	C
			CABG to improve survival is reasonable in patients with mild to moderate LV systolic dysfunction and significant multivessel CAD or proximal LAD stenosis when viable myocardium is present	IIa	B
			CABG or medical therapy is reasonable to improve morbidity and mortality for patients with severe LV dysfunction (EF < 35%), HF, and significant CAD	IIa	B
			CABG may be considered in patients with ischemic heart disease, severe LV systolic dysfunction, and operable coronary anatomy whether or not viable myocardium is present	IIb	B
2014	ESC	Myocardial revascularization	CABG is recommended for patients with significant LM stenosis and LM equivalent with proximal stenosis of both LAD and LCx arteries	I	C
			CABG is recommended for patients with significant LAD artery stenosis and multivessel disease to reduce death and hospitalization for cardiovascular causes	I	B
			Myocardial revascularization should be considered in the presence of viable myocardium	IIa	B
2016	ESC	Heart failure	Myocardial revascularization is recommended when angina persists despite treatment with anti-angina drugs	I	A

ACCF American College of Cardiology Foundation, *AHA* American Heart Association, *CABG* coronary artery bypass graft, *CAD* coronary artery disease, *ESC* European Society of Cardiology, *EF* ejection fraction, *HF* heart failure, *IHD* ischemic heart disease, *LAD* left anterior descending, *LCx* left circumflex, *LV* left ventricle, *LM* left main
[a]Class of recommendation
[b]Level of evidence

CABG 4.4%; 95% CI 2.8–6.4%) and 5-year actuarial survival (73.4%; 95% CI 68.7–77.7%) in patients with severe LVSD [20].

- However, the STICH trial demonstrated a high post-CABG mortality risk particularly within the first 30 days, and this added risk compared to medical therapy carries on for 2 years. Those with heart failure with reduced ejection fraction and CAD are likely high-risk patients who may not be considered eligible for CABG and PCI is an alternative option.

- However, the evidence for benefit of PCI is not clear since previous large RCTs excluded patients with an EF <30%. Indeed less than 2% of all patients included in the Synergy Between Percutaneous Coronary Intervention with Taxus and Cardiac Surgery (SYNTAX) had significant LVSD (EF <30%) at baseline [21, 22].

- A further meta-analysis of 19 studies from our group ($n = 4766$) found that PCI was feasible with acceptable in-hospital (1.8%; 95% CI 1.0–2.9%) and long-term (15.6%; 95% CI 11.0–20.7%) mortality and yielded similar outcomes to CABG (relative risk PCI vs. CABG 0.98; 95% CI 0.8–1.2) for patients with LVSD (EF ≤ 40%) [23].

- There is only very limited data comparing PCI with medical therapy in ICM patients. The Heart Failure Revascularisation Trial (HEART) aimed to assess the outcome in patients with EF <35% randomized to conservative management or revascularization (PCI or CABG). The study was terminated early due to recruitment difficulties and lack of funding when 138 patients were recruited out of the planned target of 800 [24]. This study was underpowered and showed no mortality difference between conservative and revascularization arms.

- The Balloon pump-assisted Coronary Intervention Study (BCIS-1) was a RCT designed to evaluate the use of elective intra-aortic balloon pump (IABP) insertion prior to high-risk PCI for severe LVSD. A total of 301 patients with impaired LV (EF <30%) and extensive myocardium at risk (BCIS-1 jeopardy score of ≥8 or target vessel supplying occluded vessel which supplied ≥40% myocardium) were enrolled. The primary outcome was the incidence of major adverse cardiac and cerebrovascular events (MACCE), defined as death, acute myocardial infarction, cerebrovascular event, or further revascularization at hospital discharge. The trial failed to show a difference in MACCE at hospital discharge (15.2% elective IABP group vs. 16.0% no planned IABP group; odds ratio [OR] elective IABP vs. no planned IABP = 0.94; 95% CI 0.51–1.76). All-cause mortality at 6 months was not significantly different (elective IABP vs. no planned IABP; OR 0.61; 95% CI 0.24–1.62) [25]. These results do not support the routine use of IABP before PCI in patients with severely impaired LV and extensive CAD. Long-term mortality data from this trial showed that all-cause mortality at a median of 51 months was 33%, demonstrating the poor prognosis of this patient group. Elective IABP was associated with a 34% reduction in long-term all-cause mortality compared with unsupported PCI [26].

- The REVascularisation for Ischaemic Ventricular Dysfunction—British Cardiovascular Intervention Society-2 (REVIVED-BCIS-2) trial is a multicenter prospective randomized open label study in the UK, which is currently enrolling to evaluate the efficacy and safety of PCI compared with medical therapy alone for patients with ICM and viable myocardium. It aims to enroll 700 patients and plans to follow up patients for 1–5.5 years, with a primary outcome of all-cause death or hospitalization for heart failure [27]. The results of REVIVED trial may provide a more robust evidence base to support revascularization with PCI in the context of ICM.

Tako-Tsubo Cardiomyopathy

- Takotsubo cardiomyopathy (TTC), also known as broken-heart syndrome, apical ballooning syndrome, or stress-induced cardiomyopathy, is a form of reversible cardiomyopathy characterized by transient ventricular systolic dysfunction immediately following a stressful event.

- First described in Japan by Sato in 1990, the Japanese word takotsubo was chosen to resemble the unusual shape assumed by the ventricle during systole. Takotsubo means "octopus pot," a contraption used for catching octopuses. Due to the increasing frequency of the condition, TTC has been incorporated into the 2006 AHA classification of cardiomyopathies [28].

- TTC accounts for 1–3% of all cases presenting with acute coronary syndrome [29]. It occurs predominantly in postmenopausal women older than 50 years with a mean age of 68 years [30, 31].

- The condition is triggered by emotional stress in approximately two-thirds of patients [32]. The clinical presentation of TTC is difficult to differentiate from MI with chest pain and dyspnea associated with ECG changes and elevated cardiac biochemical markers.

- The hallmark diagnostic feature of TTC is the extensive hypokinesia or akinesia of the apical and mid left ventricle with sparing of the basal segments that show compensatory hyperkinesis. This extensive hypokinesia of the apex leads to the characteristic apical ballooning (Fig. 19.3) resembling the octopus trap configuration, which is associated with reduced ejection fraction.

- The wall motion abnormalities usually extend beyond the distribution of a single coronary artery. Typically, there is complete recovery of ventricular function within a few days or weeks.

- In the acute setting, echocardiography and ventriculography are the most commonly used diagnostic tools. Other imaging modalities such as gated myocardial perfusion imaging, computed tomography, and magnetic resonance are complimentary for diagnosis.

- On cardiac MRI, absence of delayed gadolinium hyperenhancement is diagnostic of TTC and helps differentiate it from myocarditis and acute myocardial infarction where delayed hyperenhancement is present [33].

- Due to indistinguishable presentation from MI, most patients with TTC undergo urgent coronary angiography. Typical findings in TTC are normal or near normal coronary arteries or rarely coexistent CAD. Accordingly, TTC is a diagnosis of exclusion (Table 19.7) which can only be made after coronary angiography is performed to rule out potential coronary artery obstruction or occlusion [34].

- TTC has a favorable prognosis with near full recovery of the condition in virtually all patients. The LVEF is normalized within a

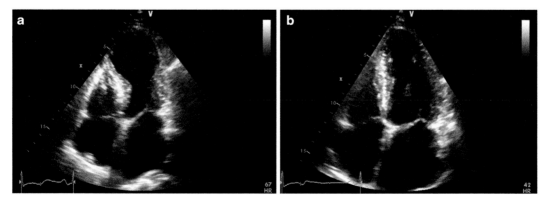

Fig. 19.3 (**a**) 63-year-old female at time of presentation, showing the characteristic "apical ballooning" of takotsubo cardiomyopathy. (**b**) Repeat echocardiogram 5 weeks later, showing recovery of left ventricular function

Table 19.7 Diagnostic criteria for Takotsubo cardiomyopathy from the Mayo Clinic [34]

Components	Mayo clinic diagnostic criteria for TTC
1	Transient hypokinesis, akinesis, or dyskinesis in the left ventricular mid segments with or without apical involvement; regional wall motion abnormalities that extend beyond a single epicardial vascular distribution; a stressful trigger is usually but not always present
2	Absence of obstructive coronary disease or angiographic evidence of acute plaque rupture
3	New electrocardiographic abnormalities (ST-segment elevation and/or T-wave inversion) or modest elevation in cardiac troponin
4	Absence of pheochromocytoma and myocarditis

ECG electrocardiography, *TTC* takotsubo cardiomyopathy

week in the majority of patients, and by the end of 4–8 weeks, nearly all patients have normalized LVEF.

- The in-hospital mortality is low at 0–2% and the long-term survival is similar to that of the general population [30, 31, 35, 36]. Only a few recurrent TTC cases have been reported. The reported 4-year recurrence rate is approximately 4–10%. The mechanisms underlying recurrence or its susceptibility are not well understood [35, 37].

- As TTC is a temporary condition, the goals of treatment are usually supportive care prior to spontaneous recovery of cardiac function. There are no specific treatments for the left ventricular failure characterizing the acute stage. Guideline-directed medical therapy for patients with left ventricular dysfunction including the short-term use (3–6 months) of cardioselective beta-blockers and ACE inhibitors are recommended by most experts.

- Although catecholamines are believed to play a putative role in the pathogenesis of TTC, inotropes are still recommended for patients with cardiogenic shock with no LV outflow tract obstruction. If cardiogenic shock is associated with LVOT obstruction, inotropes should be avoided and phenylephrine is preferred combined with beta blockade. Other supportive treatments include the use of anti-arrhythmic drugs or anticoagulants [29].

Summary

Table 19.8 Chapter summary

Key words	PCI for LV systolic dysfunction
IHD	Ischaemic heart disease is a common cause of heart failure with reduced left ventricular systolic function
ICM	Ischaemic cardiomyopathy consists of a spectrum of pathophysiological states, including myocardial stunning, hibernation, and scarring
Viability	Several imaging modalities are used to assess viability. These include dobutamine stress echocardiography, single-photon emission computed tomography, positron emission tomography, and cardiac magnetic resonance imaging
ICM treatment	The mainstay of evidence-based therapy in ICM is medical treatment as well as device therapy for heart failure
STICH extension study outcome	The STICH extension study has now shown a survival benefit for CABG compared to medical therapy alone across all clinically important outcomes after 10-year follow-up. However, there is a high postoperative mortality risk associated with CABG which is only outweighed by benefit after 2 years, and more than 60% patients in the original STICH trial have died indicating the high risk associated with this patient group
PCI vs. CABG	PCI is demonstrated to be safe with a non-inferior efficacy as compared to CABG in treating ICM, but further study is needed to evaluate its outcome compared to standard medical therapy
TTC	Takotsubo cardiomyopathy is a condition with transient ventricular systolic dysfunction driven by stress; its clinical presentation is difficult to differentiate from MI; full recovery is in general expected in all patients and the treatment involves supportive care [38]

CABG coronary artery bypass graft, *ICM* ischaemic cardiomyopathy, *IHD* ischaemic heart disease, *LV* left ventricular, *MI* myocardial infarction, *PCI* percutaneous coronary intervention, *STICH* Surgical Treatment for Ischaemic Heart Failure trial, *TTC* takotsubo cardiomyopathy

References

1. Freeman Hospital Services. [cited 2016 23 September]. http://www.newcastle-hospitals.org.uk/hospitals/freeman-hospital.aspx.
2. Ponikowski P, Voors AA, Anker SD, Bueno H, Cleland JG, Coats AJ, et al. 2016 ESC Guidelines for the diagnosis and treatment of acute and chronic heart failure: The Task Force for the diagnosis and treatment of acute and chronic heart failure of the European Society of Cardiology (ESC)Developed with the special contribution of the Heart Failure Association (HFA) of the ESC. Eur Heart J. 2016;37(27):2129–200.
3. Mostered A, Hoes AW. Clinical epidemiology of heart failure. Heart. 2007;93:1137–46.
4. Felker GM, Shaw LK, O'Connor CM. A standardized definition of ischemic cardiomyopathy for use in clinical research. J Am Coll Cardiol. 2002;39:210–8.
5. Briceno N, Schuster A, Lumley M, Perera D. Ischaemic cardiomyopathy: pathophysiology, assessment and the role of revascularisation. Heart. 2016;102(5):397–406.
6. Writing Committee Memebrs, Yancy CW, Jessup M, Bozkurt B, Butler J, Casey DE Jr, et al. 2013 ACCF/AHA guideline for the management of heart failure: a report of the American College of Cardiology Foundation/American Heart Association Task Force on Practice Guidelines. Circulation. 2013;128(16):e240–327.
7. Yao SS, Chaudhry FA. Assessment of myocardial viability with dobutamine stress echocardiography in patients with ischaemic left ventricular dysfunction. Echocardiography. 2005;22:71–83.
8. Underwood SR, Bax JJ, Vom Dahl J, et al. Imaging techniques for the assessment of myocardial hibernation: report of a study group of the European society of Cardiology. Eur Heart J. 2004;25:815–36.
9. Auerbach MA, Schöder H, Hoh C, et al. Prevalence of myocardial viability as detected by positron emission tomography in patients with ischaemic cardiomopathy. Circulation. 1999;99:2921–6.
10. Nagel E, Schuster A. Myocardial viability: dead or alive is not the question! JACC Cardiovasc Imaging. 2012;5:509–12.
11. Allman KC, Shaw LJ, Hachamovitch R, Udelson JE. Myocardial viability testing and impact of revascularization on prognosis in patients with coronary artery disease and left ventricular dysfunction: a meta-analysis. J Am Coll Cardiol. 2002;39(7):1151–8.
12. Bourque JM, Hasselblad V, Velazquez EJ, Borges-Neto S, O'Connor CM. Revascularization in patients with coronary artery disease, left ventricular dysfunction, and viability: a meta-analysis. Am Heart J. 2003;146:621–7.
13. Bonow RO, Maurer G, Lee KL, et al. STICH Trial Investigators. Myocardial viability and survival in ischaemic left ventricular dysfunction. N Engl J Med. 2011;364:1617–25.
14. Velazquez EJ, Lee KL, O'Connor CM, Oh JK, Bonow RO, Pohost GM, et al. The rationale and design of the surgical treatment for IsChemic heart failure (STICH) trial. J Thorac Cardiovasc Surg. 2007;134(6):1540–7.
15. Velazquez EJ, Lee KL, Deja MA, et al. Coronary-artery bypass surgery in patients with left ventricular dysfunction. N Engl J Med. 2011;364:1607–16.
16. Carson P, Wertheimer J, Miller A, et al. The STICH trial mode-of-death results. JACC Heart Fail. 2013;1(5):400–8.
17. Velazquez EJ, Lee KL, Jones RH, et al. Coronary-artery bypass surgery in patients with ischemic cardiomyopathy. N Engl J Med. 2016;374(16):1511–20.
18. Authors/Task Force Members, Windecker S, Kolh P, Alfonso F, Collet JP, Cremer J, et al. 2014 ESC/EACTS Guidelines on myocardial revascularization: The Task Force on Myocardial Revascularization of the European Society of Cardiology (ESC) and the European Association for Cardio-Thoracic Surgery (EACTS)Developed with the special contribution of the European Association of Percutaneous Cardiovascular Interventions (EAPCI). Eur Heart J. 2014;35(37):2541–619.
19. Hillis LD, Smith PK, Anderson JL, Bittl JA, Bridges CR, Byrne JG, et al. 2011 ACCF/AHA Guideline for Coronary Artery Bypass Graft Surgery: a report of the American College of Cardiology Foundation/American Heart Association Task Force on Practice Guidelines. Circulation. 2011;124(23):e652–735.
20. Kunadian V, Zaman A, Qiu W. Revascularization among patients with severe left ventricular dysfunction: a meta-analysis of observational studies. Eur J Heart Fail. 2011;13(7):773–84.
21. Mohr FW, Morice M-C, Kappetein AP, Feldman TE, Ståhle E, Colombo A, et al. Coronary artery bypass graft surgery versus percutaneous coronary intervention in patients with three-vessel disease and left main coronary disease: 5-year follow-up of the randomised, clinical SYNTAX trial. Lancet. 2013;381(9867):629–38.
22. Davierwala P, Mohr FW. Five years after the SYNTAX trial: what have we learnt? Eur J Cardiothorac Surg. 2013;44(1):1–3.
23. Kunadian V, Pugh A, Zaman A, Qiu W. Percutaneous coronary intervention among patients with left ventricular systolic dysfunction: a review and meta-analysis of 19 clinical studies. Coron Artery Dis. 2012;23(7):469–79.
24. Cleland JG, Calvert M, Freemantle N, Arrow Y, Ball SG, Bonser RS, et al. The Heart Failure Revascularisation Trial (HEART). Eur J Heart Fail. 2011;13(2):227–33.
25. Perera D, Stables R, Thomas M, et al. Elective intra-aortic balloon counterpulsation during high-risk percutaneous coronary intervention: a randomized controlled trial. JAMA. 2010;304(8):867–74.
26. Perera D, Stables R, Clayton T, De Silva K, Lumley M, Clack L, et al. Long-term mortality data from the balloon pump-assisted coronary intervention study (BCIS-1): a randomized, controlled trial of elective balloon counterpulsation during high-risk

percutaneous coronary intervention. Circulation. 2013;127(2):207–12.

27. REVIVED-BCIS-2 trial protocol [cited 2016 23 September]. NCT01920048. http://revived.lshtm.ac.uk.

28. Maron BJ, Towbin JA, Thiene G, Antzelevitch C, Corrado D, Arnett D, et al. Contemporary definitions and classification of the cardiomyopathies: an American Heart Association Scientific Statement From the Council on Clinical Cardiology, Heart Failure and Transplantation Committee; Quality of Care and Outcomes Research and Functional Genomics and Translational Biology Interdisciplinary Working Groups; and Council on Epidemiology and Prevention. Circulation. 2006;113(14):1807–16.

29. Parodi G, Del Pace S, Carrabba N, Salvadori C, Memisha G, Simonetti I, et al. Incidence, clinical findings, and outcome of women with left ventricular apical ballooning syndrome. Am J Cardiol. 2007;99(2):182–5.

30. Kurisu S, Sato H, Kawagoe T, Ishihara M, Shimatani Y, Nishioka K, et al. Tako-tsubo-like left ventricular dysfunction with ST-segment elevation: a novel cardiac syndrome mimicking acute myocardial infarction. Am Heart J. 2002;143(3):448–55.

31. Tsuchihashi K, Ueshima K, Uchida T, Oh-mura N, Kimura K, Owa M, et al. Transient left ventricular apical ballooning without coronary artery stenosis: a novel heart syndrome mimicking acute myocardial infarction. J Am Coll Cardiol. 2001;38(1):11–8.

32. Azzarelli S, Galassi AR, Amico F, Giacoppo M, Argentino V, Tomasello SD, et al. Clinical features of transient left ventricular apical ballooning. Am J Cardiol. 2006;98(9):1273–6.

33. Haghi D, Fluechter S, Suselbeck T, Kaden JJ, Borggrefe M, Papavassiliu T. Cardiovascular magnetic resonance findings in typical versus atypical forms of the acute apical ballooning syndrome (Takotsubo cardiomyopathy). Int J Cardiol. 2007;120(2):205–11.

34. Prasad A, Lerman A, Rihal CS. Apical ballooning syndrome (Tako-Tsubo or stress cardiomyopathy): a mimic of acute myocardial infarction. Am Heart J. 2008;155(3):408–17.

35. Elesber AA, Prasad A, Lennon RJ, Wright RS, Lerman A, Rihal CS. Four-year recurrence rate and prognosis of the apical ballooning syndrome. J Am Coll Cardiol. 2007;50(5):448–52.

36. Kurisu S, Inoue I, Kawagoe T, Ishihara M, Shimatani Y, Nakama Y, et al. Presentation of Tako-tsubo cardiomyopathy in men and women. Clin Cardiol. 2010;33(1):42–5.

37. Bybee KA, Kara T, Prasad A, Lerman A, Barsness GW, Wright RS, et al. Systematic review: transient left ventricular apical ballooning: a syndrome that mimics ST-segment elevation myocardial infarction. Ann Intern Med. 2004;141(11):858–65.

38. Ghadri J-R, Wittstein IS, Prasad A, Sharkey S, Dote K, Akashi YJ, Cammann VL, Crea F, Galiuto L, Desmet W, Yoshida T, Manfredini R, Eitel I, Kosuge M, Nef HM, Deshmukh A, Lerman A, Bossone E, Citro R, Ueyama T, Corrado D, Kurisu S, Ruschitzka F, Winchester D, Lyon AR, Omerovic E, Bax JJ, Meimoun P, Tarantini G, Rihal C, Shams Y-H, Migliore F, Horowitz JD, Shimokawa H, Lüscher TF, Templin C. International expert consensus document on Takotsubo Syndrome (Part I): clinical characteristics, diagnostic criteria, and pathophysiology. European Heart Journal. 2018;39(22):2032–46. https://doi.org/10.1093/eurheartj/ehy076.

Percutaneous Coronary Intervention: Special Considerations in Women

20

Lucy Blows and Timothy Williams

About Us The Sussex Cardiac Centre is the tertiary cardiac center for Sussex serving a population of over 1.2 million people. Located on the South Coast we have a highly varied population of all ages and socioeconomic groups. Out of 13 consultants, we have 6 interventional cardiologists performing around 1000 coronary angioplasty procedures each year, of which approximately 400 are "primary PCI" cases. We offer treatment in all areas of cardiovascular disease and also have one of the UK's largest structural heart programs having performed over 700 transcatheter aortic valve replacements since inception of the service in 2007. We have a leading research department with internationally recognized investigators, and run a number of trials with a particular interest in structural and coronary intervention.

Introduction

- Coronary artery disease (CAD) is a leading cause of death in men and women, although historically there has been more of a focus on its importance in men.
- Biological differences between the sexes impact on the nature of the disease in men and women, with implications for diagnosis and management.
- Furthermore, the unique hormonal changes resulting from pregnancy and the menopause require special consideration when managing CAD in women.

Prevalence and Outcomes

While CAD is a killer of both sexes, women are proportionally more affected, with it accounting for more deaths than from cancer, chronic respiratory disease, and Alzheimer's disease and accidents combined [1]. Although overall mortality had been in decline, the rate of CAD in young women has been increasing since 1980 [2].

The traditional cardiovascular risk factors of age, diabetes, hypertension, obesity, smoking, and dyslipidemia affect both men and women, but their impact varies between sexes.

- **Obesity** (Body Mass Index—BMI $\geq$ 30) increases the relative risk of CAD substantially more in women than simply being overweight (BMI 25–29.9). This is in contrast to men, where the relative risk of CAD from being overweight and being obese is broadly similar [3].
- **Diabetes** has a more profound effect in women than in men. In one meta-analysis the summary relative risk of fatal CAD in women with diabetes was 3.5 (95% Confidence

L. Blows (✉) · T. Williams
Sussex Cardiac Centre, Royal Sussex County
Hospital, Brighton and Sussex University Hospitals
NHS Trust, Brighton, UK
e-mail: lucy.blows@bsuh.nhs.uk

© Springer International Publishing AG, part of Springer Nature 2018
A. Myat et al. (eds.), *The Interventional Cardiology Training Manual*,
https://doi.org/10.1007/978-3-319-71635-0_20

Interval—CI 2.70–4.53), compared to 2.06 (1.81–2.34) in men [4].

- **Cigarette smoking** has traditionally been associated with up to 50% of CAD-related events in women [5]. In one study the relative risk of MI in female smokers was 2.24 (1.85–2.71), a relative risk over 1.5 times greater than the risk increase in men [6].
- **Psychological factors such as stress and anxiety** are known to contribute to overall cardiovascular risk. In women marital stress has been linked to poorer CAD prognosis [7], and depression in women has been shown to be an independent risk factor in cardiovascular disease and overall mortality [8].

Pathological Differences Are Apparent Between the Sexes

- Women generally have smaller diameter coronary vessels as seen on computed tomography coronary angiography (CTCA) than men [9]. This can impact on revascularization and treatment strategies.
- Women are more likely to have microvascular disease, rather than atheroma and endothelial dysfunction. Men have a higher atheroma burden in age-matched cases than women, and therefore have more obstructive epicardial coronary disease than women [10].
- Women being investigated for chest pain are more likely to have angiographically normal coronary arteries than men [11]. This is also true for women presenting with acute coronary syndromes (ACS), where in one report 17% of women with non-ST-segment elevation myocardial infarction (NSTEMI) were found to have no critical lesions on angiographic assessment [12]. Microvascular dysfunction is present in up to 50% of women presenting with chest pain and angiographically normal coronary arteries [13].
- Alternative mechanisms underlying a presentation of presumed ACS are therefore more common in women than men. For instance, Takotsubo or stress cardiomyopathy, which is vastly more common in women than men, can mimic an

ST-elevation myocardial infarction (STEMI) without any significant underlying CAD [14].

- Outcomes for females with CAD are worse than their male counterparts when unadjusted data is used [15]. Females have higher mortality at both 1 and 5 years after acute MI (AMI), and also present more than men with subsequent sequelae such as heart failure [16]. Much of this disparity between the sexes has been explained by the older age at presentation in women, the presence of more comorbidities, and the lower utilization of healthcare by females with CAD compared to men [17].
- Women are more likely to present with NSTEMI than STEMI [18]; however, the difference in outcome between sexes is maintained in women presenting with the latter. In the female STEMI cohort, a higher burden of comorbid disease has been blamed, together with slower "symptom to balloon" time for those treated with coronary angioplasty [19].
- In a specific analysis of patients undergoing percutaneous coronary intervention (PCI) in the UK, female gender was found to be an independent risk factor for all-cause mortality at both 30 days and 1 year [20].

Age Factors and CAD in Women

- The incidence of symptomatic CAD rises with age in both sexes, although women lag behind men by approximately 10 years [21], with the average age of first MI being 64.5 years for men and 70.3 years for women [1].
- Although the prevalence of CAD in men at younger ages is greater than in women, this gap reduces with increased age, with a surge in women presenting at advancing ages [22].
- The menopause, whether medically induced or natural, affects this disease, both directly as a result of a reduction in circulating sex hormones, but also because of the associated weight gain, increased diabetes, hypertension, and unfavorable changes in the lipid profile with an increase in low density lipoprotein cholesterol (LDL-cholesterol) and triglycerides [23–25].

Diagnostic Challenges

- Traditionally women have been considered more likely to present with "atypical" symptoms of CAD than men. This has an important bearing on the likelihood of symptoms being recognized as caused by CAD, and thus subsequent investigation and management may be hindered.
- A number of differences are present in descriptors used for symptoms of CAD by women rather than men, whereby women more commonly report [26–28]:
  – Shortness of breath
  – Back, neck, jaw, or abdominal discomfort
  – Nausea or vomiting
  – Profound fatigue
  – Lightheadedness
  – Sudden anxiety, agitation, or confusion
- Despite atypical symptoms being more common in women with respect to the description of chest pain, more similarities than differences exist, both in patients presenting with stable angina and with ACS.
- Women and men use similar words and descriptors of chest pain, including phrases such as "chest pain," "pressure," and "tightness" with similar frequency on presentation [29]. The location of pain and radiation is also similar with reports of pain in the left arm, shoulder, or back, occurring as frequently in men as in women. Women were, however, more likely to use words such as "crushing" or "pressing."
- In stable CAD with angina an association of pain with mental stress and the occurrence of regular symptoms at rest tend to be more common in women [30].
- MI in women is more likely to go unnoticed than in men. In one Icelandic study of 13,000 women, increasing frequency of ECG features of MI were noted with increasing patient age, but MI was less likely to have been clinically noted in women [31].
- In a large analysis of over one million American patients with MI, women were more likely to present without chest pain, and this difference was particularly marked at younger ages [32]. As age increased the sex difference in MI patients presenting without chest pain diminished.
- Many women presenting with symptoms of stable angina or atypical chest pain will undergo noninvasive testing. Exercise ECG testing has long been known to have lower sensitivity and specificity in women than in men, and carries a significant false positive rate [33]. This is related to anatomical and hormonal differences (particularly estrogen). It is also more common for females to exercise for a shorter duration leading to an inadequate test.
- Stress echocardiography is therefore preferred to exercise ECG testing to detect CAD in women. Sensitivity and specificity for women is comparable to men in both exercise and pharmacological stress echocardiography [33].
- Radionucleotide stress imaging also has similar levels of accuracy in women compared to men, and can be used successfully. Coronary CT calcium scoring and angiography have gained popularity over recent years. Coronary calcium score has a high negative predictive value in both sexes, and CTCA allows imaging of epicardial coronary arteries without risks associated with invasive testing [33].
- Modern multi-slice imaging allowing information to be gathered with minimum radiation exposure has attenuated previous concerns related to radiation exposure from CT imaging, particularly in younger women with exposure of breast tissue to radiation. Cardiac CT is not thought to unduly increase the risk of cancer via radiation exposure [34].
- Indications for invasive coronary angiography in women are the same as for men. In one large study, despite women being in the minority of those referred for angiography, unobstructed epicardial arteries were found significantly more commonly in women than in men [11], for both those presenting with ACS and those with stable symptoms.

Spontaneous Coronary Artery Dissection (SCAD)

- Spontaneous coronary artery dissection (SCAD) constitutes the separation of the layers of the coronary artery wall to create a false lumen between either intima and media, or

media and adventitia, without an iatrogenic or traumatic cause.

- As hemorrhage occurs into the false lumen, subsequent thrombosis can compress the true lumen of the coronary artery leading to subsequent downstream ischemia and AMI [35] (Fig. 20.1).

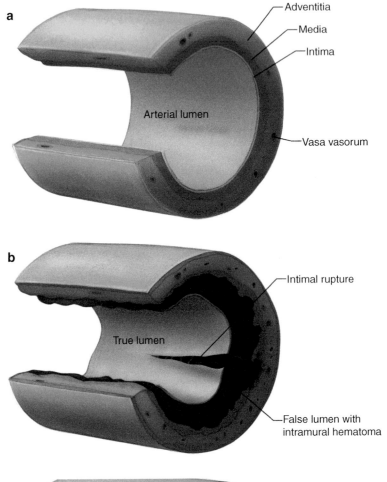

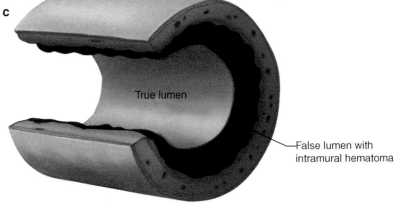

Fig. 20.1 Mechanisms of spontaneous coronary artery dissection. (**a**) Normal coronary artery. (**b**) Intimal rupture initiating tear, with intramural hematoma formation. (**c**) Spontaneous bleeding into the arterial wall, creating a false lumen filled with intramural hematoma. Reproduced with permission from Saw J, et al. J Am Coll Cardiol. 2016;68 (3):297–312

- SCAD is rare in the general population, accounting for an estimated 0.2% of cases of ACS in angiographic reports [36]. The detection of SCAD can be operator dependent, however, and the use of intracoronary imaging may lead to a higher detection of SCAD in ACS patients, with one series suggesting that in all-comers SCAD may be present in 4% of patients [37].
- Although rare, SCAD is more common in females, particularly at younger ages, and its prevalence is becoming increasingly acknowledged [38, 39]. One-quarter of females under the age of 50 presenting with ACS and undergoing angiography in one study were found to have underlying SCAD [40]. A further series suggested the incidence was as high as 36% in women presenting with ACS under the age of 60 with one or fewer traditional CAD risk factors [41].
- The pathophysiology and underlying mechanism of SCAD remain poorly understood [35, 42]. A number of conditions have been associated with SCAD, including fibromuscular dysplasia, connective tissue diseases, and the peripartum state, additional precipitants such as intense exercise and emotional stress have been demonstrated [43] (Table 20.1).
- Diagnosis of SCAD may not always be confirmed on standard coronary angiography. Intravascular imaging by either intravascular ultrasound (IVUS) or optical coherence tomography (OCT) are recommended for confirmation [35, 43–45].
- Conventional angiography tends to rely on the recognition of a radiolucent intimal flap associated with the vessel wall, and the presence of contrast staining in the wall. Relying on these findings are likely to under-diagnose SCAD in a vulnerable population, and so in young females with otherwise normal coronary arteries but an extensive, smooth, luminal narrowing, intracoronary imaging should strongly be considered [43, 44] (Figs. 20.2 and 20.3; Table 20.2).
- The optimal management of SCAD is not clear, but conservative management, PCI, and surgical revascularization are potential options [44]. Most clinicians tend to favor conservative management once SCAD has been diagnosed (assuming there is preserved luminal coronary flow) with dual antiplatelet agents being preferred. The use of beta-blockers will theoretically reduce shear stress on the vessel wall and is also

Table 20.1 Potential predisposing and precipitating factors for SCAD

Predisposing causes
Fibromuscular dysplasia
Pregnancy-related: antepartum, early postpartum, late postpartum, very late postpartum
Recurrent pregnancies: multiparity or multigravida
Connective tissue disorder: Marfan syndrome, Loeys–Dietz syndrome, Ehler–Danlos syndrome type 4, cystic medial necrosis, alpha-1 antitrypsin deficiency, polycystic kidney disease
Systemic inflammatory disease: systemic lupus erythematosus, Crohn's disease, ulcerative colitis, polyarteritis nodosa, sarcoidosis, Churg–Strauss syndrome, Wegener's granulomatosis, rheumatoid arthritis, Kawasaki, giant cell arteritis, celiac disease
Hormonal therapy: oral contraceptive, estrogen, progesterone, beta-HCG, testosterone, corticosteroids
Coronary artery spasm
Idiopathic
Precipitating stressors
Intense exercises (isometric or aerobic activities)
Intense emotional stress
Labor and delivery
Intense Valsava-type activities (e.g., retching, vomiting, bowel movement, coughing)
Recreational drugs (e.g., cocaine, amphetamines, methamphetamines)
Intense hormonal therapy (e.g., beta-HCG injections, corticosteroids injections)

Reproduced with permission from Saw J, et al. J Am Coll Cardiol. 2016;68(3):297–312

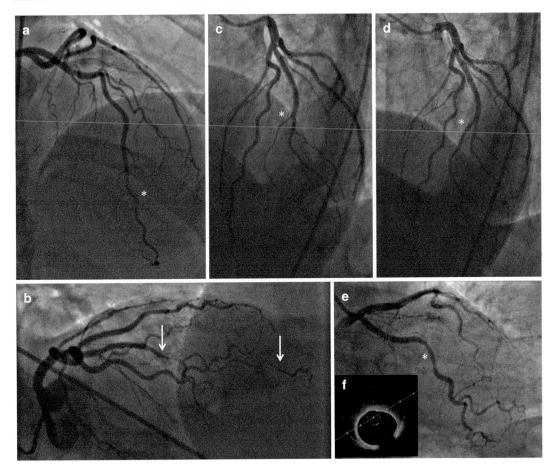

Fig. 20.2 Angiographic classification of SCAD. (**a**) Type 1 SCAD of distal left anterior descending (LAD) artery with staining of artery wall (asterisk). (**b**) Type 2A SCAD of mid-distal LAD (between arrows). (**c**) Type 2B SCAD of diagonal branch (asterisk), which healed 1 year later (asterisk in **d**). (**e**) Type 3 SCAD of mid-circumflex artery (asterisk), with corresponding optical coherence tomography showing intramural hematoma in (**f**). Reproduced with permission from Saw J, et al. J Am Coll Cardiol. 2016;68 (3):297–312

recommended. The use of glycoprotein IIbIIIa inhibitors (GPI) and fibrinolytics is not recommended [38, 42, 44].

- The role of revascularization in SCAD is controversial, and although early studies suggested benefit from revascularization more contemporary literature urges caution [38]. Both PCI and CABG are options for emergency revascularization. If there is evidence of ongoing hemodynamic instability or ischemia, then revascularization needs to be considered and will depend on the patient's anatomy and SCAD location.

- PCI is preferred for single vessel SCAD; however, in cases of left main stem or multivessel SCAD, surgical revascularization would be the preferred method [43, 44, 46] (Fig. 20.4).

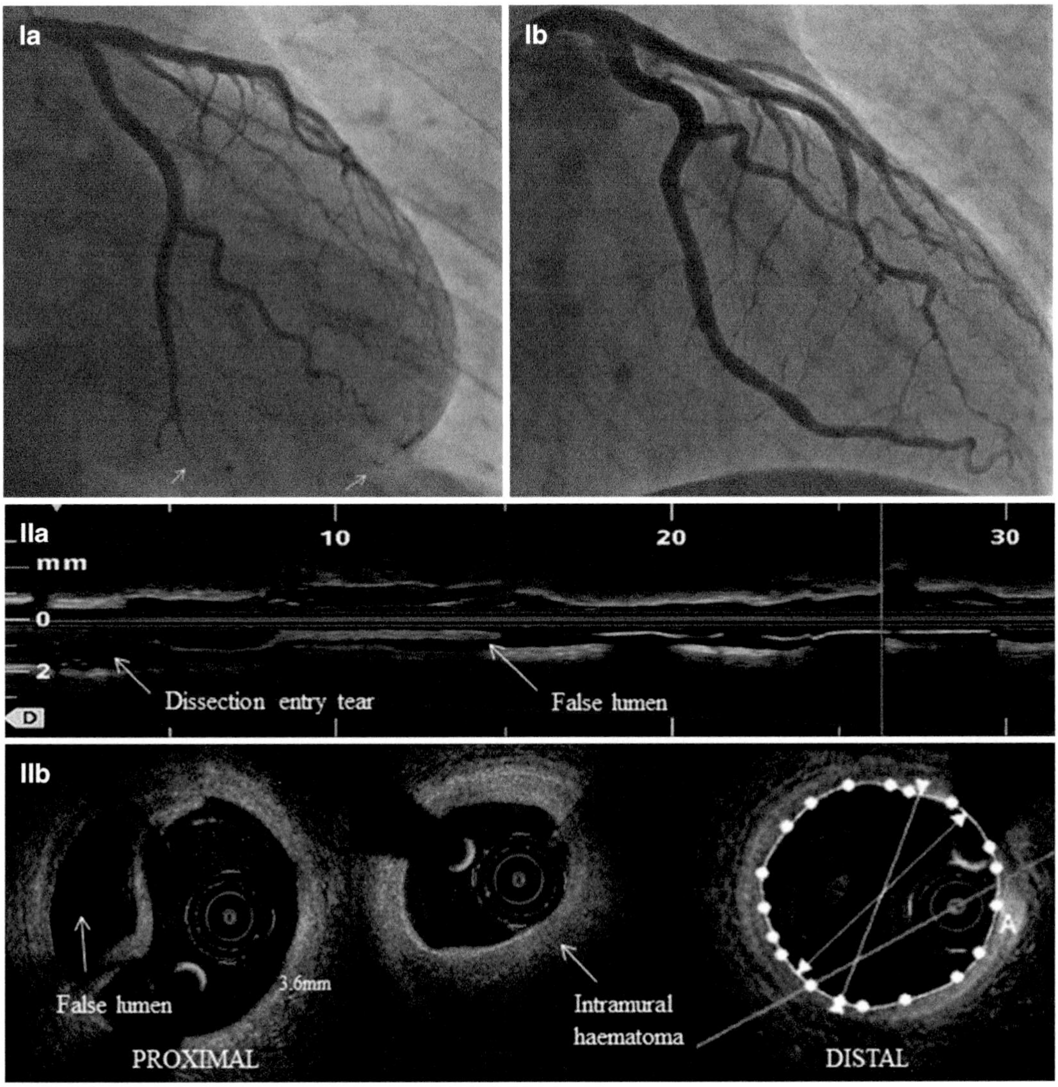

Fig. 20.3 Coronary angiographic and optical coherence tomography appearances of spontaneous coronary artery dissection. (*I*) Coronary angiographic images of spontaneous coronary artery dissection in the AV Circumflex, before (Ia - see arrows) and after (Ib) successful PCI. (*II*) Optical coherence tomography of the lesion, in long axis (IIa) and in short axis (IIb). Images courtesy of Dr. James Cockburn, Sussex Cardiac Centre, Royal Sussex County Hospital

Table 20.2 Advantages and disadvantages of intracoronary imaging for SCAD

Advantages	Disadvantages
Definitive diagnosis of SCAD	Invasive, requires anticoagulation
Confirm true lumen entry by coronary wire	Costly
Facilitate stent sizing	Not available in all laboratories
Confirm adequate stent apposition	Possible risks of extending dissection by: Guide catheter, coronary wire Imaging catheter Hydraulic extension (with OCT)
Confirm full coverage of dissected segment	Vessel occlusion (by catheter, embolization)
Facilitate diagnosis of potential arteriopathy	

Reproduced with permission from Saw J, et al. J Am Coll Cardiol. 2016;68(3):297–312

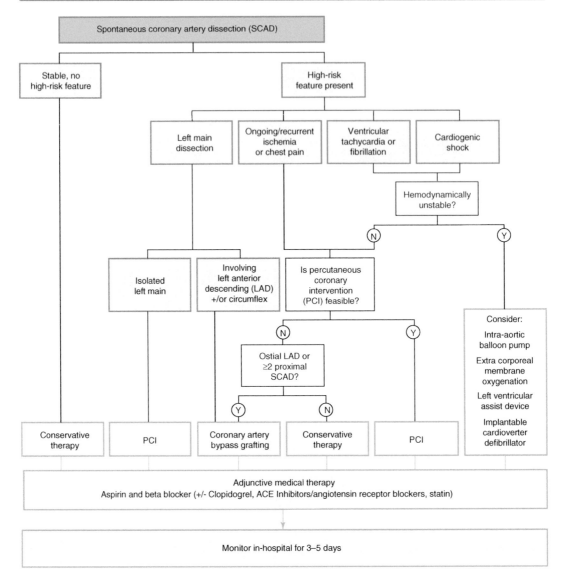

Saw, J. et al. J Am Coll Cardiol. 2016;68(3):297-312.

Fig. 20.4 Management algorithm for spontaneous coronary artery dissection. Conservative therapy is typically pursued in stable patients and those monitored in-hospital for 3–5 days. Revascularization should be considered for those with high-risk features, including PCI, if feasible. Consider intra-aortic balloon pumps, extracorporeal membranous oxygenation, left ventricular assist devices, or implantable cardioverter defibrillators in hemodynamically unstable patients. ACE = angiotensin converting enzyme; LAD = left anterior descending; PCI = percutaneous coronary intervention; SCAD = spontaneous coronary artery dissection. Reproduced with permission from Saw J, et al. J Am Coll Cardiol. 2016;68 (3):297–312

Acute Coronary Syndromes

- Non-ST elevation acute coronary syndromes (NSTEACS) include the subgroups of NSTEMI and unstable angina. Women who present with NSTEACS are older and carry more comorbidities than the equivalent male population [47].
- Data are clear that an early invasive strategy is beneficial for high-risk patients presenting with NSTEACS, especially those with positive biomarkers [48]. Despite this, women are less likely to undergo early cardiac catheterization and have worse outcomes than men. The difference in outcomes does, however, disappear when data are corrected for comorbidities and age.
- Potentially there is no benefit for low-risk women (biomarker negative) undergoing an early invasive strategy, and one study suggested a trend towards possible harm [49].
- In STEMI, primary PCI is the preferred treatment modality, with well-established evidence for its use. Key to successful implementation of primary PCI is minimizing delays in treatment, and studies have demonstrated that women are more likely to experience delays in treatment targets than men [50].
- Atypical presentations and late recognition in STEMI among female patients may be causative of this, and clearly delays in treatment need to be minimized to encourage positive outcomes.
- The longer "symptom to reperfusion time" experienced by women correlate with worse outcomes in a systematic review of prospective studies [19], in addition to their unfavorable risk profile.
- Part of the disparity in outcome in this context may reflect the underlying pathology. Women are more likely than men to have no evidence of obstructive epicardial coronary disease on angiography when presenting to hospital with ACS [51].
- Plaque rupture and ulceration were identified frequently in one study in such women after standard angiography, with alternate underlying pathologies such as vasospasm, embolism, and dissection (as discussed above) suggested to explain apparently normal findings in patients with confirmed MI on cardiac magnetic resonance imaging [51].
- Vasospasm is more frequently identified in women than in men, and requires a different approach to treatment compared to obstructive coronary disease caused by atherosclerosis [52]. Various medical therapies are suggested in cases of vasospasm, including calcium channel antagonists and nitrate preparations.

Pregnancy and Postpartum

- Historically women of child bearing age have rarely suffered from atherosclerotic CAD, although as maternal age increases and more women having children later in life, it will become more common and is likely to rise with the increasing prevalence of obesity, and related diabetes and hypertension among younger women [53].
- Although rare, 20% of maternal deaths in the UK are attributable to cardiac pathology [54]. Overall coronary vascular disease complicates 0.2–4% of pregnancies [53], and estimates from American research suggests ACS occur at a rate of 3–6.2 per 100,000 deliveries [55, 56]. The incidence was lower in a British study which identified fewer cases and gave an estimated incidence of 0.7 per 100,000 deliveries [54].
- In addition to traditional risk factors for ACS, there is higher risk in patients with eclampsia, or preeclampsia, thrombophilia, infections, or postpartum hemorrhage [55, 56].
- Spontaneous coronary artery dissection is more common in pregnant women [57], but underlying coronary atheromatous disease is also found in a significant number of patients, more commonly in women who are older during their pregnancy, and who have traditional CVD risk factors [53, 54, 57].
- The investigation of choice for pregnant women presenting with unstable angina,

NSTEMI, or STEMI remains cardiac catheterization as it is for nonpregnant women. Angiography can be performed safely with minimal exposure of the fetus to radiation, with consensus that maternal doses of radiation <50 mGy are safe, and an angiogram or PCI is usually performed with <20 mGy [58].

- An experienced operator is required to further minimize this radiation risk, and should be performed with as little fluoroscopy time as possible.
- As well as minimizing exposure time, the frame rate should be lowered to reduce radiation dose, although a balance must be found to ensure that this does not lead to a need for longer exposures or excess procedural risk. Beam size can also be adjusted and limiting the area imaged will also reduce radiation.
- Lead shielding must be used appropriately, although abdominal lead shielding only marginally reduces the radiation exposure of the fetus by approximately 2% [53, 58].
- In cases of STEMI in pregnancy, primary angioplasty remains the first line treatment, especially given the higher incidence of SCAD in this population [53]. Bare metal stents are preferred to drug eluting stents. These have the added advantage of limiting the duration of antiplatelet agents and therefore minimizes bleeding risk.
- Thrombolysis is not recommended in pregnancy as it carries significant risks of bleeding for the mother, particularly to the placental vascular bed [53], however should be considered in cases of emergency where there is no access to emergent PCI.
- As with all maternal cardiology a pragmatic approach prioritizing maternal survival is paramount. Cardiac surgery during pregnancy carries a high mortality burden (upwards of 6%), so is not preferred and should only be performed for cases of emergent need when all percutaneous options have been exhausted [58].
- Special consideration must be given to drug therapy both during and after procedures for treatment of CAD in pregnancy [59].

- Unfractionated and low molecular weight heparin do not cross the placenta and therefore do not affect the fetus. Maternal bleeding risk should, however, be taken into consideration. For the short duration of use during PCI for example, the benefits are likely to outweigh any bleeding risk.
- Bivalirudin, a direct thrombin inhibitor, is often used as an alternative in patients with heparin-induced thrombocytopenia (HIT); however, there is no data available to support its use in pregnancy and is not recommended [53].
- Fondaparinux, an alternative factor Xa inhibitor, is recommended by the American College of Obstetrics and Gynaecology for anticoagulation in cases of HIT [59].
- Aspirin is considered safe to use in pregnancy at the low maintenance doses required following MI, and must be used if PCI has been performed [59]. It can be continued at low doses for platelet inhibition during breastfeeding.
- Clopidogrel used in animal models has been shown to be safe for use in pregnancy, however concerns remain over bleeding risk. Therefore, the European Society of Cardiology (ESC) recommend limiting its use to the shortest possible duration and when strictly needed such as after PCI. There is a consensus to hold clopidogrel for 7 days prior to delivery, where possible, to reduce the risk of postpartum bleeding [59].
- There is no safety data available for newer antiplatelet agents, namely prasugrel and ticagrelor, and these should not be used.
- Glycoprotein IIbIIIa inhibitors have no safety data available, and the ESC do not recommend their use during pregnancy.

Bleeding Considerations

- Female sex is an independent risk factor for major bleeding events post coronary angiography and PCI. Evidence from trials comparing femoral versus radial access suggest that much of these risks can be mitigated by preferentially pursuing the radial route for coronary intervention [60, 61].

- Women are more likely to require crossover to the femoral route of access than men in these studies, most commonly due to radial artery spasm. This occurs significantly more often in women than men; despite this procedural success rates remain similar between men and women [60].
- Operators should be mindful of this enhanced risk of bleeding in women and take this into consideration when planning interventional procedures on females.
- Female sex is an independent risk factor for bleeding complications in ACS patients regardless of whether invasive treatment is undertaken. This area is under-explored in the literature but sex-specific variations in platelet biology have been mooted as a potential underlying cause [62].
- Dosing adjustment for weight-guided drug dosing is vital to minimize bleeding risks, particularly when GPI are used, as there is a strong association of increased bleeding complications for females treated with these drugs [62, 63].
- Lower BMI, lower creatinine clearance, and anatomical differences between men and women may also be responsible, but inappropriate weight dosing is a major driving force in bleeding risk in women.
- Clinicians are urged to carefully consider this enhanced risk when planning interventions in females, particularly to ensure appropriate drug doses are used to minimize bleeding risk.

Pharmacology

A number of drugs are used in both primary and secondary prevention of cardiovascular disease, and appropriate drug therapy is essential to the management of cardiovascular disease with a sound evidence base for improved outcomes [64]. Differences in prescribing practices exist between sexes. The EuroHeart survey of 3779 women demonstrated that although women were equally likely to be prescribed a beta-blocker as men, they were less likely to be prescribed aspirin (73% vs. 81% in men) or a statin (45% vs. 51% in men) at both hospital discharge and at 1 year, even in the presence of confirmed CAD [65].

- Aspirin should be utilized whenever a patient has presented with an acute coronary syndrome, or in confirmed cases of coronary artery disease [66, 67]. Use for primary prevention in women with at least one risk factor for cardiovascular disease is also likely to be advantageous [68].
- Benefits exist for beta-blockers and ACE inhibitors after myocardial infarction. There does not appear to be a difference in outcomes between men and women [69, 70].
- Both sexes benefit from statins for secondary prevention, with some evidence suggesting a tendency to enhanced benefit in females. The CARE trial investigating pravastatin for secondary prevention demonstrated a greater benefit in postmenopausal women included in the trial, where the use of pravastatin was associated with a 43% reduction in coronary heart disease death and nonfatal MI [71, 72]. The PROVE-IT trial investigated high-dose atorvastatin therapy compared to pravastatin in secondary prevention, demonstrating a reduction in all-cause mortality and major adverse cardiovascular events in the high-dose atorvastatin arm, and a tendency to enhanced benefit in women compared to men [73].
- The addition of a second antiplatelet drug from the thienopyridine class (clopidogrel or prasugrel), or the reversible $P2Y_{12}$ antagonist ticagrelor, reduce further ischemic events and improve outcomes in patients with acute coronary syndromes. The safety and efficacy of clopidogrel is equal between men and women, with no change in bleeding risk between sexes [74]. In an analysis of the PLATO trial of ticagrelor versus clopidogrel therapy, there was no difference in outcomes or safety between men and women [75]. Antiplatelet therapy should therefore be utilized according to guidelines and after bleeding risk assessment for both men and women.
- Although estrogen is thought to protect premenopausal women from cardiovascular

disease, and the depletion of estrogen following the menopause has been shown to increase atherosclerosis progression [76], there is no evidence to support the use of hormone replacement therapy (HRT) in the prevention of cardiovascular disease in women after the menopause. The HERS trial was a large randomized control trial to investigate the effect of HRT on prevention of cardiovascular disease, and failed to show an advantage in either short- or long-term follow-up [77, 78]. Furthermore a second large RCT suggested increased overall health risk for the use of HRT to prevent cardiovascular events [79].

Summary

- Although in principle the diagnosis and management of coronary artery disease in males and females remains the same, special considerations are needed when thinking about the female population. Women may present atypically, at a more advanced age, and different risk factors need to be taken into consideration.
- The pathology encountered is varied, with a higher prevalence of microvascular dysfunction and spontaneous coronary artery dissection found in women.
- CAD may present during pregnancy, and presents a particularly challenging circumstance where careful thought must be taken to diagnostic techniques, intervention, and subsequent management.
- Pharmacological intervention outside of pregnancy should be equal for men and women, but consideration to increased bleeding risk in women must be taken into account when weighing up benefit and risk.
- Further research is required in the future to address the discrepancy in outcomes between men and women with CAD.

References

1. Roger VL, Go AS, Lloyd-Jones DM, et al. Heart disease and stroke statistics—2012 update: a report from the American heart association. Circulation. 2012;125(1):e2–e220. https://doi.org/10.1161/CIR.0b013e31823ac046.

2. Ford ES, Capewell S. Coronary heart disease mortality among young adults in the U.S. from 1980 through 2002. J Am Coll Cardiol. 2007;50(22):2128–32. https://doi.org/10.1016/j.jacc.2007.05.056.

3. Wilson PWF, D'Agostino RB, Sullivan L, Parise H, Kannel WB. Overweight and obesity as determinants of cardiovascular risk: the Framingham experience. Arch Intern Med. 2002;162(16):1867–72. http://www.ncbi.nlm.nih.gov/pubmed/12196085. Accessed May 20, 2017.

4. Huxley R, Barzi F, Woodward M. Excess risk of fatal coronary heart disease associated with diabetes in men and women: meta-analysis of 37 prospective cohort studies. BMJ. 2006;332(7533):73–8. http://www.bmj.com/content/332/7533/73. Accessed May 20, 2017.

5. Willett WC, Green A, Stampfer MJ, et al. Relative and absolute excess risks of coronary heart disease among women who smoke cigarettes. N Engl J Med. 1987;317(21):1303–9. https://doi.org/10.1056/NEJM198711193172102.

6. Prescott E, Hippe M, Schnohr P, Hein HO, Vestbo J. Smoking and risk of myocardial infarction in women and men: longitudinal population study. BMJ. 1998;316(7137):1043–7. http://www.ncbi.nlm.nih.gov/pubmed/9552903. Accessed May 20, 2017

7. Orth-Gomér K, Wamala SP, Horsten M, Schenck-Gustafsson K, Schneiderman N, Mittleman MA. Marital stress worsens prognosis in women with coronary heart disease: the Stockholm Female Coronary Risk Study. JAMA. 2000;284(23):3008–14. http://www.ncbi.nlm.nih.gov/pubmed/11122587. Accessed May 20, 2017.

8. Wassertheil-Smoller S, Shumaker S, Ockene J, et al. Depression and cardiovascular sequelae in postmenopausal women. The Women's Health Initiative (WHI). Arch Intern Med. 2004;164(3):289–98. https://doi.org/10.1001/archinte.164.3.289.

9. Dickerson JA, Nagaraja HN, Raman SV. Gender-related differences in coronary artery dimensions: a volumetric analysis. Clin Cardiol. 2010;33(2):E44–9. https://doi.org/10.1002/clc.20509.

10. Han SH, Bae JH, Holmes DR, et al. Sex differences in atheroma burden and endothelial function in patients with early coronary atherosclerosis. Eur Heart J. 2008;29(11):1359–69. https://doi.org/10.1093/eurheartj/ehn142.

11. Sullivan AK, Holdright DR, Wright CA, Sparrow JL, Cunningham D, Fox KM. Chest pain in women: clinical, investigative, and prognostic features. BMJ. 1994;308(6933):883–6. https://doi.org/10.1136/bmj.308.6933.883.

12. Glaser R, Herrmann HC, Murphy SA, et al. Benefit of an early invasive management strategy in women with acute coronary syndromes. JAMA. 2002;288(24):3124–9. http://www.ncbi.nlm.nih.gov/pubmed/12495392. Accessed May 20, 2017.

13. Reis SE, Holubkov R, Conrad Smith AJ, et al. Coronary microvascular dysfunction is highly prevalent in women with chest pain in the absence of coronary artery disease: results from the NHLBI WISE study. Am Heart J. 2001;141(5):735–41. http://www.ncbi.nlm.nih.gov/pubmed/11320360. Accessed May 20, 2017.

14. Templin C, Ghadri JR, Diekmann J, et al. Clinical Features and Outcomes of Takotsubo (Stress) Cardiomyopathy. N Engl J Med. 2015;373(10):929–38. https://doi.org/10.1056/NEJMoa1406761.

15. Graham G. Acute coronary syndromes in women: recent treatment trends and outcomes. Clin Med Insights Cardiol. 2016;10:1–10. https://doi.org/10.4137/CMC.S37145.

16. Mehta LS, Beckie TM, DeVon HA, et al. Acute myocardial infarction in women. Circulation. 2016;133(9):916–47.

17. Bucholz EM, Butala NM, Rathore SS, Dreyer RP, Lansky AJ, Krumholz HM. Sex differences in long-term mortality after myocardial infarction: a systematic review. Circulation. 2014;30(9):757–67.

18. Hochman JS, Tamis JE, Thompson TD, et al. Sex, clinical presentation, and outcome in patients with acute coronary syndromes. N Engl J Med. 1999;341(4):226–32. https://doi.org/10.1056/NEJM199907223410402.

19. van der Meer MG, Nathoe HM, van der Graaf Y, Doevendans PA, Appelman Y. Worse outcome in women with STEMI: a systematic review of prognostic studies. Eur J Clin Invest. 2015;45(2):226–35. https://doi.org/10.1111/eci.12399.

20. Kunadian V, Qiu W, Lagerqvist B, et al. Gender differences in outcomes and predictors of all-cause mortality after percutaneous coronary intervention (Data from United Kingdom and Sweden). Am J Cardiol. 2017;119(2):210–6.https://doi.org/10.1016/j.amjcard.2016.09.052.

21. Lloyd-Jones D, Adams RJ, Brown TM, et al. Executive summary: heart disease and stroke statistics--2010 update: a report from the American Heart Association. Circulation. 2010;121(7):948–54. https://doi.org/10.1161/CIRCULATIONAHA.109.192666.

22. Lerner DJ, Kannel WB. Patterns of coronary heart disease morbidity and mortality in the sexes: a 26-year follow-up of the Framingham population. Am Heart J. 1986;111(2):383–90. http://www.ncbi.nlm.nih.gov/pubmed/3946178. Accessed February 22, 2017.

23. Gordon T, Kannel WB, Hjortland MC, McNamara PM. Menopause and coronary heart disease. The Framingham Study. Ann Intern Med. 1978;89(2):157–61. http://www.ncbi.nlm.nih.gov/pubmed/677576. Accessed February 22, 2017.

24. Muka T, Oliver-Williams C, Kunutsor S, et al. Association of age at onset of menopause and time since onset of menopause with cardiovascular outcomes, intermediate vascular traits, and all-cause mortality. JAMA Cardiol. 2016;1(7):767. https://doi.org/10.1001/jamacardio.2016.2415.

25. Mazza A, Tikhonoff V, Schiavon L, Casiglia E. Triglycerides + high-density-lipoprotein-cholesterol dyslipidaemia, a coronary risk factor in elderly women: the CArdiovascular STudy in the ELderly. Intern Med J. 2005;35(10):604–10. https://doi.org/10.1111/j.1445-5994.2005.00940.x.

26. Milner KA, Vaccarino V, Arnold AL, Funk M, Goldberg RJ. Gender and age differences in chief complaints of acute myocardial infarction (Worcester heart attack study). Am J Cardiol. 2004;93(5):606–8. https://doi.org/10.1016/j.amjcard.2003.11.028.

27. Philpott S, Boynton PM, Feder G, Hemingway H. Gender differences in descriptions of angina symptoms and health problems immediately prior to angiography: the ACRE study. Appropriateness of Coronary Revascularisation study. Soc Sci Med. 2001;52(10):1565–75. http://www.ncbi.nlm.nih.gov/pubmed/11314852. Accessed May 20, 2017.

28. Goldberg RJ, O'Donnell C, Yarzebski J, Bigelow C, Savageau J, Gore JM. Sex differences in symptom presentation associated with acute myocardial infarction: a population-based perspective. Am Heart J. 1998;136(2):189–95. https://doi.org/10.1053/hj.1998.v136.88874.

29. Kreatsoulas C, Shannon HS, Giacomini M, Velianou JL, Anand SS. Reconstructing angina: cardiac symptoms are the same in women and men. JAMA Intern Med. 2013;173(9):829. https://doi.org/10.1001/jamainternmed.2013.229.

30. Pepine CJ, Abrams J, Marks RG, Morris JJ, Scheidt SS, Handberg E. Characteristics of a contemporary population with angina pectoris. TIDES investigators. Am J Cardiol. 1994;74(3):226–31. http://www.ncbi.nlm.nih.gov/pubmed/8037126. Accessed February 26, 2017.

31. Jónsdóttir LS, Sigfusson N, Sigvaldason H, Thorgeirsson G. Incidence and prevalence of recognised and unrecognised myocardial infarction in women. The Reykjavik Study. Eur Heart J. 1998;19(7):1011–8. http://www.ncbi.nlm.nih.gov/pubmed/9717035. Accessed February 26, 2017.

32. Canto JG, Rogers WJ, Goldberg RJ, et al. Association of age and sex with myocardial infarction symptom presentation and in-hospital mortality. JAMA. 2012;307(8):813–22. https://doi.org/10.1001/jama.2012.199.

33. Stangl V, Witzel V, Baumann G, Stangl K. Current diagnostic concepts to detect coronary artery disease in women. Eur Heart J. 2008;29(6):707–17. https://doi.org/10.1093/eurheartj/ehn047.

34. Gerber TC, Carr JJ, Arai AE, et al. Ionizing radiation in cardiac imaging. Circulation. 2009;119(7):1056–65.

35. Vrints CJM. Spontaneous coronary artery dissection. Heart. 2010;96(10):801–8. https://doi.org/10.1136/hrt.2008.162073.

36. Mortensen KH, Thuesen L, Kristensen IB, Christiansen EH. Spontaneous coronary artery dissection: a Western Denmark Heart Registry Study. Catheter Cardiovasc Interv. 2009;74(5):710–7. https://doi.org/10.1002/ccd.22115.

37. Nishiguchi T, Tanaka A, Ozaki Y, et al. Prevalence of spontaneous coronary artery dissection in patients with acute coronary syndrome. Eur Heart J Acute Cardiovasc Care. 2016;5(3):263–70. https://doi.org/10.1177/2048872613504310.

38. Tweet MS, Hayes SN, Pitta SR, et al. Clinical features, management, and prognosis of spontaneous coronary artery dissection. Circulation. 2012;126(5):579–88. https://doi.org/10.1161/CIRCULATIONAHA.112.105718.

39. Thompson EA, Ferraris S, Gress T, Ferraris V. Gender differences and predictors of mortality in spontaneous coronary artery dissection: a review of reported

cases. J Invasive Cardiol. 2005;17(1):59–61. http://www.ncbi.nlm.nih.gov/pubmed/15640544. Accessed February 22, 2017.

40. Saw J, Aymong E, Mancini GBJ, Sedlak T, Starovoytov A, Ricci D. Nonatherosclerotic coronary artery disease in young women. Can J Cardiol. 2014;30(7):814–9. https://doi.org/10.1016/j.cjca.2014.01.011.

41. Motreff P, Malcles G, Combaret N, et al. How and when to suspect spontaneous coronary artery dissection? Novel insights from a single-center series on prevalence and angiographic appearance. EuroIntervention. 2017;12(18):e2236–43. https://doi.org/10.4244/EIJ-D-16-00187.

42. Alfonso F. Spontaneous coronary artery dissection. Circulation. 2012;126(6):667–70.

43. Saw J, Aymong E, Sedlak T, et al. Spontaneous coronary artery dissection: association with predisposing arteriopathies and precipitating stressors and cardiovascular outcomes. Circ Cardiovasc Interv. 2014;7(5):645–55. https://doi.org/10.1161/CIRCINTERVENTIONS.114.001760.

44. Alfonso F, Bastante T, Cuesta J, Rodríguez D, Benedicto A, Rivero F. Spontaneous coronary artery dissection: novel insights on diagnosis and management. Cardiovasc Diagn Ther. 2015;5(2):133–40. https://doi.org/10.3978/j.issn.2223-3652.2015.03.05.

45. Saw J. Coronary angiogram classification of spontaneous coronary artery dissection. Catheter Cardiovasc Interv. 2014;84(7):1115–22. https://doi.org/10.1002/ccd.25293.

46. Vanzetto G, Berger-Coz E, Barone-Rochette G, et al. Prevalence, therapeutic management and medium-term prognosis of spontaneous coronary artery dissection: results from a database of 11,605 patients. Eur J Cardiothoracic Surg. 2009;35(2):250–4. https://doi.org/10.1016/j.ejcts.2008.10.023.

47. Blomkalns AL, Chen AY, Hochman JS, et al. Gender disparities in the diagnosis and treatment of non-ST-segment elevation acute coronary syndromes: large-scale observations from the CRUSADE (Can Rapid Risk Stratification of Unstable Angina Patients Suppress Adverse Outcomes With Early Implementatio). J Am Coll Cardiol. 2005;45(6):832–7. https://doi.org/10.1016/j.jacc.2004.11.055.

48. Amsterdam EA, Wenger NK, Brindis RG, et al. 2014 AHA/ACC guideline for the management of patients with non-ST-elevation acute coronary syndromes: executive summary: a report of the American College of Cardiology/American Heart Association Task Force on Practice Guidelines. Circulation. 2014;130(25):2354–94. https://doi.org/10.1161/CIR.0000000000000133.

49. O'Donoghue M, Boden WE, Braunwald E, et al. Early invasive vs conservative treatment strategies in women and men with unstable angina and non–ST-segment elevation myocardial infarction. JAMA. 2008;300(1):71. https://doi.org/10.1001/jama.300.1.71.

50. D'Onofrio G, Safdar B, Lichtman JH, et al. Sex differences in reperfusion in young patients with ST-segment-elevation myocardial infarction: results from the VIRGO study. Circulation. 2015;131(15):1324–32. https://doi.org/10.1161/CIRCULATIONAHA.114.012293.

51. Reynolds HR, Srichai MB, Iqbal SN, et al. Mechanisms of myocardial infarction in women without angiographically obstructive coronary artery disease. Circulation. 2011;124(13):1414–25. https://doi.org/10.1161/CIRCULATIONAHA.111.026542.

52. Cenko E, Bugiardini R. Vasotonic angina as a cause of myocardial ischemia in women. Cardiovasc Drugs Ther. 2015;29(4):339–45. https://doi.org/10.1007/s10557-015-6595-4.

53. Regitz-Zagrosek V, Blomstrom Lundqvist C, Borghi C, et al. ESC Guidelines on the management of cardiovascular diseases during pregnancy: the Task Force on the Management of Cardiovascular Diseases during Pregnancy of the European Society of Cardiology (ESC). Eur Heart J. 2011;32(24):3147–97. https://doi.org/10.1093/eurheartj/ehr218.

54. Bush N, Nelson-Piercy C, Spark P, et al. Myocardial infarction in pregnancy and postpartum in the UK. Eur J Prev Cardiol. 2013;20(1):12–20. https://doi.org/10.1177/1741826711432117.

55. Ladner HE, Danielsen B, Gilbert WM. Acute myocardial infarction in pregnancy and the puerperium: a population-based study. Obstet Gynecol. 2005;105(3):480–4. https://doi.org/10.1097/01.AOG.0000151998.50852.31.

56. James AH, Jamison MG, Biswas MS, Brancazio LR, Swamy GK, Myers ER. Acute myocardial infarction in pregnancy: a United States population-based study. Circulation. 2006;113(12):1564–71. https://doi.org/10.1161/CIRCULATIONAHA.105.576751.

57. Roth A, Elkayam U. Acute myocardial infarction associated with pregnancy. J Am Coll Cardiol. 2008;52(3):171–80. https://doi.org/10.1016/j.jacc.2008.03.049.

58. Pieper PG, Hoendermis ES, Drijver YN. Cardiac surgery and percutaneous intervention in pregnant women with heart disease. Neth Heart J. 2012;20(3):125–8. https://doi.org/10.1007/s12471-012-0244-3.

59. Yarrington CD, Valente AM, Economy KE. Cardiovascular management in pregnancy: antithrombotic agents and antiplatelet agents. Circulation. 2015;132(14):1354–64. https://doi.org/10.1161/CIRCULATIONAHA.114.003902.

60. Pandie S, Mehta SR, Cantor WJ, et al. Radial versus femoral access for coronary angiography/intervention in women with acute coronary syndromes. JACC Cardiovasc Interv. 2015;8(4):505–12. https://doi.org/10.1016/j.jcin.2014.11.017.

61. Pristipino C, Pelliccia F, Granatelli A, et al. Comparison of access-related bleeding complications in women versus men undergoing percutaneous coronary catheterization using the radial versus femoral artery. Am J Cardiol. 2007;99(9):1216–21. https://doi.org/10.1016/j.amjcard.2006.12.038.

62. Wang TY, Angiolillo DJ, Cushman M, et al. Platelet biology and response to antiplatelet therapy in

women: implications for the development and use of antiplatelet pharmacotherapies for cardiovascular disease. J Am Coll Cardiol. 2012;59(10):891–900. https://doi.org/10.1016/j.jacc.2011.09.075.

63. Alexander KP, Chen AY, Newby LK, et al. Sex differences in major bleeding with glycoprotein IIb/IIIa inhibitors: results from the CRUSADE (Can Rapid Risk Stratification of Unstable Angina Patients Suppress Adverse Outcomes With Early Implementation of the ACC/AHA Guidelines) initiative. Circulation. 2006;114(13):1380–7. https://doi.org/10.1161/CIRCULATIONAHA.106.620815.

64. Mosca L, Banka CL, Benjamin EJ, et al. Evidence-based guidelines for cardiovascular disease prevention in women: 2007 update. Circulation. 2007;115(11):1481–501. https://doi.org/10.1161/CIRCULATIONAHA.107.181546.

65. Daly C. Gender differences in the management and clinical outcome of stable angina. Circulation. 2006;113(4):490–8. https://doi.org/10.1161/CIRCULATIONAHA.105.561647.

66. Collaborative overview of randomised trials of antiplatelet therapy Prevention of death, myocardial infarction, and stroke by prolonged antiplatelet therapy in various categories of patients. BMJ. 1994;308(6921):81–106. https://doi.org/10.1136/bmj.308.6921.81.

67. Antithrombotic Trialists' Collaboration. Collaborative meta-analysis of randomised trials of antiplatelet therapy for prevention of death, myocardial infarction, and stroke in high risk patients. BMJ. 2002;324(7329):71–86. http://www.ncbi.nlm.nih.gov/pubmed/11786451. Accessed March 7, 2017.

68. de Gaetano G, Collaborative Group of the Primary Prevention Project. Low-dose aspirin and vitamin E in people at cardiovascular risk: a randomised trial in general practice. Collaborative Group of the Primary Prevention Project. Lancet (London, England). 2001;357(9250):89–95. http://www.ncbi.nlm.nih.gov/pubmed/11197445. Accessed March 7, 2017.

69. Randomised trial of intravenous atenolol among 16 027 cases of suspected acute myocardial infarction: ISIS-1. First International Study of Infarct Survival Collaborative Group. Lancet (London, England). 1986;2(8498):57–66. http://www.ncbi.nlm.nih.gov/pubmed/2873379. Accessed March 7, 2017.

70. Pfeffer MA, Braunwald E, Moyé LA, et al. Effect of captopril on mortality and morbidity in patients with left ventricular dysfunction after myocardial infarction. N Engl J Med. 1992;327(10):669–77. https://doi.org/10.1056/NEJM199209033271001.

71. Lewis SJ, Sacks FM, Mitchell JS, et al. Effect of pravastatin on cardiovascular events in women after myocardial infarction: the cholesterol and recurrent events (CARE) trial. J Am Coll Cardiol. 1998;32(1):140–6. http://www.ncbi.nlm.nih.gov/pubmed/9669262. Accessed March 7, 2017.

72. Sacks FM, Pfeffer MA, Moye LA, et al. The effect of pravastatin on coronary events after myocardial infarction in patients with average cholesterol levels. N Engl J Med. 1996;335(14):1001–9. https://doi.org/10.1056/NEJM199610033351401.

73. Cannon CP, Braunwald E, McCabe CH, et al. Intensive versus moderate lipid lowering with statins after acute coronary syndromes. N Engl J Med. 2004;350(15):1495–504. https://doi.org/10.1056/NEJMoa040583.

74. Berger JS, Bhatt DL, Cannon CP, et al. The relative efficacy and safety of clopidogrel in women and men. J Am Coll Cardiol. 2009;54(21):1935–45. https://doi.org/10.1016/j.jacc.2009.05.074.

75. Husted S, James SK, Bach RG, et al. The efficacy of ticagrelor is maintained in women with acute coronary syndromes participating in the prospective, randomized, PLATelet inhibition and patient Outcomes (PLATO) trial. Eur Heart J. 2014;35(23):1541–50. https://doi.org/10.1093/eurheartj/ehu075.

76. Taddei S, Virdis A, Ghiadoni L, et al. Menopause is associated with endothelial dysfunction in women. Hypertens (Dallas, Tex 1979). 1996;28(4):576–82. http://www.ncbi.nlm.nih.gov/pubmed/8843881. Accessed March 7, 2017.

77. Hulley S, Grady D, Bush T, et al. Randomized trial of estrogen plus progestin for secondary prevention of coronary heart disease in postmenopausal women. Heart and Estrogen/progestin Replacement Study (HERS) Research Group. JAMA. 1998;280(7):605–13. http://www.ncbi.nlm.nih.gov/pubmed/9718051. Accessed March 7, 2017.

78. Grady D, Herrington D, Bittner V, et al. Cardiovascular disease outcomes during 6.8 years of hormone therapy: heart and estrogen/progestin replacement study follow-up (HERS II). JAMA. 2002;288(1):49–57. http://www.ncbi.nlm.nih.gov/pubmed/12090862. Accessed March 7, 2017.

79. Rossouw JE, Anderson GL, Prentice RL, et al. Risks and benefits of estrogen plus progestin in healthy postmenopausal women: principal results From the Women's Health Initiative randomized controlled trial. JAMA. 2002;288(3):321–33. http://www.ncbi.nlm.nih.gov/pubmed/12117397. Accessed March 7, 2017.

Coronary Intervention in the Chronic Kidney Disease, Diabetic and Elderly Populations

Sami Omar, Osama Alsanjari, and Adam de Belder

About Us The Sussex Cardiac Centre forms part of Brighton and Sussex University Hospitals NHS Trust in the UK. In our unit of 13 consultants, we have 6 interventional cardiologists typically performing approximately 1000 coronary angioplasty procedures per year, comprising of around 400 primary angioplasty activations. We have one of the UK's largest structural heart programs having performed over 700 transcatheter aortic valve replacements since its inception in 2007.

We have a strong national and international academic presence and lead industry and investigator-initiated trials for the UK. Being situated on the south coast of the UK, we cater for a relatively large local population of elderly/retired patients and have a breadth of experience in managing their acute and chronic cardiac pathologies.

Background

- Vaccinations, nutritional and medical advances have increased the longevity of life—the proportion of octogenarians is expected to triple by 2050 [1]. This has opened a new chapter in clinical cardiology—angina management of the very elderly is now daily clinical fodder [2, 3].
- Nearly a quarter of the patients presenting with acute coronary syndromes (ACS) and undergoing angiography will have diabetes mellitus (DM) [4].
- With the advent of poor lifestyle choices such as unhealthy diets and reduction in exercise, DM is likely to increase further [5].
- Chronic kidney disease (CKD), defined as an estimated glomerular filtration rate (eGFR) <60 mL/min/1.73 m^2, is a recognized global health problem [6] and is strongly associated with all-cause and cardiovascular mortality [7].
- In 2014 CKD was estimated to have a prevalence of 6.1% of the population in England [8] and about 10% of the population in the USA [9].
- CKD is frequently encountered in ACS patients, with a prevalence of 30.5% in those presenting with an ST-elevation myocardial infarction (STEMI) and 42.9% with a non-ST-elevation myocardial infarction (NSTEMI) [10].

S. Omar · O. Alsanjari · A. de Belder (✉)
Sussex Cardiac Centre, Royal Sussex County Hospital, Brighton and Sussex University Hospitals NHS Trust, Brighton, UK
e-mail: samiomar@doctors.org.uk;
osama.alsanjari@bsuh.nhs.uk;
Adam.deBelder@bsuh.nhs.uk

© Springer International Publishing AG, part of Springer Nature 2018
A. Myat et al. (eds.), *The Interventional Cardiology Training Manual*,
https://doi.org/10.1007/978-3-319-71635-0_21

Appropriateness—the Burden of Comorbidities in the Elderly

- The elderly are a different cohort of patient—they carry hazards from deteriorating vision, hearing, musculoskeletal, renal, cerebral, and cognitive function [11–13].
- When discussing prognostic significance, at what age does this become irrelevant? The resolution of cardiac symptoms with successful intervention may have a limited impact on the overall burden of other morbidities.
- When considering the option of invasive or surgical intervention in the older age group, it is important to emphasize that any favorable impact on their clinical outcome and quality of life will be limited only to the resolution of their cardiac symptoms [14–16].
- There is an age-related decline in cognition with an increasing likelihood of dementia with increasing age [11–13]. It is a difficult area—these matters are rarely binary, and the rate of decline can be very variable, but we think it would be universally accepted that invasive cardiac interventions in patients with dementia would rarely be appropriate.
- This can raise challenges in the acute setting, when patients require emergency angioplasty for STEMI or emergency pacing, when the opportunity to discuss the broader context is not available and could well lead to inappropriate procedures.
- The default position is to perform the intervention for the immediate relief of symptoms, but there are occasions where the value of the intervention to quality of life is negligible.

Clinical Presentation

- The elderly may not present with classical exertional or unstable angina pain, making the diagnosis a challenge. Often, patients presenting with unstable cardiac pain have other plausible explanations such as paroxysmal atrial fibrillation or other tachy/brady arrhythmias.

- Elevated cardiac troponins from such causes further make the correct diagnosis difficult.
- Stable angina may simply present as breathlessness on exertion, also commonly seen in patients with DM. Consequently, both these groups of patients can present later in the disease process [17].
- This is somewhat replicated in the CKD population, which have a reduction in chest pain intensity and frequency with declining renal function [18].
- ECG changes in the context of renal-related metabolic derangement poses a further challenge to diagnosis [19].
- Cardiac troponins used to risk stratify and guide treatment [20] in the majority of patients is difficult in CKD as these patients have persistently elevated levels, often misinterpreted as an acute coronary event. This persistence of circulating troponin is related to a combination of chronic nonischemic cardiac injury and poor renal clearance of the protein [21].
- In CKD patients, a troponin rise of 20% or more from baseline within 9 h is suggestive of an ischemic insult, necessitating suspicion of a coronary event [22]. A systematic review attempted to shed further light on this conundrum but concluded that a rise in troponin levels can aid in prognostication but the diagnostic utility was limited due to variations in sensitivity and specificity of the different assays and methodologies used [23].
- Revascularization strategies for patients with stable angina and ACS are based on multiple trials and are coalesced within multiple guideline recommendations from various national and international associations [24–26]. These trials are based on patients with a mean age of about 60 years.
- There are many subgroups of patients that benefit from surgical revascularization, with evidence for improved survival, but when it comes to the prospect of an octogenarian undergoing surgery, it is the morbidity and recovery that are the main stumbling blocks. For example, permanent stroke is much more likely in octogenarian patients undergoing CABG when compared with PCI (2.84% vs. 0.57%) [27],

so many of these patients undergo percutaneous coronary intervention as a suitable alternative.

- It is unknown if treatment strategies in patients with CKD are comparable to those undertaken in patients with normal renal function as the former group are either underrepresented [28] or excluded altogether [29] from the majority of the large trials. Hence, they are less likely to receive evidence-based treatment [10].
- Although the TIME trial is dated, it stands out as the only randomized controlled trial comparing medical therapy to invasive management for elderly patients with stable angina. A relatively small number of patients (305 patients >75 years) with symptomatic chronic stable angina were randomized to invasive investigation and treatment (PCI or CABG) or optimal medical therapy. The treatment group at 6 months had better symptom relief and quality of life, in addition to having less major events when compared to the medical arm (49% vs. 19%) [30].

Challenges of Complex Coronary Anatomy

- The older patient is more likely to have multi-vessel disease, calcified and tortuous coronary anatomy, chronic total occlusions, poor left ventricular (LV) function, renal impairment, and concomitant valvular disease.
- Tortuous vessels are also seen more frequently in the elderly population and those with CKD. This can provide unwelcome resistance to optimal stenting. The passage of a rigid tube around tight corners can prove problematic in some cases. Improvements in stent design, stiffer wires, and mother and child catheters have allowed resolution of most of these hurdles, but occasionally calcified tortuous angles remain defiant to stent placement.
- Fortunately, there is little coronary disease that cannot be treated by percutaneous means. The remarkable technological advances allow the modern interventional operator to deal with obstructive calcium, rigid tortuosity,

Table 21.1 Factors more prevalent in diabetic patients [4, 32–35]

Lesion characteristics
• Smaller vessel size
• Longer lesions
• Larger plaque burden with more diffuse disease
• More likely to have chronic total occlusions
Other negative systemic effects
• Higher platelet reactivity leading to a pro-thrombotic state
• Intimal hyperplasia with endothelial dysfunction
• Vascular matrix deposition
• Negative remodelling

challenging left main coronary anatomy, and chronic total occlusions, with little collateral complication [15].

- Analysis of the UK PCI database (BCIS/NICOR) show that major adverse cardiovascular event (MACE) rates for elderly patients in stable angina are low and compare favorably to a younger cohort. Often the function of intervention is resolution of difficult symptoms, and pursuing strategies for longer term mortality benefit, when one is already over 80 is difficult to justify, particularly when the intervention involves major heart surgery. There is a small literature base on highly selective patients having good mortality results from cardiac surgery, but it is often the morbidity of surgery, which leaves the older patient reeling [31].
- A combination of adverse lesion characteristics and other negative systemic effects in DM result in increased rates of early and late stent thrombosis as well as higher restenosis rates (Table 21.1) [36].
- If restenosis does occur in the diabetic patient, it is more likely to result in total occlusion, MI and/or LV dysfunction compared to those without DM [37].

Vascular Calcification

- Vascular calcification is a complex and poorly understood biological phenomenon—it is more common in patients with hypertension, diabetes, renal impairment and increases with age, and there is some data that coronary calcification is an independent predictor of mortality [38].

- Any interventional operator with a sizeable octogenarian patient group will need to be adept at managing the heavily calcified artery.
- The reduction in wall compliance can lead to inadequate lumen expansion with incomplete stent apposition leading to increased rates of stent thrombosis, and the requirement for target lesion revascularization.
- Lesion preparation with rotational atherectomy has reduced these unwelcome complications but there remains a slight noise of morbidity [39, 40].
- In a recent analysis of over 2000 patients undergoing rotational atherectomy (RA) prior to stenting within the UK, there was less procedural success when compared with a cohort of patients not requiring RA (90.3% vs. 94.6%, $p < 0.001$) and more frequent complications (9.7% vs. 5.4%, $p < 0.001$). After 2.4 ± 1.2 years follow-up, there was slightly poorer survival for patients undergoing RA even after adjustment for adverse variables and following propensity analysis [41].
- Investigation of the radial and brachial arteries of CKD patients without DM during fistula formation pre-dialysis demonstrated significant intimal hyperplasia and significantly higher calcium deposition, which in turn correlated with increased arterial stiffness. These findings are unlikely to be dissimilar from those encountered in the coronary vascular bed. All factors must be considered when undertaking PCI in this cohort of patients.
- Thus, patients with CKD are likely to have stiffer, calcified, and more diffusely diseased coronary arteries; issues and complexities need to be taken into consideration when preparing to undertake percutaneous treatment of their coronary disease.
- As most MIs are precipitated by unstable plaques, which in many cases are not significantly stenotic (<50%) lesions on angiography, coupled with the higher burden of coronary artery disease (CAD) in patients with CKD, an interventional strategy aimed

at treating the significant stenosis alone is unlikely to reduce the risk of MIs in the CKD cohort [42].

- In addition to more calcific coronary disease, which is likely to require rotablation, CKD patients are also more likely to have chronic total occlusions.
- A recent retrospective analysis of data collected prospectively suggested that CTO PCI in the hands of a skilled operator and on patients with CKD had a high success rate of 89%, improving long-term prognosis without significantly increasing the risk of contrast-induced nephropathy (CIN) [43].

Adjuvant Drug Therapies

- With age, diagnoses accumulate and the drug list grows. This is particularly so for cardiovascular conditions where optimal management for heart failure (ACE inhibitors, beta-blockers, aldosterone antagonists, diuretics), atherosclerosis (antiplatelets, statins), cardiac revascularization (dual antiplatelet therapy), atrial fibrillation (anticoagulants) all involve the prescription of multiple agents [15, 44].
- The management of cardiac disease within the older age group is riddled with the conflict of lean prescribing, in an effort to cause fewer interactions and side effects, against evidence-based prescribing of high doses of multiple agents [45].
- However, many of the trials influencing our decision-making in cardiovascular medicine are based on populations with a mean age in their early 60s, older age being a common exclusion criteria for most trials because of the increased possibility of events, which may be unrelated to the trial question. Thankfully, there are trials emerging investigating the role of medical intervention in the older age group, which will be invaluable in guiding future disease modification.
- This issue is also seen in CKD where there is limited randomized data pertaining to the use of beta-blockers and statins in ACS as these

patients were often also excluded from the landmark studies [46–50].

- Multiple observational studies have validated and support the beneficial effects of beta-blockers [46–48]. Atenolol, which is renally excreted, requires dose adjustment in this patient group.
- There is conflicting data on statins for primary prevention in CKD patients [51–53]. The large SHARP study, which included patients with CKD both on and off dialysis, did however demonstrate a benefit of the combination of simvastatin and ezetimibe [52].
- Patients with CKD not taking statins overall have poorer outcomes [54].

- Angiotensin converting enzyme inhibitors (ACEi) are recommended in patients with ACS and left ventricular ejection fraction (LVEF) <40% including patients with concomitant CKD, unless contraindicated [55, 56].
  - In patients intolerant of ACEi, angiotensin receptor blockers (ARB) should be used as a substitute [55, 56].
  - Regretfully these guidelines are not followed in patients with CKD due to concerns of worsening renal function and hyperkalemia [57].
  - This should not discourage the clinician from instigating optimal treatment. Close monitoring of renal function is of course mandatory.

Antiplatelets and Anticoagulants

- Patients with diabetes mellitus and NSTEMI have been identified as being at higher risk of MACE partly due to high platelet reactivity [34]. The use of antiplatelet agents in this cohort of patients is therefore imperative.
- Aspirin should be initiated as soon as ACS is suspected in CKD patients and continued indefinitely unless complications or contraindications to the specific therapy arise [55]. This recommendation stands despite the exclusion of CKD patients from the original trials and their propensity to bleeding and risk

of anemia. The recommendations are based on a meta-analysis of the CKD cohort in 287 randomized trials [58].

- The use of $P2Y_{12}$ receptor inhibitors in CKD patients is more contentious. This stems from their underrepresentation in the early clopidogrel trials [59]. Later trials however did suggest that clopidogrel was less efficacious as renal function declined [60, 61].
- Prasugrel was found to be more efficacious in patients with CKD [62] and ticagrelor was shown to have greater efficacy and a lower bleeding risk profile [63], which suggests that these drugs may be a better choice when considering dual antiplatelet therapy in patients with CKD.
- Although the use of the glycoprotein IIb/IIIa receptor antagonist (GPI) abciximab demonstrated significant reduction in target vessel revascularization and MACE in patients with diabetes after PCI [64], the advent of newer oral antiplatelet drugs, use of radial access, and third generation drug-eluting stents (DES) have meant the blanket use of these drugs is no longer required but may be required on a case-by-case basis [65].
- There are concerns regarding the increased risk of bleeding when GPI are combined with DAPT in patients with CKD.
  - Tirofiban and eptifibatide are eliminated via renal clearance, so their use and dose needs to be adjusted according to renal function.
  - Abciximab on the other hand does not rely on renal clearance and no dose adjustment is required. It does however cause irreversible binding and therefore longer duration of action, which may increase the risk of bleeding.
- Unfractionated heparin is only minimally excreted via the kidneys. However there is only nominal data available from the early ACS trials for patients with concomitant CKD.
- Enoxaparin is the most widely studied low molecular weight heparin (LMWH) in the setting of ACS. The guidelines recommend its use in ACS [56] despite a significant reliance on renal excretion (~ 40%).

- Fondaparinux is contraindicated in patients with CKD and an eGFR <30 as its excretion is completely reliant on renal clearance [66]. However, in a study that compared the use of enoxaparin against fondaparinux in patients with eGFR of 30–59 fondaparinux was found to be superior in the composite endpoints of death, MI, refractory ischemia, and bleeding at 30 days [67].

Contrast-Induced Nephropathy (CIN)

- Is defined as a relative increase of >25% or an absolute increase of >0.5 mg/dL in serum creatinine [68].
- Originally thought to occur 24–48 h post contrast exposure [68]; however, some data suggest that the peak rise can occur 3–6 days post exposure [69].
- Is associated with increased morbidity and mortality, and affects an estimated 20–30% of patients, particularly those with diabetes or previous renal impairment [70, 71].
- There is a direct association with the development of CIN and an increase in adverse outcomes [72]. Hence, every precaution should be taken to reduce the incidence of CIN to which patients with CKD are most susceptible.

Methods to Reduce Risk of CIN
(Table 21.2)

- Although some studies suggest that the use of N-acetyl-cysteine (NAC) protects against CIN [73, 74], others have not [75].
- Good hydration pre and post procedure is more likely to reduce the incidence of CIN [76]. This is widely recommended, but the recent AMACING trial showed no difference between prehydration and non prehydration groups; in

Table 21.2 Methods to reduce risk of CIN

Reduce contrast load, e.g., IVUS guided PCI, be frugal during angiograms
Use of IOCM instead of LOCM
Prehydration with intravenous fluids
Consider use of NAC
Consider pre-procedure statin
Consider AVERT device

fact there was potential harm due to fluid overload [77]. Furthermore, this study also excluded higher risk patients with an eGFR <30.
- The administration of statins pre-procedure significantly reduced the incidence of CIN and the need for post procedure dialysis [78]. The volume of contrast medium used has been shown to be an independent factor in the development of CIN [79]
- A device known as AVERT has been shown to significantly reduce the quantity of radiographic dye without reduction in image quality during PCI [80]. Regretfully however, this did not translate to a significant reduction in the development of CIN or an improvement in outcomes [81]. A post hoc analysis did, however, suggest that patients with moderate CKD (eGFR 40–60) demonstrated a significant reduction in the incidence of CIN.
- Several trials have demonstrated that iso-osmolar contrast medium (IOCM) was associated with lower incidence of CIN and fewer CV events when compared to a low-osmolar contrast medium (LOCM) [79, 81].
- RECOVER was a prospective randomized study comparing the nephrotoxicity of visipaque (iodixanol), a nonionic, dimeric IOCM to that of hexabrix (ioxaglate), a LOCM, conducted on 300 patients with a creatinine clearance (CrCl) of <60 mL/min undergoing coronary angiography with or without PCI. The primary endpoint was the development of CIN. The incidence of CIN was significantly lower with iodixanol compared to ioxaglate (7.9% vs. 17%; $p = 0.021$). Furthermore, the incidence of CIN was significantly lower with iodixanol in patients with severe renal impairment, concomitant diabetes, or those given ≥140 mL of contrast ($p = 0.023$, $p = 0.041$, $p = 0.038$, respectively) [79].
- Similar findings were demonstrated in a similar randomized double-blind study, where the incidence of CIN with iodixanol was significantly lower when compared to the use of iopromide (5.7% vs. 16.7%; $p = 0.011$) [82].
- In patients with advanced CKD and at high risk of CIN, PCI can be preformed effectively and without complications using IVUS and physiological guidance negating the need for contrast [83].

Which Stent: Bare Metal or Drug-Eluting?

- The emergence of first generation drug-eluting stents (SIRIUS and TAXUS) significantly reduced the incidence of restenosis in patients with DM when compared with BMS [84, 85].
- Initial trials using paclitaxel-eluting stents in patients with DM suggested a marked diminution of clinical restenosis but subsequent trials have shown inferior outcomes when compared with newer generation DES [86, 87].
- Both the neo-intimal response and the outcomes of the use of second generation DES with everolimus and zotarolimus have been found to be comparable in patients with DM [88, 89].
- There are a number of theoretical concerns about using drug-eluting stent technology in the octogenarian cohort.
  - Potential problems with compliance with dual antiplatelet therapy might increase stent thrombosis rate.
  - The increased possibility for significant bleeding complications with the longer duration of DAPT would suggest that bare metal stenting might have a role. This hypothesis was tested in the multicenter prospective XIMA trial comparing DES and BMS in an unselected group of 800 patients and found similar rates of all-cause death, stroke, and major hemorrhage, but a reduced incidence of MI and target vessel revascularization in the DES group [90]. The trial also identified the problems of doing trials in this age group as the non-cardiovascular death rates in the DES group were higher than in the BMS group skewing the final analysis.
  - More recently, the LEADERS FREE investigators compared a polymer-free Biolimus A9 drug-coated stent versus a bare metal stent in 2466 patients considered at high risk of bleeding, many of whom were elderly. What was unique about the trial is that both arms took only 1 month of dual antiplatelet therapy. There was a reduction in the primary safety endpoint for the coated stent (9.4% vs. 12.9%) with a significant reduction in target lesion revascularization as well [91].

- The SENIOR trial is comparing a 3rd generation drug-eluting stent versus a bare metal stent in 1200 patients 75 years and over undergoing coronary stenting. Both arms will receive the same length of DAPT: 1 month for stable angina and 6 months for ACS. The final results will be available in 2017 [92].
- These trials have broken new territory with inclusion of an increasing number of elderly patients helping define evidence-based decisions—it looks increasingly likely that even in this age group, the bare metal stent will be confined to history.

Acute Coronary Syndromes

NSTEMI

- The main trials that steered management of patients to an invasive strategy with a view to revascularization had a mean age of 61 years, and the concept that all patients should have coronary angiography and revascularization, if appropriate, is enshrined in cardiac practice.
- A meta-analysis has shown that the benefits were greater in the older patients within the various trials. But where does the benefit gain start to flatten out? Octogenarians are woefully underrepresented in the trial data, and where there is data, very little comes from randomized control trials, [93] and most come from large registry data sets [94, 95].
- The NSTEACS, European registries document roughly a third (27- 34%) of patients are aged ≥75 years, but not more than 20% of all patients in recent trials. Even when elderly patients are recruited into clinical trials, they are highly selected, often having substantially less comorbidity than patients encountered in daily clinical practice.
- Mortality for those aged >75 is twice that of those aged <75 and the prevalence of ACS-related complications such as heart failure, bleeding, stroke, renal failure, and infections markedly increases with age. In addition the elderly patient is less likely to be treated invasively [96].

- However, a subgroup analysis of the Treat angina with Aggrastat and determine Cost of Therapy with an Invasive or Conservative Strategy (TACTICS)-TIMI 18 trial, found that patients >75 years of age with NSTE-ACS derived the largest benefit, in terms of both relative and absolute risk reductions, from an invasive strategy at the cost of an increase in risk of major bleeding and need for transfusions [93].
- A recent important publication (After Eighty study) randomized 457 patients to early coronary angiography and revascularization if appropriate ($n = 229$) or optimal medical therapy ($n = 228$) [97]. The primary outcome (a composite of myocardial infarction, need for urgent revascularization, stroke and death) was less likely in the invasive arm (40.6%) than the conservative arm (61.4%), mainly driven by MI and urgent revascularization. There was no difference in mortality. This trial had high event rates in both groups, and the binary nature of the randomization meant that it was always likely the invasive arm would win. The real question is whether a more tailored approach to identifying the beneficiaries of revascularization would prevent the blanket approach of angiography for all.
- There are ongoing randomized prospective multicenter trials attempting to answer this very question. The Revascularisation or Medical Therapy in Elderly Patients with acute angina syndromes (the RINCAL study Clinical Trials. gov, Identifier NCT02086019) is in active recruitment and randomizes octogenarian patients with NSTEMI to initial conservative management with a view to invasive assessment and treatment if conservative measures fail versus invasive assessment for all, thus including angiography as part of the management whatever the clinical circumstance. The primary endpoint is death from cardiovascular cause and myocardial infarction at 1 year.
- An early revascularization strategy in the management of all patients with NSTEMI is clearly superior to a more conservative strategy [98]; an early revascularization strategy is advocated even more in patients

with coexistent DM [20]. However, the optimal revascularization strategy of PCI vs. CABG remains unclear.
- DM in itself is a major procedural risk factor in either form of revascularization (PCI or CABG) [99].
- DM is a predictor of poor outcome in patients presenting with ACS and treated with PCI [100]. A pooled analysis of 6 studies comparing the effects of DM on the frequency of adverse events (over 1 year) in patients with ACS and undergoing PCI demonstrated that patients presenting with STEMI and concomitant DM had the highest rates of all-cause mortality, followed by those presenting with NSTEMI and DM, then those with STEMI without DM, and finally those with NSTEMI and no DM (13.4%, 10.3%, 6.4% and 4.4%, respectively) [101].

STEMI

- Immediate PCI for patients with STEMI is now the treatment of choice, if appropriate expertise is available to perform the procedure in a timely manner. Older patients have more to gain from primary angioplasty, but they can provide a challenge to the interventionalist—they are more likely to be sicker, have less ventricular function to work with, have an increased likelihood of significant comorbidity, and have more challenging coronary anatomy to deal with.
- The ESC guidelines on the management of AMI in patients presenting with persistent ST-segment elevation offer no specific guidance for octogenarians, other than to acknowledge that they are at higher risk of side effects from medical treatment, including the risk of bleeding with antiplatelet agents and anticoagulants, and also hypotension, bradycardia, and renal failure. In addition to the intrinsic bleeding risk of the elderly, as a group older patients are more frequently exposed to excessive doses of antithrombotic drugs that are excreted by the kidney [8, 20].

- For what it is worth, our practice is to activate the primary angioplasty team for all STEMI patients, and the only time to step away from intervening urgently is when the patient has arrived in the catheter laboratory and been clinically assessed.

CABG Versus PCI in Multivessel Coronary Disease

- The BARI trial first suggested that patients with DM were better served by CABG rather than percutaneous balloon angioplasty as long as they received at least 1 arterial conduit [102]. Despite advances over the last three decades from simple balloon angioplasty to 2nd generation drug-eluting stents a meta-analysis of 14 studies comparing multivessel PCI to CABG in patients with DM suggested that the outcomes have not significantly changed with a persistence of 30% all-cause mortality favoring CABG [103].
- The underpowered CARDIA was designed to compare PCI (a mixture of bare metal and first generation DES) to CABG in patients with diabetes and multivessel coronary disease. There was little difference in death and CVA, but the requirement for further revascularization and the incidence of MI was increased in the PCI group [104].
- There is evidence for less morbidity associated with PCI—the ACUITY trial demonstrated that patients suffering from DM and presenting with ACS and concomitant multivessel disease had less bleeding and AKI when treated with PCI rather than CABG. The rates of MI, stroke, and death were comparable. PCI was only inferior with regard to the need for repeat target vessel revascularization [105].
- The much larger FREEDOM study, a two-arm superiority trial designed to pit PCI against CABG in the diabetic patient cohort in the hope of settling this debate, confirmed the better longer term outcomes with surgery for the diabetic cohort albeit at the expense of greater immediate comorbidity [106].

- The SYNTAX score II study intimated that it may not be the presence of DM per se that differentiates the outcomes between PCI and CABG, postulating that associated conditions such as advanced CAD and renal dysfunction that impact the perceived better outcomes with CABG [107].

Conclusion

Our practice has evolved to become comfortable in routinely treating an aging population, together with their rising comorbidities, such as DM and CKD. Whether the patients' have one or all three of these challenges, there is a significant overlap in their coronary pathology, optimal treatment plan, and long-term outcomes with percutaneous revascularization. They commonly have an increase in the prevalence of calcific/complex atherosclerotic disease, tortuous anatomy, and risk of CIN. The evolution of second and third generation DES has resulted in significantly improved patient outcomes in this cohort. Results observed from more recent studies is beginning to show that these high risk patient groups which we have discussed equally benefit from treatment of their symptomatic coronary disease, comparably to those studied in the landmark PCI trials which often excluded CKD patients and the elderly.

References

1. Centers for Disease Control and Prevention (CDC). Trends in aging—United States and worldwide. MMWR Morb Mortal Wkly Rep. 2003;52(6): 101–4, 106.
2. Rich MW. Epidemiology, clinical features, and prognosis of acute myocardial infarction in the elderly. Am J Geriatr Cardiol. 2006;15(1):7–11. quiz 12
3. Kozlov KL, Bogachev AA. Coronary revascularization in the elderly with stable angina. J Geriatr Cardiol. 2015;12(5):555–68.
4. Smith SC Jr, et al. Prevention conference VI: diabetes and cardiovascular disease: writing group VI: revascularization in diabetic patients. Circulation. 2002;105(18):e165–9.
5. Zimmet P, et al. Diabetes mellitus statistics on prevalence and mortality: facts and fallacies. Nat Rev Endocrinol. 2016;12(10):616–22.

6. Couser WG, et al. The contribution of chronic kidney disease to the global burden of major noncommunicable diseases. Kidney Int. 2011;80(12):1258–70.

7. Chronic Kidney Disease Prognosis, Consortium, et al. Association of estimated glomerular filtration rate and albuminuria with all-cause and cardiovascular mortality in general population cohorts: a collaborative meta-analysis. Lancet. 2010;375(9731): 2073–81.

8. England PH. Chronic Kidney Disease (CKD) prevalence model – YHPHO. http://www.yhpho.org.uk/ resource/view.aspx?RID=204692. 2014.

9. Promotion, N.C.f.C.D.P.a.H. National chronic kidney disease fact sheet. 2014.

10. Fox CS, et al. Use of evidence-based therapies in short-term outcomes of ST-segment elevation myocardial infarction and non-ST-segment elevation myocardial infarction in patients with chronic kidney disease: a report from the National Cardiovascular Data Acute Coronary Treatment and Intervention Outcomes Network registry. Circulation. 2010; 121(3):357–65.

11. Linden T, et al. Visual neglect and cognitive impairment in elderly patients late after stroke. Acta Neurol Scand. 2005;111(3):163–8.

12. Deal JA, et al. Hearing impairment and incident dementia and cognitive decline in older adults: the health ABC study. J Gerontol A Biol Sci Med Sci. 2017;72(5):703–9.

13. Lo Coco D, Lopez G, Corrao S. Cognitive impairment and stroke in elderly patients. Vasc Health Risk Manag. 2016;12:105–16.

14. Kaehler J, Meinertz T, Hamm CW. Coronary interventions in the elderly. Heart. 2006;92(8):1167–71.

15. Task Force on Myocardial Revascularization of the European Society of Cardiology, et al. Guidelines on myocardial revascularization. Eur Heart J. 2010; 31(20):2501–55.

16. de Boer SP, et al. Mortality and morbidity reduction by primary percutaneous coronary intervention is independent of the patient's age. JACC Cardiovasc Interv. 2010;3(3):324–31.

17. Umachandran V, et al. The perception of angina in diabetes: relation to somatic pain threshold and autonomic function. Am Heart J. 1991;121(6 Pt 1): 1649–54.

18. Szummer K, et al. Relation between renal function, presentation, use of therapies and in-hospital complications in acute coronary syndrome: data from the SWEDEHEART register. J Intern Med. 2010;268(1):40–9.

19. Herzog CA, et al. Clinical characteristics of dialysis patients with acute myocardial infarction in the United States: a collaborative project of the United States Renal Data System and the National Registry of Myocardial Infarction. Circulation. 2007;116(13): 1465–72.

20. Authors/Task Force, members, et al. 2014 ESC/ EACTS Guidelines on myocardial revascularization: The Task Force on Myocardial Revascularization of the European Society of Cardiology (ESC) and the European Association for Cardio-Thoracic Surgery (EACTS)Developed with the special contribution of the European Association of Percutaneous Cardiovascular Interventions (EAPCI). Eur Heart J. 2014;35(37):2541–619.

21. Newby LK, et al. ACCF 2012 expert consensus document on practical clinical considerations in the interpretation of troponin elevations: a report of the American College of Cardiology Foundation task force on Clinical Expert Consensus Documents. J Am Coll Cardiol. 2012;60(23):2427–63.

22. Group, N.W, et al. National Academy of Clinical Biochemistry laboratory medicine practice guidelines: use of cardiac troponin and B-type natriuretic peptide or N-terminal proB-type natriuretic peptide for etiologies other than acute coronary syndromes and heart failure. Clin Chem. 2007;53(12):2086–96.

23. Stacy SR, et al. Role of troponin in patients with chronic kidney disease and suspected acute coronary syndrome: a systematic review. Ann Intern Med. 2014;161(7):502–12.

24. Hannan EL, et al. Appropriateness of coronary revascularization for patients without acute coronary syndromes. J Am Coll Cardiol. 2012;59(21):1870–6.

25. Graham MM, et al. Quality of life after coronary revascularization in the elderly. Eur Heart J. 2006;27(14):1690–8.

26. Cohen DJ, et al. Quality of life after PCI with drug-eluting stents or coronary-artery bypass surgery. N Engl J Med. 2011;364(11):1016–26.

27. Dacey LJ, et al. Long-term survival after surgery versus percutaneous intervention in octogenarians with multivessel coronary disease. Ann Thorac Surg. 2007;84(6):1904–11. discussion 1904-11

28. Coca SG, et al. Underrepresentation of renal disease in randomized controlled trials of cardiovascular disease. JAMA. 2006;296(11):1377–84.

29. Charytan D, Kuntz RE. The exclusion of patients with chronic kidney disease from clinical trials in coronary artery disease. Kidney Int. 2006;70(11): 2021–30.

30. Investigators T. Trial of invasive versus medical therapy in elderly patients with chronic symptomatic coronary-artery disease (TIME): a randomized trial. Lancet. 2001;358(9286):951–7.

31. Alexander KP, et al. Outcomes of cardiac surgery in patients age ≥80 years: results from the National Cardiovascular Network. J Am Coll Cardiol. 2000; 35(3):731–8.

32. Aronson D, Bloomgarden Z, Rayfield EJ. Potential mechanisms promoting restenosis in diabetic patients. J Am Coll Cardiol. 1996;27(3):528–35.

33. West NE, et al. Clinical and angiographic predictors of restenosis after stent deployment in diabetic patients. Circulation. 2004;109(7):867–73.

34. De Servi S, et al. Relationship between diabetes, platelet reactivity, and the SYNTAX score to one-year clinical outcome in patients with non-ST-segment elevation acute coronary syndrome

undergoing percutaneous coronary intervention. EuroIntervention. 2016;12(3):312–8.

35. Eckel RH, et al. Prevention conference VI: diabetes and cardiovascular disease: writing group II: pathogenesis of atherosclerosis in diabetes. Circulation. 2002;105(18):e138–43.

36. Holmes DR Jr, et al. Restenosis after percutaneous transluminal coronary angioplasty (PTCA): a report from the PTCA Registry of the National Heart, Lung, and Blood Institute. Am J Cardiol. 1984; 53(12):77C–81C.

37. Mak KH, Faxon DP. Clinical studies on coronary revascularization in patients with type 2 diabetes. Eur Heart J. 2003;24(12):1087–103.

38. Schenker MP, et al. Interrelation of coronary calcification, myocardial ischemia, and outcomes in patients with intermediate likelihood of coronary artery disease: a combined positron emission tomography/computed tomography study. Circulation. 2008;117(13):1693–700.

39. Abdel-Wahab M, et al. High-speed rotational atherectomy before paclitaxel-eluting stent implantation in complex calcified coronary lesions: the randomized ROTAXUS (Rotational Atherectomy Prior to Taxus Stent Treatment for Complex Native Coronary Artery Disease) trial. JACC Cardiovasc Interv. 2013;6(1):10–9.

40. Parikh K, et al. Safety and feasibility of orbital atherectomy for the treatment of calcified coronary lesions: the ORBIT I trial. Catheter Cardiovasc Interv. 2013;81(7):1134–9.

41. Cockburn J, et al. Contemporary clinical outcomes of patients treated with or without rotational coronary atherectomy—an analysis of the UK central cardiac audit database. Int J Cardiol. 2014;170(3):381–7.

42. Charytan DM, et al. Angiographic characteristics of coronary arterial segments progressing to myocardial infarction in patients with and without chronic kidney disease. Clin Exp Nephrol. 2013;17(2):232–9.

43. Liu Y, et al. Percutaneous coronary intervention for chronic total occlusion improved prognosis in patients with renal insufficiency at high risk of contrast-induced nephropathy. Sci Rep. 2016; 6:21426.

44. McMurray JJ, et al. ESC Guidelines for the diagnosis and treatment of acute and chronic heart failure 2012: The task force for the diagnosis and treatment of acute and chronic heart failure 2012 of the European Society of Cardiology. Developed in collaboration with the heart failure association (HFA) of the ESC. Eur Heart J. 2012;33(14): 1787–847.

45. Chrischilles EA, et al. Association between preadmission functional status and use and effectiveness of secondary prevention medications in elderly survivors of acute myocardial infarction. J Am Geriatr Soc. 2016;64(3):526–35.

46. Wright RS, et al. Acute myocardial infarction and renal dysfunction: a high-risk combination. Ann Intern Med. 2002;137(7):563–70.

47. Keough-Ryan TM, et al. Outcomes of acute coronary syndrome in a large Canadian cohort: impact of chronic renal insufficiency, cardiac interventions, and anemia. Am J Kidney Dis. 2005;46(5):845–55.

48. Berger AK, Duval S, Krumholz HM. Aspirin, beta-blocker, and angiotensin-converting enzyme inhibitor therapy in patients with end-stage renal disease and an acute myocardial infarction. J Am Coll Cardiol. 2003;42(2):201–8.

49. de Lemos JA, et al. Early intensive vs a delayed conservative simvastatin strategy in patients with acute coronary syndromes: phase Z of the A to Z trial. JAMA. 2004;292(11):1307–16.

50. Scandinavian Simvastatin Survival Study Group. Randomised trial of cholesterol lowering in 4444 patients with coronary heart disease: the Scandinavian Simvastatin Survival Study (4S). Lancet. 1994; 344(8934):1383–9.

51. Holdaas H, et al. Effect of fluvastatin on cardiac outcomes in renal transplant recipients: a multicentre, randomized, placebo-controlled trial. Lancet. 2003;361(9374):2024–31.

52. Baigent C, et al. The effects of lowering LDL cholesterol with simvastatin plus ezetimibe in patients with chronic kidney disease (study of heart and renal protection): a randomized placebo-controlled trial. Lancet. 2011;377(9784):2181–92.

53. Fellstrom BC, et al. Rosuvastatin and cardiovascular events in patients undergoing hemodialysis. N Engl J Med. 2009;360(14):1395–407.

54. Lim SY, et al. Effect on short- and long-term major adverse cardiac events of statin treatment in patients with acute myocardial infarction and renal dysfunction. Am J Cardiol. 2012;109(10):1425–30.

55. O'Gara PT, et al. 2013 ACCF/AHA guideline for the management of ST-elevation myocardial infarction: a report of the American College of Cardiology Foundation/American Heart Association Task Force on Practice Guidelines. Circulation. 2013;127(4): e362–425.

56. Jneid H, et al. 2012 ACCF/AHA focused update of the guideline for the management of patients with unstable angina/non-ST-elevation myocardial infarction (updating the 2007 guideline and replacing the 2011 focused update): a report of the American College of Cardiology Foundation/American Heart Association Task Force on Practice Guidelines. J Am Coll Cardiol. 2012;60(7):645–81.

57. Ahmed A, et al. A propensity score analysis of the impact of angiotensin-converting enzyme inhibitors on long-term survival of older adults with heart failure and perceived contraindications. Am Heart J. 2005; 149(4):737–43.

58. Antithrombotic Trialists C. Collaborative meta-analysis of randomized trials of antiplatelet therapy for prevention of death, myocardial infarction, and stroke in high risk patients. BMJ. 2002;324(7329):71–86.

59. Yusuf S, et al. Effects of clopidogrel in addition to aspirin in patients with acute coronary syndromes

without ST-segment elevation. N Engl J Med. 2001; 345(7):494–502.

60. Best PJ, et al. The efficacy and safety of short- and long-term dual antiplatelet therapy in patients with mild or moderate chronic kidney disease: results from the clopidogrel for the Reduction of Events During Observation (CREDO) trial. Am Heart J. 2008;155(4):687–93.

61. Sabatine MS, et al. Addition of clopidogrel to aspirin and fibrinolytic therapy for myocardial infarction with ST-segment elevation. N Engl J Med. 2005;352(12):1179–89.

62. Wiviott SD, et al. Prasugrel versus clopidogrel in patients with acute coronary syndromes. N Engl J Med. 2007;357(20):2001–15.

63. Wallentin L, et al. Ticagrelor versus clopidogrel in patients with acute coronary syndromes. N Engl J Med. 2009;361(11):1045–57.

64. Marso SP, et al. Optimizing the percutaneous interventional outcomes for patients with diabetes mellitus: results of the EPISTENT (evaluation of platelet IIb/IIIa inhibitor for stenting trial) diabetic sub study. Circulation. 1999;100(25):2477–84.

65. Hillegass WB. Diabetes is not sufficient justification for IIb/IIIa use in percutaneous coronary intervention. Catheter Cardiovasc Interv. 2015;86(3):376–7.

66. Samama MM, Gerotziafas GT. Evaluation of the pharmacological properties and clinical results of the synthetic pentasaccharide (fondaparinux). Thromb Res. 2003;109(1):1–11.

67. Fifth Organization to Assess Strategies in Acute Ischemic Syndromes, Investigators, et al. Comparison of fondaparinux and enoxaparin in acute coronary syndromes. N Engl J Med. 2006;354(14):1464–76.

68. James MT, et al. Contrast-induced acute kidney injury and risk of adverse clinical outcomes after coronary angiography: a systematic review and meta-analysis. Circ Cardiovasc Interv. 2013;6(1):37–43.

69. Budano C, et al. Impact of contrast-induced acute kidney injury definition on clinical outcomes. Am Heart J. 2011;161(5):963–71.

70. Mehran R, et al. A simple risk score for prediction of contrast-induced nephropathy after percutaneous coronary intervention: development and initial validation. J Am Coll Cardiol. 2004;44(7):1393–9.

71. McCullough PA, et al. Contrast-Induced Nephropathy (CIN) consensus working panel: executive summary. Rev Cardiovasc Med. 2006;7(4):177–97.

72. Narula A, et al. Contrast-induced acute kidney injury after primary percutaneous coronary intervention: results from the HORIZONS-AMI substudy. Eur Heart J. 2014;35(23):1533–40.

73. Pezeshgi A, et al. Evaluation of the protective effect of N-acetylcysteine on contrast media nephropathy. J Renal Inj Prev. 2015;4(4):109–12.

74. Marenzi G, et al. N-acetylcysteine and contrast-induced nephropathy in primary angioplasty. N Engl J Med. 2006;354(26):2773–82.

75. Aslanger E, et al. Intrarenal application of N-acetylcysteine for the prevention of contrast medium-induced nephropathy in primary angioplasty. Coron Artery Dis. 2012;23(4):265–70.

76. Jurado-Roman A, et al. Role of hydration in contrast-induced nephropathy in patients who underwent primary percutaneous coronary intervention. Am J Cardiol. 2015;115(9):1174–8.

77. Nijssen EC, Rennenberg RJ, Nelemans PJ, et al. Prophylactic hydration to protect renal function from intravascular iodinated contrast material in patients at high risk of contrast-induced nephropathy (AMACING): a prospective, randomized, phase 3, controlled, open-label, non-inferiority trial. Lancet. 2017;389(10076):1312–22. https://doi.org/10.1016/S0140-6736(17)30057-0.

78. Khanal S, et al. Statin therapy reduces contrast-induced nephropathy: an analysis of contemporary percutaneous interventions. Am J Med. 2005;118(8):843–9.

79. Jo SH, et al. Renal toxicity evaluation and comparison between visipaque (iodixanol) and hexabrix (ioxaglate) in patients with renal insufficiency undergoing coronary angiography: the RECOVER study: a randomized controlled trial. J Am Coll Cardiol. 2006;48(5):924–30.

80. Kaye DM, et al. Reducing iodinated contrast volume by manipulating injection pressure during coronary angiography. Catheter Cardiovasc Interv. 2014;83(5):741–5.

81. Effect of the AVERT™ contrast modulation system on contrast dose reduction and acute kidney injury after coronary angiography and PCI, in EuroPCR. Paris. 2016.

82. Nie B, et al. A prospective, double-blind, randomized, controlled trial on the efficacy and cardiorenal safety of iodixanol vs. iopromide in patients with chronic kidney disease undergoing coronary angiography with or without percutaneous coronary intervention. Catheter Cardiovasc Interv. 2008;72(7):958–65.

83. Ali ZA, et al. Imaging- and physiology-guided percutaneous coronary intervention without contrast administration in advanced renal failure: a feasibility, safety, and outcome study. Eur Heart J. 2016;7(40):3090–5.

84. Moussa I, et al. Impact of sirolimus-eluting stents on outcome in diabetic patients: a SIRIUS (SIRolImUS-coated Bx velocity balloon-expandable stent in the treatment of patients with de novo coronary artery lesions) sub study. Circulation. 2004;109(19):2273–8.

85. Hermiller JB, et al. Outcomes with the polymer-based paclitaxel-eluting TAXUS stent in patients with diabetes mellitus: the TAXUS-IV trial. J Am Coll Cardiol. 2005;45(8):1172–9.

86. Dibra A, et al. Paclitaxel-eluting or sirolimus-eluting stents to prevent restenosis in diabetic patients. N Engl J Med. 2005;353(7):663–70.

87. Kaul U, et al. Paclitaxel-eluting versus everolimus-eluting coronary stents in diabetes. N Engl J Med. 2015;373(18):1709–19.

88. Park KW, et al. Everolimus-eluting Xience v/Promus versus zotarolimus-eluting resolute stents in patients with diabetes mellitus. JACC Cardiovasc Interv. 2014;7(5):471–81.

89. Won H, et al. Neointimal response to second-generation drug-eluting stents in diabetic patients with de-novo coronary lesions: intravascular ultrasound study. Coron Artery Dis. 2015;26(3):212–9.

90. de Belder A, et al. A prospective randomized trial of everolimus-eluting stents versus bare-metal stents in octogenarians: the XIMA trial (Xience or Vision Stents for the Management of Angina in the Elderly). J Am Coll Cardiol. 2014;63(14):1371–5.

91. Urban P, et al. Polymer-free drug-coated coronary stents in patients at high bleeding risk. N Engl J Med. 2015;373(21):2038–47.

92. Varenne O, et al. The SYNERGY II Everolimus elutiNg stent In patients Older than 75 years undergoing coronary Revascularization associated with a short dual antiplatelet therapy (SENIOR) trial: rationale and design of a large-scale randomized multicentre study. EuroIntervention. 2017;12(13):1614–22.

93. Bach RG, et al. The effect of routine, early invasive management on outcome for elderly patients with non-ST-segment elevation acute coronary syndromes. Ann Intern Med. 2004;141(3):186–95.

94. Barywani SB, et al. Acute coronary syndrome in octogenarians: association between percutaneous coronary intervention and long-term mortality. Clin Interv Aging. 2015;10:1547–53.

95. Fach A, et al. Comparison of outcomes of patients with ST-segment elevation myocardial infarction treated by primary percutaneous coronary intervention analyzed by age groups (<75, 75 to 85, and >85 years); (Results from the Bremen STEMI Registry). Am J Cardiol. 2015;116(12):1802–9.

96. Rosengren A, et al. Age, clinical presentation, and outcome of acute coronary syndromes in the Euroheart acute coronary syndrome survey. Eur Heart J. 2006;27(7):789–95.

97. Tegn N, Abdelnoor M, Aaberge L, et al. for the After Eighty study investigators. Invasive versus conservative strategy in patients aged 80 years or older with non-ST-elevstion myocardial infarction or unstable angina pectoris (after eighty study): an open-label randomized controlled trial. Lancet. 2016;387:1057–65.

98. Mehta SR, et al. Routine vs selective invasive strategies in patients with acute coronary syndromes: a collaborative meta-analysis of randomized trials. JAMA. 2005;293(23):2908–17.

99. Banning AP, et al. Diabetic and nondiabetic patients with left main and/or 3-vessel coronary artery disease: comparison of outcomes with cardiac surgery and paclitaxel-eluting stents. J Am Coll Cardiol. 2010;55(11):1067–75.

100. Ritsinger V, et al. High event rate after a first percutaneous coronary intervention in patients with diabetes mellitus: results from the Swedish coronary angiography and angioplasty registry. Circ Cardiovasc Interv. 2015;8(6):e002328.

101. Piccolo R, et al. Effect of diabetes mellitus on frequency of adverse events in patients with acute coronary syndromes undergoing percutaneous coronary intervention. Am J Cardiol. 2016;118(3):345–52.

102. Influence of diabetes on 5-year mortality and morbidity in a randomized trial comparing CABG and PTCA in patients with multivessel disease: the Bypass Angioplasty Revascularization Investigation (BARI). Circulation. 1997;96(6):1761–9.

103. Herbison P, Wong CK. Has the difference in mortality between percutaneous coronary intervention and coronary artery bypass grafting in people with heart disease and diabetes changed over the years? A systematic review and meta-regression. BMJ Open. 2015;5(12):e010055.

104. Kapur A, et al. Randomized comparison of percutaneous coronary intervention with coronary artery bypass grafting in diabetic patients. 1-year results of the CARDia (Coronary Artery Revascularization in Diabetes) trial. J Am Coll Cardiol. 2010;55(5):432–40.

105. Ben-Gal Y, et al. Surgical versus percutaneous coronary revascularization for multivessel disease in diabetic patients with non-ST-segment-elevation acute coronary syndrome: analysis from the Acute Catheterization and Early Intervention Triage Strategy trial. Circ Cardiovasc Interv. 2015;8(6):e002032.

106. Bansilal S, et al. The Future REvascularization Evaluation in patients with Diabetes mellitus: Optimal management of Multivessel disease (FREEDOM) trial: clinical and angiographic profile at study entry. Am Heart J. 2012;164(4):591–9.

107. Farooq V, et al. Anatomical and clinical characteristics to guide decision making between coronary artery bypass surgery and percutaneous coronary intervention for individual patients: development and validation of SYNTAX score II. Lancet. 2013;381(9867):639–50.

Stent Thrombosis

22

Javier Cuesta, Marcos García-Guimaraes,
Fernando Rivero, Teresa Bastante,
and Fernando Alfonso

About Us The Interventional Cardiology Unit of the Hospital Universitario de La Princesa in Madrid is devoted to excellence in patient care, under- and postgraduate teaching and clinical research. Diagnostic procedures, coronary interventions, pacemaker implantation, and structural heart procedures are performed by a team of experienced interventional cardiologists. The unit is fully integrated within the Cardiac Department where joint clinical and research meetings are held. Heart Team meetings with the cardiac surgery team are considered an important part of the clinical decision-making process for patients with complex coronary or valve disease. Students from the Universidad Autónoma de Madrid and cardiac registrars are trained in the Cardiac Department. Research is organized under the auspices of La Princesa Research Institute. The unit is mainly focused on clinical care but also in advancing knowledge in new interventional and diagnostic procedures. In particular, intracoronary imaging and physiology are areas of intensive research. In addition, mechanisms of stent failure also represent a major area of interest.

The team has participated in joint European efforts on stent thrombosis (PRESTIGE). In addition, the unit is leading and coordinating different nationwide studies on in-stent restenosis (The RIBS program). Original observational studies, prospective registries, and randomized clinical trials are being designed and developed to address different areas of clinical interest. Participation in multicenter international studies are also part of the research agenda. Research is considered indispensable to improve clinical practice and patient care.

Introduction

- Coronary stents constitute the default strategy during percutaneous coronary intervention (PCI) as they provide improved safety and efficacy compared with balloon angioplasty alone [1, 2].
- Stents reduce restenosis rates compared to balloon angioplasty predominantly as a result of a larger acute gain that translates into a greater minimal lumen diameter at follow-up. Although neointimal proliferation is increased after bare metal stent (BMS) implantation, eventually the net lumen gain at follow-up is larger than that obtained with balloon angioplasty.
- Drug-eluting stents (DES) significantly reduced neointimal proliferation and the need for

J. Cuesta · M. García-Guimaraes · F. Rivero
T. Bastante · F. Alfonso (✉)
Department of Cardiology, Hospital Universitario
de La Princesa, Universidad Autónoma de Madrid,
Madrid, Spain

© Springer International Publishing AG, part of Springer Nature 2018
A. Myat et al. (eds.), *The Interventional Cardiology Training Manual*,
https://doi.org/10.1007/978-3-319-71635-0_22

reinterventions as compared with BMS. In addition, the safety of PCI improved after the introduction of coronary stents that drastically reduced the incidence of abrupt vessel closure. However, stent thrombosis (ST) still remains an important and feared complication. This entity has a wide chronological spectrum encompassing anywhere from intra-procedural to many years after implantation.

Definitions of Stent Thrombosis

- In order to standardize definitions for patients enrolled in cardiovascular trials, universal definitions were agreed upon in 2007 by a group of experts known as the Academic Research Consortium (ARC) [3].
- The ARC proposed two distinct classifications of ST incorporating both levels of evidence as

well as timing of events (Table 22.1). In clinical practice, due to differences in pathophysiology and predisposing risk factors, ST is frequently divided into 2 major groups: early ST ($\leq$30 days) and late ST (>30 days).

Incidence of Stent Thrombosis

- Assessing the true "real-world" incidence of ST is challenging as angiographic or pathologic confirmation remain necessary to fulfill the criteria of definite ST.
- Overall, the current incidence of ST is very low (1–2%) but this entity remains a dreadful complication associated with a high mortality rate (around 30%).
- Generally, early ST is more frequent than late ST although due to increasing number of patients with implanted stents, the absolute

Table 22.1 Definition of stent thrombosis according to the academic research consortium [3]

Level of certainty
Definite ST: Angiographic confirmation
Presence of a thrombus that originates in the stent or in the segment 5 mm proximal or distal to the stent and presence of at least one of the following criteria within a 48-h time window:
– Acute onset of ischemic symptoms at rest
– New ischemic electrocardiographic changes that suggest acute ischemia
– Typical rise and fall in cardiac biomarkers
– Nonocclusive thrombus
– Intracoronary thrombus
– Occlusive thrombus
– TIMI 0 or TIMI 1 intra-stent or proximal to a stent up to the most adjacent proximal side branch or main branch
Definite ST: Pathological confirmation
Evidence of recent thrombus within the stent determined at autopsy or via examination of tissue retrieved following thrombectomy
Probable ST
Considered to have occurred after intracoronary stenting in the following cases:
– Any unexplained death within the first 30 days
– Irrespective of the time after the index procedure, any myocardial infarction that is related to documented acute ischemia in the territory of the implanted stent without angiographic confirmation of stent thrombosis and in the absence of any other obvious cause
Possible ST
Considered to have occurred with any unexplained death from 30 days after intracoronary stenting until end of trial follow-up

Timing of events	
Acute	0–24 h after stent implantation
Subacute	24 h–30 days after stent implantation
Late	30 days–1 year after stent implantation
Very late	1 year after stent implantation

number of cases presenting with late ST (prevalence) is increasing.

- The initial analysis of a large observational registry of Swedish patients reported an increase in mortality with first-generation DES which only became apparent 6 months after the procedure [4]. At that time, the incidence of late and very late ST associated with DES versus BMS was called into question.
- Two years after the initial report from the Swedish registry, Lagerqvist et al. [5] published an extensive analysis comparing the incidence of ST with different types of stents. During the observational period, the overall risk of ST was lower after DES than after BMS implantation. However, from 6 months after stent implantation and onward, the risk for ST was higher with first-generation DES compared with BMS.
- Recent large-scale registries showed that with contemporary antithrombotic therapies and modern generation DES, the rate of early ST is <1%, and beyond 30 days is 0.2–0.6% per year [6]. Indeed, accumulating evidence strongly suggest that new-generation DES are not only safer than first-generation DES but also significantly safer than currently available BMS.

Clinical Presentation and Diagnosis

- The most frequent manifestation of ST is as an acute ST-segment elevation myocardial infarction (STEMI). However, ST can also present as sudden death, non-ST-segment elevation myocardial infarction (NSTEMI) or may even be diagnosed incidentally in asymptomatic patients with well-developed collateral vessels.
- Coronary angiography remains a useful tool to detect thrombus within the stent as a filling defect or simply occluding the stent completely (diameter stenosis 100%, TIMI flow grade 0).
- Previous studies have also demonstrated the importance of intracoronary imaging to complement the angiographic information. Intravascular ultrasound (IVUS) may be used to detect the underlying mechanism of ST (underexpansion, malapposition, edge dissection) [7]. More recently, optical coherence tomography (OCT), with its unique resolution enabling the detection of small thrombus not visualized by angiography or IVUS, has gained widespread clinical acceptance as an attractive diagnostic tool in this challenging scenario [8–10].

Causes of Stent Thrombosis

- A multitude of mechanisms may lead to the occurrence of ST. Accordingly, it is useful to classify potential risk factors as patient-, procedure-, or device-specific (Table 22.2).
- These may predispose to ST by one of the following pathophysiological mechanisms:
  - Exposure of blood flow to prothrombotic subendothelial components such as stent struts and/or polymer material, which are able to activate the extrinsic pathway of the coagulation cascade;
  - Slow coronary flow and low shear stress leading to activation of the intrinsic pathway;
  - Inadequate inhibition of platelet activation (insufficient antiaggregation or premature discontinuation of dual antiplatelet therapy [DAPT]); or
  - Patient-related factors leading to a prothrombotic state (malignancy, acute coronary syndrome, etc.).

Table 22.2 Risk factors for stent thrombosis

Patient-related factors
– PCI for acute coronary syndrome/ST-segment elevation MI
– Low ejection fraction
– Malignancy
– Renal failure
– Diabetes mellitus
Procedural factors
– Inadequate stent expansion/sizing
– Incomplete stent apposition
– Inflow/outflow disease
– Residual edge dissection
Antithrombotic drug factors
– Premature cessation of DAPT
– Nonresponse to antiplatelets

Early Stent Thrombosis

- Early ST occurs within 30 days after stent implantation where technical and procedural risk factors appear to play a critical role.
- In these patients, suboptimal procedural results (stent underexpansion, areas of malapposition, slow flow, residual edge dissections or residual proximal or distal disease) are considered important predictors of ST.
- In addition, patient-related risk factors, like malignancy, index PCI in the setting of acute MI, reduced left ventricular function, insulin-requiring diabetes mellitus, and renal insufficiency, are also important risk factors for early ST.
- Finally, impaired response to ADP-antagonist therapy or early discontinuation of DAPT may have catastrophic consequences. Many studies have focused on the value of monitoring the response to ADP-antagonist therapy. However to date, no trial has yet been able to demonstrate clinical benefit when results of platelet function tests are used to optimize antithrombotic therapy.
- The most important predictor of ST remains discontinuation of antiplatelet therapy in the initial 30 days after stent implantation [11].

Late and Very Late Stent Thrombosis

- ST >30 days after stent implantation is associated with several pathophysiological factors including ongoing vessel inflammation, persistent fibrin deposition, and, very importantly, delayed endothelial coverage. Re-endothelization is significantly delayed with DES compared with BMS.
- Malapposition is often observed in these patients. Late stent malapposition appears to play an important pathophysiological role. Persistent late malapposition is a result of a malapposed stent at the time of deployment. However, late malapposition may also be the consequence of positive vessel wall remodeling in cases where the stent was well apposed at the time of implantation (late acquired malapposition).

- Resolution of an underlying thrombus remains another possibility. This phenomenon is more common among DES and previous studies have associated it with an increased risk of very late ST [12].
- Patient-related risk factors also remain important. These include reduced left ventricular function, low response to ADP-antagonist therapy, and diabetes mellitus.
- Finally, stent-related factors should be also considered. As previously mentioned a decade ago a major controversy was generated about the possibility that first-generation DES would increase the risk of ST. Thanks to anatomic-pathological studies, the inflammatory reaction caused by the durable polymer coatings of the first-generation DES was identified as the main cause of this increased risk.
- New-generation DES, with thinner struts and more biocompatible polymer coatings, have solved this problem and, in fact, current data suggest that they are safer than BMS [5, 13, 14].
- Finally, neoatherosclerosis (intra-stent fibro-atheroma with or without calcification) has been observed in both BMS and DES. Several studies have suggested that neoatherosclerosis appears earlier in DES compared to BMS [15]. Importantly, it has been demonstrated that the presence of neoatherosclerosis with neointimal rupture is an important cause of late and very late ST [16, 17].

Management

- Most cases of ST present as an acute MI with a TIMI flow <3 (TIMI 0 in 60–80% of patients). Thus, emergent cardiac catheterization with restoration of coronary flow is the mainstay of acute management [18].
- Evidence regarding the best interventional strategy in these patients is limited and largely based on observational studies. In a report from the CathPCI Registry, involving more than 7000 cases of ARC definite ST, aspiration thrombectomy was performed in one-third of patients and a new stent was implanted in 64% of them [18].
- Treatment should be individualized. Every particular case may require a specific treatment

depending on the predominant cause of ST. Clinical practice guidelines recommend intracoronary imaging to detect underlying mechanical problems and risk factors for ST such as stent malapposition, stent underexpansion, edge dissections, neoatherosclerosis, or stent fracture. This information may help to guide revascularization and future management.

- Antiplatelet therapy is also an important consideration. In general, the use of potent ADP-antagonist such as prasugrel or ticagrelor (especially if the event occurred on clopido-

grel treatment) is recommended in patients suffering from ST.

Stent Malapposition

- The presence of a separation between the stent struts and the vessel wall is frequently detected in these patients and has been considered as a risk factor for ST (Fig. 22.1).
- In these cases, angioplasty with appropriately sized balloons is enough to resolve the problem.

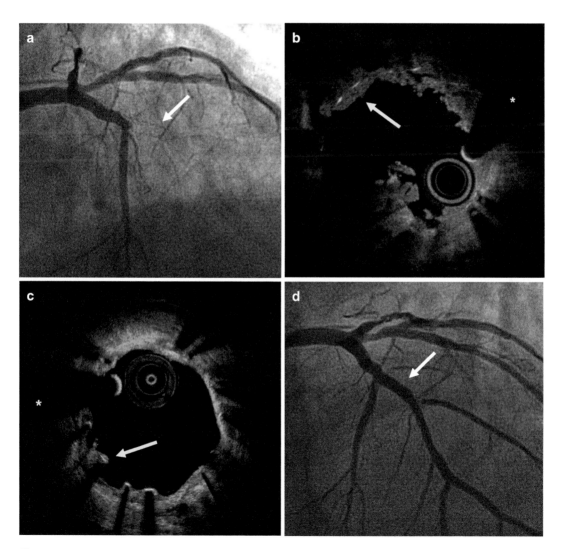

Fig. 22.1 A 65-year-old man was admitted with an anterior myocardial infarction. Coronary angiography showed an occlusion of the stent implanted 1 year before at the mid segment of the left anterior descending coronary artery (**a, white arrow**). Optimal coherence tomog-

raphy revealed areas of malapposition with thrombus (**b** and **c, yellow arrows**). Angioplasty with noncompliant balloon post-dilatation was performed with an excellent angiographic result (**d**). (* = indicates guide wire artifact)

IVUS and OCT provide additional help to select the size of the balloon by accurately measuring the diameter and area of the reference vessel and by monitoring the results of balloon dilation [10].

- In some patients with calcified plaques or complex anatomy residual malapposition may be impossible to correct.

Stent Underexpansion

- This is a frequent mechanism of ST due to highly calcified and rigid arteries that do not allow adequate expansion of the stent at the time of implantation. Alternatively, this problem may be consequence of an inadequate initial stent deployment.
- IVUS and OCT represent the best tools for the diagnosis of underexpansion (Fig. 22.2).
- This phenomenon should be aggressively tackled with high-pressure dilations using noncompliant balloons. The size of the balloon

must be chosen according to the diameter of the reference segment determined by intracoronary imaging. The systematic implantation of a new stent is not advised as it does not solve the problem of underexpansion and might predispose to a new episode of ST.

Edge Dissection

- In many cases these cannot be detected by angiography but are easily diagnosed with IVUS or OCT.
- In these cases, a new stent should be implanted to seal the dissection, obtain a larger residual lumen, and restore coronary flow [19].

Neoatherosclerosis

- Neoatherosclerosis with neointimal rupture and thrombus (complicated neoatherosclerosis) has been established as a cause of ST.

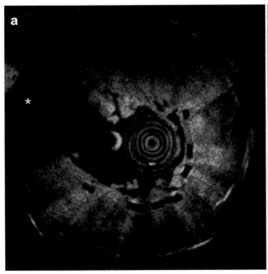
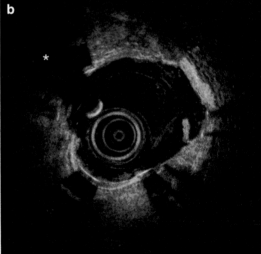

Fig. 22.2 (**a**) A 68-year-old man with in-stent restenosis was treated with a bioresorbable vascular scaffold (BVS). Two days later he suffered a ST. OCT revealed severe underexpansion of the BVS (black rectangular boxes). (**b**) A drug-eluting stent (2.5 × 12 mm) was implanted in a patient with a severe calcified lesion at the distal segment of the left anterior descending coronary artery. One week later, the patient suffered a ST. OCT revealed severe stent underexpansion (minimal stent diameter 1.8 mm). (* = indicates guide wire artifact)

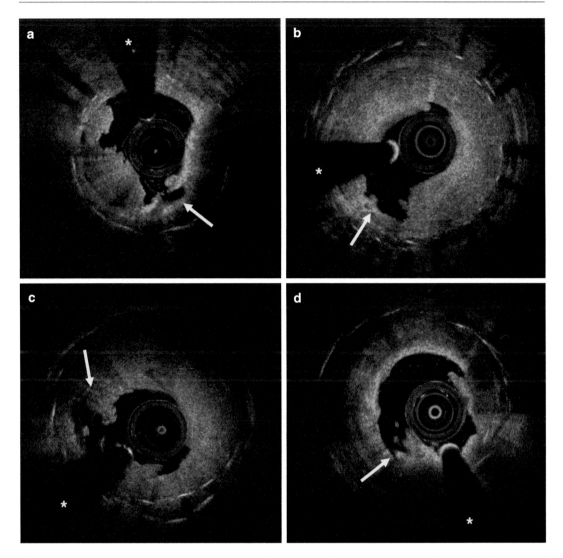

Fig. 22.3 Optical coherence tomography images of different cases of neoatherosclerosis with neointimal rupture and associated thrombus (**yellow arrows**). (* = indicates guide wire artifact)

In these cases, OCT rather than IVUS is of great help to make the diagnosis (Fig. 22.3).

- The best treatment for patients presenting with ST as a result of neoatherosclerosis remains unknown. Many investigators suggest that after flow restoration these patients should be managed as other patients with in-stent restenosis.
- Implantation of a new stent might be an adequate solution. However, using a drug-coating balloon may also be a good alternative to avoid the implantation of a new metallic layer [20].

Stent Fracture

- Stent fracture has been associated with right coronary artery location, excessive tortuosity or angulation of the vessel, overlapping stents, and long stents.
- Stent fracture may cause damage to the endothelium and trigger ST. Stent fracture may also stimulate the occurrence of in-stent restenosis.
- Implantation of a new stent is frequently used to address this complication.

Prevention of Stent Thrombosis

- Given the poor outcomes of ST despite early recognition and adequate treatment, the most important step in the treatment of this complication is prevention.
- Unfortunately, risk factors related to patient history and anatomy are non-modifiable. Diabetes mellitus is present in a large number of patients undergoing PCI and these patients have poor clinical outcomes compared with nondiabetic patients [21]. Prasugrel significantly reduces the incidence of ST in diabetic patients, so ensuring an optimal antiplatelet therapy in these patients remains essential [22].
- Another important aspect in relation to the prevention of ST is the duration of DAPT after DES implantation. Discontinuation of DAPT is the most powerful predictor of ST during the first 6 months after PCI [23]. Thus, clinical practice guidelines recommend a prolonged duration of DAPT of >6 months in stable patients and at least 12 months for patients with acute coronary syndrome.
- In addition, it is also important deferring whenever possible elective surgical procedures for at least 1 year. If there are major reasons to interrupt DAPT this should be postponed as long as possible after stenting and aspirin should be continued.
- The technique at the time of stent implantation is also very important. An optimal procedural result is essential to minimize the risk of ST. Adequate stent expansion and apposition should be achieved, avoiding residual edge dissections. Imaging techniques such as IVUS or OCT are important to guide stent implantation.

Bioresorbable Vascular Scaffolds (BVS)

- BVS are new devices that offer the advantages of DES without the requirement of a permanent metal layer on/within the coronary artery wall (see also Chap. 11). Moreover, these devices offer the potential benefit of restoration of normal vasomotor tone.

- Efficacy and safety results with BVS in early observational studies and randomized clinical trials were comparable with those obtained with new-generation DES.
- Recently, however, adverse safety and efficacy signals have been identified. In fact, several studies have been recently published suggesting a significantly higher incidence of ST with BVS compared with new-generation DES [24, 25]. It is important to emphasize, however, that the majority of cases of ST in the group of BVS occurred in complex lesions (calcified lesions, STEMI) and the use of intracoronary imaging was not mandatory in these studies.
- Thus, assessing whether meticulous imaging-guided BVS implantation may overcome device-related late complications will require prospective evaluation.
- Likewise, the optimal strategy and duration of DAPT in these patients must be refined. New-generation polymeric BVS, with thinner struts, enhanced expansive capability, and improved resorption kinetics will be soon available. Hopefully, novel BVS devices will be safer and more effective than first-generation BVS.

Conclusion

ST is an uncommon but dreadful complication of PCI with high mortality rates. The use of coronary imaging in these patients is important during the diagnosis as well as to guide treatment and optimize final results. Recognition and management of risk factors remains essential in the prevention of this fearsome complication.

References

1. Fischman DL, Leon MB, Baim DS. A randomized comparison of coronary stent placement and balloon angioplasty in the treatment of coronary artery disease. N Engl J Med. 1994;331:496–501.
2. Serruys PW, de Jaegere P, Kiemeneij F. A comparison of balloon-expandable stent implantation with balloon angioplasty in patients with coronary artery disease. N Engl J Med. 1994;331:489–95.
3. Cultip DE, Windecker S, Mehran R. Academic Research Consortium. Clinical end points in coronary stent

trials: a case for standardized definitions. Circulation. 2007;115:1208–13.

4. Lagerqvist B, James SK, Stenestrand U. SCAAR Study Group. Long-term outcomes with drug-eluting stents versus bare-metal stents in Sweden. N Engl J Med. 2007;356:1009–19.

5. Lagerqvist B, Carlsson J, Fröbert O. Stent thrombosis in Sweden: a report from the Swedish Coronary Angiography and Angioplasty Registry. Circ Cardiovasc Interv. 2009;2:401–8.

6. Levine GN, Bates ER, Blankenship JC. ACCF/AHA/SCAI guideline for percutaneous coronary intervention: a report of the American College of Cardiology Foundation/American Heart Association Task Force on Practice Guidelines and the Society for Cardiovascular Angiography and Interventions. J Am Coll Cardiol. 2011;58:e44–e122.

7. Alfonso F, Suarez A, Angiolillo DJ. Findings of intra-vascular ultrasound during acute stent thrombosis. Heart. 2004;90:1455–9.

8. Kubo T, Imanishi T, Takarada S. Assessment of cul-prit lesion morphology in acute myocardial infarction: ability of optical coherence tomography compared with intravascular ultrasound and coronary angios-copy. J Am Coll Cardiol. 2007;50:933–9.

9. Cuesta J, Rivero F, Alfonso F. Ongoing stent thrombo-sis: optical coherence tomography findings. Rev Esp Cardiol. 2015;68:1024.

10. Alfonso F, Dutary J, Paulo M. Combined use of optical coherence tomography and intravascular ultrasound imaging in patients undergoing coronary interven-tions for stent thrombosis. Heart. 2012;98:1213–20.

11. Iakovou I, Schmidt T, Bonizzoni E. Incidence, pre-dictors, and outcome of thrombosis after success-ful implantation of drug-eluting stents. JAMA. 2005;293:2126–30.

12. Cook S, Wenaweser P, Togni M. Incomplete stent appo-sition and very late stent thrombosis after drug-eluting stent implantation. Circulation. 2007;115:2426–34.

13. Tada T, Byrne RA, Simunovic I. Risk of stent throm-bosis among bare-metal stents, first-generation drug-eluting stents, and second-generation drug-eluting stents: results from a registry of 18,334 patiens. JACC Cardiovasc Interv. 2013;6:1267–74.

14. Raber L, Magro M, Stefanini GG. Very late coronary stent thrombosis of a newer-generation everolimus-eluting stent compared with early-generation drug-eluting stents: a prospective cohort study. Circulation. 2012;125:1110–21.

15. Nakazawa G, Vorpahl M, Finn AV, Narula J, Virmani R. One step forward and two steps back with drug-eluting stents: from preventing restenosis to causing late thrombosis and nouveau atherosclerosis. JACC Cardiovasc Imaging. 2009;2:625–8.

16. Alfonso F, Fernandez-Viña F, Medina M. Neoathero-sclerosis: the missing link between very late stent thrombosis and very late in-stent restenosis. J Am Coll Cardiol. 2013;61:155.

17. Bastante T, Rivero F, Cuesta J. Bioresorbable vascu-lar scaffold for very late stent thrombosis resulting from ruptured neoatherosclerosis. Rev Port Cardiol. 2015;34:779.

18. Armstrong EJ, Feldman DN, Wang TY. Clinical presentation, management, and outcomes of angio-graphically documented early, late and very late stent thrombosis. JACC Cardiovasc Interv. 2012;5:131–40.

19. Biondi-Zoccai GG, Agostoni P, Sangiorgi GM. Incidence, predictors, and outcomes of coronary dis-sections left untreated after drug-eluting stent implan-tation. Eur Heart J. 2006;27:540–6.

20. Alfonso F, Bastante T, Cuesta J. Drug-coated balloon treatment of very late stent thrombosis due to com-plicated neoatherosclerosis. Arq Bras Cardiol. 2016; 106:541–3.

21. Berry C, Tardif JC, Bourassa MG. Coronary heart dis-ease in patient with diabetes. Part II: recent advances in coronary revascularization. J Am Coll Cardiol. 2007;49:643–56.

22. Wiviott SD, Braunwald E, Angiolillo DJ. Greater clinical benefit of more intensive oral antiplatelet therapy with prasugrel in patients with diabetes mel-litus in the trial to assess improvement in therapeutic outcomes by optimizing platelet inhibition with pra-sugrel – thrombolysis in myocardial infarction 38. Circulation. 2008;118:1626–36.

23. Dangas GD, Claessen BE, Mehran R. Stent thrombo-sis after primary angioplasty for STEMI in relation to non-adherence to dual antiplatelet therapy over time: results of the HORIZONS-AMI trial. Euro-Intervention. 2013;8(9):1033.

24. Ellis SG, Kereiakes DJ, Metzger DC, ABSORB III Investigators. Everolimus-eluting bioresorbable scaf-folds for coronary artery disease. N Engl J Med. 2015; 373(20):1905–15.

25. Toyota T, Morimoto T, Shiomi H. Very late scaffold thrombosis of bioresorbable vascular scaffold: sys-tematic review and a meta-analysis. JACC Cardiovasc Interv. 2017;10:27–37.

Cardiogenic Shock and Mechanical Circulatory Support

23

Stephen P. Hoole and Alain Vuylsteke

About Us

Royal Papworth Hospital in Cambridgeshire is a regional (East of England) and national center caring for patients with heart and lung disease and is one of the leading cardiothoracic specialist hospitals in the United Kingdom. Royal Papworth Hospital currently treats around 24,400 inpatients and day patients and sees over 73,600 outpatients per year. It has over 1800 staff, 289 beds, and an annual budget of over £110 million. Royal Papworth Hospital was one of the first 20 hospitals in England to be granted NHS Foundation Trust status in 2004.

Royal Papworth Hospital is:

- One of five designated centers for Respiratory ECMO in the UK
- One of the three designated centers for ventricular assist devices in the UK
- The largest heart and lung transplant center in the UK, performing the first heart-lung transplant in the UK
- The designated National Pulmonary Hypertension Centre and the only UK center performing pulmonary endarterectomy and balloon pulmonary angioplasty

S. P. Hoole (✉) · A. Vuylsteke
Royal Papworth Hospital, Cambridge, UK
e-mail: s.hoole@nhs.net

- The largest cardiac surgical unit in the UK
- The regional heart attack center performing >2000 PCI and 700 primary PCI annually
- The regional TAVI center

A full summary of the key clinical milestones achieved at Papworth over its 90 year history and details of the New Papworth Hospital, due to complete in 2018, can be found on the hospital website http://www.royalpapworth.nhs.uk/index.php.

Cardiogenic Shock

- Cardiogenic shock (CS) is sustained hypotension with inadequate tissue perfusion in spite of adequate left ventricular filling pressure. This is manifested by tissue hypoperfusion and organ dysfunction.
- The natural history of cardiogenic shock is a downward spiral of ischemic left ventricular (LV) systolic dysfunction and worsening end-organ perfusion, leading to death (Fig. 23.1).
- The diagnosis of CS is based on clinical and hemodynamic criteria as shown in Table 23.1. The causes of cardiogenic shock are summarized in Table 23.2.
- The commonest cause of CS is acute myocardial infarction (MI), complicating approximately 2–3% of acute MI (BCIS database 2014) [1]. The prognosis is poor, despite instigating

Fig. 23.1 The downward spiral of hemodynamic effects as a result of untreated cardiogenic shock

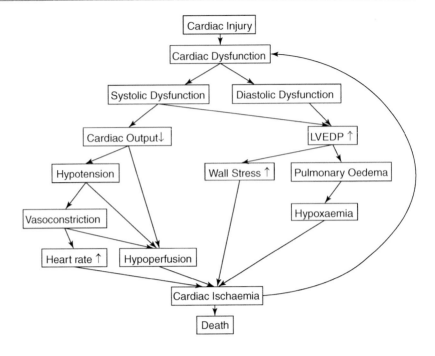

Table 23.1 Cardiogenic shock diagnostic criteria

Clinical criteria	Systolic blood pressure < 90 mmHg for >30 min Heart rate > 100 bpm Impaired end-organ perfusion (oliguria, altered consciousness, elevated lactate)
Hemodynamic criteria	Cardiac index <1.8 L/min/m² without pharmacological support Cardiac index <2.2 L/min/m² with pharmacological support Capillary wedge pressure > 15 mmHg Absence of low left and right sided intracardiac filling pressures

Table 23.2 Causes of cardiogenic shock

Pump failure
Acute myocardial infarction
Large (anterior) infarction
Smaller infarction with preexisting LV dysfunction
Right ventricular infarction
Acute myocarditis
End-stage cardiomyopathy
Myocardial contusion
Septic shock with myocardial depression
Cardiotoxic drugs, e.g., beta-blocker overdose
Electrical complications
Intractable (ventricular) arrhythmia
Mechanical complications
Papillary muscle rupture and acute severe mitral regurgitation
Aortic dissection and acute severe aortic regurgitation
Ventricular septal defect
Cardiac rupture and tamponade

supportive treatment, and the mortality rate is greater than 50%.

- The SHOCK trial registry [2] has confirmed that CS usually occurs within the first 24 h of an acute MI with three-quarters due to LV failure and the remainder due to acute mechanical complications such as mitral regurgitation, ventricular septal defect, tamponade and cardiac rupture or intractable arrhythmia.
- The SHOCK trial demonstrated that emergency revascularization for acute MI complicated by CS decreased mortality at 1 year by 13% when compared with a strategy of conservative therapy.
- This chapter will review the treatment of CS including the role of mechanical circulatory support after acute MI and/or for patients requiring high-risk percutaneous coronary intervention (PCI).

Treatment

Interventional Therapies

- This should always be considered as early reperfusion of ischemic myocardium has been shown to provide long-term survival benefit in the setting of CS associated with acute MI.
- The SHOCK trial registry confirmed that early and complete coronary revascularization improved survival at 6 months and 1 year when compared to medical optimization alone (50% vs. 37%; $p = 0.027$ and 47% vs. 34%; $p = 0.025$, respectively) [3].
- The European Society of Cardiology (ESC) guideline recommends early revascularization by PCI or CABG [4].
- Mechanical circulatory support might be required to support tissue perfusion while reperfusion is performed.

Medical Treatment

- There is no drug to treat cardiogenic shock.
- Thrombolytic agents can help re-establishing perfusion of the myocardium.
- Inotropic drugs such as catecholamines, phosphodiesterase inhibitors, or calcium sensitizers will increase cardiac contractility and help maintain organ perfusion. But these drugs will increase myocardial oxygen demand and potentially exacerbate myocardial ischemia. In addition, inotropic drugs will modify vasomotor tone, causing either vasoconstriction or vasodilation.
- The combination of these effects can be used to improve organ perfusion and hemodynamic indices but their use has failed to decrease mortality in patients presenting with acute MI complicated by CS.
- There is no evidence to use one drug preferentially. Most clinicians will combine drugs to balance their various effects. The best combination of drugs can be selected by monitoring the cardiac output, hemodynamic parameters, and end-organ perfusion indices.

- In severe cardiogenic shock, we believe that the pulmonary artery flotation catheter remains the most accurate method to measure cardiac output but great care should be given to the interpretation of the numbers obtained; *they must never be interpreted in isolation.*

Mechanical Circulatory Support

- Mechanical circulatory support can be used to support organs while a definitive intervention is performed, or if time is required to allow cardiac recovery or to bridge the patient to transplantation.
- The correct mechanical support option must be deployed at the correct time and clinician and institutional experience will influence the choice of support. A long-term treatment strategy should be agreed and in place before mechanical support is instigated as the only chance of survival to discharge from hospital are through recovery, implantation of a durable left ventricular assist device or heart transplantation. Careful patient selection is therefore essential.

Intra-aortic Balloon Pump (IABP) Counterpulsation

- IABP counterpulsation is a method of temporary mechanical circulatory support that attempts to create a more favorable balance of myocardial oxygen supply and demand by using the concepts of systolic unloading and diastolic augmentation.
- As a consequence, cardiac output, ejection fraction, and coronary perfusion are increased, with a concomitant decrease in LV wall stress, systemic resistance to LV ejection, and pulmonary capillary wedge pressure [5].
- The dominant effect is to decrease afterload and LV wall stress and myocardial oxygen demand; the augmentation of coronary flow has been inconsistently demonstrated, particularly when there is significant coronary disease.

Practicalities

- An appropriately sized catheter with a polyethylene balloon at its tip is inserted usually via the femoral artery using a Seldinger technique. The radioopaque tip of the catheter is positioned at the level of the tracheal carina, 1–2 cm distal to the left subclavian artery to avoid cerebral embolic complications (Fig. 23.2a). The caudal end of the polyethylene balloon is then approximately at the level of the renal arteries.

- The balloon inflation can be triggered from an ECG trace or a pressure waveform and is usually set initially for 1:1 inflation-deflation to each cardiac cycle at 100% augmentation, although this can be titrated according to response.

- The augmented pressure waveform during an appropriately synchronized inflation-deflation cycle should increase diastolic pressure by up to 30% during inflation and reduce systolic pressure during deflation (Fig. 23.2b). However, improper timing can lead to inefficient LV

support and counteract the intended purpose of therapy.

- Inflation too early, before aortic valve closure, resulting in fusion with the dicrotic notch, will increase LVEDP and wall stress, whereas inflation too late (or deflation too early) fails to augment diastolic pressure and possibly coronary flow. Late balloon deflation results in LV ejection against an increased afterload, worsening wall stress.

- Optimal support depends on the balloon's position in the aorta, the blood displacement volume, balloon diameter in relation to aortic diameter, the timing of balloon inflation and deflation, and the patient's own heart rate, blood pressure and vascular resistance.

- An IABP can be used for up to several months if required to reach definitive treatment such as heart transplantation. It requires anticoagulation if used for prolonged periods of time in patients restricted to bed rest.

- Its use is associated with vascular injury, limb ischemia and embolization, stroke, bleeding,

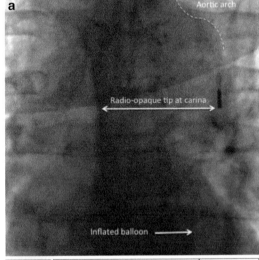

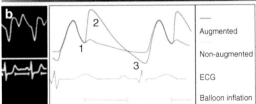

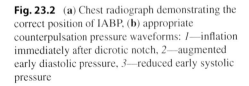

Fig. 23.2 (**a**) Chest radiograph demonstrating the correct position of IABP, (**b**) appropriate counterpulsation pressure waveforms: *1*—inflation immediately after dicrotic notch, *2*—augmented early diastolic pressure, *3*—reduced early systolic pressure

infection, and thrombocytopenia. The contra-indications to IABP insertion are summarized in Table 23.3.

Evidence and Guidelines

- The SHOCK trial registry demonstrated that treating CS with IABP support reduced inhospital mortality compared to those receiving thrombolytic therapy alone to treat STEMI (47% vs. 63%, $p < 0.0001$) [2].
- However, this benefit has not been corroborated in the era of primary PCI [6] and the IABP-SHOCK II trial [7] did not demonstrate an improvement in all-cause mortality at 30 days after primary PCI with IABP counterpulsation compared to primary PCI alone (39.7% vs. 41.3%, RR 0.96 (0.79–1.17), $p = 0.69$).
- The CRISP-AMI also failed to observe a reduction in anterior infarction size in the IABP supported group treated by primary PCI [8].
- The ESC 2012 guidelines have given the routine use of IABP in CS a grade III, LOE A recommendation, increasing to grade IIa, LOE C in cases of CS associated with mechanical complications [4].
- The IABP remains the workhorse circulatory support device used by cardiovascular specialists due to the simplicity/rapidity of insertion, but the device provides only modest hemodynamic support.

Table 23.3 Contraindications to IABP

Absolute
Moderate/severe aortic regurgitation
Aortic dissection
Relative
Sepsis
Peripheral vascular disease
Coagulopathy

- The efficacy of counterpulsation critically depends on intrinsic ventricular function, which is not always sufficient to maintain adequate cardiac output in extreme cases of CS due to LV failure. For this reason, additional support devices have been introduced to provide superior hemodynamic support (Table 23.4) [9].

Peripheral (Percutaneous) Ventricular Assist Device (VAD)

- Impella™ (Abiomed) and the Percutaneous Heart Pump (Thoratec) are trans-valvular devices that provide direct unloading of the LV using an integrated pump and catheter system. A catheter carrying the pump housing sits across the aortic valve and pulls blood volume from the LV and ejects it into the ascending aorta.
- The smallest device can provide flow rates up to 2.5 L/min; larger devices are available providing up to 3.5 L/min and 5 L/min (although the 5 L device often requires surgical implantation).
- It has been used for temporary support in the setting of high-risk PCI and as a bridge to recovery in acute MI (Fig. 23.3a).
- TandemHeart™ (CardiacAssist) provides left atrial-to-femoral artery bypass and can be inserted under fluoroscopy in the cardiac catheterization laboratory without surgical implantation.
- It requires a transseptal cannula that allows direct unloading of the left heart, and, by providing a cardiac output independent of ventricular stroke volume, this device can provide support only exceeded by traditional surgically implanted ventricular assist devices. An external centrifugal pump provides flow rates up to 4 L/min (Fig. 23.3b).

Table 23.4 Comparison of percutaneous mechanical support devices

	TandemHeart™	Impella 2.5	CP®	5.0	ECLS
Catheter size (F)	–	9	9	9	–
Cannula size (F)	21 (v)	12	14	21	17–21 (v)
	12–19 (a)				16–19 (a)
Flow (L/min)	4.0	2.5	4.0	5.0	7.0
LV unloading	++	+	++	++	–
Duration of use	Hours-days	Hours-days	Days-weeks		

Fig. 23.3 Percutaneous
VADs: (**a**) Impella™ and
(**b**) TandemHeart™
(Reprinted with
permission from
Abiomed and
CardiacAssist)

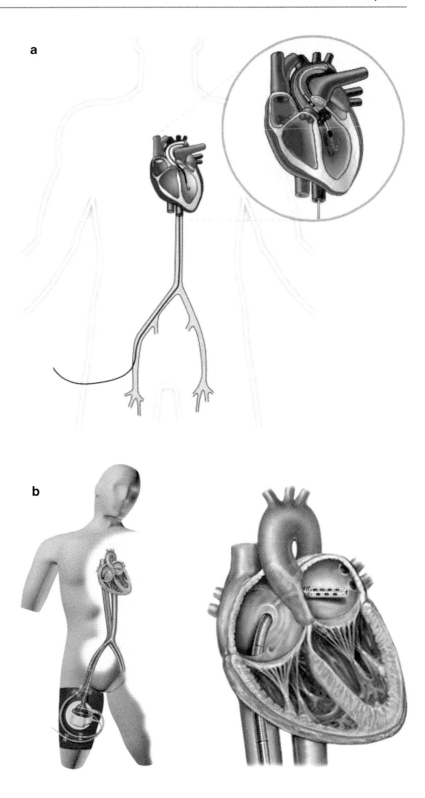

Practicalities

- In contrast to IABP, the percutaneous VAD systems have a greater diameter and require larger bore access (Table 23.4). These devices are not suitable if there is significant peripheral vascular disease.
- The use of Impella is contraindicated if there is severe aortic valve stenosis or regurgitation, a mechanical aortic valve replacement or mural LV thrombus.
- The potential complications from percutaneous VADs include vascular injury and access site bleeding, limb ischemia, stroke, tamponade, and hemolysis.
- In addition, entanglement with the mitral subvalvular apparatus can cause severe mitral regurgitation and exacerbate pulmonary congestion. For these reasons a detailed echocardiographic examination is required before and after implantation.
- Implantation of the TandemHeart is complex and requires advanced interventional techniques to perform the transseptal puncture with an insertion time of up to 1 h. Displacement of the cannula during patient transport or if the leg is moved can be problematic and must be avoided as displacement into the right atrium results in massive right to left shunting. Cannula migration into a pulmonary vein can also lead to pump malfunction.

Evidence

- The ISAR-SHOCK trial confirmed that Impella provided superior hemodynamic support to IABP [10]. The Protect II study compared Impella 2.5-L system to IABP in preventing major adverse events during and after non-emergent high-risk PCI and found that the 30-day incidence of major adverse clinical events was not different for patients with IABP or Impella 2.5 hemodynamic support (Impella 35.1% vs. IABP 40.1%, $p = 0.227$) [11].
- However, the lower CS mortality than previously reported in both groups perhaps suggests that those in extremis (and perhaps most likely to benefit from Impella) were not included.

- A randomized trial of 41 patients supported with IABP or TandemHeart demonstrated no difference in mortality (HR 0.95 (0.48–1.90)) despite marked improvement in hemodynamics in the group allocated to the TandemHeart [12]. There was an increased risk of bleeding and a signal of excess limb ischemia in the TandemHeart treated group.

Extracorporeal Life Support (ECLS)

Venoarterial extracorporeal membrane oxygenation (VA-ECMO) provides cardiopulmonary support for patients whose hearts no longer provide adequate tissue blood flow and tissue oxygenation.

Practicalities

- Peripheral VA-ECMO requires cannulation of the femoral artery and vein to establish a circuit—removing deoxygenated blood from the inferior vena cava and returning oxygenated blood to the aorta (Fig. 23.4a).
- Central VA-ECMO is similar to peripheral, but requires direct cannulation of the ascending aorta via a sternotomy to establish the circuit (Fig. 23.4b).
- VA-ECMO can be placed without fluoroscopy at the patient's bedside in an emergency. It allows rapid restoration of the circulation in patients in preterminal CS. VA-ECMO decreases pulmonary artery pressure, augments systemic perfusion, and achieves adequate tissue oxygenation. It can be used to support both left and right ventricular failure.
- Cannulae are inserted by Seldinger technique (peripheral) or by direct central cannulation via sternotomy or thoracotomy.
- Systemic anticoagulation is required prior to cannula placement. This prevents clotting within the circuit due to blood-surface interaction and formation of intravascular thrombus probably due to blood stagnating or flowing in an opposite direction in the aorta (in the case of peripheral VA ECMO).

Fig. 23.4 VA ECMO:
(**a**) peripheral and (**b**)
central (Reprinted with
permission from The
Intensive Care Society
2012)

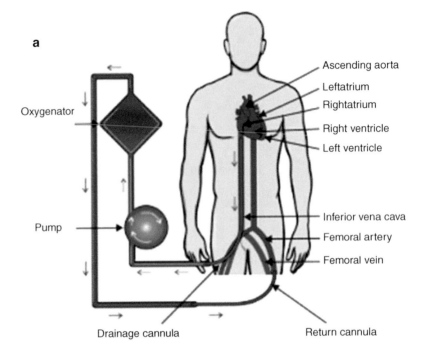

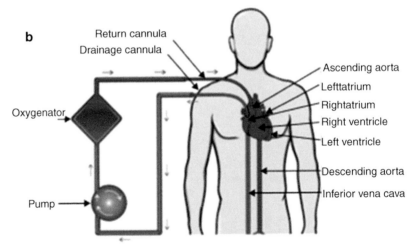

- The femoral artery may become significantly occluded by the 24F cannula required for peripheral VA ECMO, resulting in leg ischemia. A separate perfusion line is always required in the distal superficial femoral artery to prevent this.
- Peripheral VA-ECMO increases LV afterload causing an increase in LVEDP, LV walls stress, and oxygen demand. It does not unload the ventricle and may increase filling pressure and volume.

- Placement of a left ventricular vent should be considered to decompress and rest the ventricle. In extreme circumstances the afterload may be so high as to close the aortic valve, stagnating blood in the LV and ascending aorta that significantly increases the risk of thrombus formation and stroke.
- Both ECMO flow and output from the left ventricle contribute to the total systemic blood flow. Similarly, the relative flows and their associated oxygen saturations determine

systemic oxygen saturation. It is important to realize that these circulations may compete.

- A patient with reasonable cardiac function but impaired lung function may present with differential circulations. The poorly oxygenated blood from the left ventricle preferentially supplies the cerebral and coronary circulations, while well-oxygenated blood from the femoral arterial cannula supplies the lower body (named the Harlequin syndrome). For this reason, oxygenation should be monitored from the right radial artery to avoid and quickly address hypoxemia.

- *Peripheral VA ECMO should be used in patients with reasonable respiratory function, while central VA ECMO is more appropriate in patients with combined cardiorespiratory failure as oxygenated blood will be distributed to the whole body.*

- The optimal ECMO blood flow is the lowest flow rate required to provide adequate cardiopulmonary support without risk of thrombus forming in the circuit.

- The Extracorporeal Life Support (ELSO) general guidelines define adequate support as that which achieves an arterial saturation greater than 80% and venous saturation greater than 70% [13].

- For central VA ECMO, the optimal pump flow is achieved by adjusting the flow until the pulmonary arterial pulse pressure is at least 10 mmHg in order to maintain continuous flow through the heart and pulmonary circulation.

- In patients with limited or no LV ejection, inotropic drugs may be used to maintain contractility during cardiac ECMO. This prevents valve fusion and reduces the risk of ventricular thrombosis. Usually flows of 3–6 L/min in average-size adults are sufficient for ECMO.

- The amount of anticoagulation is less than during conventional cardiopulmonary bypass due to the lack of blood/air interface in the reservoir and the use of heparin-bonded circuits in the newer-generation pumps.

- The complications of ECMO can be summarized as cannula, circuit or patient-based (Table 23.5). Severe peripheral vascular disease is a contraindication to peripheral VA ECMO.

Table 23.5 ECMO complications

Cannula-based
Limb ischemia
Venous thrombosis
Bleeding (including retroperitoneal)
Circuit-based
Air in the circuit and gas embolization[a]
Tube rupture and catastrophic hemorrhage[a]
Low flow due to hypovolemia
Membrane oxygenator thrombosis
Obstructed cannulae and/or tubing
Patient-based
Bleeding due to coagulopathy and/or thrombocytopenia
Intracerebral
Harlequin syndrome or differential circulation
Thrombosis and emboli
Infection

[a]Treated by immediate circuit clamping of inflow and outflow pipes

Evidence

- The use of VA-ECMO in CS is based on case-reports and case-series. There is no evidence to support its routine use in CS. Despite this, its use is increasing as enthusiastic clinicians believe it can provide emergency circulatory support while a definitive solution is sought.

- In a single-center, retrospective study, 219 patients with CS post MI treated with PCI and adjunctive ECMO had a higher 30-day survival than an historical control group of 115 patients without ECMO (60% vs. 35%) [14]. Others have reported around 50% survival in patients with cardiogenic shock supported with ECMO.

Surgical Ventricular Assist Device

- These are longer-term solutions to cardiac support and require surgery to be implanted. The VAD commonly consists of a power-source (external) and motorized pump (external or internal) with pipes from the pump inserted directly into the LV apex and aorta (for an LVAD) (Fig. 23.5). Biventricular support can be offered if required.

Fig. 23.5 Surgical
VAD—HeartMate 3™
(Reprinted with
permission from
Thoratec Corporation)

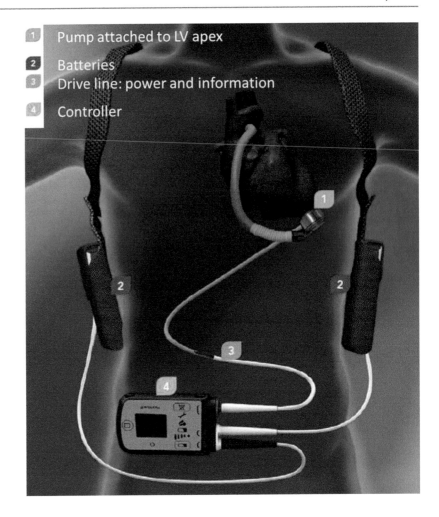

- These pumps can be used a bridge-to-transplant, a bridge-to-recovery in patients with a reversible ventricular insult or as a destination therapy.

Practicalities
- The pumps used in VADs provide pulsatile or continuous flow. In the former, positive displacement propels blood forward whereas the latter relies on centrifugal or axial flow propelled by a magnetized spinning rotor. Continuous flow pumps tend to be smaller and more durable.
- Possible complications include bleeding secondary to the anticoagulation required for the device, VAD-related infection that can be challenging to eradicate, device thrombosis, hemolysis, and stroke.

Evidence
The HeartMate II trial has demonstrated that a continuous-flow LVAD provides effective hemodynamic support for at least 18 months in patients awaiting transplantation, with improved functional status and quality of life [15].

Cardiac Transplantation

- When the heart is irrevocably damaged, then cardiac transplantation may be considered, although demand (those on the transplant waiting list) outstrips supply (donor hearts) by at least a ratio of 2:1.
- Ischemic and dilated cardiomyopathy remain the commonest indications for cardiac trans-

Table 23.6 Eligibility for cardiac transplantation

Indications for cardiac transplantation include
Irreversible NYHA class III/IV heart failure
Prognosis: Estimated 1-year survival of <80%, by a validated heart failure risk prediction tool
Contraindications to cardiac transplantation
Comorbidities that increase the risk of transplant failure
Age > 65 years (relative contraindication)
Body mass index (BMI) >35 kg/m^2/metabolic syndrome
Renal dysfunction: eGFR <30 mL/min/1.73 m^2
Severe symptomatic cerebrovascular disease
Frailty
Active systemic disease, e.g., collagen vascular disease or sickle cell disease
Pulmonary vascular disease that can cause RV failure in the donor heart if transplanted
Fixed pulmonary vascular resistance of greater than 4 wood units (320 dynes cm^{-5}) that doesn't respond to VAD or medical therapy
Issues that affect immunosuppression
Active systemic infection
Active malignancy—patients with malignancies who have demonstrated a 3- to 5-year disease-free interval may be considered, depending on the tumor type
An ongoing history of substance abuse (e.g., alcohol, drugs, or tobacco)
Psychosocial instability
Inability to comply with medical follow-up care

plantation. Two hundred heart transplants are carried out annually in the UK.
- Due to the limited supply of donor hearts case selection is important and strict criteria must be met to be eligible for cardiac transplantation [16] (Table 23.6).
- The 1-year survival rate after cardiac transplantation is as high as 81.8%, with a 5-year survival rate of 69.8%. Patients report a good quality of life.

Summary

- The treatment of cardiogenic shock is challenging particularly in the setting of acute MI. Inotropic drugs and mechanical devices have been shown to improve hemodynamic endpoints but not survival.

- Many patients with CS will only survive if they can be bridged from short-term support to longer term ventricular assist device or heart transplantation.

References

1. http://www.bcis.org.uk/pages/page_box_contents.asp?PageID=824
2. Sanborn TA, Sleeper LA, Bates ER, et al. Impact of thrombolysis, intra-aortic balloon pump counterpulsation, and their combination in cardiogenic shock complicating acute myocardial infarction: a report from the SHOCK Trial Registry. SHould we emergently revascularize Occluded Coronaries for cardiogenic shocK? J Am Coll Cardiol. 2000;36(3 Suppl A):1123–9.
3. Hochman JS, Sleeper LA, Webb JG, et al. Early revascularization in acute myocardial infarction complicated by cardiogenic SHOCK. SHOCK Investigators. SHould we emergently revascularize Occluded Coronaries for cardiogenic shocK. N Engl J Med. 1999;341(9):625–34.
4. Windecker S, Kohl P, Alfonso F, et al. 2014 ESC/EACTS guidelines on myocardial revascularization: The Task Force on Myocardial Revascularization of the European Society of Cardiology (ESC) and the European Association for Cardio-Thoracic Surgery (EACTS) developed with the special contribution of the European Association of Percutaneous Cardiovascular Interventions (EAPCI). Eur Heart J. 2014;35(37):2541–619.
5. Kern MJ. Intra-aortic balloon counterpulsation. Coron Artery Dis. 1991;2(6):649–60.
6. Sjauw KD, Engstrom AE, Vis MM, et al. A systematic review and meta-analysis of intra-aortic balloon pump therapy in ST-elevation myocardial infarction: should we change the guidelines? Eur Heart J. 2009;30(4):459–68.
7. Thiele H, Zeymer U, Neumann FJ, et al. Intraaortic balloon support for myocardial infarction with cardiogenic shock. N Engl J Med. 2012;367(14):1287–96.
8. Patel MR, Smalling RW, Thiele H, et al. Intra-aortic balloon counterpulsation and infarct size in patients with acute anterior myocardial infarction without shock: the CRISP AMI randomized trial. JAMA. 2011;306(12):1329–37.
9. Cheng JM, den Uil SE, van der Ent M, et al. Percutaneous left ventricular assist devices vs. intra-aortic balloon pump counterpulsation for treatment of cardiogenic shock: a meta-analysis of controlled trials. Eur Heart J. 2009;30:2102–8.
10. Seyfarth M, Sibbing D, Bauer I, et al. A randomized clinical trial to evaluate the safety and efficacy of a percutaneous left ventricular assist device versus intra-aortic balloon pumping for treatment of cardiogenic

S. P. Hoole and A. Vuylsteke

326

shock caused by myocardial infarction. J Am Coll Cardiol. 2008;52(19):1584–8.

11. O'Neill WW, Kleiman NS, Moses J, et al. A prospective, randomized clinical trial of hemodynamic support with Impella 2.5 versus intra-aortic balloon pump in patients undergoing high-risk percutaneous coronary intervention: the PROTECT II study. Circulation. 2012;126(14):1717–27.

12. Thiele H, Sick P, Boudriot E, Diederich KW, et al. Randomized comparison of intra-aortic balloon support with a percutaneous left ventricular assist device in patients with revascularized acute myocardial infarction complicated by cardiogenic shock. Eur Heart J. 2005;26:1276–83.

13. Extracorporeal Life Support Organization. General Guidelines for all ECLS cases Version 1:1. April 2009. http://www.elso.med.umich.edu/WordForms/ELSO%20Guidelines%20General%20All%20ECLS%20Versio n1.1.pdf

14. Sheu JJ, Tsai TH, Lee FY, et al. Early extracorporeal membrane oxygenator-assisted primary percutaneous coronary intervention improved 30-day clinical outcomes in patients with ST-segment elevation myocardial infarction complicated with profound cardiogenic shock. Crit Care Med. 2010;38(9):1810–7.

15. Miller LW, Pagani FD, Russell SD, et al. Use of a continuous-flow device in patients awaiting heart transplantation. N Engl J Med. 2007;357(9):885–96.

16. Mehra MR, Canter CE, Hannan MM, et al. The 2016 International Society for Heart Lung Transplantation listing criteria for heart transplantation: a 10-year update. J Heart Lung Transplant. 2016;35(1):1–23.

Ian Webb, Rafal Dworakowski,
and Philip MacCarthy

About Us

King's College Hospital is one of the largest and busiest teaching hospitals in the UK, forming part of the King's Health Partners Academic Health Sciences Centre. Situated in south east London, it serves an immediate population of over 800,000 residents, and provides a major trauma center and tertiary and quaternary services for south east England. The Cardiovascular Division provides subspecialty expertise and runs in parallel to the King's College London British Heart Foundation Centre of Excellence. King's College Hospital has had a 24-h primary percutaneous coronary intervention (PCI) service since 2003 and is a major Heart Attack Centre in London, treating more than 1000 patients per year on the primary PCI pathway in addition to 150 survivors of out-of-hospital cardiac arrest. King's has a proactive Out-of-Hospital Cardiac Arrest program, designed with the London Ambulance and Emergency Care Services, which includes evidence-based, rapid triage pathways, selective therapeutic hypothermia and advanced left ventricular support. In 2015, more than 50 patients were supported with either Impella or venoarterial extracorporeal membrane oxygen-

ation (ECMO). It is supported by dedicated ICU teams, rehabilitation services, and a brain injury program. King's has instigated and participated in a large number of trials/studies which support the evidence base in this patient group.

Out-of-Hospital Cardiac Arrest: The Facts

- Mortality from out-of-hospital cardiac arrest (OOHCA) remains exceptionally high, in spite of advances in prehospital and hospital care. All-comer survival in patients actively resuscitated is approximately 10% [1, 2], with significant regional variabilities worldwide driven by geography, public health measures (e.g., basic life support education and use of automated cardiac defibrillators in public areas), and expertise of both "first responders" and receiving hospital centers [3].
- Demographic factors and arrest details associated with an improved outcome are outlined in Table 24.1. Those with so-called "Utstein" criteria are thought to have the best prognosis, and are defined as:
  - Patients with a witnessed cardiac arrest.
  - Patients suffering an arrest due to presumed underlying heart disease.
  - Those with a presenting ventricular fibrillation (VF) rhythm [4].

I. Webb · R. Dworakowski · P. MacCarthy (✉)
Department of Cardiology, King's College Hospital,
King's Health Partners, London, UK
e-mail: philip.maccarthy@nhs.net

© Springer International Publishing AG, part of Springer Nature 2018
A. Myat et al. (eds.), *The Interventional Cardiology Training Manual*,
https://doi.org/10.1007/978-3-319-71635-0_24

Table 24.1 Multivariate predictors of an improved outcome from out-of-hospital cardiac arrest (modified from Refs. [21, 75])

Younger age
Lower patient comorbidity
Non-diabetic
Cardiac arrest in public location
Bystander CPR
Early return of spontaneous circulation (ROSC)
VF or VT as presenting rhythm with early defibrillation
STEMI ECG pattern
Prehospital airway protection
Absence of cardiogenic shock or need for inotropes
Therapeutic hypothermia

- Indeed, advances in survival and prognosis over the past 15 years have almost exclusively been in this select group of patients with presenting shockable rhythms.
- Where patients are successfully admitted to hospital with return of spontaneous circulation (ROSC), survival to discharge increases to approximately 25% [5, 6].
- The likelihood of survival appears to correlate with the number of OOHCA cases treated by any individual institute [7, 8]. This is driven in part by multidisciplinary goal-directed therapies as part of a "Bundle of Care" approach, which includes more aggressive post-resuscitation care, mild therapeutic hypothermia, access to early coronary angiography, and revascularization of culprit coronary disease where appropriate [9–12].
- Effective post-resuscitation pathways also impact on rates of complications from multiorgan failure and brain injury with subsequent favorable neurological outcomes [13–15].
- Immediate or early hospital mortality in OOHCA survivors is usually due to primary pump failure (either due to the extent of myocardial necrosis or global myocardial ischemia sustained during the resuscitation attempt) or arrhythmia, whereas in the later phase of hospital care it is commonly a complication of brain injury and poor neurological recovery [16, 17].
- There are currently very little randomized controlled trial data in managing OOHCA survivors, perhaps with the exception of therapeutic hypothermia. Most of the evidence in the available literature is from retrospective studies and registries and consequent interpretation of these data is difficult. Extrapolation of data that guides therapeutic intervention from existing acute coronary syndromes (ACS) trials (the overwhelming majority of which specifically exclude comatose patients) may be reasonable in some situations.
- However, there are important differences between comatose and non-comatose patients, ranging from the presenting history through to absorption kinetics and adjunctive pharmacological interventions.

Early Coronary Angiography in OOHCA Survivors

Evidence for Coronary Disease Being a Causative Factor

- Postmortem and acute angiographic findings in selected OOHCA patients suggest that obstructive coronary disease (often defined as a luminal obstruction of ≥50%) is found in over 70% of cases [18–20]. Where patients are appropriately triaged and referred on for emergency angiography, fresh occlusive coronary lesions are found in 48–67% of cases [19, 20], with critical non-flow limiting disease present in another 26% [20].
- The positive predictive value of finding culprit coronary disease in OOHCA patients with ST-segment elevation on ECG (with or without chest pain) is 0.87–0.96, with a negative predictive value of 0.42–0.61 [19, 21].
- Accordingly, there is little debate about the need for immediate coronary angiography in this group. However, patients without ST-segment elevation on their ECG are much more heterogeneous and when studied, will have a large number of etiologies for their cardiac arrest.
- Despite this, many comprehensive retrospective studies show that the incidence of significant coronary disease in this non-STEMI group of OOHCA survivors is also very high—variably found in 26–58% of patients [21, 22].
- The key issue for the clinician is whether this coronary disease has *caused* the cardiac arrest, and, secondarily, how to treat it. Many argue

that patients without an obvious noncoronary cause for OOHCA should proceed to emergency angiography, particularly when survival and a good functional recovery are otherwise anticipated.

Evidence for Early Coronary Intervention

- The 2012 European Society of Cardiology guidelines on ST-segment elevation myocardial infarction (STEMI) suggest that all OOHCA survivors with ECG evidence of STEMI undergo immediate coronary angiography with a view to primary PCI, as well as those patients with a high index of suspicion for ongoing ischemia, even where there is no clear ST-segment elevation [23]. This is now supported in expert consensus guidance published more recently by the European Association for Percutaneous Cardiovascular Interventions (EAPCI) [24].

- There is an established evidence base to support an early invasive strategy in ACS patients. However, this is not the case in comatose OOHCA survivors, particularly in those with non-STEMI ECG pattern in whom there may be additional diagnostic and prognostic considerations.

- Among the key questions that remain are the exact timing of coronary angiography, the benefits of "early" or "delayed" revascularization versus medical therapy alone, and the pharmacotherapy strategy employed, where intervention is deemed appropriate.

- Multiple observational studies looking at the use of an early invasive strategy in OOHCA have been published over the past decade [12, 25–42], with a synoptic overview of these studies confirming this approach as feasible and safe (Table 24.2).

- A meta-analysis of 3981 selected OOHCA patients from the United States, of whom 19% and 17% underwent coronary angiography

Table 24.2 Key observational studies over the past decade assessing use of an early invasive strategy in OOHCA survivors

Author	Year	N	STEMI (%)	PCI (%)	PCI success (%)	Survival (%)	Good neurological recovery (%)
Quintero-Moran [26]	2006	27	27 (100)	27 (100)	23 (85)	18 (67)	N/A
Sunde [12]	2007	47	N/A	30 (64)	N/A	N/A	N/A
Garot [27]	2007	186	186 (100)	186 (100)	161 (87)	103 (70)	89 (48)
Markusohn [28]	2007	25	25 (100)	25 (100)	22 (88)	19 (76)	17 (68)
Werling [29]	2007	24	N/A	13 (54)	N/A	16 (67)	N/A
Valente [30]	2008	31	31 (100)	31 (100)	N/A	23 (74)	N/A
Mager [31]	2008	21	21 (100)	21 (100)	N/A	18 (86)	N/A
Peels [32]	2008	44	44 (100)	44 (100)	38 (86)	22 (50)	N/A
Merchant [33]	2008	30	13 (43)	30 (100)	17 (57)	22 (80)	N/A
Reynolds [34]	2009	96	42 (44)	N/A	N/A	52 (54)	N/A
Lettieri [35]	2009	99	99 (100)	99 (100)	79 (80)	77 (78)	72 (73)
Pan [36]	2010	49	49 (100)	49 (100)	42 (86)	31 (63)	N/A
Batista [37]	2010	20	10 (50)	20 (100)	N/A	8 (40)	6 (30)
Dumas [21]	2010	435	134 (31)	202 (46)	177 (88)	171 (39)	160 (37)
Tomte [25]	2011	252	N/A	N/A	N/A	140 (56)	N/A
Mollman [38]	2011	65	36 (55)	65 (100)	64 (98)	46 (71)	N/A
Nanjayya [39]	2012	35	31 (89)	21 (60)	N/A	20 (57)	14 (40)
Bro-JepPeson [40]	2012	360	116 (32)	198 (55)	101 (83)	219 (61)	207 (58)
Zanuttini [41]	2012	93	32 (34)	N/A	N/A	50 (54)	36 (39)
Zimmerman [42]	2013	48	48 (100)	44 (92)	37 (84)	32 (67)	16 (33)

Modified from Noc et al. [24]

N/A not available, *OOHCA* out-of-hospital cardiac arrest, *PCI* percutaneous coronary intervention, *STEMI* ST-segment elevation acute myocardial infarction

and PCI within 24 h of admission, respectively, confirmed that a favorable neurological outcome was independently associated with early coronary angiography and reperfusion [43].

- A more recent meta-analysis confirmed this trend by showing an overall survival in the acute angiography group of 58.8% vs. 30.9% in the control group, with improved neurological outcomes (58.0% vs. 35.8%; OR 2.20, 95% CI 1.46–3.32) [44].
- Unfortunately, these data are confounded: In all observational OOHCA studies published it is acknowledged there is considerable bias of patients selected for angiography. Generally speaking, these patients are clinically selected and are younger, more likely to fulfill Utstein criteria and have better peri-arrest neurological scores. Moreover, they are more likely to have been treated in high volume units, which have been shown to achieve better outcomes for a variety of reasons.
- Therefore, even where angiography and revascularization are independently associated with improved outcomes, there are highly likely to

be additional confounding variables. Nevertheless, this association cannot be ignored and these studies act as an important reinforcement of good clinical assessment and risk stratification.

Optimal Timing of Angiography and Other Frontline Diagnostic Tests

- The concept and principles of early revascularization in OOHCA survivors are no different from patients without OOHCA—namely, the early restoration of coronary flow, securing of unstable coronary lesions and reduction of ischemia/necrosis as a substrate for arrhythmia and pump failure.
- Unless there is a clear alternative explanation for the patient's cardiac arrest, all OOHCA survivors to hospital admission should at least be *considered* for early angiography in their early triage.
- The ECG remains the frontline diagnostic tool to start the decision process (Fig. 24.1). For the reasons rehearsed above, all OOHCA survivors with clear ST-segment elevation on the

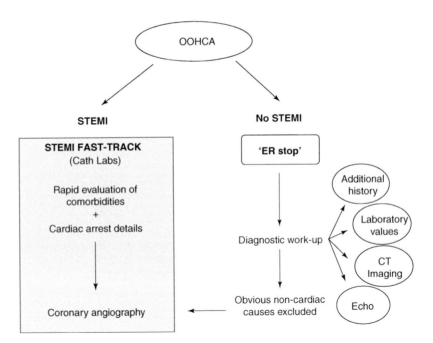

Fig. 24.1 Management of survivors of OOHCA. Patients successfully resuscitated with evidence of ST-segment elevation myocardial infarction on ECG should proceed directly to coronary angiography. All other patients should first be assessed in the emergency room ("ER stop") for further diagnostic workup before being considered for coronary angiography. Reproduced with permission from Nerla R et al. [76]

post-resuscitation ECG should be considered for immediate coronary angiography and transferred directly to the catheter laboratory of a designated Heart Attack Centre for further management.

- Patients with a presumed coronary cause for the OOHCA but without ST-segment elevation should ideally undergo early angiography after immediate assessment. For this reason, many argue that it is best to transport such patients to a unit that has the facility to do this at all times (i.e., a Heart Attack Centre).
- The initial assessment of this patient group is considered crucial in enabling careful assessment by a multidisciplinary team to exclude other possible causes of OOHCA and decide on the most sensible sequence of immediate investigations (Fig. 24.1). These patients would be directed to the Emergency Room for the initial triage—the so-called "ER-stop."
- In the case of diagnostic uncertainty, routine CT imaging of the brain, thorax, and abdomen may be considered depending on the clinical scenario. All patients should also undergo early bedside echocardiography to assess the following features: ventricular function, regional wall motion abnormalities, valvular heart disease, tamponade, aortic root dissection, or acute right ventricular changes due to massive pulmonary embolism.
- CT brain imaging should not delay coronary investigation unless a cerebrovascular event is suspected as a cause of the cardiac arrest, or trauma involving the head raises the possibility of intracranial bleeding. In either case, this should then be considered the first and possibly only diagnostic procedure. However, the difference between a cerebral and cardiac catastrophe can occasionally be more difficult than expected, particularly as the former can result in significant ECG change.
- Once obvious confounding diagnoses are excluded, all remaining patients should then proceed directly to coronary angiography as

soon as possible according to guidelines for high-risk non-ST-segment-elevation ACS (NSTE-ACS) [45].

Interventional Considerations

- There is a paucity of data addressing different revascularization strategies in relation to angiographic characteristics, completeness of revascularization, and adjunctive therapies in this patient group. It is nevertheless recommended that "clear culprit" lesions defined variably by acute occlusion, evidence of thrombus or correlation with ECG and echocardiographic data, are managed immediately by PCI (just as they would be in other scenarios), in order to decrease the incidence of recurrent cardiac arrest, to reduce infarct size and to improve hemodynamic stability [24].
- Contemporary ACS data suggest mortality and morbidity benefits from multivessel or "complete" revascularization during index hospitalization [46–48]. Whether this is undertaken immediately or in a staged fashion is likely to be dependent on patient characteristics, cardiac arrest details, and hemodynamic/electrical stability in the acute phase.
- Coronary anatomy complexity is also an important determinant, and may additionally guide modality of revascularization—in our experience emergency surgical grafting, for example, should not be undertaken when the neurological outcome is uncertain, though interval coronary artery bypass grafting (CABG) after neurological recovery, with or without initial PCI as a hybrid approach, is feasible and safe.
- Current guidelines suggest that moderate lesions with TIMI III flow may be considered for interval revascularization, once the patient's prognosis is more secure and additional investigations available (such as formal echocardiography, stress testing in a select group, neurological recovery, etc.) [45]. This approach acknowledges both diagnostic and

prognostic uncertainty in the acute patient without ST-segment elevation, but allows immediate coronary risk stratification.

Left Ventricular Support Devices (See Also Chap. 23)

- Cardiogenic shock is present in 30–40% of OOHCA survivors, and typically develops within 4–6 h of the arrest. Pump failure can occur from the myocardial necrosis sustained from the index coronary occlusion, global myocardial hypoxia incurred during the resuscitation attempt, or both.
- In our experience, global LV systolic impairment "in excess" of the territory supplied by an occluded infarct-related artery is a poor prognostic sign. Left ventricular support may be required to help bridge the patient's hemodynamics pending definitive revascularization, supporting the stunned myocardium and improving peripheral tissue and other organ perfusion.

- Nevertheless, as with all cardiogenic shock trials, irrespective of preceding arrest, no device has yet been shown definitively to alter prognosis.
- A number of support devices are in routine clinical practice (Fig. 24.2). Among these, only the intra-aortic balloon pump (IABP) has been investigated in this clinical setting. Its feasibility and safety have been demonstrated in comatose survivors of OOHCA with cardiogenic shock [49], but no prognostic benefit was demonstrated in the SHOCK II IABP trial, in which approximately 40% of patients were resuscitated OOHCA survivors [50].
- Second-generation devices include extracorporeal membrane oxygenation (ECMO) circuits, Impella and the TandemHeart. Each of these has unique technical features, physiological effects, and potential hazards, as summarized in Table 24.3.
- There are a number of small observational case series confirming their safety and feasibility, including prehospital ECMO [51], although larger, multicenter randomized controlled studies will be required to determine if

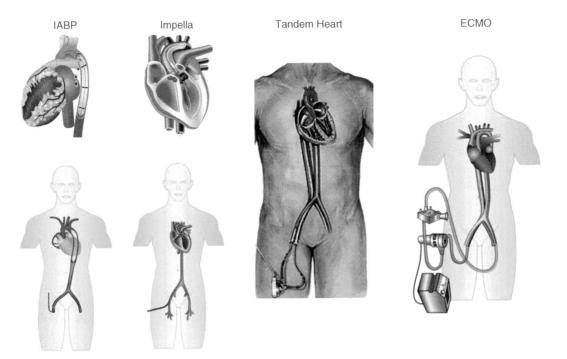

IABP   Impella   Tandem Heart   ECMO

Fig. 24.2 Commonly used left ventricular support devices for cardiogenic shock. Modified with permission from Werdan et al. [77]

Table 24.3 Hemodynamic effects of the major LV support devices

	Hemodynamic support	Afterload	LV stroke volume	Coronary perfusion	LV preload	PCW pressure	PT perfusion	Active cooling
IABP	0.5–1.0 L/min	↓	↑	↑	↓	↓	–	No
Impella	2.5–5.0 L/min	–	↓	↑?	↓↓	↓↓	↑	No
TandemHeart	4.0 L/min	↑	↓	Unknown	↓↓↓	↓↓↓	↑	(Yes)
ECMO	>4.5 L/min	↑	↓	Unknown	↓↓↓	↓↓↓	↑	Yes

Reproduced with permission from Nerla R et al. [76]

ECMO extracorporeal membrane oxygenation, *IABP* intra-aortic balloon pump, *LV* left ventricular, *PCW* pulmonary capillary wedge, *PT* peripheral tissues

these complex support systems enhance patient outcomes in the wider population.

- At present, such devices have to be tailored to individual patients according to the clinical scenario and local expertise. At King's we hold a "mini-multidisciplinary meeting" with our intensive care colleagues to make such decisions. If diminished coronary flow is an ongoing problem, we favor the IABP, whereas in cases where brief proximal coronary occlusion has caused massive myocardial territory damage but been fully restored during primary PCI, an Impella or ECMO may be more appropriate.

Automated CPR Devices

- Coronary angiography and PCI can be undertaken while the patient remains in cardiac arrest. Cardiopulmonary resuscitation devices, such as the Lucas™ device or Autopulse® can be initiated by first responders, and are capable of providing efficient massage to support the circulation until a definitive intervention is performed, or until such time as the patient can be established onto ECMO.
- Operating under these conditions is difficult, due to restricted visibility on fluoroscopy and patient motion. Nevertheless, when initiated early after a cardiac arrest, this can be an effective bridge to therapy in selected patients.

Pharmacotherapy

- Effective anticoagulation and antiplatelet therapy are major considerations in OOHCA

patients undergoing emergency coronary revascularization. Acute stent thrombosis occurs in up to 10% of ACS patients complicated by cardiac arrest [52, 53], with an odds ratio of 12.9 compared to ACS patients without arrest (95%CI 1.3–124.6; $p = 0.027$) [53]. This carries a substantial additional mortality risk [54].

- Likely causative factors include:
  - Non-administration of drugs.
  - Malabsorption and altered metabolism.
  - A highly procoagulant and inflammatory state.
  - The adverse hemodynamic status of the patient [53, 54].
- Where intervention is performed, aspirin and adjunctive antiplatelets should be administered as quickly as possible via nasogastric tube. Second- and third-line $P2Y_{12}$ inhibitors (prasugrel and ticagrelor) have improved pharmacokinetics, but still have a substantial delay until effective platelet inhibition is achieved.
- There may be a benefit from bridging with an intravenous glycoprotein receptor inhibitor (eptifibatide, tirofiban, or abciximab) or novel intravenous $P2Y_{12}$ inhibitor (cangrelor). Indeed, there is recent evidence that administration of eptifibatide in this setting results in profound platelet inhibition measured both by the VerifyNow IIb/IIIa and the Multiplate TRAP tests for at least 22 h [55].
- Similarly, in STEMI patients without cardiac arrest, a single up-front bolus of abciximab without additional infusion might be sufficient to bridge the delayed effect of oral agents [56]. Key pharmacological properties of the antiplatelet agents are summarized in Table 24.4.

Table 24.4 Principle pharmacokinetic characteristics of commonly used antiplatelet agents in emergency PCI

Drug	ROA	Loading dose	Time to EPI (min)	Time to PFR (h)	Cooling interaction
Aspirin	Oral, IV	300 mg (200 mg i.v.)	60	96	Mild
Clopidogrel	Oral	600 mg	360	120	Relevant
Prasugrel	Oral	60 mg	90–120	168	Mild
Ticagrelor	Oral	180 mg	60–120	48–120	Mild to moderate
Cangrelor	IV	30 µg/kg (bolus)	2	0.5	None?
Abciximab	IV	0.25 mg/kg (bolus)	15	24–48	None
Tirofiban	IV	180 µg/kg (bolus)	15–30	4	None
Eptifibatide	IV	10 µg/kg (bolus)	15–30	4	None

Reproduced with permission from Nerla R et al. [76]

BW body weight, *EPI* effective platelet inhibition (i.e., platelet function inhibited in more than 50% of subjects), *IV* intravenous, *PCI* percutaneous coronary intervention, *PFR* platelet function recovery, *ROA* route of administration

- The benefits of profound inhibition of platelet reactivity should be weighed against the increased risk of bleeding due to arterial access, post-CPR chest wall injuries, and declared and occult head injury. Post hoc analysis from the TTM trial suggest that patients undergoing early coronary angiography (+/− PCI) had significantly higher rates of bleeding (22% vs. 14%; OR 1.62 $p = 0.01$), driven primarily by access site complications (10% vs. 4%; OR 2.42 $p = 0.007$) [57]. To what extent radial access can minimize complications in this patient group is unclear, but data from non-comatose ACS patients would support this approach where possible [58–60].

Adjunctive Patient Support

Targeted Therapeutic Hypothermia (TTM)

- A major concern in survivors of OOHCA is neurological recovery. Transient interruption of cerebral blood flow for only a few minutes triggers an almost immediate cascade of deleterious molecular pathways, which can ultimately lead to cerebral injury [61]. Cooling slows down cellular metabolism at a rate of 6–7% for each 1 °C decrease in temperature [62, 63], attenuating cell membrane destruction, pathological calcium release, and reactive oxygen formation.

- Two randomized controlled trials have demonstrated significant gains in mortality reduction and neurological recovery for OOHCA patients with shockable heart rhythms treated by early mild hypothermia for 12–24 h [63, 64]. This has also subsequently shown to be beneficial in less-selective OOHCA patient subgroups [65].

- TTM is now widely employed worldwide, although the extent of hypothermia required to gain a benefit is no longer thought to be so crucial. A recent study in OOHCA survivors randomized patients to either 33 °C or 36 °C [57]; survival to discharge and good neurologic outcomes did not differ significantly between groups. Furthermore, post hoc analysis has demonstrated more profound hemodynamic alterations in the 33 °C group, with decreased heart rate, elevated levels of lactate, and greater vasopressor support, all of which have independently been associated with increased mortality [66].

- TTM can be achieved through a variety of techniques, from nasal cooling (e.g., Rhinchill®), through to surface cooling devices (including ice packs) and intravenous catheter systems (e.g., Thermogard XP®).

- No one system has been randomized against another in head-to-head comparisons of technical or clinical efficacy, although intravenous rather than surface cooling techniques achieve more rapid cooling of core body temperature [67].

- The European Resuscitation Council Guidelines currently recommend hypothermia for all comatose OOHCA survivors regardless of the initial rhythm, although the weaker evidence base for patients presenting with non-shockable heart rhythm is recognized [68].
- Many centers still do not follow these guidelines and use of TTM has decreased after recent negative trials [57]. There are four stages of hypothermia:
  - Initiation
  - Maintenance
  - Rewarming
  - Return to normothermia (Fig. 24.3) [69]

- If it is to be used, hypothermia should be initiated as soon as possible, since a 20% increase in mortality has been described for every hour of delay [70]. Several liters of cooled intravenous saline will decrease temperatures by 1 °C within 30 min [70], help to prevent post-resuscitation hypotension, and can be delivered simply by first responders or emergency room personnel. Ice bags and cooling blankets are simple and effective, but are difficult to titrate to target temperature, whereas temperature-regulated surface and endovascular devices allow easier temperature control during the maintenance phase, and prevent rapid temperature changes during rewarming.
- Hypothermia is generally considered contraindicated in intracranial or severe extracranial hemorrhage, refractory hypotension, severe sepsis, and pregnancy.

Neuro-Rehabilitation

- Providing appropriate neuro-rehabilitation care and determining functional recovery after OOHCA remains challenging for both patients and families. Prognostic neurological assessment relies on physical examination, electroencephalography (EEG), neuroimaging, sensory stimulatory evoked potentials (SSEP's), and to a lesser extent currently through use of biomarkers.
- The positive and negative predictive values of these tests are variable and ill-defined, such that the presence of an early abnormality does not always indicate a poor long-term prognosis, and vice versa. However, some data suggest that two abnormal findings, such as incomplete recovery of brainstem reflexes and bilaterally absent SSEP's, have a higher specificity for poor neurological recovery [71].
- A recent meta-analysis identified a series of early predictors of poor neurological outcome in comatose patients resuscitated from OOHCA treated using therapeutic hypothermia [72]. Among these, the presence of either burst-suppression or electrographic status epilepticus evolving from burst-suppression appeared most prognostic.

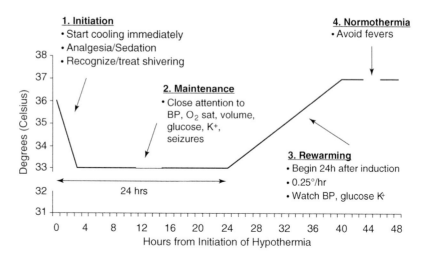

Fig. 24.3 Stages of therapeutic hypothermia in clinical practice. Reproduced with permission from Scirica BM [69]

- Current AHA guidelines recommend that neurological prognostication should be delayed until at least 72 h after the return to normothermia [11].

Implantable Cardiac Defibrillator (ICD) Therapy

- Patients who survive OOHCA due to VF/VT arrest, without a reversible cause and with good functional and neurological prognosis, should be considered for implantable ICD therapy before discharge. This includes patients with structural cardiomyopathies (e.g., hypertrophic or dilated cardiomyopathies) and the "channelopathies" such as Brugada or long QT syndrome.
- Revascularized STEMI patients with or without VT/VF arrest have similar long-term prognoses, assuming left ventricular function is not significantly impaired [23]. For this reason, current STEMI guidelines do not recommend routine ICD therapy in patients with OOHCA survivors with VT or VF in the context of acute infarction up to 48 h.
- Much of this data derives from the thrombolysis era. However, a recent study including 4653 consecutive PCI-treated STEMI patients has supported this approach in contemporary practice, with no negative influence of VT/VF in the acute phase of STEMI on the long-term prognosis [73].
- A meta-analysis of three major randomized ICD studies, which included a large number of OOHCA survivors of various cardiac etiologies, has demonstrated a 27% reduction in the relative risk of dying (absolute reduction of 3.5% per year) associated with ICD implantation; this was due almost entirely to a 50% reduction in arrhythmic death, most notably in patients with patients with LVEF ≤35% [74].
- In successfully revascularized ACS patients it is anticipated that there will be some interval functional recovery of LV function. Since no ICD trial has shown prognostic benefit of early predischarge intervention in this group

(patients with poor LVEF treated with ICD do have less arrhythmic death, but higher pump-failure related death), it is standard practice in many centers to reassess ventricular function, scar burden, and telemetry-detected arrhythmias at 6–12 weeks and then reconsider ICD +/− cardiac resynchronization therapy in addition to optimal heart failure management.
- Nevertheless, patients at very high risk—such as those with recurrent arrhythmia as an inpatient, extreme low LVEF and likely transplant candidates may be considered early for pre-discharge ICD therapy.

Conclusions

- OOHCA is a major cause of mortality and morbidity and its incidence is increasing due to more effective ambulance and bystander resuscitation.
- Important predictors of a favorable outcome include early life-support measures and facilitated transfer to hospital where a comprehensive assessment of the patient can be made and early interventions undertaken.
- Patients with clear ST-elevation on the post-resuscitation ECG, with a reasonable expectation of survival, should be offered emergency coronary angiography and revascularization, where appropriate. Those who fulfill Utstein criteria and are therefore very likely to have a coronary cause for their arrest should be treated similarly.
- Those without ST-elevation or those in whom the diagnosis remains uncertain should be assessed at the "ER-stop" with clinical review and systematic imaging, where indicated, including bedside echocardiography. If no obvious cause is found, these patients should then undergo emergency coronary angiography.
- Protocolized multidisciplinary goal-directed therapies are likely to improve patient survival and support a favorable neurological recovery, but randomized controlled data to support many of these interventions are sparse.

References

1. Berdowski J, Berg RA, Tijssen JG, Koster RW. Global incidences of out-of-hospital cardiac arrest and survival rates: systematic review of 67 prospective studies. Circ Cardiovasc Qual Outcomes. 2010;81:1479–87.
2. Sasson C, Rogers MAM, Dahl J, Kellermann AL. Predictors of survival from out-of-hospital cardiac arrest: a systematic review and meta-analysis. Circ Cardiovasc Qual Outcomes. 2010;3:63–81.
3. Perkins GD, Cooke MW. Variability in cardiac arrest survival: the NHS ambulance service quality indicators. Emerg Med J. 2012;29:3–5.
4. Cummins RO, Chamberlain DA, Abramson NS, et al. Recommended guidelines for uniform reporting of data from out-of-hospital cardiac arrest: the Utstein Style. A statement for health professionals from a task force of the American Heart Association, the European Resuscitation Council, the Heart and Stroke Foundation of Canada, and the Australian Resuscitation Council. Circulation. 1991;84:960–75.
5. Herlitz J, Engdahl J, Svensson L, Angquist KA, Silfverstolpe J, Holmberg S. Major differences in 1-month survival between hospitals in Sweden among initial survivors of out-of-hospital cardiac arrest. Resuscitation. 2006;70:404–9.
6. Mashiko K, Otsuka T, Shimazaki S, Kohama A, Kamishima G, Katsurada K, Sawada Y, Matsubara I, Yamaguchi K. An outcome study of out-of-hospital cardiac arrest using the Utstein template: a Japanese experience. Resuscitation. 2002;55:241–6.
7. Carr BG, Kahn JM, Merchant RM, Kramer AA, Neumar RW. Inter-hospital variability in post-cardiac arrest mortality. Resuscitation. 2009;80:30–34.66.
8. Callaway CW, Schmicker R, Kampmeyer M, Powell J, Rea TD, Daya MR, Aufderheide TP, Davis DP, Rittenberger JC, Idris AH, Nichol G. Receiving hospital characteristics associated with survival after out-of-hospital cardiac arrest. Resuscitation. 2010;81:524–9.
9. Kirves H, Skrifvars MB, Vahakuopus M, Ekstrom K, Martikainen M, Castren M. Adherence to resuscitation guidelines during prehospital care of cardiac arrest patients. Eur J Emerg Med. 2007;14:75–81.
10. Gaieski DF, Band RA, Abella BS, Neumar RW, Fuchs BD, Kolansky DM, Merchant RM, Carr BG, Becker LB, Maguire C, Klair A, Hylton J, Goyal M. Early goal-directed hemodynamic optimization combined with therapeutic hypothermia in comatose survivors of out-of-hospital cardiac arrest. Resuscitation. 2009;80:418–24.
11. Peberdy MA, Callaway CW, Neumar RW, Geocadin RG, Zimmerman JL, Donnino M, Gabrielli A, Silvers SM, Zaritsky AL, Merchant R, Vanden Hoek TL, Kronick SL. 2010 American Heart Association guidelines for cardiopulmonary resuscitation and emergency cardiovascular care science. Circulation. 2010;122:S768–86.
12. Sunde K, Pytte M, Jacobsen D, Mangschau A, Jensen LP, Smedsrud C, Draegni T, Steen PA. Implementation of a standardised treatment protocol for post resuscitation care after out-of-hospital cardiac arrest. Resuscitation. 2007;73:29–39.
13. Neumar RW, Nolan JP, Adrie C, Aibiki M, Berg RA, Bottiger BW, Callaway C, Clark RS, Geocadin RG, Jauch EC, Kern KB, Laurent I, Longstreth WT Jr, Merchant RM, Morley P, Morrison LJ, Nadkarni V, Peberdy MA, Rivers EP, Rodriguez-Nunez A, Sellke FW, Spaulding C, Sunde K, Vanden Hoek T. Post-cardiac arrest syndrome: epidemiology, pathophysiology, treatment, and prognostication. A consensus statement from the International Liaison Committee on Resuscitation (American Heart Association, Australian and New Zealand Council on Resuscitation, European Resuscitation Council, Heart and Stroke Foundation of Canada, InterAmerican Heart Foundation, Resuscitation Council of Asia, and the Resuscitation Council of Southern Africa); the American Heart Association Emergency Cardiovascular Care Committee; the Council on Cardiovascular Surgery and Anesthesia; the Council on Cardiopulmonary, Perioperative, and Critical Care; the Council on Clinical Cardiology; and the Stroke Council. Circulation. 2008;118:2452–83.
14. Safar P. Resuscitation from clinical death: pathophysiologic limits and therapeutic potentials. Crit Care Med. 1988;16:923–41.
15. Skrifvars MB, Pettila V, Rosenberg PH, Castren M. A multiple logistic regression analysis of in-hospital factors related to survival at six months in patients resuscitated from out-of-hospital ventricular fibrillation. Resuscitation. 2003;59:319–28.
16. Schoenenberger RA, von Planta M, von Planta I. Survival after failed out-of-hospital resuscitation. Are further therapeutic efforts in the emergency department futile? Arch Intern Med. 1994;154:2433–7.
17. Laver S, Farrow C, Turner D, Nolan J. Mode of death after admission to an intensive care unit following cardiac arrest. Intensive Care Med. 2004;30:2126–8.
18. Davies MJ. Anatomic features in victims of sudden coronary death: coronary artery pathology. Circulation. 1992;85:119–24.
19. Spaulding CM, Joly LM, Rosenberg A, Monchi M, Weber SN, Dhainaut JF, Carli P. Immediate coronary angiography in survivors of out-of-hospital cardiac arrest. N Engl J Med. 1997;336:1629–33.
20. Zeliaś A, Stępińska J, Andres J, Trąbka-Zawicki A, Sadowski J, Żmudka K. Ten-year experience of an invasive cardiology centre with out-of-hospital cardiac arrest patients admitted for urgent coronary angiography. Kardiol Pol. 2014;72(8):687–99.
21. Dumas F, Cariou A, Manzo-Silberman S, Grimaldi D, Vivien B, Rosencher J, Empana JP, Carli P, Mira JP, Jouven X, Spaulding C. Immediate percutaneous coronary intervention is associated with better survival after out-of-hospital cardiac arrest. Insights from the PROCAT registry. Circ Cardiovasc Interv. 2010;3:200–7.

22. Hollenbeck RD, McPherson JA, Mooney MR, Unger BT, Patel NA, McMullan PW, Hsu C-H, Seder DB, Kern KB. Early cardiac catheterisation is associated with improved survival in comatose survivors of cardiac arrest without STEMI. Resuscitation. 2014;85:88–95.

23. Steg PG, James SK, Atar D, Badano LP, Blömstrom-Lundqvist C, Borger MA, Di Mario C, Dickstein K, Ducrocq G, Fernandez-Aviles F, Gershlick AH, Giannuzzi P, Halvorsen S, Huber K, Juni P, Kastrati A, Knuuti J, Lenzen MJ, Mahaffey KW, Valgimigli M, Van 'thof A, Widimsky P, Zahger D, Task Force on the management of ST-segment elevation acute myocardial infarction of the European Society of Cardiology (ESC). ESC guidelines for the management of acute myocardial infarction in patients presenting with ST-segment elevation. Eur Heart J. 2012;33:2569–619.

24. Noc M, Fajadet J, Lassen JF, Kala P, MacCarthy P, Olivecrona GK, Windecker S, Spaulding C. Invasive coronary treatment strategies for out-of-hospital cardiac arrest: a consensus statement from the European Association for Percutaneous Cardiovascular Interventions (EAPCI)/Stent for Life (SFL) groups. EuroIntervention. 2014;10:31–7.

25. Tømte O, Andersen GØ, Jacobsen D, Drægni T, Auestad B, Sunde K. Strong and weak aspects of an established post-resuscitation treatment protocol—a five-year observational study. Resuscitation. 2011;82:1186–93.

26. Quintero-Moran B, Moreno R, Villarreal S, Perez-Vizcayno MJ, Hernandez R, Conde C, Vazquez P, Alfonso F, Banuelos C, Escaned J, Fernandez-Ortiz A, Aycona L, Macaya C. Percutaneous coronary intervention for cardiac arrest secondary to ST-elevation acute myocardial infarction. Influence of immediate paramedical/medical assistance on clinical outcome. J Invasive Cardiol. 2006;18:269–72.

27. Garot P, Lefevre T, Eltchaninoff H, Morice MC, Tamion F, Abry B, Lesault PF, Tarnec JY, Pouges C, Margenet A, Monchi M, Laurent I, Dumas P, Garot J, Louvard Y. Six-month outcome of emergency percutaneous coronary intervention in resuscitated patients after cardiac arrest complicating ST-elevation myocardial infarction. Circulation. 2007;115:1354–62.

28. Markushon E, Roguin A, Sebbag A, Aronson D, Dragu R, Amikam S, Boulus M, Grenadier E, Kerner A, Nikolsky E, Markiewicz W, Hammerman H, Kapeliovich M. Primary percutaneous coronary intervention after out-of-hospital cardiac arrest: patients and outcomes. Isr Med Assoc J. 2007;9:257–9.

29. Werling M, Thoren AB, Axelsson C, Herlitz J. Treatment and outcome in post-resuscitation care after out-of-hospital cardiac arrest when a modern therapeutic approach was introduced. Resuscitation. 2007;73:40–5.

30. Valente S, Lazzeri C, Saletti E, Chiostri M, Gensini GF. Primary percutaneous coronary intervention in comatose survivors of cardiac arrest with ST-elevation acute myocardial infarction: a single-center experi-ence in Florence. J Cardiovasc Med (Hagerstown). 2008;9:1083–7.

31. Mager A, Kornowski R, Murninkas D, Vaknin-Assa H, Ukabi S, Brosh D, Battler A, Assali A. Outcome of emergency percutaneous coronary intervention for acute ST-elevation myocardial infarction complicated by cardiac arrest. Coron Artery Dis. 2008;19(8):615.

32. Peels HO, Jessurun GA, van der Horst IC, Arnold AE, Piers LH, Zijlstra F. Outcome in transferred and nontransferred patients after primary percutaneous coronary intervention for ischaemic out-of-hospital cardiac arrest. Catheter Cardiovasc Interv. 2008;71:147–51.

33. Merchant RM, Abella BS, Khan M, Huang KN, Beiser DB, Neumar RW, Carr BG, Becker LB, Vanden Hoek TL. Cardiac catheterization is underutilized after in-hospital cardiac arrest. Resuscitation. 2008;79:398–403.

34. Reynolds JC, Callaway CW, El Khoudary SR, Moore CG, Alvarez RJ, Rittenberger JC. Coronary angiography predicts improved outcome following cardiac arrest: propensity-adjusted analysis. J Intensive Care Med. 2009;24:179–86.

35. Lettieri C, Savoritto S, De Servi S, Guagliumi G, Repetto A, Piccaluga E, Politi A, Ettori F, Castiglioni B, Fabbiocchi F, De Cesare N, Sangiorgi G, Musumechi G, D'Urbano M, Pirelli S, Zanini R, Klugmann S, Lombard I MA Study Group. Emergency percutaneous coronary intervention in patients with ST-elevation myocardial infarction complicated by out-of-hospital cardiac arrest: early and medium-term outcome. Am Heart J. 2009;157:569–75.

36. Pan W, Yang SS, Wang LF, Sun YM, Li ZQ, Zhou LJ, Li Y, Li WM. Outcome of patients with ST-elevation myocardial infarction complicated by pre-hospital cardiac arrest underwent emergency percutaneous coronary intervention. Zhonghua Xin Xue Guan Bing Za Zhi. 2010;38:875–9.

37. Batista LM, Lima FO, Januzzi JL Jr, Donahue V, Snydeman C, Greer DM. Feasibility and safety of combined percutaneous coronary intervention and therapeutic hypothermia following cardiac arrest. Resuscitation. 2010;81:398–403.

38. Möllmann H, Szardien S, Liebetrau C, Elsässer A, Rixe J, Rolf A, Nef H, Weber M, Hamm C. Clinical outcome of patients treated with an early invasive strategy after out-of-hospital cardiac arrest. J Int Med Res. 2011;39:2169–77.

39. Nanjayya VB, Nayyar V. Immediate coronary angiogram in comatose survivors of out-of-hospital cardiac arrest—an Australian study. Resuscitation. 2012;83:699–704.

40. Bro-Jeppesen J, Kjaergaard J, Wanscher M, Pedersen F, Holmvang L, Lippert FK, Møller JE, Køber L, Hassager C. Emergency coronary angiography in comatose cardiac arrest patients: do real-life experiences support the guidelines? Eur Heart J Acute Cardiovasc Care. 2012;1:291–301.

41. Zanuttini D, Armellini I, Nucifora G, Carchietti E, Trillò G, Spedicato L, Bernardi G, Proclemer

A. Impact of emergency coronary angiography on in-hospital outcome of unconscious survivors after out-of-hospital cardiac arrest. Am J Cardiol. 2012;110:1723–8.

42. Zimmermann S, Flachskampf FA, Schneider R, Dechant K, Alff A, Klinghammer L, Rittger H, Achenbach S. Mild therapeutic hypothermia after out-of-hospital cardiac arrest complicating ST-elevation myocardial infarction: long-term results in clinical practice. Clin Cardiol. 2013;36:414–21.

43. Callaway CW, Schmicker RH, Brown SP, Albrich JM, Andrusiek DL, Aufderheide TP, Christenson J, Daya MR, Falconer D, Husa RD, Idris AH, Ornato JP, Rac VE, Rea TD, Rittenberger JC, Sears G, Stiell IG, Investigators ROC. Early coronary angiography and induced hypothermia are associated with survival and functional recovery after out-of-hospital cardiac arrest. Resuscitation. 2014;85:657–63.

44. Camuglia AC, Randhawa VK, Lavi S, Walters DL. Cardiac catheterization is associated with superior outcomes for survivors of out of hospital cardiac arrest: review and meta-analysis. Resuscitation. 2014;85:1533–40.

45. Hamm CW, Bassand JP, Agewall S, Bax J, Boersma E, Bueno H, Caso P, Dudek D, Gielen S, Huber K, Ohman M, Petrie MC, Sonntag F, Uva MS, Storey RF, Wijns W, Zahger D, ESC Committee for Practice Guidelines. ESC guidelines for the management of acute coronary syndromes in patients presenting without persistent ST-segment elevation: The Task Force for the management of acute coronary syndromes (ACS) in patients presenting without persistent ST-segment elevation of the European Society of Cardiology (ESC). Eur Heart J. 2011;32:2999–3054.

46. Gershlick AH, Khan JN, Kelly DJ, Greenwood JP, Sasikaran T, Curzen N, Blackman DJ, Dalby M, Fairbrother KL, Banya W, Wang D, Flather M, Hetherington SL, Kelion AD, Talwar S, Gunning M, Hall R, Swanton H, McCann GP. Randomized trial of complete versus lesion-only revascularization in patients undergoing primary percutaneous coronary intervention for STEMI and multivessel disease: the CvLPRIT trial. J Am Coll Cardiol. 2015;65(10):963–72.

47. Wald DS, Morris JK, Wald NJ, Chase AJ, Edwards RJ, Hughes LO, Berry C, Oldroyd KG, PRAMI Investigators. Randomized trial of preventive angioplasty in myocardial infarction. N Engl J Med. 2013;369(12):1115–23.

48. Engstrøm T, Kelbæk H, Helqvist S, Høfsten DE, Kløvgaard L, Holmvang L, Jørgensen E, Pedersen F, Saunamäki K, Clemmensen P, De Backer O, Ravkilde J, Tilsted HH, Villadsen AB, Aarøe J, Jensen SE, Raungaard B, Køber L, DANAMI-3—PRIMULTI Investigators. Complete revascularisation versus treatment of the culprit lesion only in patients with ST-segment elevation myocardial infarction and multi-vessel disease (DANAMI-3 Primulti): an open-label, randomised controlled trial. Lancet. 2015;386(9994):665–71.

49. Hovdenes J, Laake JH, Aaberge L, Haugaa H, Bugge JF. Therapeutic hypothermia after out-of-hospital cardiac arrest: experiences with patients treated with percutaneous coronary intervention and cardiogenic shock. Acta Anaesthesiol Scand. 2007;51:137–42.

50. Thiele H, Zeymer U, Neumann FJ, Ferenc M, Olbrich HG, Hausleitner J, Richard G, Hennersdorf M, Empen K, Fuernau G, Desch S, Eitel I, Hambrecht R, Fuhrmann J, Bohm M, Ebelt H, Schneider S, Schuller G, Werdan K, IABP-SHOCK II Trial Investigators. Intra-aortic balloon support for myocardial infarction with cardiogenic shock. N Engl J Med. 2012;367:1287–96.

51. Stub D, Bernard S, Pellegrino V, Smith K, Walker T, Sheldrake J, Hockings L, Shaw J, Duffy S, Burrell A, Cameron P, De Villiers S, Kaye D. Refractory cardiac arrest treated with mechanical CPR, hypothermia, ECMO and early reperfusion (the CHEER trial). Resuscitation. 2015;86:88–94.

52. Shah N, Garg J, Agarwal V, Mehta K, Jacobs L, Patel N, Freudenberger R. Stent thrombosis is not increased in cardiac arrest patients undergoing therapeutic hypothermia: an analysis of 15,079 procedures. J Am Coll Cardiol. 2015;65:A167 (10 Suppl)

53. Joffre J, Varenne O, Bougouin W, Rosencher J, Mira JP, Cariou A. Stent thrombosis: an increased adverse event after angioplasty following resuscitated cardiac arrest. Resuscitation. 2014;85(6):769–73.

54. Buchanan GL, Basavarajaiah S, Chieffo A. Stent thrombosis: incidence, predictors and new technologies. Thrombosis. 2012;2012:956962.

55. Steblovnik K, Blinc A, Bozic-Mijovski M, Kranjec I, Melkic E, Noc M. Platelet reactivity in comatose survivors of cardiac arrest undergoing percutaneous coronary intervention and hypothermia. EuroIntervention. 2015;10(12):1418–24.

56. Valgimigli M, Campo G, Tebaldi M, Monti M, Gambetti S, Scalone A, Parinello G, Ferrari R. Fabolus Synchro (facilitation through abciximab by dropping infusion Line in patients undergoing coronary stenting. Synergy with clopidogrel at high loading dose regimen) Investigators. Randomized double-blind comparison of effects of abciximab bolus only vs. on-label regimen on ex vivo inhibition of platelet aggregation in responders to clopidogrel undergoing coronary stenting. J Thromb Haemost. 2010;8:1903–11.

57. Nielsen N, Wetterslev J, et al. for the TTM Trial Investigators. Targeted temperature management at 33°C versus 36°C after cardiac arrest. N Engl J Med. 2013;369:2197–206.

58. Bernat I, Horak D, Stasek J, Mates M, et al. ST-segment elevation myocardial infarction treated by radial or femoral approach in a multicenter randomized clinical trial: The STEMI-RADIAL Trial. J Am Coll Cardiol. 2014;63(10):964–72.

59. Jolly SS, Yusuf S, Cairns J, Niemelä K, et al. for the RIVAL trial group. Radial versus femoral access for coronary angiography and intervention in patients with acute coronary syndromes (RIVAL): a ran-

domised, parallel group, multicentre trial. Lancet. 2011;377(9775):1409–20.

60. Romagnoli E, Biondi-Zoccai G, Sciahbasi A, Politi L, Rigattieri S, Pendenza G, Summaria F, Patrizi R, Borghi A, Di Russo C, Moretti C, Agostoni P, Loschiavo P, Lioy E, Sheiban I, Sangiorgi G. Radial versus femoral randomized investigation in ST-segment elevation acute coronary syndrome: the RIFLE-STEACS (Radial Versus Femoral Randomized Investigation in ST-Elevation Acute Coronary Syndrome) study. J Am Coll Cardiol. 2012;60(24):2481–9.

61. Eleff SM, Maruki Y, Monsein LH, Traystman RJ, Bryan RN, Koehler RC. Sodium, ATP, and intracellular pH transients during reversible complete ischemia of dog cerebrum. Stroke. 1991;22:233–41.

62. Nolan JP, Morley PT, Hoek TL, Hickey RW. Advancement Life support Task Force of the International Liaison committee on Resuscitation Therapeutic hypothermia after cardiac arrest An advisory statement by the Advancement Life support Task Force of the International Liaison committee on Resuscitation. Resuscitation. 2003;57:231–5.

63. The Hypothermia after Cardiac Arrest Study Group. Mild therapeutic hypothermia to improve the neurologic outcome after cardiac arrest. N Engl J Med. 2002;346:549–56.

64. Bernard SA, Gray TW, Buist MD, Jones BM, Silvester W, Gutteridge G, Smith K. Treatment of comatose survivors of out-of-hospital cardiac arrest with induced hypothermia. N Engl J Med. 2002;346:557–63.

65. Kim YM, Yim HW, Jeong SH, Klem ML, Callaway CW. Does therapeutic hypothermia benefit adult cardiac arrest patients presenting with non-shockable initial rhythms? A systematic review and meta-analysis of randomized and non-randomized studies. Resuscitation. 2012;83:188–96.

66. Bro-Jeppesen J, Annborn M, Hassager C, Wise MP, Pelosi P, Nielsen N, Erlinge D, Wanscher M, Friberg H, Kjaergaard J, TTM Investigators. Hemodynamics and vasopressor support during targeted temperature management at 33°C versus 36°C after out-of-hospital cardiac arrest: a post hoc study of the target temperature management trial. Crit Care Med. 2015;43(2):318–27.

67. Yenari MA, Colbourne F, Hemmen TM, Han HS, Krieger D. Therapeutic hypothermia in stroke. Stroke Res Treat. 2011;Article ID 157969.

68. Deakin CD, Nolan JP, Soar J, Sunde K, Koster RW, Smith GB, Perkins GD. European resuscitation council guidelines for resuscitation 2010 section 4: adult advanced life support. Resuscitation. 2010;81:1305–52.

69. Scirica BM. Therapeutic hypothermia after cardiac arrest. Circulation. 2013;127:244–50.

70. Moore TM, Callaway CW, Hostler D. Core temperature cooling in healthy volunteers after rapid intravenous infusion of cold and room temperature saline solution. Ann Emerg Med. 2008;51:153–9.

71. Rossetti AO, Oddo M, Logroscino G, Kaplan PW. Prognostication after cardiac arrest and hypothermia: a prospective study. Ann Neurol. 2010;67:301–7.

72. Sandroni C, Cavallaro F, Callaway CW, D'Arrigo S, Sanna T, Kuiper MA, Biancone M, Della Marca G, Farcomeni A, Nolan JP. Predictors of poor neurological outcome in adult comatose survivors of cardiac arrest: a systematic review and meta-analysis. Part 2: Patients treated with therapeutic hypothermia. Resuscitation. 2013;84:1324–38.

73. Demirel F, Rasoul S, Elvan A, Ottervanger JP, Dambrink JH, Gosselink AM, Hoorntje JC, Ramdat Misier AR, van 't Hof AW. Impact of out-of-hospital cardiac arrest due to ventricular fibrillation in patients with ST-elevation myocardial infarction admitted for primary percutaneous coronary intervention: impact of ventricular fibrillation in STEMI patients. Eur Heart J Acute Cardiovasc Care. 2015;4(1):16–23.

74. Connolly SJ, Hallstrom AP, Cappato R, Schron EB, Kuck KH, Zipes DP, Greene HL, Boczor S, Domanski M, Follmann D, Gent M, Roberts RS. Meta-analysis of the implantable cardioverter defibrillator secondary prevention trials. AVID, CASH and CIDS studies. Antiarrhythmics vs Implantable Defibrillator study. Cardiac Arrest Study Hamburg. Canadian Implantable Defibrillator Study. Eur Heart J. 2000;21:2071–8.

75. Iqbal MB, Al-Hussaini A, Rosser G, Salehi S, Phylactou M, Rajakulasingham R, Patel J, Elliott K, Mohan P, Green R, Whitbread M, Smith R, Ilsley C. Predictors of survival and favorable functional outcomes after an out-of-hospital cardiac arrest in patients systematically brought to a dedicated heart attack center (from the Harefield Cardiac Arrest Study). Am J Cardiol. 2015;115(6):730–7.

76. Nerla R, Webb I, MacCarthy P. Out-of-hospital cardiac arrest: contemporary management and future perspectives. Heart. 2015;101:1505–16.

77. Werdan K, Gielen S, Ebelt H, Hochman JS. Mechanical circulatory support in cardiogenic shock. Eur Heart J. 2014;35:156–67.

Mechanical Complications of Acute Myocardial Infarction

Andras Peter Durko, Wouter Jacob van Leeuwen, and Arie Pieter Kappetein

About Us

Erasmus MC, located in Rotterdam, the Netherlands, is among the country's largest hospitals and Europe's leading medical faculties. The Thoraxcentrum of EMC integrates cardiology, pulmonology, and cardiothoracic surgery. With approximately 1800 PCIs and 1200 open heart surgeries performed annually, the Thoraxcentrum embraces the full-spectrum of cardiothoracic surgery and invasive cardiology: from pediatric heart transplantation to complex percutaneous structural heart interventions. Besides excellence in patient care, Thoraxcentrum is aiming to distinguish itself in research by playing a principal role in clinical trials shaping the future of chest medicine, such as SYNTAX, EXCEL, and SURTAVI trials.

Quick Reference to Recommendations

	C-O-R	L-O-E	Ref.
Recommendations (acute/subacute setting)			
Emergency invasive evaluation is indicated in patients with acute heart failure or cardiogenic shock complicating ACS	I	B	[1]
Emergency revascularization with either PCI or CABG is recommended in suitable patients with cardiogenic shock due to pump failure after STEMI irrespective of the time delay from MI onset	I	B	[2]
(In patients with acute heart failure in the setting of ACS), emergency echocardiography is indicated to assess LV and valvular function and exclude mechanical complications	I	C	[1]
IABP insertion should be considered in patients with hemodynamic instability/cardiogenic shock due to mechanical complications	IIa	C	[1]

(continued)

A. P. Durko · W. J. van Leeuwen · A. P. Kappetein (✉)
Erasmus Medical Centre, University Medical Center
Rotterdam, Rotterdam, The Netherlands
e-mail: a.durko@erasmusmc.nl; w.j.vanleeuwen@
erasmusmc.nl; a.kappetein@erasmusmc.nl

© Springer International Publishing AG, part of Springer Nature 2018
A. Myat et al. (eds.), *The Interventional Cardiology Training Manual*,
https://doi.org/10.1007/978-3-319-71635-0_25

(continued)

	C-O-R	L-O-E	Ref.
The use of intra-aortic balloon pump (IABP) counterpulsation can be useful for patients with cardiogenic shock after STEMI who do not quickly stabilize with pharmacological therapy	IIa	B	[2]
Short-term mechanical circulatory support in ACS patients with cardiogenic shock may be considered	IIb	C	[1]
(After STEMI), alternative LV assist devices for circulatory support may be considered in patients with refractory cardiogenic shock	IIb	C	[2]
Patients with mechanical complication after acute myocardial infarction require immediate discussion by the Heart Team	I	C	[1]
Emergency surgery for mechanical complications of acute myocardial infarction is indicated in case of hemodynamic instability	I	C	[1]
CABG is recommended in patients with STEMI at time of operative repair of mechanical defects	I	B	[2]
Percutaneous repair of VSD may be considered after discussion by the Heart Team	IIb	C	[1]
Recommendations (chronic setting)			
LV aneurysmectomy during CABG should be considered in patients with a large LV aneurysm, if there is a risk of rupture, large thrombus formation, or the aneurysm is the origin of arrhythmias	IIa	C	[1]
CABG with surgical ventricular restoration may be considered in patients with scarred LAD territory, especially if a postoperative LVESV index <70 mL/m² can be predictably achieved	IIb	B	[1]

ACS acute coronary syndrome, *PCI* percutaneous coronary intervention, *CABG* coronary artery bypass grafting, *LV* left ventricle, *IABP* intra-aortic balloon pump, *STEMI* ST-elevation myocardial infarction, *VSD* ventricular septal defect, *LVESV* left ventricular end systolic volume, *C-O-R* class of recommendation, *L-O-E* level of evidence

Relevant guidelines:

1. 2014 ESC/EACTS Guidelines on myocardial revascularization [1]
2. 2013 ACCF/AHA Guideline for the Management of ST-Elevation Myocardial Infarction [2]

Introduction and Epidemiology

- Mechanical complications are rare, however dreaded, and potentially lethal consequences of acute myocardial infarction (AMI). They manifest as a tear (rupture) of the necrotic myocardium with ventricular septal rupture (VSR), free wall rupture, and/or ischemic mitral regurgitation (IMR) as a consequence.
- The introduction and routine use of primary reperfusion therapies such as thrombolysis and especially primary PCI in the management of AMI have reduced the incidence of excessive myocardial necrosis and the subsequent rupture of the acutely ischemic myocardium. However clinicians can still expect to encounter this life-threatening entity in a minority (around 1%) of patients following AMI [3].
- As survival of medically treated patients is extremely poor, diagnosis of an acute/subacute event requires urgent surgical referral, and in most cases necessitates life-saving emergency surgery.
- Mortality after surgical treatment, however, is also high, rendering decision-making in this condition often complex and not always straightforward.
- Typically, mechanical complications following AMI most often affect the left ventricle and are classified based on the timing of onset after the primary event:
  - Acute/subacute (within days to weeks after AMI):
    Ventricular septal rupture (VSR); anterior or posterior, manifested as acute left-to-right shunting on the ventricular level
    Papillary muscle rupture (PMR); partial or total, manifested as acute severe mitral regurgitation

Free wall rupture (FWR)
– Chronic (within weeks to years after AMI):
Ventricular pseudoaneurysm
Ventricular aneurysm
- Features of different mechanical complications are discussed later in this chapter, but all combinations can be encountered in clinical practice.

Acute and Subacute Complications

Presentation

- Although mechanical complications most commonly present as an emergency case, symptoms can vary from very mild, as shortness of breath, to severe and even sudden death. Moreover, rapid deterioration of patients with initially minor symptoms can occur.
- Older and hypertensive patients without previous myocardial infarction are more prone to develop mechanical complications after AMI.

Common Mechanism and Usual Timing After the Acute Event

- Mechanical complications can be anticipated after large, transmural myocardial infarctions. The mechanism involves the full-thickness coagulation necrosis of ischemic myocardial tissue, followed by neutrophil infiltration.
- Apoptosis of neutrophils and release of lytic enzymes contribute to the disintegration of the tissue. Local extravasation followed by intramural hematoma formation, dissecting into the necrotic tissue further contributes to the rupture of injured myocardium [4].
- Some controversy exists around the exact time of presentation, but it follows a bimodal peak: most acute ruptures occur within the first 24 h, and the remainder within 1 week after AMI.

Presentation as an Urgent Case at the Emergency Department

- In general, new onset of cardiac failure (asthma cardiale, shock, collapse, or sudden death) with the diagnosis of a recent myocardial infarction

should always raise the suspicion of a mechanical complication in a patient presenting at the emergency department.
- However, mechanical complications can also occur as a first presentation of a previously undetected silent AMI. The most common initial symptoms are described in detail below.

Special Considerations in Prehospital Care

- Ideally, unstable patients with the signs and symptoms of a mechanical complication after AMI in a prehospital setting should be transferred urgently to centers not only capable of primary PCI but also having the possibility of advanced mechanical circulatory support (MCS) and cardiac surgery [5].

In-hospital Presentation as a Complication After (Delayed) PCI

- Patients with mechanical complications might also be encountered on a cardiology ward with sudden deterioration of clinical status, often after delayed PCI for AMI.

Diagnosis

- **Presenting symptoms**: include restlessness, chest pain, abrupt onset of shortness of breath, arrhythmia, hypotension, syncope, pulmonary edema, oligo-anuria, shock, or sudden death
- **Physical examination**: new onset of usually harsh holosystolic murmur, signs of pulmonary congestion on auscultation (suggestive for papillary muscle rupture)
- **ECG**: as after STEMI; no specific signs exist suggestive of mechanical complications
- **Chest X-ray (CXR)**: enlarged cardiac silhouette (a specific sign in cardiac tamponade), signs of pulmonary congestion can be present
- **Lab**: as after STEMI; no specific examination exists suggestive for mechanical complications
- **TTE**: Echocardiography is the cornerstone of diagnosis. Pericardial effusion, signs of tamponade (in free wall rupture), left-to-right shunting on the ventricular level (Fig. 25.1),

Fig. 25.1 Transthoracic echocardiography of ventricular septal rupture. A high velocity jet can be seen across the ruptured interventricular septum

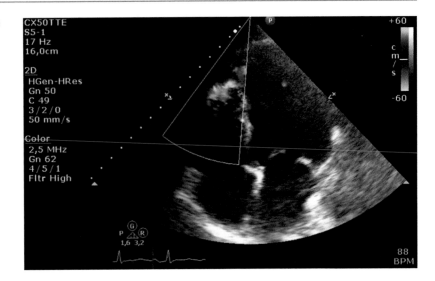

severe mitral regurgitation with mitral prolapse or flail, decreased left ventricular function, and signs of right ventricular failure and dilatation (in ventricular septal rupture and papillary muscle rupture) are the key findings. If TTE is inconclusive, transesophageal echocardiography (TEE) might be necessary.

Additional clues:
- **Pericardiocentesis**: when performing emergency pericardiocentesis to relieve tamponade, obtaining blood should raise the suspicion for FWR.
- **Coronary angiography**: if stable enough, the patient should undergo urgent coronary angiography.

Role of IABP or ECLS Before Surgery

- As patients with mechanical complications can present with, or quickly develop, overt cardiac failure, mechanical circulatory support is often necessary.
- Insertion of an intra-aortic balloon pump (IABP) should be considered in patients with cardiogenic shock and mechanical complication following AMI [6].
- In refractory circulatory collapse, more advanced means of extracorporeal life support (ECLS) such as prompt percutaneous initiation of extracorporeal membrane oxygenation

(ECMO) might be needed to stabilize the patient until definitive treatment [7].

Indication for Operation and Timing of Surgery

- Mechanical complications following AMI require immediate action. As patients can deteriorate suddenly, prompt surgical referral and Heart Team discussion is vital.
- Prognosis with maintained medical therapy alone is extremely poor, however surgical repair carry also a substantial risk of inhospital mortality.

The following should be considered in decision-making:

1. The risk of mortality is higher if surgery is carried out on an emergency or salvage basis [8].
2. However, the high mortality observed in emergent cases is most likely attributed to the initial bad condition of the patient.
3. From a technical viewpoint, delayed surgery can prevent sutures tearing through necrotic, not yet scarred tissue, which increases the chance of a successful repair.
4. Initially stable patients can deteriorate rapidly, necessitating salvage surgery with obviously higher risk.

- In a nutshell, the risk of early surgery must be weighed against the unpredictable consequences of postponing surgery [9]. Decision-making is even more complex in sedated/ventilated patients, when neurological status cannot be assessed.
- In summary, giving a straightforward or absolute guidance on the proper timing of surgery in mechanical complications after AMI is impossible.
- Careful, case-based, bedside multidisciplinary Heart Team decision-making, with frequent re-evaluation of clinical status, is mandatory and is the only way to optimize outcomes.

Role of Concomitant Myocardial Revascularization

- Although questioned by some, concomitant myocardial revascularization along with repair of mechanical complications of AMI can improve outcomes [10–13].
- Generally, revascularization of all stenotic and graftable vessels is advisable. However, technically, it is often not possible to graft the culprit vessel as they are often incorporated in the surgical suture line or excised along with the necrotic myocardium, or covered with the patch used for repair.

Postinfarction Ventricular Septal Rupture

Definition
- Postinfarction ventricular septal rupture (VSR) is a tear of the interventricular septum, causing acute left-to-right shunting, pulmonary overcirculation, and biventricular failure.

General Features
- Primary reperfusion in AMI has significantly decreased VSR occurrence: currently, it is around 0.2% of all AMI cases [9].
- Most commonly, the left anterior descending (LAD) artery and the posterior descending branch of the right coronary artery (RCA-PD)

are affected. Total occlusions are often associated with VSRs.
- The location of the culprit lesion will determine the site of the VSR: apical and anterior VSRs are associated with LAD occlusion, while posterior VSRs with RCA infarcts.
- Posterior VSRs are more complex in morphology, difficult to expose and are often associated with pronounced right ventricular dysfunction, and have a worse prognosis [14].

Preoperative Considerations
- Patients presenting with VSR are often critically ill. Apparently stable patients can deteriorate rapidly, therefore close observation on ICU is necessary.
- Medical management should aim to reduce left ventricular filling pressures and afterload: inotropes, diuretics, and placement of an IABP should be considered.
- In cases of refractory cardiogenic shock, percutaneous ECLS might be necessary. Immediate surgical referral and Heart Team discussion is essential.

Overview of Operative Technique
- Repair of a postinfarction VSR is challenging. The operation is performed on total cardiopulmonary bypass with cardioplegic arrest. Proper myocardial protection is of paramount importance.
- Typically, defects are approached by a left ventricular incision through the infarct area. However, alternative right ventricular or even right atrial approaches have also been described [15, 16].
- The main concept of repair is covering the defect with an oversized pericardial or Dacron patch, anchored to the adjacent nonischemic myocardial tissue (Figs. 25.2 and 25.3).
- In cases of anterior VSR, the patch can remain totally intraventricular (infarct exclusion), or it can be externalized and incorporated in the left ventricular suture line [17]. Suture lines are usually reinforced with strips and pledgets of teflon-felt to prevent sutures from tearing through (Fig. 25.2).
- Reconstruction of a posterior VSR can be even more demanding: infarct exclusion is a

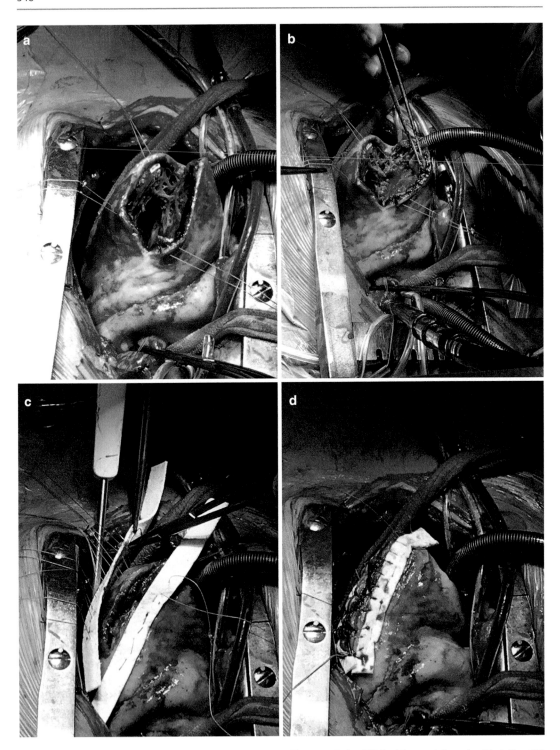

Fig. 25.2 Operative repair of an antero-apical ventricular septal rupture (VSR). (**a**) Left ventricular (LV) incision through the infarct area. (**b**) The VSR is covered with a patch of autologous pericardium, from the LV side. (**c**) Closure of the LV incision, reinforced with teflon-felt strips. The edge of the patch is incorporated to the suture line. (**d**) Completed repair, LV incision closed

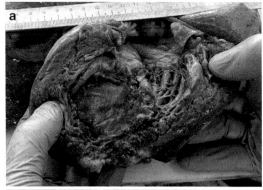

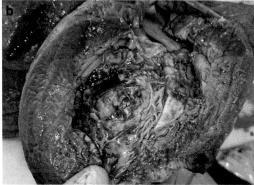

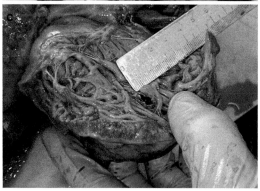

Fig. 25.3 Section of the heart after ventricular septal rupture repair (VSR). (**a**) Left ventricle (LV) opened, pericardial patch covering the septum. Note the marked LV hypertrophy. (**b**) Patch removed to visualize VSR from the LV side. Extensive myocardial necrosis around the defect. (**c**) VSR, as seen from the right ventricular (RV) side. Note the trabeculated RV architecture

feasible option; however occasionally extensive patch reconstruction of the ventricular wall or septum might also be required [18–21].

Percutaneous Options

- The first attempts at percutaneous closure of a ventricular septal defect date back to the late 1980s [22]. Since then, a series of retrospective studies have demonstrated the efficacy and feasibility of this method even in cases of postinfarction septal rupture [23–25]. Definitive closure of small or medium-sized defects has been reported.

- Even if only partially successful, percutaneous intervention can also buy time. Decreasing the shunt and stabilizing the circulation enables delay of definitive surgical closure until scarring occurs. This option can be considered during a Heart Team discussion, on a case-based decision-making.

Outcome

- Chance of survival without intervention is minimal. However, surgical reconstruction also carries a considerable risk of mortality. Early mortality in smaller series range between 26 and 41%, while data from the STS National Database on 2876 contemporary-era VSR patients demonstrated an average 43% inhospital/30-day mortality [8, 26–29].

- Long-term survival of inhospital survivors is also compromised, with a reported five-year survival between 65 and 79% [27–29]. Transcatheter closure can claim comparable short-term results with an average 32% inhospital/30-day mortality, as summarized in a recent review [30].

Papillary Muscle Rupture

Definition

- Papillary muscle rupture (PMR) after AMI is defined as a partial or total tear of one ischemic papillary muscle anchoring the mitral subvalvular apparatus. PMR results in acute severe mitral regurgitation (MR) and subsequent pulmonary edema.

General Features

- The two papillary muscles have a different blood supply. Usually, the anterolateral receives blood from two coronary arteries (LAD and LCx), while the posteromedial has only one feeding artery (LCX or RCA), and is much more prone to ischemia caused by coronary artery occlusion.
- Therefore, PMR tends to affect the postero-medial papillary muscle most frequently [13, 31, 32]. As a result, the posterior-medial commissure (PC), A2-A3 and P2-P3 are the commonly involved segments in the resulting regurgitation.
- The severity of cardiac failure symptoms, related to the severity of MR, is the key determinant in timing of surgery. Cases of total rupture resulting in sudden, excessive MR are typically poorly tolerated and often lead to sudden death before any intervention can take place. In a series of 50 patients, 65% needed salvage or emergent surgery, and only 10% were operated on an elective basis [33].

Key Preoperative Issues

- Critically ill patients developing severe pulmonary edema and cardiac failure can benefit from immediately initiated percutaneous ECLS. IABP insertion should also be considered. After establishing the diagnosis, urgent surgical referral and Heart Team discussion is essential.

Overview of Operative Technique

- The possibilities of surgical management are highly influenced by the extent of rupture. Cases of total rupture with bileaflet prolapse or flail are less amenable for mitral valve repair (Fig. 25.4). In this case valve replacement is the preferred option.
- In cases of partial or incomplete rupture however, valve repair can also be considered with acceptable results [32, 34]. Valve repair techniques in the setting of PMR include commissuroplasty, chordal transposition, papillary muscle head reimplantation, and quadrangular resection, completing the procedure with a downsized annuloplasty.
- Naturally, surgical expertise, the general condition of the patient, timing (emergency, urgent or elective surgery), and the universal need to decrease further ischemic injury by minimizing cross-clamp time are also key factors influencing the decision between valve replacement or repair in PMR.

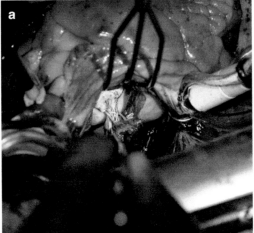
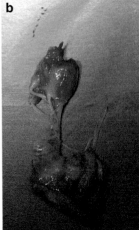

Fig. 25.4 Total papillary muscle rupture (PMR), anterior leaflet flail. (**a**) Mitral valve exposed through a standard left atrial incision. Note the ruptured papillary muscle head in the left atrial cavity. (**b**) Excised anterior mitral leaflet with the ruptured papillary muscle head

Percutaneous Options

- In extreme high-risk patients, MitraClip can be considered in the setting of PMR also [35]. Although initial reports with very limited number of subjects are promising, currently this approach can only be advised as a bail-out strategy for critically ill patients unfit for surgery [36, 37].

Outcome

- Scarce data exists on outcomes in large patient cohorts. However, inhospital mortality after mitral valve replacement or repair in PMR is around 20–25%, and overall survival can be expected around 70–80%, 65%, and 30–50% at 1, 5, and 10 years, respectively [13, 33, 38, 39].

Ventricular Free Wall Rupture

Definition
- Ventricular free wall rupture (FWR) following myocardial infarction is defined as transmural necrosis and subsequent disruption of the ischemic myocardium.
- Active bleeding into the pericardial space ultimately leads to pericardial tamponade.

General Features
- From a surgical viewpoint, two distinct groups of acute FWR can be identified:
  - The "oozing type," without obvious source of bleeding and blood slowly accumulating in the pericardial sac.
  - The "blow-out type" when a macroscopic defect on the myocardium is visible, with high-volume bleeding causing abrupt pericardial tamponade [40].
- This variability is reflected in the clinical presentation also: initial symptoms can range from minimal to severe chest pain to collapse and sudden death [41]. In the vast majority of cases, LAD and the LCx are identified as culprit vessels [42].

- Most clinical signs seen in FWR are rather more specific for cardiac tamponade than for FWR, however electromechanical dissociation without preceding overt cardiac failure in STEMI patients is believed to be highly specific for FWR [43].

Key Preoperative Issues
- After initial stabilization of the patient, primary tasks of the perioperative caregiver are:
  1. To organize urgent surgical referral.
  2. To obtain and send blood samples for essential preoperative examinations (blood group, hematology, hemostasis, ions, and electrolytes).
  3. To transfer the patient to operating theater as soon as possible.
- In manifest tamponade and circulatory collapse percutaneous relief by pericardiocentesis can be attempted, however clot might be expected in the pericardial cavity.

Overview of Surgical Technique
- The extremely fragile, necrotic myocardial wall "does not hold the sutures" and a surgeon can easily face uncontrollable bleeding if attempting direct closure of the defect. Therefore, the two most commonly utilized techniques are:
  - The "classic method" involves the wide excision of the adjacent necrotic myocardium (infarctectomy) followed by patch-reconstruction of the left ventricular wall on cardiopulmonary bypass [44].
  - More recently, a less-invasive option is to cover the affected region with an oversized pericardial patch, reinforced by glue, with or without suture anchoring. The use of local hemostatic medicated sponges (such as TachoSil®) has also proven to be beneficial. The procedure can also be carried out off-pump [45–47]. The off-pump technique confers the advantage of avoiding heparinization, cardiopulmonary bypass, and cardioplegic arrest of the already ischemic myocardium.

Outcome

- According to the SHOCK Trial Registry data, expected overall inhospital mortality after FWR is around 60%, being the worst among all mechanical complications after AMI [42].

After Surgery

Mechanical Circulatory Support After Surgery

- Due to the gross myocardial necrosis and the additional ischemic time during cross-clamping, difficulties in weaning from cardiopulmonary bypass can occur.
- Usual practice includes leaving the operating theater with IABP support, however employing more advanced means of temporary MCS or the use of extracorporeal membrane oxygenation (ECMO) might also be necessary.

Postoperative Course and Long-Term Outcome

- The severity of the underlying disease and the complexity of the operation are reflected in the postoperative course: prolonged ICU stay, often complicated with low cardiac output, respiratory or renal failure can be expected.
- Naturally, long-term outcome of inhospital survivors will be influenced by the permanent consequences of the massive myocardial necrosis.

Late Complications

Left Ventricular Aneurysm

Definition

- By definition, a true aneurysm is an abnormal protrusion of the vascular wall, containing all layers of the original structure. In the absence of timely revascularization after large trans-

mural AMIs, extensive myocardial necrosis can occur.
- As the acute phase passes, the necrotic myocardium is gradually replaced by fibrotic scar tissue unable to contribute to active myocardial contraction. Consequently, the affected ventricular segments exhibit paradoxical outward movement during systole (dyskinesia) and tend to dilate, ultimately leading to aneurysm formation.

General Features

- Normally, aneurysms of the heart affect the left ventricle (LV). In the majority of cases (85%) the location is antero-apical or apical [48]. As dyskinetic left ventricular regions are interfering with normal cardiac function, symptoms of heart failure can occur in the presence of a large LV aneurysm.
- LV aneurysms tend to calcify and are often filled with mural thrombi. Persisting ST-segment elevation on the ECG, enlarged cardiac silhouette, or calcifications seen on the CXR might be suggestive signs of a LV aneurysm.
- In preoperative planning, however, the use of more advanced imaging techniques (such as cardiac MRI) and assessment of myocardial viability are highly advisable [49].

Indications for Surgery

- The rationale of surgical treatment is:
  - To decrease heart failure symptoms by restoring LV geometry and excluding the noncontractile segment of the left ventricle, consequently improving ejection fraction.
  - To prevent the possible complications caused by the presence of the aneurysm: rupture, thromboembolic events, or arrhythmias.
- Contrary to expectations, the Surgical Treatment for Ischemic Heart Failure (STICH) trial has failed to demonstrate any improvement in symptoms or survival when comparing CABG with surgical ventricular

reconstruction (SVR) to CABG alone in patients with coronary artery disease, LV aneurysm, and decreased left ventricular ejection fraction [50].

- Of note, STICH is highly criticized for having major flaws in study design and other large series reported improved survival and symptomatic status after SVR [49, 51, 52].
- Therefore, LV aneurysm repair is indicated in the presence of a large LV aneurysm and heart failure symptoms. Other indications include a high risk of rupture, large thrombus formation, or when the aneurysm is the origin of arrhythmias [1].

Overview of Surgical Technique

- Surgical treatment of left ventricular aneurysms has undergone a significant evolution since its inception in the 1950s [53]. From the numerous techniques described during the past decades the two most commonly employed are linear closure and patch ventriculoplasty ("endoventricular circular patch plasty repair" or "endoaneurysmorrhaphy") [54]. Both methods employ cardiopulmonary bypass.
- Linear closure, suggested by Denton Cooley in 1958, is a simple resection of the scar tissue forming the aneurysm. The continuity of the left ventricular wall is restored by a double linear suture line reinforced by teflon-felt strips [55].
- Patch ventriculoplasty was first described separately by Vincent Dor and Adib Jatene in the 1980s, introducing an entirely new concept to aneurysm repair (Fig. 25.5) [56, 57]. Although the technique underwent subsequent modifications, the main concept is the following:
  - The left ventricle is entered through the aneurysm and thrombectomy is performed when indicated.
  - The margin of viable myocardium is identified and a circular purse-string suture is inserted and tied at the rim of viable tissue to narrow the orifice of the aneurysm and restore physiological LV shape.

- The narrowed orifice is closed by an adequately sized (prosthetic or prosthetic-pericardial) patch.
  - For the last step, the left ventricular wall is closed above the patch (Fig. 25.6) [58, 59].
- Theoretically, when compared to linear closure, patch ventriculoplasty or "surgical ventricular restoration" confers the advantage of achieving a more physiologic LV cavity, permits exclusion of the septal akinetic segments, and finally it allows extensive subendocardial scar excision if necessary [56].
- As LV aneurysm is a consequence of ischemic heart disease, concomitant surgical myocardial revascularization or mitral valve surgery to address chronic ischemic mitral regurgitation is often required.

Outcome

- 30-day mortality after SVR is expected to be around 5–7%, but can be even as low as 2% [49–52].
- According to the RESTORE SVR registry data, 5-year overall survival is around 70% after SVR [52].

Left Ventricular Pseudoaneurysm

Definition

- Left ventricular pseudoaneurysm formation is a late consequence of an undiscovered or unoperated myocardial free wall rupture.
- Due to pericardial adhesions or quick hematoma formation, the process is self-limiting: bleeding to the pericardial cavity causes only a local hemopericardium, not manifest tamponade.
- As a result, a pseudoaneurysm is created: unlike true aneurysms, the wall is constituted of mural thrombi and the parietal pericardium alone.

Diagnosis and General Features

- Left ventricular pseudoaneurysms can develop not only after a contained rupture of

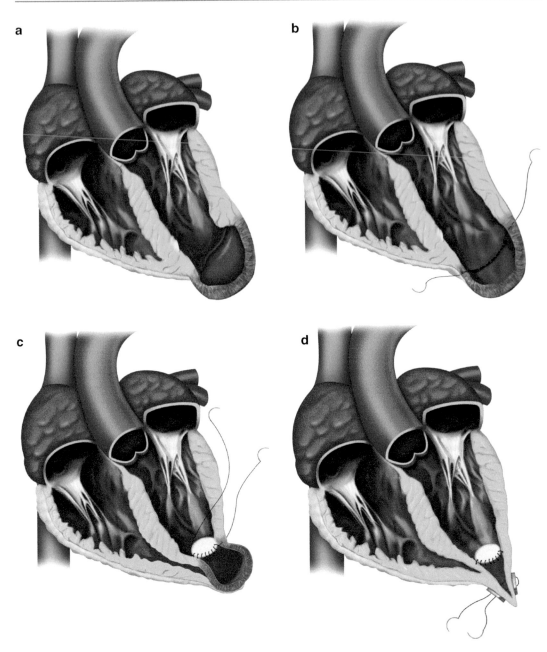

Fig. 25.5 The concept of "Surgical Ventricular Restoration." (**a**) Cross section of the heart, with a large left ventricular (LV) aneurysm. (**b**) The aneurysm incised and a circular purse-string suture inserted at the border of scar and viable myocardium to narrow the ori- fice. (**c**) Purse-string tightened and the remaining defect on the LV apex is closed with a patch, restoring a more physiological LV cavity. (**d**) The aneurysm is closed above the patch, suture line is reinforced with strips of teflon-felt

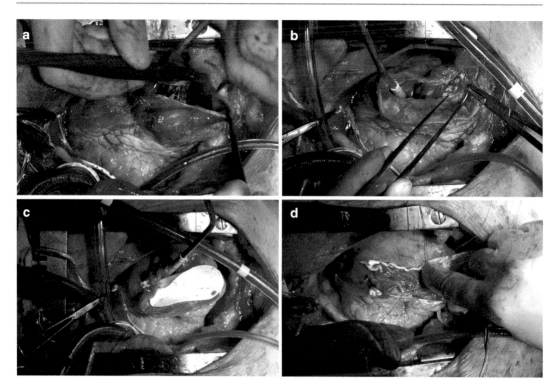

Fig. 25.6 "Surgical Ventricular Restoration," operative technique. (**a**) Left ventricular aneurysm incised. (**b**) Inserting the purse-string suture to narrow the neck of the aneurysm. (**c**) Reconstructing the LV cavity with a prosthetic patch. (**d**) Closure of the LV, reinforced with teflon-felt strips

the myocardial wall following AMI. They have also been described after infective endocarditis, chest trauma, or mitral valve surgery. These entities are not discussed here.

- Unlike true aneurysms, left ventricular pseudoaneurysms are more common on the lateral or diaphragmatic surface (Fig. 25.7) [60, 61].

- As pseudoaneurysms are believed to have a higher tendency for progressive growth and rupture compared to "true" left ventricular aneurysms, an urgent surgical referral is indicated after establishing the diagnosis [61].

- However, differentiating between true and false aneurysms can be challenging. Echocardiography is sometimes inconclusive, necessitating the use of more advanced imaging modalities such as cardiac CT or MRI [62].

Surgical Technique

- In some cases, size or location of the pseudoaneurysm can render conventional sternotomy challenging. Therefore, preparedness for rapid, peripheral institution of cardiopulmonary bypass is advisable.

- After exposing the pseudoaneurysm, repair follows the main steps described for left ventricular aneurysm repair.

Percutaneous Options

- Recently, cases of successful percutaneous closure of left ventricular pseudoaneurysms have been reported in patients at high risk for conventional surgery, demonstrating the feasibility and efficacy of transcatheter approaches in this condition [63].

- Of note, these procedures have only been carried out by highly skilled and experienced structural interventionists, rendering the widespread applicability of these techniques limited [64].

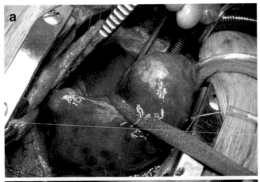

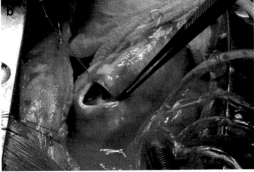

Fig. 25.7 Left ventricular (LV) pseudoaneurysm. (**a**) LV pseudoaneurysm exposed. Note the lateral location. (**b**) LV pseudoaneurysm incised. Note the narrow neck

Conclusions

- Although their incidence is significantly decreased in the primary PCI era, mechanical complications can still be encountered after AMI.
- Development of an early mechanical complication after AMI represents a life-threatening situation and necessitates prompt action.
- Patients with the suspicion of a mechanical complication require ICU admission. Early echocardiography is essential.
- As serious circulatory compromise can be expected, mechanical circulatory support should be considered early.
- Urgent surgical referral and Heart Team discussion are essential to optimize outcomes. Proper timing of the intervention is a key determinant of success.
- Besides open heart surgery, percutaneous options are also emerging. Decisions regarding treatment timing and modality require multidisciplinary discussion and should be individualized.

- Late mechanical complications of AMI include LV aneurysms and pseudoaneurysms. The differential diagnosis is challenging and advanced imaging is required.
- SVR should be considered in large LV aneurysms, decreased LV function, and heart failure symptoms, or to prevent complications.
- LV pseudoaneurysms carry a higher risk of rupture and require urgent surgical referral.

Acknowledgement Disclosure statement: No conflicts of interest to report.

References

1. Authors/Task Force Members, Windecker S, Kolh P, Alfonso F, Collet JP, Cremer J, et al. 2014 ESC/EACTS Guidelines on myocardial revascularization: The Task Force on Myocardial Revascularization of the European Society of Cardiology (ESC) and the European Association for Cardio-Thoracic Surgery (EACTS)Developed with the special contribution of the European Association of Percutaneous Cardiovascular Interventions (EAPCI). Eur Heart J. 2014;35(37):2541–619.
2. O'Gara PT, Kushner FG, Ascheim DD, Casey DE, Chung MK, de Lemos JA, et al. ACCF/AHA guideline for the management of ST-elevation myocardial infarction. Circulation. 2013;127(4):e362. https://doi.org/10.1161/CIR0b013e3182742cf6.
3. Magalhães P, Mateus P, Carvalho S, Leão S, Cordeiro F, Moreira JI. Relationship between treatment delay and type of reperfusion therapy and mechanical complications of acute myocardial infarction. Eur Heart J Acute Cardiovasc Care. 2016;5(5):468–74. https://doi.org/10.1177/2048872616637038.
4. Birnbaum Y, Fishbein MC, Blanche C, Siegel RJ. Ventricular septal rupture after acute myocardial infarction. N Engl J Med. 2002;347(18):1426–32. https://doi.org/10.1056/NEJMra020228.
5. Beygui F, Castren M, Brunetti ND, Rosell-Ortiz F, Christ M, Zeymer U, et al. Pre-hospital management of patients with chest pain and/or dyspnoea of cardiac origin. A position paper of the Acute Cardiovascular Care Association (ACCA) of the ESC. Eur Heart J Acute Cardiovasc Care. 2015. https://doi.org/10.1177/2048872615604119
6. Kettner J, Sramko M, Holek M, Pirk J, Kautzner J. Utility of intra-aortic balloon pump support for ventricular septal rupture and acute mitral regurgitation complicating acute myocardial infarction. Am J Cardiol. 2013;112(11):1709–13.
7. McLaughlin A, McGiffin D, Winearls J, Tesar P, Cole C, Vallely M, et al. Veno-arterial ECMO in the setting

of post-infarct ventricular septal defect: a bridge to surgical repair. Heart Lung Circ. 2016;25(11):1063–6.

8. Arnaoutakis GJ, Zhao Y, George TJ, Sciortino CM, McCarthy PM, Conte JV. Surgical repair of ventricular septal defect after myocardial infarction: outcomes from the society of thoracic surgeons national database. Ann Thorac Surg. 2012;94(2):436–44. https://doi.org/10.1016/j.athoracsur.2012.04.020.

9. Jones BM, Kapadia SR, Smedira NG, Robich M, Tuzcu EM, Menon V, et al. Ventricular septal rupture complicating acute myocardial infarction: a contemporary review. Eur Heart J. 2014;35(31):2060–8. https://doi.org/10.1093/eurheartj/ehu248.

10. Dalrymple-Hay MJ, Langley SM, Sami SA, Haw M, Allen SM, Livesey SA, et al. Should coronary artery bypass grafting be performed at the same time as repair of a post-infarct ventricular septal defect? Eur J Cardiothorac Surg. 1998;13(3):286–92.

11. Hochman JS, Buller CE, Sleeper LA, Boland J, Dzavik V, Sanborn TA, et al. Cardiogenic shock complicating acute myocardial infarction—etiologies, management and outcome: a report from the SHOCK Trial Registry. Should we emergently revascularize occluded coronaries for cardiogenic shocK? J Am Coll Cardiol. 2000;36(3 Suppl A):1063–70.

12. Barker TA, Ramnarine IR, Woo EB, Grayson AD, Au J, Fabri BM, et al. Repair of post-infarct ventricular septal defect with or without coronary artery bypass grafting in the northwest of England: a 5-year multi-institutional experience. Eur J Cardiothorac Surg. 2003;24(6):940–6.

13. Chevalier P, Burri H, Fahrat F, Cucherat M, Jegaden O, Obadia J-F, et al. Perioperative outcome and long-term survival of surgery for acute post-infarction mitral regurgitation. Eur J Cardio-Thorac Surg. 2004;26(2):330–5. https://doi.org/10.1016/j.ejcts.2004.04.027.

14. Crenshaw BS, Granger CB, Birnbaum Y, Pieper KS, Morris DC, Kleiman NS, et al. Risk factors, angiographic patterns, and outcomes in patients with ventricular septal defect complicating acute myocardial infarction. Circulation. 2000;101(1):27. https://doi.org/10.1161/01.CIR.101.1.27.

15. Massetti M, Babatasi G, Le Page O, Bhoyroo S, Saloux E, Khayat A. Postinfarction ventricular septal rupture: early repair through the right atrial approach. J Thorac Cardiovasc Surg. 2000;119(4):784–9.

16. Isoda S, Imoto K, Uchida K, Hashiyama N, Yanagi H, Tamagawa H, et al. "Sandwich technique" via right ventricle incision to repair postinfarction ventricular septal defect. J Card Surg. 2004;19(2):149–50.

17. David TE, Dale L, Sun Z. Postinfarction ventricular septal rupture: repair by endocardial patch with infarct exclusion. J Thorac Cardiovasc Surg. 1995;110(5):1315–22.

18. Daggett WM, Guyton RA, Mundth ED, Buckley MJ, McEnany MT, Gold HK, et al. Surgery for post-myocardial infarct ventricular septal defect. Ann Surg. 1977;186(3):260–70.

19. Daggett WM, Buckley MJ, Akins CW, Leinbach RC, Gold HK, Block PC, et al. Improved results of surgical management of postinfarction ventricular septal rupture. Ann Surg. 1982;196(3):269–77.

20. Nakajima M, Tsuchiya K, Inoue H, Naito Y, Mizutani E. Modified Daggett's technique for early repair of postinfarct posterior ventricular septal rupture. Ann Thorac Surg. 2003;75(1):301–2.

21. Pett SB, Follis F, Allen K, Temes T, Wernly JA. Posterior ventricular septal rupture: an anatomical reconstruction. J Card Surg. 1998;13(6):445–50.

22. Lock JE, Block PC, McKay RG, Baim DS, Keane JF. Transcatheter closure of ventricular septal defects. Circulation. 1988;78(2):361. https://doi.org/10.1161/01.CIR.78.2.361.

23. Maltais S, Ibrahim R, Basmadjian A-J, Carrier M, Bouchard D, Cartier R, et al. Postinfarction ventricular septal defects: towards a new treatment algorithm? Ann Thorac Surg. 2009;87(3):687–92.

24. Calvert PA, Cockburn J, Wynne D, Ludman P, Rana BS, Northridge D, et al. Percutaneous closure of post-infarction ventricular septal defect: in-hospital outcomes and long-term follow-up of UK experience. Circulation. 2014;129:2395. https://doi.org/10.1161/CIRCULATIONAHA.113.005839.

25. Assenza GE, McElhinney DB, Valente AM, Pearson DD, Volpe M, Martucci G, et al. Transcatheter closure of post-myocardial infarction ventricular septal rupture. Circ Cardiovasc Interv. 2013;6(1):59. https://doi.org/10.1161/CIRCINTERVENTIONS.112.972711.

26. Poulsen SH, Præstholm M, Munk K, Wierup P, Egeblad H, Nielsen-Kudsk JE. Ventricular septal rupture complicating acute myocardial infarction: clinical characteristics and contemporary outcome. Ann Thorac Surg. 2008;85(5):1591–6. https://doi.org/10.1016/j.athoracsur.2008.01.010.

27. Prêtre R, Ye Q, Grünenfelder J, Lachat M, Vogt PR, Turina MI. Operative results of "repair" of ventricular septal rupture after acute myocardial infarction. Am J Cardiol. 1999;84(7):785–8.

28. Papadopoulos N, Moritz A, Dzemali O, Zierer A, Rouhollapour A, Ackermann H, et al. Long-term results after surgical repair of postinfarction ventricular septal rupture by infarct exclusion technique. Ann Thorac Surg. 2009;87(5):1421–5.

29. Jeppsson A, Liden H, Johnsson P, Hartford M, Radegran K. Surgical repair of post infarction ventricular septal defects: a national experience. Eur J Cardiothorac Surg. 2005 Feb;27(2):216–21.

30. Schlotter F, de Waha S, Eitel I, Desch S, Fuernau G, Thiele H. Interventional post-myocardial infarction ventricular septal defect closure: a systematic review of current evidence. EuroIntervention. 2016;12(1):94–102.

31. Tanimoto T, Imanishi T, Kitabata H, Nakamura N, Kimura K, Yamano T, et al. Prevalence and clinical significance of papillary muscle infarction detected by late gadolinium-enhanced magnetic resonance imaging in patients with ST-segment elevation myocardial infarction. Circulation.

2010;122(22):2281.   https://doi.org/10.1161/
CIRCULATIONAHA.109.935338.

32. Jouan J, Tapia M, Cook RC, Lansac E, Acar
C. Ischemic mitral valve prolapse: mechanisms and
implications for valve repair. Eur J Cardio-Thorac
Surg. 2004;26(6):1112–7. https://doi.org/10.1016/j.
ejcts.2004.07.049.

33. Bouma W, Wijdh-den Hamer IJ, Koene BM, Kuijpers
M, Natour E, Erasmus ME, et al. Long-term survival
after mitral valve surgery for post-myocardial infarction papillary muscle rupture. J Cardiothorac Surg.
2015;10:11.

34. Bouma W, Wijdh-den Hamer IJ, Klinkenberg TJ,
Kuijpers M, Bijleveld A, van der Horst ICC, et al.
Mitral valve repair for post-myocardial infarction
papillary muscle rupture. Eur J Cardio-Thorac Surg.
2013;44(6):1063–9.   https://doi.org/10.1093/ejcts/
ezt150.

35. Grover FL, Vemulapalli S, Carroll JD, Edwards FH,
Mack MJ, Thourani VH, et al. 2016 annual report of
The Society of Thoracic Surgeons/American College
of Cardiology Transcatheter Valve Therapy Registry.
J Am Coll Cardiol. 2017;69(10):1215–30.

36. Estévez-Loureiro R, Arzamendi D, Freixa X,
Cardenal R, Carrasco-Chinchilla F, Serrador-Frutos
A, et al. Percutaneous mitral valve repair for acute
mitral regurgitation after an acute myocardial infarction. J Am Coll Cardiol. 2015;66(1):91–2.

37. Adamo M, Curello S, Chiari E, Fiorina C, Chizzola G,
Magatelli M, et al. Percutaneous edge-to-edge mitral
valve repair for the treatment of acute mitral regurgitation complicating myocardial infarction: a single
centre experience. Int J Cardiol. 2017;234:53–7.

38. Chen Q, Darlymple-Hay MJ, Alexiou C, Ohri SK,
Haw MP, Livesey SA, et al. Mitral valve surgery for
acute papillary muscle rupture following myocardial
infarction. J Heart Valve Dis. 2002 Jan;11(1):27–31.

39. Tavakoli R, Weber A, Vogt P, Brunner HP, Pretre R,
Turina M. Surgical management of acute mitral valve
regurgitation due to post-infarction papillary muscle rupture. J Heart Valve Dis. 2002;11(1):20–5; discussion 6

40. Bashour T, Kabbani SS, Ellertson DG, Crew J, Hanna
ES. Surgical salvage of heart rupture: report of two
cases and review of the literature. Ann Thorac Surg.
1983;36(2):209–13.

41. Balakumaran K, Verbaan CJ, Essed CE, Nauta J, Bos
E, Haalebos MMP, et al. Ventricular free wall rupture: sudden, subacute, slow, sealed and stabilized
varieties. Eur Heart J. 1984;5(4):282–8. https://doi.
org/10.1093/oxfordjournals.eurheartj.a061653.

42. Slater J, Brown RJ, Antonelli TA, Menon V, Boland
J, Col J, et al. Cardiogenic shock due to cardiac free-
wall rupture or tamponade after acute myocardial
infarction: a report from the SHOCK Trial Registry.
J Am Coll Cardiol. 2000;36(3 Suppl 1):1117. https://
doi.org/10.1016/S0735-1097(00)00845-7.

43. Figueras J, Curós A, Cortadellas J, Soler-Soler
J. Reliability of electromechanical dissociation
in the diagnosis of left ventricular free wall rup-

ture in acute myocardial infarction. Am Heart J.
1996;131(5):861–4.

44. Reardon MJ, Carr CL, Diamond A, Letsou GV, Safi
HJ, Espada R, et al. Ischemic left ventricular free wall
rupture: prediction, diagnosis, and treatment. Ann
Thorac Surg. 1997;64(5):1509–13.

45. Sakaguchi G, Komiya T, Tamura N, Kobayashi
T. Surgical treatment for postinfarction left ventricular free wall rupture. Ann Thorac Surg.
2008;85(4):1344–6.

46. Zoffoli G, Battaglia F, Venturini A, Asta A, Terrini A,
Zanchettin C, et al. A novel approach to ventricular
rupture: clinical needs and surgical technique. Ann
Thorac Surg. 2012;93(3):1002–3.

47. Pocar M, Passolunghi D, Bregasi A, Donatelli
F. TachoSil® for postinfarction ventricular free
wall rupture. Interact Cardiovasc Thorac Surg.
2012;14(6):866–7.   https://doi.org/10.1093/icvts/
ivs085.

48. Olearchyk AS, Lemole GM, Spagna PM. Left ventricular aneurysm. Ten years' experience in surgical treatment of 244 cases. Improved clinical status,
hemodynamics, and long-term longevity. J Thorac
Cardiovasc Surg. 1984;88(4):544–53.

49. Dor V, Civaia F, Alexandrescu C, Sabatier M,
Montiglio F. Favorable effects of left ventricular
reconstruction in patients excluded from the Surgical
Treatments for Ischemic Heart Failure (STICH) trial.
J Thorac Cardiovasc Surg. 2011;141(4):905–16.e4.

50. Jones RH, Velazquez EJ, Michler RE, Sopko G, Oh
JK, O'Connor CM, et al. Coronary bypass surgery
with or without surgical ventricular reconstruction.
N Engl J Med. 2009;360(17):1705–17. https://doi.
org/10.1056/NEJMoa0900559.

51. Skelley NW, Allen JG, Arnaoutakis GJ, Weiss ES,
Patel ND, Conte JV. The impact of volume reduction
on early and long-term outcomes in surgical ventricular restoration for severe heart failure. Ann Thorac
Surg. 2011;91(1):104–11; discussion 11–2

52. Athanasuleas CL, Buckberg GD, Stanley AW, Siler
W, Dor V, Di Donato M, et al. Surgical ventricular
restoration in the treatment of congestive heart failure
due to post-infarction ventricular dilation. J Am Coll
Cardiol. 2004;44(7):1439–45.

53. Likoff W, Bailey CP. Ventriculoplasty: excision of
myocardial aneurysm: report of a successful case. J
Am Med Assoc. 1955;158(11):915–20. https://doi.
org/10.1001/jama.1955.02960110021006.

54. Mukaddirov M, Demaria RG, Perrault LP, Frapier J-M,
Albat B. Reconstructive surgery of postinfarction left
ventricular aneurysms: techniques and unsolved problems. Eur J Cardio-Thorac Surg. 2008;34(2):256–61.
https://doi.org/10.1016/j.ejcts.2008.03.061.

55. Cooley DA, Collins HA, Morris GC Jr, Chapman
DW. Ventricular aneurysm after myocardial
infarction: surgical excision with use of temporary cardiopulmonary bypass. J Am Med Assoc.
1958;167(5):557–60.   https://doi.org/10.1001/
jama.1958.02990220027008.

56. Dor V, Saab M, Coste P, Kornaszewska M, Montiglio F. Left ventricular aneurysm: a new surgical approach. Thorac Cardiovasc Surg. 1989;37(1):11–9.

57. Jatene AD. Left ventricular aneurysmectomy. Resection or reconstruction. J Thorac Cardiovasc Surg. 1985 Mar;89(3):321–31.

58. Dor V, Sabatier M, Di Donato M, Maioli M, Toso A, Montiglio F. Late hemodynamic results after left ventricular patch repair associated with coronary grafting in patients with postinfarction akinetic or dyskinetic aneurysm of the left ventricle. J Thorac Cardiovasc Surg. 1995;110(5):1291–301.

59. Athanasuleas CL, Stanley AWH Jr, Buckberg GD, Dor V, DiDonato M, Blackstone EH. Surgical anterior ventricular endocardial restoration (SAVER) in the dilated remodeled ventricle after anterior myocardial infarction. J Am Coll Cardiol. 2001;37(5):1199–209.

60. Brown SL, Gropler RJ, Harris KM. Distinguishing left ventricular aneurysm from pseudoaneurysm. A review of the literature. Chest. 1997;111(5):1403–9.

61. Frances C, Romero A, Grady D. Left ventricular pseudoaneurysm. J Am Coll Cardiol. 1998;32(3):557–61.

62. Konen E, Merchant N, Gutierrez C, Provost Y, Mickleborough L, Paul NS, et al. True versus false left ventricular aneurysm: differentiation with MR imaging—initial experience. Radiology. 2005;236(1):65–75. https://doi.org/10.1148/radiol.2361031699.

63. Dudiy Y, Jelnin V, Einhorn BN, Kronzon I, Cohen HA, Ruiz CE. Percutaneous closure of left ventricular pseudoaneurysm. Circ Cardiovasc Interv. 2011;4(4):322. https://doi.org/10.1161/CIRCINTERVENTIONS.111.962464.

64. Kapadia SR, Tuzcu EM. Plugging holes. Circ Cardiovasc Interv. 2011;4(4):308. https://doi.org/10.1161/CIRCINTERVENTIONS.111.964387.

James Cockburn, Osama Alsanjari, and David Hildick-Smith

About Us

The Sussex Cardiac Centre is the tertiary cardiac center for Sussex serving a population of over 1.2 million people. It offers treatment in all areas of cardiovascular disease. The unit has a big research department, with particular interests in coronary and structural heart intervention. The BBC ONE trial comparing single- vs. two-stent strategies to treat bifurcation disease was run from the Sussex Cardiac Centre, as is the current EBC MAIN trial. This chapter is based on treatment strategies used within this center and reflects current local practice.

What Is a Bifurcation?

A bifurcation lesion is a lesion occurring at or adjacent to a significant division of a major epicardial coronary artery [1]. Bifurcations represent 10–15% of all lesions treated by percutaneous coronary intervention (PCI).

J. Cockburn · O. Alsanjari · D. Hildick-Smith (✉)
Sussex Cardiac Centre, Brighton and Sussex
University Hospitals NHS Trust, Brighton, UK
e-mail: james.cockburn@bsuh.nhs.uk; david.
hildick-smith@bsuh.nhs.uk

Planning a Bifurcation Lesion Procedure

The Evidence

- To date the evidence from randomized control trials of single- vs. two-stent strategies suggests that using a single-stent strategy where possible offers the best outcome to patients.
- Two-stent techniques are associated with higher rates of major adverse cardiovascular events (MACE), largely driven by higher rates of peri-procedural myocardial infarction (PMI).
- Most recently, the 5-year survival from a patient-level pooled analysis of the Nordic Bifurcation Study and the British Bifurcation Coronary Study was published confirming a provisional single-stent approach was associated with lower long-term mortality than a systematic two-stent technique [2].

The Anatomy and the Medina Classification

- Refer to a bifurcation lesion using standardized anatomical jargon.
- The proximal main vessel (PMV), distal main vessel (DMV), and the side branch (SB).
- The Medina classification (Fig. 26.1) is a simple and now universal classification of

© Springer International Publishing AG, part of Springer Nature 2018
A. Myat et al. (eds.), *The Interventional Cardiology Training Manual*,
https://doi.org/10.1007/978-3-319-71635-0_26

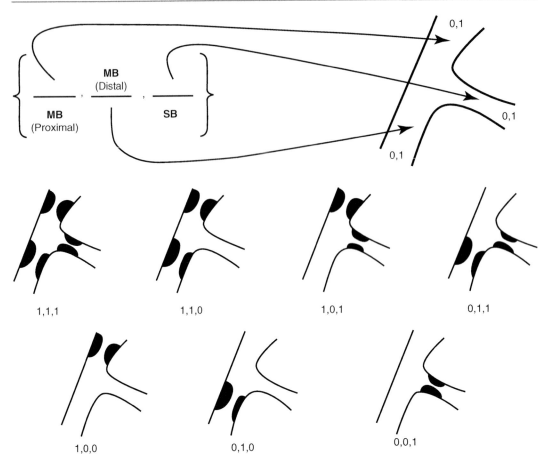

Fig. 26.1 The Medina classification of coronary bifurcation lesions. Reproduced with permission from Medina A, de Lezo JS, Pan M. Rev Esp Cardiol. 2006;59(2),183–4

bifurcation lesions that offers a standardized way to describe and hence interpret treatment of bifurcations [3].

- Limitations of the Medina classification do exist since it does not consider:
  - Bifurcation angles
  - Extent of calcification
  - Lesion lengths
  - Functional significance of the lesions
  - Plaque distribution and plaque burden as seen directly by intracoronary imaging such as intravascular ultrasound (IVUS)
  - Fate of the side branch (SB) upon dilatation of the main vessel (MV)

Murray's Law

- This is a useful law to help determine vessel size and therefore stent choice when undertaking bifurcation stenting.
- Finet's adaptation of Murray's law suggests that the proximal vessel diameter is the sum of the distal main vessel and the side branch vessel diameters multiplied by 0.678.
- This approximation holds good for most coronary vessel diameters [4].
- $D_{mother} = 0.678 \times (D_{daughter1} + D_{daughter2})$, where D_{mother} = proximal main vessel, $D_{daughter1}$ = distal main vessel, and $D_{daughter2}$ = side branch vessel

Catheter Choice and Access Site

- Bifurcations, including left main stem (LMS) lesions, can be adequately treated using six French guiding catheters, which allows two wires and two balloons to track without issue.
- New radial sheaths, such as glidesheath slender (Terumo Inc., Japan), offer the ability to upsize to 7F if required (6F to 7F).
- The access site should, however, be at the operator's discretion.

The Provisional or Single-Stent Technique

- This should be considered the standard approach for treating bifurcations, and is endorsed by the European Bifurcation Club (EBC) [5].
- Points to consider:
  - Wiring of the SB should be considered unless losing it is considered irrelevant, or the side branch is large caliber and undiseased at its ostium. Most of the MACE related to bifurcation procedures results from periprocedural myocardial infarction (PMI).
  - A narrow angle between the MV and SB, ostial SB disease and small SB vessels are markers of possible SB occlusion after MV stenting.
  - Adequate MV lesion preparation should be performed using adjunctive techniques if

required, and may have to be conducted up-front if impossible to wire the SB.
  - Use coronary wires that the operator is most familiar with, but recrossing may be helped with hydrophilic wires.
  - Drug-eluting stents (DES) are recommended for bifurcation stenting, and should be chosen on their ability to accommodate expansion to the proximal MV diameter, but should also be sized with consideration paid to the distal MV diameter.
  - 30 s inflations are recommended to achieve adequate stent expansion.
- There are four main steps and another 4 if the side branch requires attention (see Fig. 26.2)
  - Step 1: Wire both branches
  - Step 2: Pre-dilatation and MV stenting using a stent diameter according to the distal MV reference.
  - Step 3: Proximal optimization technique (POT).
  - Step 4: If Thrombolysis in Myocardial Infarction (TIMI) III flow is present into the SB, the procedure can be stopped.
- If the SB needs attention (e.g., significant flow limitation, <TIMI III flow), the following steps are required:
  - Step 5: Rewire the SB through the MV distal strut, ideally via "pullback rewiring" from MV to SB.
  - Step 6: Remove jailed SB wire (watch for guide catheter deep-throating).

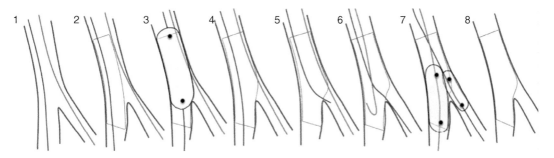

Fig. 26.2 Provisional bifurcation stenting. Steps 1–4 represent the main steps involved in stenting of the main vessel. Steps 5–8 indicate the maneuvers involved if the side branch also requires attention

- Step 7: Kissing balloon inflation, ideally with short noncompliant balloons in order to avoid SB dissection and stent distortion.
- Step 8: Further proximal post-dilatation or re-POT to account for MV stent distortion from the kissing balloon inflation.
• Issues to note when considering SB intervention:
  - How large and how hemodynamically significant does the SB appear to be?
  - At what angle does the SB come out from the MV (see Fig. 26.3)?

- Is there significant ostial or proximal SB disease?
- Will the SB be difficult to wire?
- Comorbid state and risk profile of the patient and will this impact upon the importance of the SB?
- The level of MV disease and degree of plaque burden.
• Routine SB pre-dilatation should be avoided but considered in the presence of severe ostial SB disease. While this may facilitate rewiring, there is a risk of dissecting the SB and therefore failure to rewire.

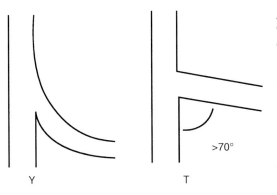

Fig. 26.3 Side branch angulation and morphology. Y-shaped angulation: coronary wire access relatively straightforward but risk of plaque shift much greater. T-shaped angulation: coronary wire access more difficult but risk of plaque shift less

The Proximal Optimization Technique (POT)

• The POT was devised by Darremont, and relates to a method of expanding the stent up to and including the carina, using a balloon sized to the proximal vessel diameter (Fig. 26.4).
• This produces a curved expansion of the stent into the bifurcation point and facilitates recrossing, distal recrossing, kissing inflations, and ostial stent coverage of the side branch (Fig. 26.5).
• Noncompliant or semi-compliant balloons should be used.

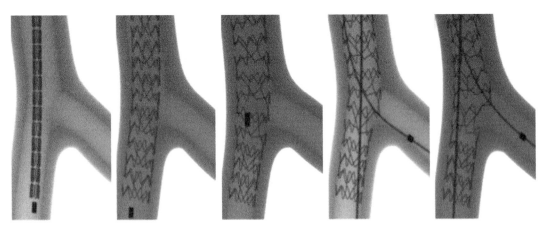

Fig. 26.4 The Proximal Optimization Technique (POT). From left to right—the stent size is selected according to the diameter of the distal main vessel. Once deployed the stent in the main vessel is fully apposed distally (beyond the bifurcation) but not proximally. The POT is performed with a balloon sized to the proximal main vessel diameter, with the distal balloon marker placed just proximal to the carina. Once performed, the POT facilitates wire access through the distal strut (see Fig. 26.5), which, after kissing balloon inflation, allows for good side branch scaffolding. Reproduced with permission from Sawaya et al. J Am Coll Cardiol Intv 2016;9:1861–78

Proximal crossing   Distal crossing

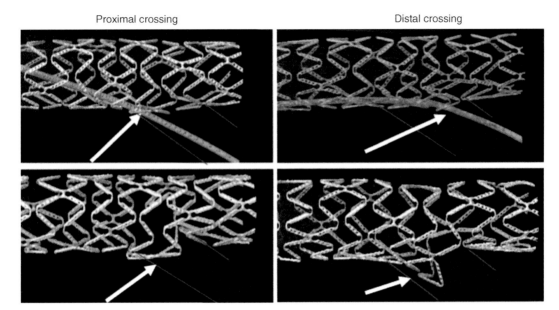

Fig. 26.5 The importance of distal cell recrossing close to the carina after main vessel stenting. Appropriately performed proximal optimization of the main vessel stent facilitates recrossing of the coronary wire through the strut closest to the carina. This in turn allows for improved scaffolding of the side branch ostium compared to proxi- mal recrossing of the wire, which tends to push the struts inward toward the main vessel lumen. The white arrow indicates the location of wire recrossing and its effect on side branch scaffolding. Reproduced with permission from Sawaya et al. J Am Coll Cardiol Intv 2016;9:1861–78

Kissing Balloon Inflations in Simple Stenting

- Nordic III has established that there is no systematic clinical advantage to a routine kissing strategy when a single-stent treatment is used, despite theoretical advantages, but also no systematic disadvantage [6].

Side Branch Stenting Technique in a Provisional Strategy

- In essence SB stenting in a provisional strategy is a "bail-out" and should be considered when there is:
  - Significant compromise to SB flow
  - Presence of a major SB dissection
  - When the SB is significantly diseased and large enough to lead to significant residual ischemia
- T-stenting of the SB can be used in the majority of cases when SB dilatation is per-

formed properly through a distal strut (Fig. 26.6).
- If the angle is close to 90°, modified T-stenting (also known as T and protrude— i.e., TAP) should be considered, as other techniques are associated with a high risk of stent mal-apposition. This requires precise deployment of the SB stent at the ostium (Fig. 26.7).
- Therefore knowledge of where a stent sits relative to its proximal marker is key to this (and varies by manufacturer) as well as finding an optimal view to avoid too much protrusion inside the MV stent or worse still a gap between the two stents.
- If the SB ostium is not properly covered by the MV stent, an overlapping technique is necessary, and we usually use the culotte.
- Crush stenting is a non-provisional technique, which commits the operator to a two-stent technique at the outset, the results of which were inferior to culotte in the NORDIC II trial (Fig. 26.8).

Fig. 26.6 T-stenting technique of the side branch. Reproduced with permission from Iakovou et al. J Am Coll Cardiol 2005;46:1446–55

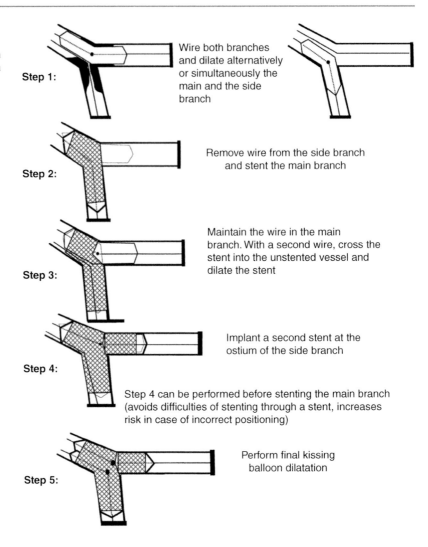

Step 1: Wire both branches and dilate alternatively or simultaneously the main and the side branch

Step 2: Remove wire from the side branch and stent the main branch

Step 3: Maintain the wire in the main branch. With a second wire, cross the stent into the unstented vessel and dilate the stent

Step 4: Implant a second stent at the ostium of the side branch

Step 4 can be performed before stenting the main branch (avoids difficulties of stenting through a stent, increases risk in case of incorrect positioning)

Step 5: Perform final kissing balloon dilatation

When to Use Two-Stent Techniques

- The aim should be to start most procedures with a single-stent strategy.
- However the recent EBC II trial, which compared a single- vs. two-stent technique with the culotte in a large SB (>2.5 mm diameter and >5 mm length ostial stenosis) found no specific benefit to the two-stent technique [7].

What Technique?

- The aim as a trainee should be to become competent with single-stent bifurcations and then to aim to become well trained in one complex strategy. Intuitively it is much better to be able to perform one complex strategy well rather than two or more poorly.
- Bifurcations treated with two stents, despite refinements in technique such as POT and kissing balloon inflations, remain higher risk for early stent thrombosis. Therefore, as a department we would recommend the culotte technique and T protrusion stenting (discussed above).
- Crush stenting by name alone does not sound a sensible thing to do to a stent. Crushing makes recrossing more difficult and success rates are lower. The DK-crush technique is superior but requires more instrumentation (Fig. 26.9).

Fig. 26.7 Modified T-stenting of the side branch. Reproduced with permission from Iakovou et al. J Am Coll Cardiol 2005;46:1446–55

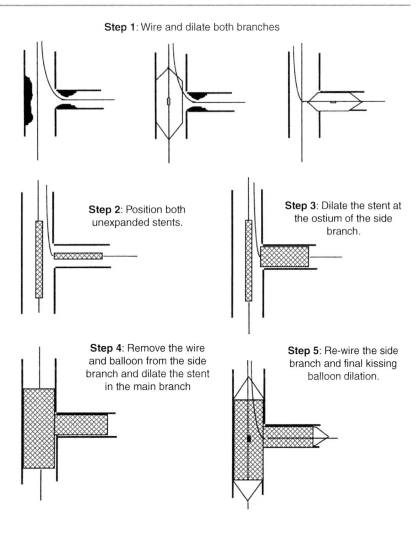

Step 1: Wire and dilate both branches

Step 2: Position both unexpanded stents.

Step 3: Dilate the stent at the ostium of the side branch.

Step 4: Remove the wire and balloon from the side branch and dilate the stent in the main branch

Step 5: Re-wire the side branch and final kissing balloon dilation.

How to Perform a Culotte

- The culotte technique efficacy has been documented in many trials (Nordic I, II, IV and BBC-1) [1]. The only limitation to this technique can be significant size discrepancy between the PMV and the SB (Fig. 26.10).
- Two steps are considered mandatory. Firstly, stent platform selection needs to be based on expansion characteristics in order to avoid major mal-apposition in the MV.
- Secondly, the POT is mandatory to correct for any suspected mal-apposition occurring in the MV during the procedure.

- Step 1: Wire the MV and SB
- Step 2: Pre-dilate and stent SB with SB stent extending back into MV
- Step 3: POT SB stent (aim to use NC balloon sized to proximal main vessel)
- Step 4: Rewire MV via SB stent and then remove jailed MV wire
- Step 5: Dilate MV through stent struts and stent MV (stent size chosen on basis of DMV reference diameter)
- Step 6: POT MV stent (aim to use NC balloon at least 0.5–1 mm greater than stent reference diameter)
- Step 7: Recross into SB through distal cell where possible and then remove trapped SB wire.
- Step 8: Pre-dilatation of SB stent to reopen ostium
- Step 9: Kissing balloon inflation, ideally with short noncompliant balloons, sized to the SB and DMV respectively. Individual

Fig. 26.8 Crush stenting technique of the side branch. Reproduced with permission from Iakovou et al. J Am Coll Cardiol 2005;46:1446–55

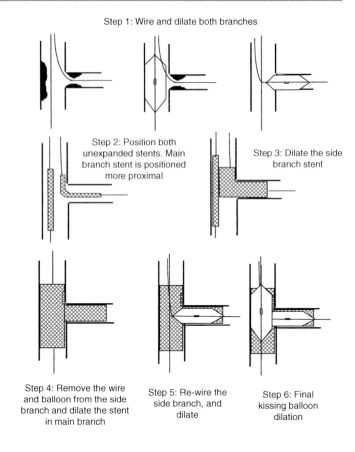

Step 1: Wire and dilate both branches

Step 2: Position both unexpanded stents. Main branch stent is positioned more proximal

Step 3: Dilate the side branch stent

Step 4: Remove the wire and balloon from the side branch and dilate the stent in main branch

Step 5: Re-wire the side branch, and dilate

Step 6: Final kissing balloon dilation

high-pressure dilatation prior to the kissing inflation is recommended.

- Step 10: Further proximal post-dilation or re-POT to account for MV stent distortion from kiss

Imaging and Bifurcations

- Angiographic assessment of bifurcations has several limitations and therefore may be aided by intracoronary imaging.
- Optical coherence tomography (OCT) is a high resolution imaging technique, which allows for superior imaging of the luminal surface, calcium, stent positions, wires, and the SB ostium from both MV and SB pullbacks, relative to IVUS.
- However OCT may increase the use of contrast and can be suboptimal in very large vessels and aorto-ostial assessment [8].
- IVUS, by way of contrast, has better depth penetration allowing better characterization of

plaque burden and does not require optimal vessel flushing during acquisition.

- Both modalities enable lesion assessment, evaluation of pre-dilatation, reference sizing and evaluation of adequate vessel and stent expansion after stenting [9–13].
- Probably the most beneficial aspect of imaging in complex two-stent interventions is evaluation of wire positions after stent rewiring to ensure optimal SB recrossing [14–16].

Left Main Stem Bifurcations (See Also Chap. 27)

- There is increasing evidence to suggest that PCI with DES is a non-inferior revascularization option relative to the "gold standard" of coronary artery bypass grafting (CABG) in patients with significant LMS disease.

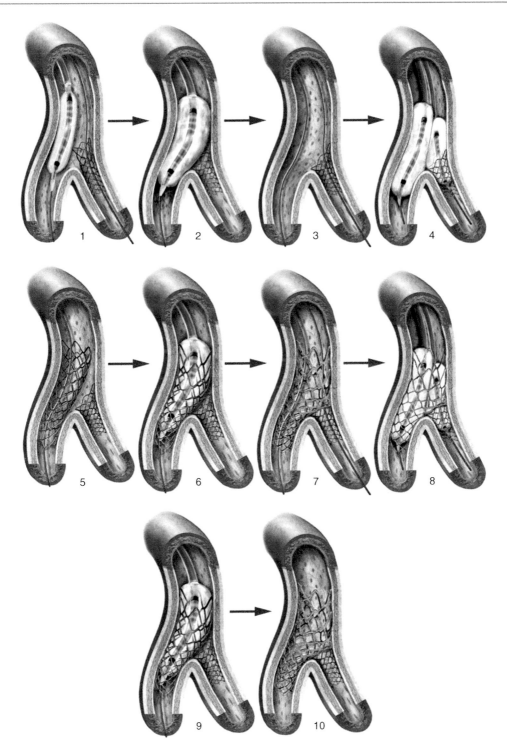

Fig. 26.9 The double kissing (DK) crush technique. (*1*) Side branch (SB) stenting with short main vessel (MV) protrusion. (*2*) Ostial SB stent balloon crush. (*3*) Recross SB with coronary wire. (*4*) First kissing balloon inflation. (*5*) Remove SB wire and stent MV across the ostium of the SB. (*6*) Perform a proximal optimization of the MV stent (see also Fig. 26.4). (*7*) Rewire the SB via the MV stent and the crushed SB stent. (*8*) Second kissing balloon inflation. (*9*) Second proximal optimization of the MV stent. (*10*) Final result. Reproduced with permission from Sawaya et al. J Am Coll Cardiol Intv 2016;9:1861–78

Fig. 26.10 The culottes stenting technique. Reproduced with permission from Iakovou et al. J Am Coll Cardiol 2005;46:1446–55

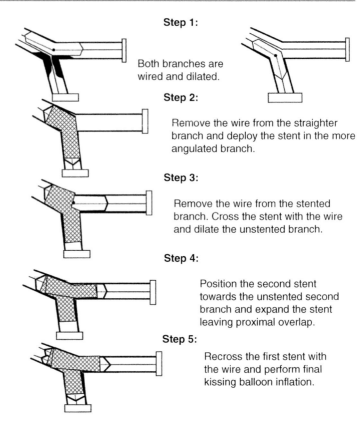

Step 1:

Both branches are wired and dilated.

Step 2:

Remove the wire from the straighter branch and deploy the stent in the more angulated branch.

Step 3:

Remove the wire from the stented branch. Cross the stent with the wire and dilate the unstented branch.

Step 4:

Position the second stent towards the unstented second branch and expand the stent leaving proximal overlap.

Step 5:

Recross the first stent with the wire and perform final kissing balloon inflation.

- The left main stem (LMS) is the largest bifurcation of the coronary tree and has a number of unique features:
  - The myocardium subtended by the LMS generally accounts >50% of the total myocardial mass
  - The PMV reference diameter generally measures between 4.5 and 5.5 mm
  - The SB is always a major epicardial coronary artery
  - The left circumflex artery (LCx) is often considered the SB
  - Occlusion of the LCx is not acceptable as it supplies a large myocardial territory

LMS Treatment and Techniques

- As for all bifurcation lesions, a provisional or single-stent approach is recommended in most cases, as data from observational non-randomized studies suggest that this technique where feasible has a higher rate of target lesion revascularization relative to two-stent techniques.

- Most issues arising from LMS bifurcations can be overcome by sensible stent selection and positioning, and by use of the POT technique.
- If a two-stent technique is required and the vessels are of similar size, then a culotte may be feasible.
- If there is an angle of or close to 90° (T-shape angulation), the T or TAP would be recommended in the majority of double-stenting cases.
- The randomized European Bifurcation Club Left Main (EBC MAIN) study is currently recruiting and is looking specifically at whether a single- or two-stent strategy is best for true bifurcation LMS disease, with respect to death, target lesion revascularization (TLR), and myocardial infarction at 1 year, and angina status, stent thrombosis, death, myocardial infarction, and TLR at three- and five-year clinical follow-up.

Bioresorbable Vascular Scaffolds and Bifurcations

- Bioresorbable stents (BRS) may offer potential advantages compared with metallic DES for bifurcation PCI, particularly as there is potential for "un-jailing" of the SB ostium as the device resorbs.
- However there are limitations to this technology currently, in particular strut thickness and limited expansion capacity, as well as the signals for increased early and late scaffold thrombosis, particularly in small vessels.
- If BRS is to be used for bifurcations, then clearly the provisional strategy remains the default technique.

Important Points to Consider When Using BRS in Bifurcations

- Appropriate vessel sizing (confirmed by intracoronary imaging, ideally OCT or equivalent) is required to facilitate correct size of scaffold as the expansion capacity of the Absorb BRS allows post-dilatation up to 0.5 mm above the nominal diameter.
- Lesion preparation is key and often 1:1 balloon sizing is required with noncompliant (NC) balloons to confirm adequate vessel expansion.
- There is no data yet to determine if BRS sizing should be made on the basis of DMV or PMV diameter.
- POT is mandatory with an NC balloon within 0.5 mm of the scaffold diameter.
- Routine use of kissing balloons is not recommended due to the risk of scaffold fracture, but if required, a low-pressure KISS or "SNUGGLE" technique can be used.
- All procedural results should be checked and confirmed for distal dissection, underexpansion, and mal-apposition with intracoronary imaging.
- Currently the ABC-1 trial, performed in our department, is looking at the provisional strategy with ABSORB (ABSORB scaffold, Abbott Vascular, USA) in bifurcations, with randomization to proximal or distal vessel sizing.

Two-Stent Techniques Using Absorb BRS

- It is the feeling of the department that, while technically feasible, any form of two-stent strategy with BRS should only be considered as part of a clinical trial, especially due to a late signal of potential scaffold thrombosis in these patients.

Dedicated Bifurcation Stents

- Dedicated bifurcation devices remain a niche area, mainly because of the fact that they are not "user friendly."
- Two main dedicated systems are commercially available—the Tryton (Tryton Medical, USA) and Axxess systems (Biosensors, Switzerland), respectively.
- Data for the Tryton stent is encouraging in some respects but the device remains limited by the fact that it is not drug-eluting.

Medina Classification 0,0,1 Treatment

- Rarely do these lesions require intervention as most often any symptoms can be adequately treated with optimal medical therapy.
- If required, a pressure wire study to determine fractional flow reserve can be useful to confirm physiological impairment to flow from the anatomical obstruction.
- One always needs to be careful to make sure that any treatment does not have a negative effect on the MV.
- Other possible techniques have involved the use of drug-eluting balloons but there remains a lack of head-to-head trial data in this group of patients.

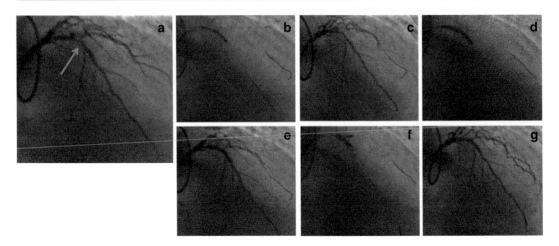

Fig. 26.11 Provisional bifurcation stenting. Plates (**a–g**): (**a**) diagnostic angiogram revealing a critical stenosis of the proximal left anterior descending (LAD) artery involving the first diagonal side branch bifurcation (arrow); (**b**) both the LAD and D1 have been wired followed by pre-dilatation of the LAD; (**c**) angiogram following pre-dilatation with Thrombolysis In Myocardial Infarction (TIMI) 3 flow in the side branch; (**d**) stent deployment in the proximal LAD across the ostium of the D1 side branch; (**e**) angiogram post stent deployment demonstrating "pinching" of the D1 ostium; (**f**) kissing balloon inflations of both the proximal LAD and ostial D1; (**g**) final angiographic result with TIMI 3 flow down the LAD and D1

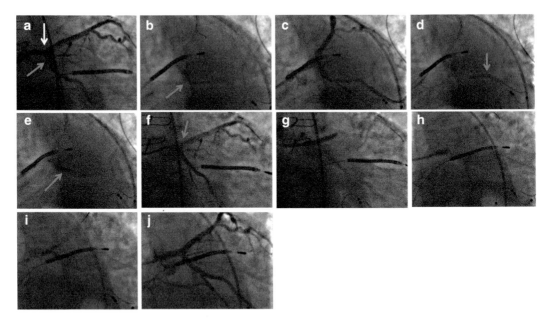

Fig. 26.12 T-stenting. Plates (**a–j**): (**a**) Diagnostic angiogram showing significant distal left main stem (LMS—white arrow) extending into proximal left circumflex (LCx—blue arrow) disease; (**b**) wiring of both the left anterior descending (LAD) artery and pre-dilatation of the LCx (arrow); (**c**) angiogram after pre-dilatation; (**d**) first stent deployed into mid-LCx (arrow); (**e**) second stent deployed to cover ostial LCx (arrow); (**f**) positioning of LMS-LAD stent (arrow); (**g**) stent deployed to LMS-LAD; (**h**) proximal optimisation (POT) positioning distal balloon marker at the carina; (**i**) sequential high pressure inflations followed by final kissing balloon inflation; (**j**) final angiographic result

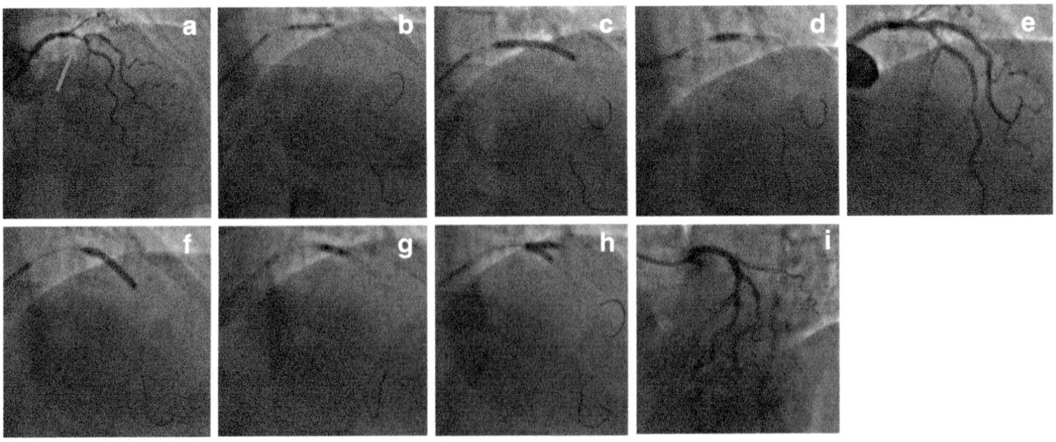

Fig. 26.13 Culotte stenting. Plates (**a–i**): (**a**) diagnostic angiogram demonstrating a critical stenosis at the LAD/D1 bifurcation; (**b**) pre-dilatation of the diagonal which is shown to be a relatively large vessel in comparison with the LAD; (**c**) stent deployment into diagonal; (**d**) proximal optimisation of the D1 stent to prepare for re-crossing into LAD. The distal marker of the balloon loaded onto the diagonal wire is positioned at the carina; (**e**) angiogram after proximal optimisation. Re-crossing of the coronary wire from D1 stent into LAD; (**f**) second stent deployed into LAD, the proximal segment of both stents now overlapping at the bifurcation; (**g**) proximal optimisation of the LAD stent; (**h**) kissing balloon inflations after performing sequential high pressure inflations to both stented vessels; (**i**) final angiographic result

Conclusions

- When treating bifurcations, where possible, aim to use a single-stent technique.
- Systematic use of the Medina classification is recommended, despite its limitations.
- The provisional single-stent technique should be the default strategy for most bifurcations.
- The POT technique should be considered a standard step in bifurcation treatment.
- When using a provisional technique, kissing inflations are not considered mandatory.
- When using a provisional technique and a side branch stent is required, T, TAP and culotte are all potentially good techniques.
- OCT and IVUS may help guide bifurcation treatment, in particular optimizing SB rewiring position (Figs. 26.11, 26.12, and 26.13).

References

1. Hildick-Smith D, Lassen JF, Albiero R, Lefevre T, Darremont O, Pan M, Ferenc M, Stankovic G, Louvard Y, European Bifurcation Club. Consensus from the 5th European Bifurcation Club meeting. EuroIntervention. 2010;6:34–8.
2. Behan MW, Holm NR, de Belder AJ, Cockburn J, Erglis A, Curzen NP, Niemelä M, Oldroyd KG, Kervinen K, Kumsars I, Gunnes P, Stables RH, Maeng M, Ravkilde J, Jensen JS, Christiansen EH, Cooter N, Steigen TK, Vikman S, Thuesen L, Lassen JF, Hildick-Smith D. Coronary bifurcation lesions treated with simple or complex stenting: 5-year survival from patient-level pooled analysis of the Nordic Bifurcation Study and the British Bifurcation Coronary Study. Eur Heart J. 2016;37:1923–8.
3. Medina A, Suarez de Lezo J, Pan M. A new classification of coronary bifurcation lesions. Rev Esp Cardiol. 2006;59:183.
4. Murray CD. The physiological principle of minimum work applied to the angle of branching of arteries. J Gen Physiol. 1926;9:835–41.

5. Lassen JF, Holm NR, Banning A, Burzotta F, Lefèvre T, Chieffo A, Hildick-Smith D, Louvard Y, Stankovic G. Percutaneous coronary intervention for coronary bifurcation disease: 11th consensus document from the European Bifurcation Club. EuroIntervention. 2016;12:38–46.

6. Niemelä M, Kervinen K, Erglis A, Holm NR, Maeng M, Christiansen EH, Kumsars I, Jegere S, Dombrovskis A, Gunnes P, Stavnes S, Steigen TK, Trovik T, Eskola M, Vikman S, Romppanen H, Mäkikallio T, Hansen KN, Thayssen P, Aberge L, Jensen LO, Hervold A, Airaksinen J, Pietilä M, Frobert O, Kellerth T, Ravkilde J, Aarøe J, Jensen JS, Helqvist S, Sjögren I, James S, Miettinen H, Lassen JF, Thuesen L, Nordic-Baltic PCI Study Group. Randomized comparison of final kissing balloon dilatation versus no final kissing balloon dilatation in patients with coronary bifurcation lesions treated with main vessel stenting: the Nordic-Baltic Bifurcation Study III. Circulation. 2014;123:79–86.

7. Hildick-Smith D, Behan MW, Lassen JF, Chieffo A, Lefèvre T, Stankovic G, Burzotta F, Pan M, Ferenc M, Bennett L, Hovasse T, Spence MJ, Oldroyd K, Brunel P, Carrie D, Baumbach A, Maeng M, Skipper N, Louvard Y. The EBC TWO Study (European Bifurcation Coronary TWO): a randomized comparison of provisional T-stenting versus a systematic 2 stent Culotte strategy in large caliber true bifurcations. Circ Cardiovasc Interv. 2016;9(9).

8. Fujino Y, Bezerra HG, Attizzani GF, Wang W, Yamamoto H, Chamie D, Kanaya T, Mehanna E, Tahara S, Nakamura S, Costa MA. Frequency-domain optical coherence tomography assessment of unprotected left main coronary artery disease—a comparison with intravascular ultrasound. Catheter Cardiovasc Interv. 2013;82:E173–83.

9. Mintz GS, Nissen SE, Anderson WD, Bailey SR, Erbel R, Fitzgerald PJ, Pinto FJ, Rosenfield K, Siegel RJ, Tuzcu EM, Yock PG. American College of Cardiology Clinical Expert Consensus Document on Standards for Acquisition, Measurement and Reporting of Intravascular Ultrasound Studies (IVUS). A report of the American College of Cardiology Task Force on Clinical Expert Consensus Documents. J Am Coll Cardiol. 2001;37:1478–92.

10. Tearney GJ, Regar E, Akasaka T, Adriaenssens T, Barlis P, Bezerra HG, Bouma B, Bruining N, Cho JM, Chowdhary S, Costa MA, de Silva R, Dijkstra J, Di Mario C, Dudek D, Falk E, Feldman MD, Fitzgerald P, Garcia-Garcia HM, Gonzalo N, Granada JF, Guagliumi G, Holm NR, Honda Y, Ikeno F, Kawasaki M, Kochman J, Koltowski L, Kubo T, Kume T, Kyono H, Lam CC, Lamouche G, Lee DP, Leon MB, Maehara A, Manfrini O, Mintz GS, Mizuno K, Morel MA, Nadkarni S, Okura H, Otake H, Pietrasik A, Prati F, Raber L, Radu MD, Rieber J, Riga M, Rollins A, Rosenberg M, Sirbu V, Serruys PW, Shimada K, Shinke T, Shite J, Siegel E, Sonoda S, Suter M, Takarada S, Tanaka A, Terashima M, Thim T, Uemura S, Ughi GJ, van Beusekom HM, van der Steen AF, Van Es GA, van Soest G, Virmani R, Waxman S, Weissman NJ, Weisz G, International Working Group for Intravascular Optical Coherence Tomography (IWG-IVOCT). Consensus standards for acquisition, measurement, and reporting of intravascular optical coherence tomography studies: a report from the International Working Group for Intravascular Optical Coherence Tomography Standardization and Validation. J Am Coll Cardiol. 2012;59:1058–72.

11. Prati F, Guagliumi G, Mintz GS, Costa M, Regar E, Akasaka T, Barlis P, Tearney GJ, Jang IK, Arbustini E, Bezerra HG, Ozaki Y, Bruining N, Dudek D, Radu M, Erglis A, Motreff P, Alfonso F, Toutouzas K, Gonzalo N, Tamburino C, Adriaenssens T, Pinto F, Serruys PW, Di Mario C. Expert's OCT Review Document. Expert review document part 2: methodology, terminology and clinical applications of optical coherence tomography for the assessment of interventional procedures. Eur Heart J. 2012;33:2513–20.

12. Motreff P, Rioufol G, Gilard M, Caussin C, Ouchchane L, Souteyrand G, Finet G. Diffuse atherosclerotic left main coronary artery disease unmasked by fractal geometric law applied to quantitative coronary angiography: an angiographic and intravascular ultrasound study. EuroIntervention. 2010;5:709–15.

13. Habara M, Nasu K, Terashima M, Kaneda H, Yokota D, Ko E, Ito T, Kurita T, Tanaka N, Kimura M, Ito T, Kinoshita Y, Tsuchikane E, Asakura K, Asakura Y, Katoh O, Suzuki T. Impact of frequency-domain optical coherence tomography guidance for optimal coronary stent implantation in comparison with intravascular ultrasound guidance. Circ Cardiovasc Interv. 2012;5:193–201.

14. Holm NR, Tu S, Christiansen EH, Reiber JH, Lassen JF, Thuesen L, Maeng M. Use of three-dimensional optical coherence tomography to verify correct wire position in a jailed side branch after main vessel stent implantation. EuroIntervention. 2011;7:528–9.

15. Alegria-Barrero E, Foin N, Chan PH, Syrseloudis D, Lindsay AC, Dimopolous K, Alonso-Gonzalez R, Viceconte N, De Silva R, Di Mario C. Optical coherence tomography for guidance of distal cell recrossing in bifurcation stenting: choosing the right cell matters. EuroIntervention. 2012;8:205–13.

16. Okamura T, Onuma Y, Yamada J, Iqbal J, Tateishi H, Nao T, Oda T, Maeda T, Nakamura T, Miura T, Yano M, Serruys PW. 3D optical coherence tomography: new insights into the process of optimal rewiring of side branches during bifurcational stenting. EuroIntervention. 2014;10:907–15.

Left Main Coronary Artery Intervention

27

Giovanni Luigi De Maria and Adrian Paul Banning

About Us

Professor Adrian Banning is Consultant Cardiologist at the John Radcliffe Hospital—Oxford University Hospitals NHS Trust and Professor of Interventional Cardiology at Oxford University. Dr. Giovanni Luigi De Maria works at the John Radcliffe Hospital as Fellow in Interventional Cardiology. The John Radcliffe Hospital performs 1400 percutaneous coronary interventions per year with a catchment area of approximately one million people. The center has an established TAVI and CTO program and has been a live site for the TCT and PCR meetings. We are currently involved in multicenter randomized trials in the field of multivessel and left main coronary artery PCI (European top enroller for the EXCEL study, Co PI for SYNTAX II study, involvement in NOBLE, IDEAL left main, FAME 3, and the EBC MAIN studies).

G. L. De Maria · A. P. Banning (✉)
Oxford Heart Centre, John Radcliffe Hospital,
Oxford University Hospital NHS Trust, Oxford, UK
e-mail: adrian.banning@ouh.nhs.uk

Introduction

- The left main coronary artery (LMCA) supplies the majority of blood to the left ventricle. This fact alone explains why untreated obstructive LMCA disease is associated with a poor prognosis.
- Coronary artery bypass grafting (CABG) has a clear indication with a proven mortality benefit and it has been conventionally regarded as the gold standard treatment for LMCA disease.
- However, thanks to evolving technologies and technique, trials have progressively supported the alternative use of coronary stents in certain patient subsets with LMCA disease.
- In left main disease particularly, stringent technique is essential to obtain an optimal and durable result. Rigorous procedural planning, application of appropriate procedural imaging and lesion preparation together with careful patient-selection, are crucial in LMCA intervention.
- The aim of this chapter is to guide the reader through the main aspects that need attention when dealing with LMCA disease and provides a practical algorithm to apply in the catheterization laboratory.

© Springer International Publishing AG, part of Springer Nature 2018
A. Myat et al. (eds.), *The Interventional Cardiology Training Manual*,
https://doi.org/10.1007/978-3-319-71635-0_27

Is Stenosis of the Left Main Coronary Artery a "Big Deal?"

- LMCA disease has a relatively low incidence accounting for approximately 4% of all coronary angiograms, with isolated LMCA disease in only 5–10% of these cases [1].
- There are four main reasons why LMCA disease requires special attention:
  - **Prognostic:** LMCA provides blood to 84% of the left ventricle in patients with a right-dominant system and 100% in patients with a left-dominant system, meaning that LMCA disease or LMCA injury during PCI can lead to catastrophic and rapid hemodynamic deterioration. Unsurprisingly an acutely occluded LMCA with cardiogenic shock has a 70% mortality at 24 h [2].
  - **Anatomical:** detection and quantification of LMCA stenosis is complex because of its short length, the diffuse nature of the disease, and the concomitant atherosclerosis in adjacent vessels [3] which can make it difficult to obtain a "normal" proximal reference.
  - **Histological:** LMCA is in direct communication with the ascending aorta. LMCA atherosclerosis is similar to aortic disease (an elastic artery) rather than in the remaining segments of the coronary tree (muscular arteries), presenting with less necrotic core, less thin fibrous cap atheroma, and a higher fibrotic and calcific component [4, 5]. This means the LMCA disease is "tougher" and therefore needs lesion preparation before stenting.
  - **Technical:** LMCA atherosclerosis usually involves the bifurcation in the vast majority of cases (up to 80% of cases), meaning that PCI to LMCA requires the skills used during bifurcation percutaneous coronary intervention (PCI) (see also Chap. 26) [3].

CABG or PCI: The Evidence from Clinical Trials

- The CASS study was the first trial reporting a prognostic benefit of CABG over medical treatment for LMCA disease [6], with a well described 98% patency rate of the left internal mammary artery (LIMA) graft to LAD at 10 years [7].
- After the promising clinical results obtained with drug-eluting stents (DES), PCI is progressively becoming an attractive alternative to CABG for LMCA. Four large studies have initially supported PCI as a therapeutic option for LMCA disease in specific clinical scenarios (Table 27.1) [8–11].
- Of these four trials the SYNTAX study included 705 patients with LMCA disease. The study showed a similar rate of major adverse cardiac and cerebrovascular events (MACCE) at 1 year in PCI and CABG groups (15.8% vs. 13.7%, $p = 0.48$) with a higher rate of repeat revascularization (11.8% vs. 6.5%, $p = 0.02$) and lower rate of stroke (0.3% vs. 2.7%, $p = 0.009$) in the PCI group [9]. However, when patients were stratified according to the anatomic complexity, expressed by the SYNTAX score, it did appear clear that patients with LMCA disease associated with low (SYNTAX score <22) or intermediate (SYNTAX score >22 and <32) complexity presented similar outcomes at 1 and 3 years with both PCI and CABG, while CABG presented a clear benefit over PCI only in the group of patients with LMCA disease and a high anatomic complexity (SYNTAX score >32) [9, 12].
- The results of the SYNTAX study has led to a change in the current European guidelines giving the following indications [13]:
  - LMCA disease with SYNTAX Score <22 = IA for both CABG and PCI
  - LMCA disease with SYNTAX Score >22 and <32 = IB for CABG and IIaB for PCI
  - LMCA disease with SYNTAX Score >32 = IB for CABG and IIIB for PCI

Table 27.1 Main studies supporting PCI in LMCA disease

	Year of publication	Patients enrolled	Follow-up (years)	LMCA disease definition	Drug-eluting stent	Primary endpoint	Event rate		p
							PCI	CABG	
LE MANS	2009	105	1	Angio diameter stenosis >50%	BMS and 1st generation (paclitaxel DES and Sirolimus DES)	Change in ejection fraction	3.3 ± 6.7%	0.5 ± 0.8%	0.047
SYNTAX	2010	705	1	Angio diameter stenosis >50%	1st generation (paclitaxel DES)	Death, MI, TVR, CVA	15.8%	13.7%	0.48
Boudriot et al.	2011	201	1	Angio diameter stenosis >50%	1st generation (Sirolimus DES)	Death, MI, TVR	19.0%	13.9%	0.19 (non-inferiority p value)
PRECOMBAT	2011	600	1	Angio diameter stenosis >50%	1st generation (Sirolimus DES)	Death, MI, TVR, CVA	8.7%	6.7%	0.01 (non-inferiority p value)
EXCEL	2016	1905	3	Angio diameter stenosis >70% / Angio diameter stenosis >50% but <70% **And** Noninvasive ischemia *or* FFR <0.80 *or* IVUS MLA <6 mm^2 (LMCA) *or* IVUS MLA <4 mm^2 (LAD or LCx)	2nd generation Everolimus DES	Death, MI, CVA	15.4%	14.7%	0.02 (non-inferiority p value)
NOBLE	2016	1200	Projected 5	Angio diameter stenosis >50% or FFR <0.80	2nd generation Biolimus DES / All 2nd generation CE-marked DES Allowed	Death, MI, TVR, CVA	29%	19%	0.0066

The table summarizes the main features of the principal completed studies comparing PCI and CABG for LMCA disease. What should strike the reader is the evolution of the definition of LMCA disease over the past 10 years. Notably the definition of significant LMCA disease does not rely only on the coronary angiogram anymore, but also on data derived from FFR and intravascular imaging. Similarly, the gradual transition from first to second generation drug-eluting stent use should be noted.

Key: *BMS* bare metal stent, *CVA* cerebrovascular accident, *DES* drug-eluting stent, *FFR* fractional flow reserve, *IVUS* intravascular ultrasound, *LAD* left anterior descending, *LCx* left circumflex, *LMCA* left man coronary artery, *MI* myocardial infarction, *MLA* minimal lumen area, *PCI* percutaneous coronary intervention, *TVR* target vessel revascularization

- However the results of SYNTAX have to be interpreted with caution for the following reasons:
  - SYNTAX was not a LMCA study, primarily recruiting patients with multivessel disease. Only 13% of patients had isolated LMCA disease.
  - SYNTAX was a negative study overall and the data on LMCA should only be seen as the result of a subgroup analysis of a negative study.
  - In SYNTAX coronary artery disease was assessed only by angiography. It is recognized that especially in LMCA disease, further investigations with intravascular imaging and/or functional assessment are usually required.
  - SYNTAX patients in the PCI group were treated with first generation DES.

- The interventional cardiology community has therefore welcomed the results of both the NOBLE and EXCEL studies. They represent the first two dedicated LMCA clinical trials, randomizing patients to "state of the art" PCI versus CABG [14].
- The Nordic-Baltic-British left main revascularization (NOBLE) study was a non-inferiority study randomizing 1201 patients with LMCA disease to percutaneous revascularization with mainly biolimus-eluting stents (BES) versus CABG over a period of 6 years (from December 2008 to January 2015) [15].
- LMS disease was defined according to an angiographic stenosis ≥50% and/or a fractional flow reserve (FFR) ≤0.80. Notably, although a SYNTAX score ≤32 was not a prespecified inclusion criterion, no more than three additional noncomplex coronary lesions were permitted in addition to the LMS lesion.
- The projected MACCE rate at 5 years favored CABG (HR 1.48 [1.11–1.96], $p = 0.007$ for superiority), mainly as consequence of a significantly higher rate of non-procedural myocardial infarction (7% vs. 2%, $p = 0.004$) and higher repeat revascularization (16% vs. 10%, $p = 0.03$) in the PCI group.
- Conversely, the Evaluation of Xience versus CABG for effectiveness of left main revascularization (EXCEL) trial was the largest randomized clinical trial comparing PCI versus surgery specifically for the treatment of LMS disease randomizing 1905 patients with LMCA disease to CABG versus PCI with 2nd generation cobalt-chromium everolimus-eluting stents (EES) over a period of nearly 3 years (from September 2010 to March 2014) [16].

- As in NOBLE, LMCA disease was defined according to an angiographic stenosis ≥70% or an angiographic stenosis between 50 and 70% in the presence of an invasive (FFR) or noninvasive documentation of inducible ischemia. However, only in EXCEL, but not in NOBLE, enrolled patients had a low-intermediate SYNTAX Score (≤32) as inclusion criterion.
- The EXCEL study has showed that PCI was non-inferior to CABG in terms of MACCE rate at 3 years (15.4% in the PCI arm vs. 14.7% in the CABG arm, $p = 0.02$ for non-inferiority).
- MACCE definition in EXCEL differed from that in NOBLE including only all-cause mortality, myocardial infarction, and stroke. However, when ischemia-driven revascularization was added to the composite endpoint in EXCEL, no significant differences in events were found between those undergoing PCI vs. CABG (23.1% vs. 19.1%, $p = 0.01$ for non-inferiority).
- Although important, we do not expect a paradigm shift in LMCA revascularization guideline recommendations in the aftermath of the NOBLE and EXCEL trials.
- Limitations of the NOBLE study were:
  - A higher than expected rate of stent thrombosis.
  - Adoption of first generation drug-eluting stents in 7.4% of PCI patients.
  - Exclusion of procedural MI from the primary MACCE endpoint.
  - An unexplained high rate of stroke in the PCI arm.
- The "catch up" phenomenon observed after the PCI arm of the EXCEL study advised caution before considering superiority of stenting over surgery in every LMCA case in the low-intermediate SYNTAX score tertile.
- A consistent message across the studies is the crucial role of the Heart Team, which remains central in the decision-making process con-

cerning LMCA revascularization. Careful individual patient review is pivotal to highlight particular anatomic or clinical features that will favor a particular revascularization approach. The two trials and following meta-analysis on the topic [17] have also the merit to contribute to increase the amount of information that the physician can provide to patients in the discussion about the best revascularization option for severe LMCA. Such decision remains indeed strictly connected not also with coronary anatomy, any medical comorbidities, and local expertise but also with personal patient preferences [18].

- In the discussion between CABG versus PCI for patients with LMCA disease, the potential of hybrid coronary revascularization should not be forgotten. This approach may combine the benefits of minimally invasive direct coronary artery bypass grafting (MIDCAB), i.e., long-lasting patency of LIMA to LAD, and PCI (avoidance of sternotomy, cardiopulmonary bypass and aortic manipulation with consequent reduced risk of stroke, bleeding, infection, pulmonary complications and truncated recovery time) [19].

- This could be an attractive option for complex patients, such as the elderly and/or morbidly obese patients especially those with diffuse disease of the LAD. In most centers this technique is not a realistic therapeutic option [20].

Risk Stratification and the Heart Team

- Understanding which patients should be considered for PCI or CABG and understanding what is the best timing for such intervention is the first decision that the operator has to take when faced with significant LMCA disease.

- The clinical presentation is the first parameter to take into account. A patient with LMCA disease presenting with stable angina as an elective case is completely different from a patient with LMCA disease/thrombosis in the setting of an ST-elevation myocardial infarction (STEMI) with ongoing chest pain and eventual hemodynamic instability.

- The mortality rate associated with acute LMCA occlusion (defined as complete obstruction or stenosis >70% with compromised TIMI flow) is extremely high and requires a prompt intervention [2]. In this situation PCI to LMCA is definitely the first-line approach; however, having the cardiac surgeon on board and involved in the discussion is very helpful in this situation in order to keep open the possibility of "bail-out" CABG.

- Moreover, because of the rapid hemodynamic deterioration related to acute LMCA occlusion, the cardiac surgeon may represent a good ally to establish a cardiopulmonary bypass circuit when high intensity circulatory support (namely Impella or extracorporeal membrane oxygenation—ECMO) is not available.

- A total different approach should instead be employed when LMCA disease is diagnosed in a non-emergent setting. As a general rule, whenever LMCA is detected in a patient with stable angina or ACS without any ongoing symptoms and/or ECG signs of profound ischemia, the best strategy is to discuss the case with colleagues within the Heart Team.

- Even though its specific application in patients with LMCA disease has been challenged recently, by the NOBLE and EXCEL studies, the SYNTAX score still represents a potentially useful tool to facilitate the patient selection process and optimal decision-making within the Heart Team [21].

- However, The SYNTAX score takes into account only variables related to the complexity of the coronary anatomy, without considering clinical parameters. For this reason, within the Heart Team discussion, it is highly recommended to consider two other risk scores [22], namely the EuroScore (both additive and logistic) [23] and the Society of Thoracic Surgeon (STS) score [24].

- The recently developed SYNTAX II score is an updated version of the SYNTAX score, taking into account bedside coronary anatomy complexity (still expressed by the SYNTAX score itself) plus clinical variables (age, gender, ejection fraction, renal function, lung disease, and peripheral vascular disease) [25]. It is very likely that it will be incorporated for future patient selection and risk stratification within the Heart Team discussion, but currently it has not been prospectively validated yet [26].

How to Assess Left Main Coronary Artery Disease for PCI

- The first consideration for the operator is to determine the extent of disease and especially whether there is relevant disease involving the bifurcation. The procedural complexity, the immediate and long-term success rates are related to this crucial variable [27]. A careful and appropriate assessment of the LMCA anatomy and atherosclerosis distribution must precede the actual intervention. There are four main tools to fulfill this purpose.

Coronary Angiography

- Angiography represents the first-line assessment tool for LMCA disease. Caudal views (LAO35°CRA35°, LAO0°CRA20°, LAO20°CRA20°) are helpful for good visualization of the LMCA body and bifurcation, while cranial views (especially LAO20°CRA20°) might be adopted to confirm ostial LMCA disease, as in the case of pressure damping during intubation or poor back-spilling of contrast dye into the aorta during injection.
- When the atherosclerotic burden is very high with involvement of all the branches of the bifurcation, then the coronary angiogram itself might be enough for overall planning of the procedure (bifurcation vs. non-bifurcation PCI, single- versus two-stent technique). In this specific scenario FFR and intravascular imaging can be adopted for better delineation of the PCI details.
- However, in most of the cases the true anatomy and plaque distribution of the LMCA cannot fully be derived from the coronary angiogram and additional diagnostic tools are necessary to properly plan the intervention.

Fractional Flow Reserve

- Three technical aspects have to be considered when performing an FFR study of the LMCA:
  - The pressure wire should be equalized in the aorta or within the disengaged guiding catheter especially in the case of possible ostial LMCA disease.
  - Guide catheter has to be appropriately disengaged to avoid aortic pressure damping during FFR measurement (possible risk of false negative FFR).
  - Intravenous adenosine infusion is preferred as it assures steady hyperemia and allows pressure wire pullback.
- There are two specific situations in which FFR can aid the operator's decision while planning and performing a LMCA PCI:
  - Pre-stenting: LMCA angiographic intermediate disease in the context of further disease involving more distally the LAD and/or the LCx.
  - Post-stenting: Pinched LAD or LCx ostium secondary to plaque or carina shift after provisional stenting.
- The first scenario is a quite common situation, since LMCA atherosclerosis is often observed in the context of diffuse involvement of the whole coronary tree. In this situation it might be tricky for the operator to define to what degree the LMCA contributes to the total ischemic burden [28].
- If only one of the bifurcation limbs is diseased distally, the operator can perform an FFR study on the non-diseased/least diseased branch. In such cases an FFR ≤0.80 would confirm a significant contribution of LMCA to the ischemic burden, conversely the operator can limit the treatment only to the clearly diseased branch without embarking on LMCA PCI if FFR is >0.80.
- If both LAD and LCx are distally diseased, no FFR study can be done to strictly identify the contribution of the LMCA disease, until one (or both) of the two branches has been treated. In this case the suggestion is to treat the most diseased branch and after that to perform the FFR study on the just treated branch to unmask the ischemic potential of the residual LMCA disease (Fig. 27.1).

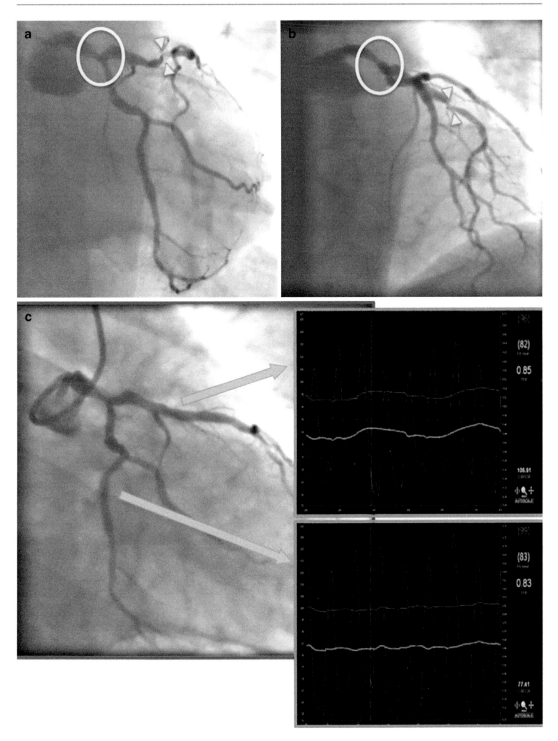

Fig. 27.1 FFR-guided PCI to the left main coronary artery. Example of LMCA bifurcation disease (Panel **a** and **b**) in a patient admitted for an elective angiogram for stable angina. Significant disease of the LAD artery was also observed (orange arrowheads in Panel **a** and **b**). Stenting to LAD was performed (Panel **c**) and then FFR was assessed to unmask the ischemic burden of the LMCA bifurcation disease. Both LAD and left circumflex presented a FFR value >0.80 and therefore no intervention to LMCA bifurcation was indicated. Key: *FFR* fractional flow reserve, *LAD* left anterior descending, *LMCA* left main coronary artery

- Alternatively a pre-procedure FFR study with pressure wire pullback on both branches can be considered to selectively unmask the LMCA disease contribution (Fig. 27.2).
- When LMCA bifurcation disease is approached with provisional stenting, it is not uncommon to have a pinched ostium of the side branch (usually LCx) secondary to plaque or carina shift. FFR on the side branch can aid the operator in deciding if kissing inflation or conversion to a two-stent technique should be performed. This approach is supported by two small studies showing how less than one-third of the angiographic jailed LCx ostia were ultimately functionally significant (FFR < 0.80) [29, 30].

Intravascular Imaging

- Intravascular imaging has to be considered a mandatory tool for any PCI to LMCA with IVUS currently a IIaB indication in the European Guidelines [13] for the following reasons:

- Better definition of LMCA anatomy and atherosclerosis distribution
- Better definition of plaque burden and any calcific component
- Stent sizing
- Stent optimization

Intravascular Ultrasound

- IVUS is the imaging technique with the largest amount of data supporting application in LMCA PCI. In the pre-FFR era, IVUS was originally used to identify at what degree of stenosis (measured as residual minimal lumen area—MLA) intervention to LMCA can safely be deferred.
- The initial cutoff of MLA ≤ 9.0 mm^2 [31] has been progressively reduced up to the currently accepted value of 6 mm^2, initially validated against FFR in a small study by Jasti et al. [32] and then clinically confirmed in the larger LITRO trial which showed no difference in 2 year mortality in patients with deferred PCI to LMCA compared to revascularized ones [33].

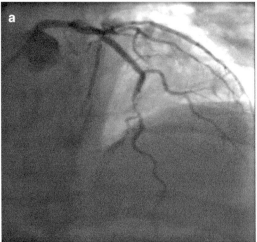
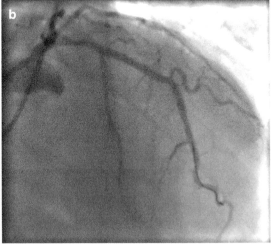

Fig. 27.2 FFR and OCT assessment of the LMCA. Example of angiographically silent LMCA disease unmasked by combination of FFR and OCT in patient referred for coronary angiogram because of stable angina. After treatment of angiographically significant mid LAD disease (Panel **a** and **b**), moderate residual disease of the proximal LAD and LMCA was investigated by using FFR (Panel **c**). A positive FFR was detected and at pullback it was noted that the bigger jump was across the ostium of the LAD (angiographically silent). OCT was performed confirming the presence of consistent atherosclerotic burden extending from the proximal LAD back to the distal LMCA. PCI to LMCA-LAD with provisional stenting technique was then performed. Key: *FFR* fractional flow reserve, *OCT* optical coherence tomography, *LAD* left anterior descending, *LMCA* left main coronary artery

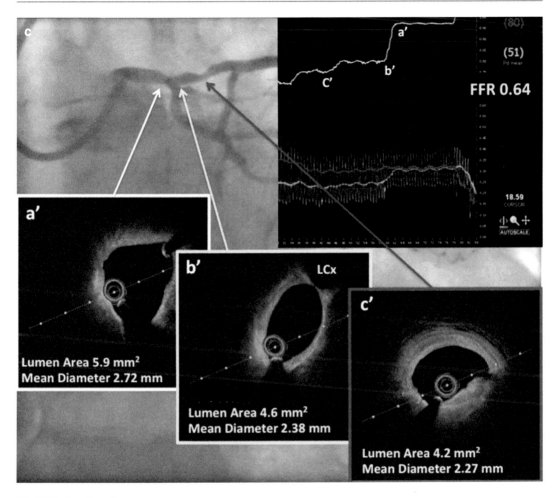

Fig. 27.2 (continued)

- Smaller cutoffs (4.8 and 4.5 mm^2) have been proposed and validated with FFR by other groups, but since referring specifically to Asian populations [34, 35], they should not be applied in other ethnic groups and for this reason current practice is to defer PCI to LMCA when MLA >6 mm^2.
- With the current availability of FFR in defining "when" PCI to LMCA is indicated, IVUS has a major role in defining "how" PCI to LMCA should be performed. IVUS can help to identify the real distribution of atherosclerosis at the site of bifurcation (Fig. 27.3) especially unmasking angiographically undetected disease of the LAD or LCx ostia.
- In this regard an IVUS study has showed "the diffuse nature" of LMCA disease extending to

the LAD in the 90% of cases, to the LCx in the 66.4% of cases and to both branches in the 62% of cases with consistent sparing of the carina [36].
- This information is important when
  - FFR interpretation is tricky because of diffuse atherosclerosis in both LAD and LCx.
  - A decision has to be taken about provisional versus a two-stent strategy to treat the LMCA bifurcation.
- The ability of IVUS to easily identify calcific plaque may help the operator in deciding up front the degree of lesion preparation before stenting, for instance to perform aggressive predilation with noncompliant balloons or rotablation.

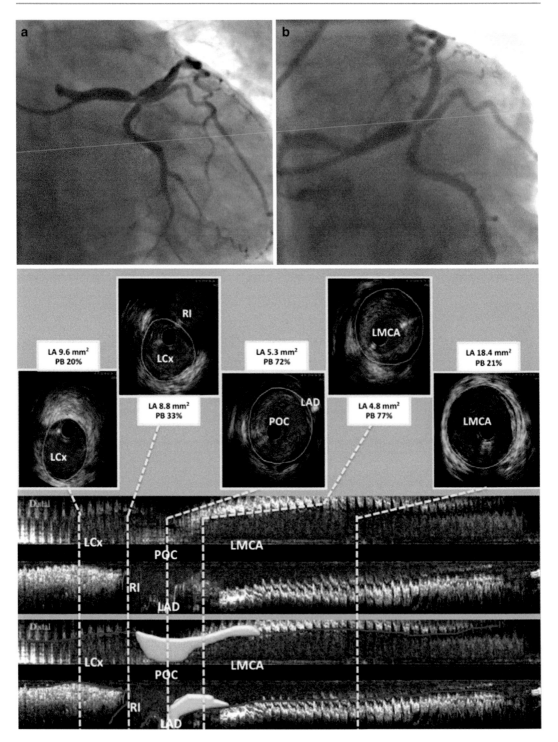

Fig. 27.3 IVUS assessment of the LMCA. This is an example of IVUS assessment of LMCA anatomy and atherosclerotic burden distribution. Patient referred for stable angina. Coronary angiogram detected significant disease of distal LMCA involving the trifurcation with clear disease extension toward the LAD (Panel **a** and **b**). Involvement of the RI and LCx ostia was unclear according to coronary angiogram. IVUS was performed with such purpose, confirming LMCA disease extending toward the LAD and the POC of the bifurcation with nonsignificant disease at the ostia of both LCx and RI. Excluding LCx and RI disease allowed the operator to proceed to treat this trifurcation with provisional single-stent technique of the LAD toward the LMCA. Key: *LA* lumen area, *LAD* left anterior descending, *LCx* left circumflex, *POC* polygon of convergence, *RI* ramus intermediate

- The longitudinal and circumferential extension together with the depth of the calcific plaque component are all parameters to take into account when planning how to prepare the lesion before stenting.
- By facilitating identification of non-diseased references, IVUS can facilitate stent selection in terms of both diameter and length, thus minimizing the risk of stent under/oversizing as well as the chance of incomplete disease coverage, geographical miss, or landing into diseased segments.
- Finally IVUS is a valuable tool post-PCI to check and optimize the final result by favoring detection of stent under-expansion and malapposition [28]. In such regard cutoff values for minimal stent area to prevent in-stent restenosis have been proposed by Kang et al. [37] (Fig. 27.4):
  - >5 mm² ostium LCx
  - >6 mm² ostium LAD
  - >7 mm² polygon of confluence
  - >8 mm² LMCA
- Even if no large randomized clinical trial has been performed to assess ad hoc whether intravascular imaging-guided PCI to LMCA is associated with a better long-term clinical outcome, convincing data from large registries suggest a long-term mortality benefit in patients undergoing IVUS-guided compared to angio-guided PCI to LMCA [38, 39]. In this regard "IVUS-optimization" is based on individual operator's discretion and not yet on prespecified and prospectively validated criteria.
- Useful technical aspects to consider when performing LMCA IVUS include:
  - Mechanical pullback is preferred over manual pullback in order to obtain information about length of disease/stent
  - Manual pullback can be useful for assessment of LMCA ostium
  - Appropriate guiding-catheter engagement and placing of the guidewire and IVUS catheter beyond the bifurcation is advised in order to favor IVUS catheter co-axiality. An oblique image, because of poor co-axiality, can lead to overestimation of the true lumen area.

Optical Coherence Tomography

- Because of its high spatial resolution, OCT is an appealing imaging tool to guide LMCA PCI [40]. Indeed stent malapposition and stent edge dissection can be better assessed by OCT than IVUS [41] (Fig. 27.5). Similarly at follow-up OCT allows a better identification of stent coverage than IVUS [42].
- However, as it is a relatively new technology, the amount of data on OCT in LMCA PCI is smaller than for IVUS. As such the latter is typically preferred for LMCA interrogation.
- As for IVUS, there are no established criteria to guide the optimization of the final stenting result when using OCT. Moreover, the operator has to be aware that the luminal measures obtained with OCT are usually smaller than those obtained with IVUS, meaning that IVUS cutoffs may not work as well for OCT [43]. This should be taken into account in case OCT is adopted for stent sizing.
- Two technical aspects should be considered when investigating the LMCA with OCT:
  - Light depth penetration is lower than ultrasound penetration.
  - Lumen needs to be cleared from blood by contrast dye injection.
- Otherwise the implications are that:
  - Large size LMCA may not be appropriately imaged by OCT.
  - OCT can be applied to assess LMCA bifurcation and eventually LMCA body but not the LMCA ostium [44].

Left Main Coronary Artery Stenting Techniques

LMCA Ostium/Body Disease

- When considering an ostium/body LMCA lesion with no involvement of the bifurcation, some important procedural aspects need to be considered:
  - Appropriate lesion preparation. Predilatation should always be performed. IVUS

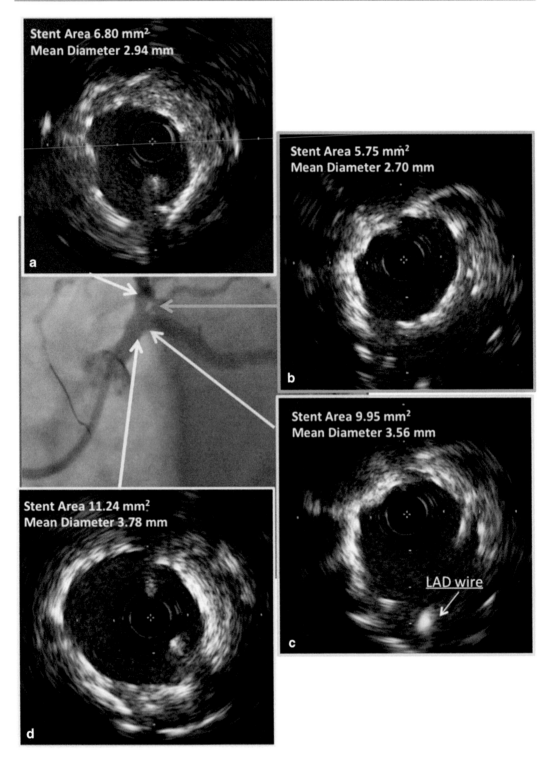

Fig. 27.4 Post-stenting IVUS assessment of the LMCA. IVUS was performed on both LAD and LCx after LMCA stenting. IVUS detected good stent expansion and apposition in all the segments of the bifurcation. Notably achieved stent area fulfilled the Kang's criteria in each segment of the bifurcation (LAD >6 mm², LCx >5 mm²; Polygon of Convergence >7 mm², LMCA>8 mm²). Key: *IVUS* intravascular ultrasound, *LAD* left anterior descending, *LCx* left circumflex, *LMCA* left main coronary artery

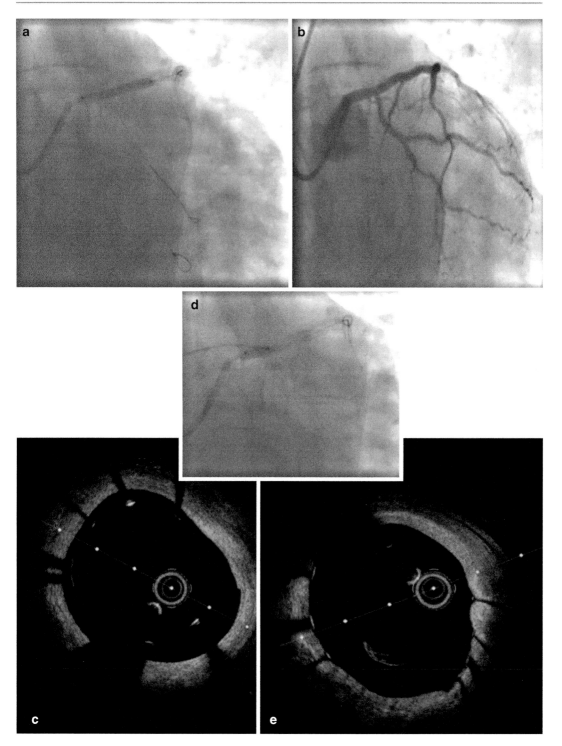

Fig. 27.5 OCT-guided provisional stenting for LMCA disease. Here the LMCA was stented with a 3.5 × 30 mm drug-eluting stent (Panel **a**), and then potted with a 3.5 × 8 mm non compliant balloon. An apparent good angiographic result on both LAD and LCx was observed angiographically (Panel **b**). OCT detected however a significant segment of malapposition in the LMCA (Panel **c**), requiring further POT at high pressure with a 4.0 × 8 mm non compliant balloon, achieving full stent expansion and apposition in the LMCA as confirmed at the final OCT run (Panel **e**). Key: *OCT* optical coherence tomography, *LAD* left anterior descending, *LCx* left circumflex, *LMCA* left main coronary artery, *POT* proximal optimization technique

should aid calcific plaque detection and the operator is advised to have a low threshold for use of rotablation.

- Accurate stent sizing (preferably intravascular imaging-guided).
- Appropriate coverage of the ostium. Working in a cranial view (LAO20° CRA30°) may help.
- Accurate assessment of stenting result with intravascular imaging with eventual further postdilatation if necessary.
- Flaring of the most proximal part of the stent covering the ostium ensuring opening of the stents struts toward the aortic root.
- Careful handling of the guiding catheter and careful removal of deflated balloons are warranted in order to avoid LMCA deep intubation with consequent risk of stent longitudinal compression at the ostium.

LMCA Bifurcation Disease

- As for non-LMCA bifurcation, provisional main branch stenting should be considered as the default approach when treating LMCA bifurcation disease. However LMCA bifurcation presents specific features that make it unique and different from any other bifurcation in the coronary tree [3]:
  - The side branch (usually LCx) is often large in diameter and subtends a large territory of myocardium.
  - The bifurcation angle is usually large (>70°) making the side branch rewiring difficult after main branch stenting.
  - The size of the proximal main branch is large (4–5 mm), and sometimes beyond the size of commonly available stents. This implies that the operator should be familiar with the maximum range of diameters achievable after postdilatation for each stent available on the shelf [45].
  - Trifurcation disease might be encountered in a nontrivial percentage of cases (10%).
- For all these reasons it is important and crucial for the operator to identify in advance those

scenarios where the provisional approach is feasible and likely to be successful and those where a two-stent technique may be preferred.

Provisional Stenting for LMCA Bifurcation: Technical Aspects

- Provisional stenting should be considered in case of [46]:
  - Nonsignificant angiographic (and possibly confirmed at IVUS/OCT) disease of the side branch (LCx) ostium. A cutoff of MLA >3.7 mm² or plaque burden <56% in the LCx ostium has been suggested to exclude the possibility of an FFR <0.8 in the side branch after provisional stenting of the main vessel [29].
  - LCx nondominant or small in size (<2.5 mm).
  - Very large angle between LAD and LCx.

Side Branch Wiring

- When provisional stenting it is advised to wire the side branch in order to protect it in case of potential plaque or carina shift following predilation and/or stenting. Side branch wiring allows protection via:
  - Widening the angle between LAD and LCx.
  - Keeping a ready access to the side branch in case of rapid hemodynamic deterioration following abrupt side branch obstruction.
- Moreover if side branch rewiring is necessary after stenting as in the case of final kissing inflation (FKI) or conversion to two-stent strategy, the jailed wire can aid the operator to identify the ostium of the side branch and eventually favoring rewiring through a more distal strut allowing better side branch scaffolding (see also Chap. 26) [47].
- Even though distal wiring is challenging to assess with angiography, recent data support OCT application with 3D reconstruction for this aim, introducing a potential new indication for OCT in LMCA bifurcation PCI [48].

Proximal Optimization Technique (POT)

- As for any bifurcation, the stent should be sized according to the distal main vessel diameter, and for this reason, after main vessel stenting proximal optimization technique (POT) should be performed in order to [49] (Fig. 27.5):
  - Reshape the proximal part of the stent, ensuring complete stent expansion and apposition in the proximal main branch (i.e., in the LMCA)
  - Opening the stent strut toward the ostium of the side branch with consequent better side branch ostium scaffolding
  - Easier side branch rewiring (if needed)
- It is important to note that when performing POT, the balloon has to be kept away from the distal main vessel to avoid a worsening of carina shift during inflation. We advocate placing the distal marker right in front of the carina as a way to achieve this goal.
- There is no real consensus at the moment about the choice of removing or keeping the jailed side branch wire before the POT. The arguments for removing it are to reduce the chance of wire trapping, snapping or deep guiding catheter intubation with possible stent longitudinal compression while pulling the wire.
- Conversely keeping the wire offers the choice of ready access to the side branch and better visualization of the side branch ostium to favor distal rewiring.
- A possible compromise is to keep only a short segment of the jailed wire during the POT.

Final Kissing Balloon Inflation (FKI)

- The role for systematic FKI after provisional stenting is still not well defined, with small retrospective and observational studies not confirming so far a role in terms of better clinical outcome [50, 51].
- In our opinion FKI should be performed when a suboptimal result has been achieved on the side branch, as an eventual preliminary step before considering to switch to bail-out double stenting (Fig. 27.6).
- Notably there will be upcoming evidence suggesting that FKI should be followed by a second POT in order to reshape the proximal main branch in a circular fashion [52].

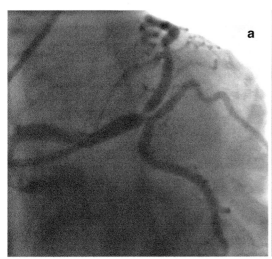
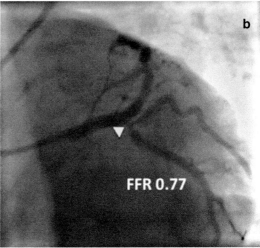

Fig. 27.6 Side branch handling after provisional stenting. After provisional stenting of the LMCA, angiographic stenosis of the side branch (namely LCx) is a possible consequence secondary to plaque or carina shift. Distal LMCA disease into a tight ostial LAD lesion noted (Panel **a**). After stenting of LAD toward LMCA, LCx pinching was observed (Panel **b**—yellow arrowhead) with patient starting to complain of chest discomfort. FFR noted to be abnormal in the LCx. IVUS had been performed pre-stent and was then repeated on the LCx, showing a reduction in lumen area from 8.8 mm^2 (Panel **c**) reduced to 5.6 mm^2 (Panel **d**) likely to be related to carina shift. Kissing balloon inflation was then performed (Panel **e**) achieving good final angiographic (Panel **f**) and IVUS (Panel **g**) results. Key: *IVUS* intravascular ultrasound, *FFR* fractional flow reserve, *LAD* left anterior descending, *LCx* left circumflex, *LMCA* left main coronary artery

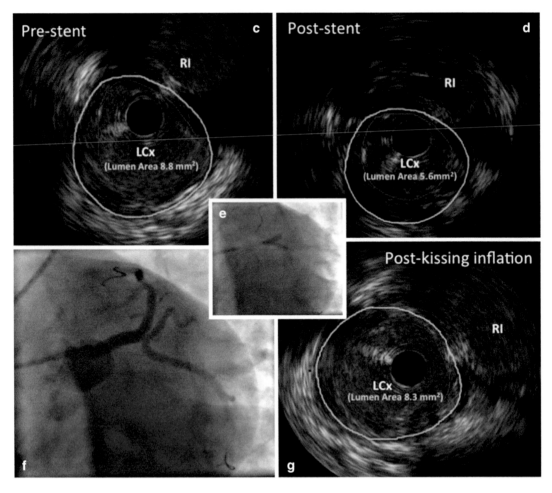

Fig. 27.6 (continued)

Conversion to Bail-Out Two-Stent Strategy

- A residual angiographic stenosis of the side branch ostium after main vessel stenting is not a condition that should alone induce the operator to convert to double stenting unless there is:
  - Flow impairment down the side branch
  - Persistency of symptoms and signs of ongoing ischemia
  - FFR on the side branch ≤0.80
- Possible double-stenting techniques to consider when converting from provisional stenting to LMCA are predominantly:
  - T-stenting or T with a small protrusion (TAP)
  - Culotte

- The angle between LAD and LCx and the operator's familiarity with a specific technique should be the main factors in driving the choice, bearing in mind that T stenting or TAP are a good option when there is a very wide angle between LAD and LCx.
- If double stenting is performed, FKI with eventual re-POT are strongly recommended as a final step of the procedure.

Double Stenting for LMCA Bifurcation: Technical Aspects

- By intention double stenting for LMCA bifurcation should be considered in case of [46]:

– Significant angiographic (and possibly confirmed at IVUS/OCT) disease of the side branch (LCx) ostium.
– LCx dominant or large in size (>2.5 mm)
– Narrow angle between LAD and LCx

Which Branch Should Be Stented First?

• There is no real consensus here.
• Three parameters should be considered when taking this decision:
  – Which is the most diseased branch?
  – Which is the largest branch?
  – Which is the branch that is potentially more difficult to recross?
• Considering that rewiring is usually easier for the LAD, the general rule should be to stent the most diseased vessel first [3], which otherwise could be further compromised by possible carina or plaque shift if approached later.
• Stenting the LCx first should be strongly considered in case of a very wide angle between

(>90°), making an eventual rewiring through stent struts extremely difficult.

Which Double-Stenting Technique?

• There is no consensus with regard to a technique performing better than the others in LMCA PCI and all techniques have been showed to be feasible, safe, and overall effective.
• The DK Crush III study has been the only one showing a clinical superiority of double kissing crush (DK crush) technique over culotte in LMCA PCI [53].
• The bottom line is that each double-stenting technique has points of strength and points of weakness (Table 27.2), and probably the best advice to give to the reader is to be proficient with one- or two-stent techniques to apply routinely when needed to approach a LMCA bifurcation [54].
• It should be highlighted that in critical situations with a very unstable patient because of

Table 27.2 Strengths and weaknesses of different two-stent techniques for LMCA bifurcation intervention

	Pros	Cons	When should be preferred for LMCA
Culotte	• 6Fr guiding catheter compatible • Theoretically applicable for any LAD/LCx angle • Predictable scaffolding	• Long and potentially complex, requiring two "rewiring" steps • Temporary loss of control of main branch during second stent implantation • Possible abrupt occlusion of main branch • Long segment with a double layer of stent struts in the proximal main vessel	Better results when there is no extremely wide LAD–LCx angle: • Better scaffolding • Appropriate carina coverage
Crush	• Relatively quick • Low risk of side branch occlusion • Good side branch ostium coverage	• Difficult rewiring in view of FKI • Long segment with a triple layer of stent struts in the proximal MV	Better results when there is no extremely wide LAD–LCx angle: • Better scaffolding • Appropriate carina coverage
Mini-crush	• Low amount of multiple layers of struts • Good scaffolding of side branch ostium • Easier rewiring and FKI	• Short segment with a triple layer of stent struts in the proximal MV	Better results when there is no extremely wide LAD–LCx angle: • Better scaffolding • Appropriate carina coverage
DK-crush	• Good carina coverage • Good scaffolding of side branch • Easier FKI	• Long and potentially complex, requiring multiple "rewiring" and kissing inflations	Theoretically applicable in all anatomies in the setting of a stable patient

Table 27.2 (continued)

	Pros	Cons	When should be preferred for LMCA
SKS	• Quick and easy • No chance of loss of one of the branches • No rewiring needed	• Not 6Fr compatible • Long metallic neo-carina • Possible overstretching of proximal MV • Difficult access in case of need of reintervention at follow-up	Emergent LMCA occlusion/subocclusion in the context of severe hemodynamic instability
T-stenting/TAP	• Excellent scaffolding of side branch for 90° angles	• Possible non coverage of side branch ostium (conventional T stenting) • Protrusion of side branch stent into the proximal main vessel (TAP)	To be considered for anatomy with 90° angles

LMCA occlusion or subocclusion, the simultaneous kissing stents (SKS) technique allows a rapid restoration of LMCA patency without embarking on a longer and more complex double-stenting technique.

• The SKS technique should be regarded more as a bail-out approach, rather than an elective approach because of the occurrence of a diaphragmatic membrane formed by the two overlapped stents in the lumen of the LMCA [55].

• However, irrespective of the stenting technique adopted, what is truly important is to be aware that when double stenting is performed for LMCA PCI:

– POT should always be performed to facilitate rewiring.
– FKI with eventual second POT should always be performed (Fig. 27.7).
– Final result should always be checked with intravascular imaging.

Conclusions

Please refer to our comprehensive algorithm to approach LMCA in daily practice (Fig. 27.8).

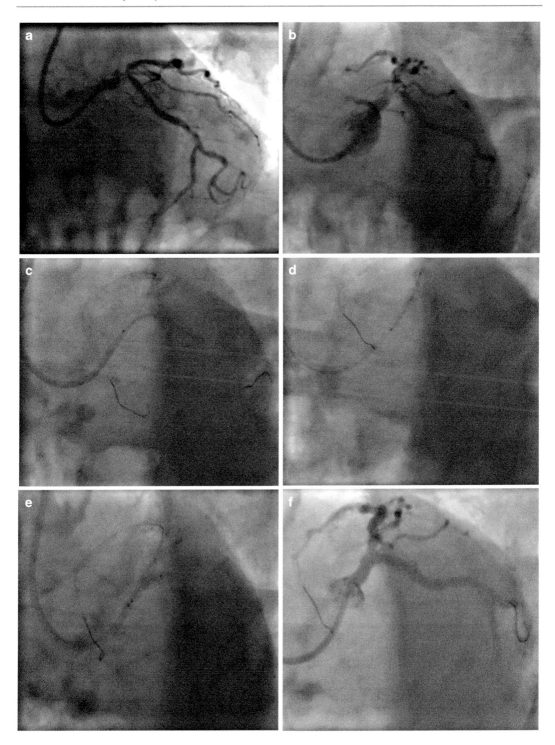

Fig. 27.7 Double-stent technique for LMCA. Patient with stable angina presented with significant angiographic disease of the LMCA involving the bifurcation (Medina 1,1,1) (Panels **a**, **b**). Because of the critical disease in a large side branch (left circumflex), by intention a double-stent technique (Culotte) was adopted in this case (see also Chap. 26). After stenting both branches (Panels **c**, **d**), final kissing balloon inflation (Panel **e**) was performed achieving a good final angiographic result (Panel **f**)

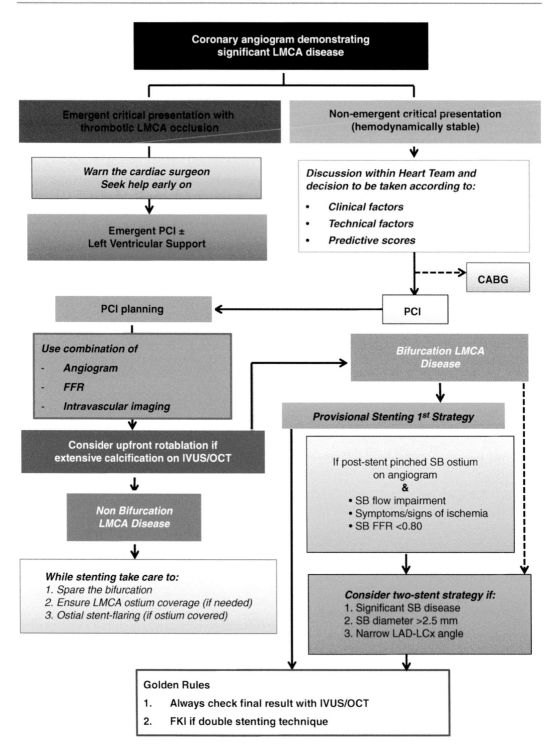

Fig. 27.8 A general algorithm for left main coronary artery intervention. Key: *CABG* coronary artery bypass grafting, *FFR* fractional flow reserve, *FKI* final kissing inflation, *IVUS* intravascular ultrasound, *LAD* left anterior descending, *LCx* left circumflex, *LMCA* left main coronary artery, *OCT* optical coherence tomography, *PCI* percutaneous coronary intervention, *SB* side branch, *SKS* simultaneous kissing stent

References

1. Giannoglou GD, Antoniadis AP, Chatzizisis YS, Damvopoulou E, Parcharidis GE, Louridas GE. Prevalence of narrowing >or=50% of the left main coronary artery among 17,300 patients having coronary angiography. Am J Cardiol. 2006;98:1202–5.
2. Patel N, De Maria GL, Kassimis G, et al. Outcomes after emergency percutaneous coronary intervention in patients with unprotected left main stem occlusion: the BCIS national audit of percutaneous coronary intervention 6-year experience. JACC Cardiovasc Interv. 2014;7:969–80.
3. Lefèvre T, Girasis C, Lassen JF. Differences between the left main and other bifurcations. EuroIntervention. 2015;11 Suppl:106–10.
4. Wykrzykowska JJ, Mintz GS, Garcia-Garcia HM, et al. Longitudinal distribution of plaque burden and necrotic core-rich plaques in nonculprit lesions of patients presenting with acute coronary syndromes. JACC Cardiovasc Imaging. 2012;5(3 Suppl):10–8.
5. Mercado N, Moe TG, Pieper M, et al. Tissue characterisation of atherosclerotic plaque in the left main: an in vivo intravascular ultrasound radiofrequency data analysis. EuroIntervention. 2011;7:347–52.
6. Chaitman BR, Fisher LD, Bourassa MG, et al. Effect of coronary bypass surgery on survival patterns in subsets of patients with left main coronary artery disease. Report of the Collaborative Study in Coronary Artery Surgery (CASS). Am J Cardiol. 1981;48:765–77.
7. Shah PJ, Durairaj M, Gordon I, et al. Factors affecting patency of internal thoracic artery graft: clinical and angiographic study in 1434 symptomatic patients operated between 1982 and 2002. Eur J Cardiothorac Surg. 2004;26:118–24.
8. Buszman PE, Buszman PP, Kiesz RS, et al. Early and long-term results of unprotected left main coronary artery stenting: the LE MANS (Left Main Coronary Artery Stenting) registry. J Am Coll Cardiol. 2009;54:1500–11.
9. Morice MC, Serruys PW, Kappetein AP, et al. Outcomes in patients with de novo left main disease treated with either percutaneous coronary intervention using paclitaxel-eluting stents or coronary artery bypass graft treatment in the Synergy Between Percutaneous Coronary Intervention with TAXUS and Cardiac Surgery (SYNTAX) trial. Circulation. 2010;121:2645–53.
10. Boudriot E, Thiele H, Walther T, et al. Randomized comparison of percutaneous coronary intervention with sirolimus-eluting stents versus coronary artery bypass grafting in unprotected left main stem stenosis. J Am Coll Cardiol. 2011;57:538–45.
11. Park SJ, Kim YH, Park DW, et al. Randomized trial of stents versus bypass surgery for left main coronary artery disease. N Engl J Med. 2011;364:1718–27.
12. Kappetein AP, Feldman TE, Mack MJ, et al. Comparison of coronary bypass surgery with drug-eluting stenting for the treatment of left main and/or three-vessel disease: 3-year follow-up of the SYNTAX trial. Eur Heart J. 2011;32:2125–34.
13. Windecker S, Kolh P, Alfonso F, et al. 2014 ESC/EACTS guidelines on myocardial revascularization: The Task Force on Myocardial Revascularization of the European Society of Cardiology (ESC) and the European Association for Cardio-Thoracic Surgery (EACTS)Developed with the special contribution of the European Association of Percutaneous Cardiovascular Interventions (EAPCI). Eur Heart J. 2014;35:2541–619.
14. Campos CM, Christiansen EH, Stone GW, Serruys PW. The EXCEL and NOBLE trials: similarities, contrasts and future perspectives for left main revascularisation. EuroIntervention. 2015;11(Suppl V):115–9.
15. Mäkikallio T, Holm NR, Lindsay M, et al. Percutaneous coronary angioplasty versus coronary artery bypass grafting in treatment of unprotected left main stenosis (NOBLE): a prospective, randomised, open-label, non-inferiority trial. Lancet. 2016;388:2743–52.
16. Stone GW, Sabik JF, Serruys PW, et al. Everolimus-eluting stents or bypass surgery for left main coronary artery disease. N Engl J Med. 2016;375:2223–35.
17. Giacoppo D, Colleran R, Cassese S, Frangieh AH, Wiebe J, Joner M, Schunkert H, Kastrati A, Byrne RA. Percutaneous coronary intervention vs coronary artery bypass grafting in patients with left main coronary artery stenosis: a systematic review and meta-analysis. JAMA Cardiol. 2017;2:1079–88.
18. Ruel M, Verma S, Bhatt DL. What is the optimal revascularization strategy for left main coronary stenosis? JAMA Cardiol. 2017;2:1061–2.
19. Delhaye C, Sudre A, Lemesle G, et al. Hybrid revascularization, comprising coronary artery bypass graft with exclusive arterial conduits followed by early drug-eluting stent implantation, in multivessel coronary artery disease. Arch Cardiovasc Dis. 2010;103:502–11.
20. Kappetein AP, Head SJ. CABG, stents, or hybrid procedures for left main disease? EuroIntervention. 2015;11(Suppl V):111–4.
21. Capodanno D, Di Salvo ME, Cincotta G, Miano M, Tamburino C, T C. Usefulness of the SYNTAX score for predicting clinical outcome after percutaneous coronary intervention of unprotected left main coronary artery disease. Circ Cardiovasc Interv. 2009;2:302–8.
22. Garg S, Stone GW, Kappetein AP, JFrd S, Simonton C, Serruys PW. Clinical and angiographic risk assessment in patients with left main stem lesions. JACC Cardiovasc Interv. 2010;3:891–901.
23. Roques F, Nashef SA, Michel P, et al. Risk factors and outcome in European cardiac surgery: analysis of the EuroSCORE multinational database of 19030 patients. Eur J Cardiothorac Surg. 1999;15:816–22.
24. Mehta RH, Grab JD, O'Brien SM, et al. Bedside tool for predicting the risk of postoperative dialysis in patients undergoing cardiac surgery. Circulation. 2006;114:2208–16.
25. Farooq V, van Klaveren D, Steyerberg EW, et al. Anatomical and clinical characteristics to guide

decision making between coronary artery bypass surgery and percutaneous coronary intervention for individual patients: development and validation of SYNTAX score II. Lancet. 2013;381:639–50.

26. Campos CM, van Klaveren D, Farooq V, et al. Long-term forecasting and comparison of mortality in the Evaluation of the Xience Everolimus Eluting Stent vs. Coronary Artery Bypass Surgery for Effectiveness of Left Main Revascularization (EXCEL) trial: prospective validation of the SYNTAX Score II. Eur Heart J. 2015;36:1231–41.

27. Tiroch K, Mehilli J, Byrne RA, et al. Impact of coronary anatomy and stenting technique on long-term outcome after drug-eluting stent implantation for unprotected left main coronary artery disease. JACC Cardiovasc Interv. 2014;7:29–36.

28. Bing R, Yong AS, Lowe HC. Percutaneous transcatheter assessment of the left main coronary artery current status and future directions. JACC Cardiovasc Interv. 2015;8:1529–39.

29. Kang SJ, Ahn JM, Kim WJ, et al. Functional and morphological assessment of side branch after left main coronary artery bifurcation stenting with cross-over technique. Catheter Cardiovasc Interv. 2014;83:545–52.

30. Nam CW, Hur SH, Koo BK, et al. Fractional flow reserve versus angiography in left circumflex ostial intervention after left main crossover stenting. Korean Circ J. 2011;41:304–7.

31. Nissen SE, Yock P. Intravascular ultrasound: novel pathophysiological insights and current clinical applications. Circulation. 2001;103:604–16.

32. Jasti V, Ivan E, Yalamanchili V, Wongpraparut N, Leesar MA. Correlations between fractional flow reserve and intravascular ultrasound in patients with an ambiguous left main coronary artery stenosis. Circulation. 2004;110:2831–6.

33. de la Torre Hernandez JM, Hernández Hernandez F, Alfonso F, et al. Prospective application of predefined intravascular ultrasound criteria for assessment of intermediate left main coronary artery lesions results from the multicenter LITRO study. J Am Coll Cardiol. 2011;58:351–8.

34. Kang SJ, Lee JY, Ahn JM, et al. Intravascular ultrasound-derived predictors for fractional flow reserve in intermediate left main disease. JACC Cardiovasc Interv. 2011;4:1168–74.

35. Park SJ, Ahn JM, Kang SJ, et al. Intravascular ultrasound-derived minimal lumen area criteria for functionally significant left main coronary artery stenosis. JACC Cardiovasc Interv. 2014;7:868–74.

36. Oviedo C, Maehara A, Mintz GS, et al. Intravascular ultrasound classification of plaque distribution in left main coronary artery bifurcations: where is the plaque really located? Circ Cardiovasc Interv. 2010;3:105–12.

37. Kang SJ, Ahn JM, Song H, et al. Comprehensive intravascular ultrasound assessment of stent area and its impact on restenosis and adverse cardiac events in 403 patients with unprotected left main disease. Circ Cardiovasc Interv. 2011;4:562–9.

38. Park SJ, Kim YH, Park DW, et al. Impact of intravascular ultrasound guidance on long-term mortality in stenting for unprotected left main coronary artery stenosis. Circ Cardiovasc Interv. 2009;2:167–77.

39. de la Torre Hernandez JM, Baz Alonso JA, Gómez Hospital JA, et al. Clinical impact of intravascular ultrasound guidance in drug-eluting stent implantation for unprotected left main coronary disease: pooled analysis at the patient-level of 4 registries. JACC Cardiovasc Interv. 2014;7:244–54.

40. Lowe HC, Narula J, Fujimoto J, Jang IK. Intracoronary optical diagnostics: current status, limitations and potential. J Am Coll Cardiol Interv. 2011;4:1257–70.

41. Fujino Y, Bezerra HG, Attizzani GF, et al. Frequency-domain optical coherence tomography assessment of unprotected left main coronary artery disease-a comparison with intravascular ultrasound. Catheter Cardiovasc Interv. 2013;82:173–83.

42. Capodanno D, Prati F, Pawlowsky T, et al. Comparison of optical coherence tomography and intravascular ultrasound for the assessment of in-stent tissue coverage after stent implantation. EuroIntervention. 2009;5:538–43.

43. Kubo T, Akasaka T, Shite J, et al. OCT compared with IVUS in a coronary lesion assessment: the OPUS-CLASS study. JACC Cardiovasc Imaging. 2013;6:1095–104.

44. Burzotta F, Dato I, Trani C, et al. Frequency domain optical coherence tomography to assess non-ostial left main coronary artery. EuroIntervention. 2015;10:e1.

45. Ng J, Foin N, Ang HY, et al. Over-expansion capacity and stent design model: an update with contemporary DES platforms. Int J Cardiol. 2016;221:171–9.

46. Park SJ, Ahn JM, Foin N, Louvard Y. When and how to perform the provisional approach for distal LM stenting. EuroIntervention. 2015;11(Suppl V):120–4.

47. Mylotte D, Routledge H, Harb T, et al. Provisional side branch-stenting for coronary bifurcation lesions: evidence of improving procedural and clinical outcomes with contemporary techniques. Catheter Cardiovasc Interv. 2013;82:437–45.

48. Okamura T, Onuma Y, Yamada J, et al. 3D optical coherence tomography: new insights into the process of optimal rewiring of side branches during bifurcational stenting. EuroIntervention. 2014;10:907–15.

49. Lassen JF, Holm NR, Banning A, et al. Percutaneous coronary intervention for coronary bifurcation disease: 11th consensus document from the European Bifurcation Club. EuroIntervention. 2016;12:38–46.

50. Niemelä M, Kervinen K, Erglis A, et al. Randomized comparison of final kissing balloon dilatation versus no final kissing balloon dilatation in patients with coronary bifurcation lesions treated with main vessel stenting: the Nordic-Baltic Bifurcation Study III. Circulation. 2011;123:79–86.

51. Gao Z, Xu B, Yang YJ, et al. Effect of final kissing balloon dilatation after one-stent technique at left-main bifurcation: a single center data. Chin Med J. 2015;128:733–9.

52. Derimay F, Souteyrand G, Motreff P, et al. Sequential proximal optimizing technique in provisional bifurcation stenting with Everolimus-eluting bioresorbable vascular scaffold: fractal coronary bifurcation bench for comparative test between absorb and XIENCE Xpedition. JACC Cardiovasc Interv. 2016;9:1397–406.

53. Chen SL, Xu B, Han YL, et al. Comparison of double kissing crush versus Culotte stenting for unprotected distal left main bifurcation lesions: results from a multicenter, randomized, prospective DKCRUSH-III study. J Am Coll Cardiol. 2013;61:1482–8.

54. Roh JH, Santoso T, Kim YH. Which technique for double stenting in unprotected left main bifurcation coronary lesions? EuroIntervention. 2015;11(Suppl V):125–8.

55. Siotia A, Morton AC, Malkin CJ, Raina T, Gunn J. Simultaneous kissing drug-eluting stents to treat unprotected left main stem bifurcation disease: medium term outcome in 150 consecutive patients. EuroIntervention. 2012;8:691–700.

Chronic Total Occlusions

28

Rohit Sirohi, Amerjeet Banning,
and Anthony H. Gershlick

About Us

University Hospitals of Leicester remains one of the most innovation-driven cardio-thoracic centers in the UK, notable "firsts" being ECMO, vascular-brachytherapy, first drug eluting stent (2002), first absorbable stent (2010), first TAVI (2006), first world live LMS course (2005). It presented to TCT in 2005 and to the National Live course in 2013.

The center serves a total catchment area of just under one million population and has provided 24/7 STEMI PCI since 2008. Complex percutaneous pediatric procedures, EP and devices are a routine part of the service provided in five cardiac cath labs.

UHL has run its CTO live course for 14 years, and has been a lead investigational center for >15 international multicenter PCI studies, and has devised, run and reported four major interventional trials. It has an Interventional Fellow appointment. It has strong links through the recent Biomedical Research Center with the University of Leicester.

R. Sirohi · A. Banning · A. H. Gershlick (✉)
Glenfield Hospital, University Hospitals of Leicester
NHS Trust, Leicester, UK
e-mail: amerjeet.banning@doctors.org.uk;
agershlick@aol.com

Introduction

- Chronic total occlusion (CTO) intervention remains a challenge in terms of percutaneous coronary intervention (PCI). Traditionally average success rates (60–70% British Cardiovascular Interventional Society—BCIS data), procedure duration, radiation exposure, procedural complications and specialized operator training and maintenance of procedure volume have led to negative perceptions on the value of CTO PCI.

- Absence of robust data proving hard end point clinical benefit also raise questions over cost efficacy when traditional markers such an incremental cost-effectiveness ratio (ICER) are used.

- However in the right patients with real-life debilitating symptoms despite medical therapy, CTO PCI can transform a patient's quality of life—being able to walk and exercise with friends and family without having to stop because of angina can be life changing.

- We know there are a significant number of patients who have life-limiting angina despite medication and who can languish with poor quality of life for many years. CTO PCI done to a high standard so as to get good results, can change that.

- Recent advances in techniques including the retrograde approach as well as newer

© Springer International Publishing AG, part of Springer Nature 2018
A. Myat et al. (eds.), *The Interventional Cardiology Training Manual*,
https://doi.org/10.1007/978-3-319-71635-0_28

generation stents have yielded better results and renewed interest in CTO treatment.

- Therefore, it is beholden to the trainee/new consultant or other interventionist becoming interested in CTO PCI to ensure the following:
  - Learn the technique in a structured formal progressive manner, preferably under the mentorship of another more experienced CTO operator.
  - Do cases in conjunction with experienced colleagues.
  - Become totally familiar with antegrade techniques first.
  - Audit their data including success rates.
  - Look to proctorship when they consider techniques/kit they are not familiar with.
  - Attend live interactive courses as part of their summative experiential learning curve.
  - Understand the principles behind the various techniques and are aware of the complications associated with this sometimes technically demanding procedure.
  - Are fully aware of the issues around contrast-induced nephropathy and especially around radiation protection.
- This chapter will detail ways of ensuring best practice with most likely chance of success for PCI-CTO. It will provide the evidence base where available and include tips and tricks for best clinical practice.

Definition

- For a lesion to be deemed a CTO requires it to have been present by definition for 3 months although this may be difficult to define.
- A CTO is often considered present when there has been no obvious acute event. It is often the anatomical nature at angiography that suggests chronicity—the presence of an occlusion (TIMI 0 flow) and the presence of antegrade or retrograde collaterals.
- The Euro CTO club consensus document [1] suggests the occlusion duration can be divided into three levels of certainty:

- **Certain**—angiographically confirmed TIMI 0 flow in a previous angiogram more than 3 months ago.
- **Likely**—clinically confirmed with objective evidence of an acute myocardial infarction in the territory of the occluded vessel more than 3 months ago.
- **Undetermined**—CTO with TIMI 0 flow and angiographic anatomy suggestive of long-standing occlusion with stable angina symptoms unchanged in the last 3 months.
- Such definitions probably do not serve a useful purpose other than for ensuring tight inclusion criteria for trials involving CTO patients.

Prevalence

- The true prevalence of CTO is unknown as there is no routine screening. Most data are derived from diagnostic coronary angiography databases.
- It is estimated that CTO account for up to a third of coronary artery lesions [1–3]. Despite the apparent high prevalence the proportion of patients undergoing PCI for CTO is only between 8 and 15% [4, 5].

Indications for PCI

- Since there are no robust data suggesting mortality benefit, the primary purpose of CTO revascularization is improvement in angina symptoms and overall prognosis [6–8].
- That said the BCIS registry has clearly indicated that there may be mortality benefit from *successful* intervention in CTO [9] (Fig. 28.1).
- CTO PCI should be considered an important therapeutic option when patients present with:
  - Clinical evidence of ischemia such as angina symptoms or breathlessness
  - Where there is objective evidence of moderate to severe ischemia (>10% ischemic burden on myocardial perfusion scan, >3 segments on stress echocardiography) with viability in the territory supplied by the occluded vessel, even in the absence of symptoms

Fig. 28.1 Impact of successful recanalization of chronic total occlusion on mortality. Kaplan-Meier plot demonstrating differences in mortality between those procedures with successful and failed CTO PCI. Success was associated with a decrease in mortality. Reproduced with permission from George S et al. JACC 2014; 64: 235–243 [9]. Key: *CTO* chronic total occlusion, *PCI* percutaneous coronary intervention

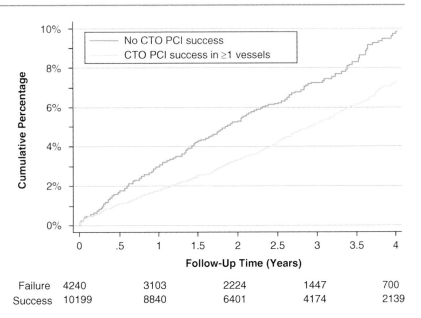

Failure	4240	3103	2224	1447	700
Success	10199	8840	6401	4174	2139

– Cardiac MRI can be particularly helpful in determining viability utilizing late gadolinium enhancement

• While the evidence is not particularly robust it has been suggested that in addition to providing symptom relief, CTO revascularization may also offer other benefits such as improvement in left ventricular function [10–14], improvement of myocardial functional tests [15, 16], a reduction in need for coronary artery bypass grafting (CABG) [17], and weak evidence (registry data) for an overall improvement in mortality [18–21].

• It has been shown that in patients presenting with STEMI who have a CTO in a non-infarct-related artery, there is a significant increase in mortality and further cardiac events, as compared to patients with either single vessel culprit disease or multivessel disease with no bystander CTO lesion [22, 23].

Patient Selection: Who Should Have CTO PCI?

• Patient selection is important. PCI CTO is more costly than routine PCI in terms of time invested, financial outlay and risk to patient from extra radiation and contrast load.

• Careful history and examination to ascertain symptom burden is mandatory. Patients should have ongoing symptoms despite optimal medical therapy before being further investigated.

• Functional assessment should be undertaken to assess viability and ischemia burden. An ischemic burden/viability of $\geq 10\%$ in the territory of the occluded artery has been widely adopted as an appropriate cutoff for CTO PCI [24].

• Suitable CTO PCI cases may be considered for discussion at a multidisciplinary team (MDT) meeting, although if the criteria above are established and the CTO practice is mature this need not be mandated.

• Success rates of CTO PCI are dependent on:
  – Careful patient selection.
  – The complexity of the CTO lesion. The J-CTO score (Multicentre CTO Registry of Japan score) can be used to classify CTO lesion complexity into easy, intermediate, difficult to very difficult [25] (Fig. 28.2). The J-CTO score is strongly predictive of procedural success [26].
  – The clinical skills and experience of the operator.
  – In relation to success in the most complex lesions, the interaction at procedure between two scrubbed operators (although this does not mandate two operators are required per case).

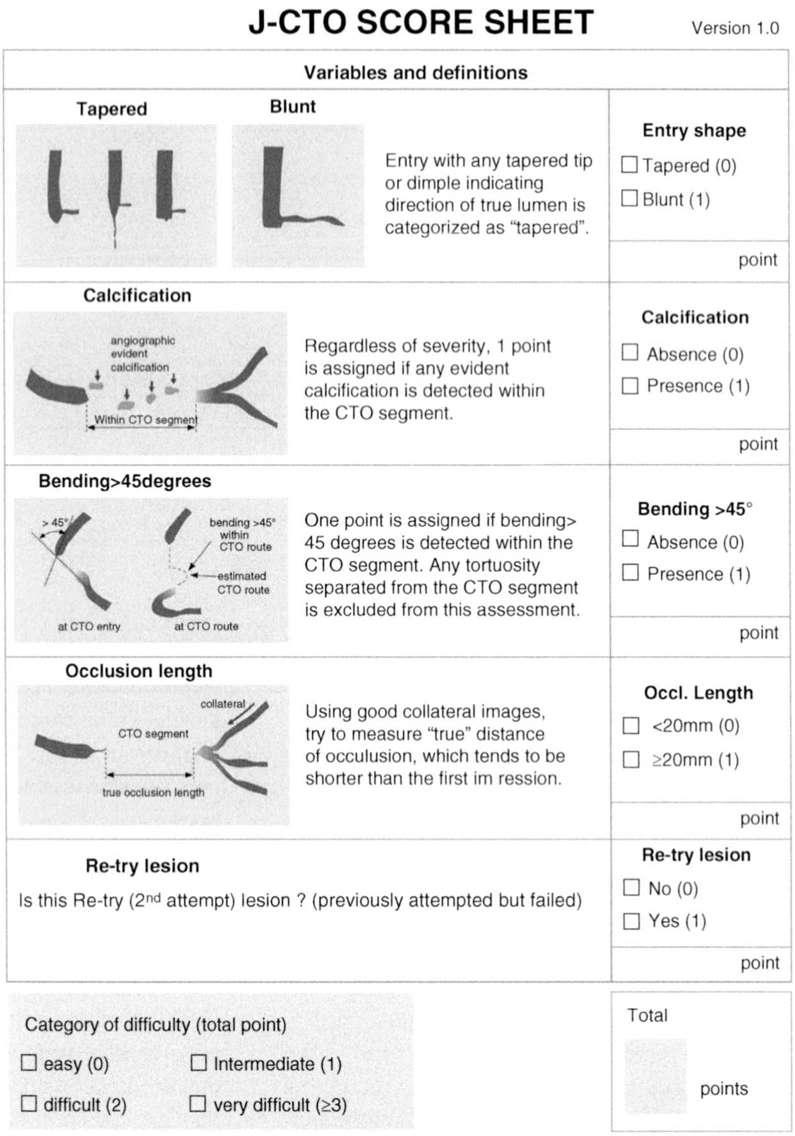
J-CTO SCORE SHEET
Version 1.0
Variables and definitions
Tapered
Blunt
Entry with any tapered tip or dimple indicating direction of true lumen is categorized as "tapered".
Entry shape
☐ Tapered (0)
☐ Blunt (1)
point
Calcification
angiographic evident calcification
Within CTO segment
Regardless of severity, 1 point is assigned if any evident calcification is detected within the CTO segment.
Calcification
☐ Absence (0)
☐ Presence (1)
point
Bending>45degrees
> 45°
bending >45° within CTO route
estimated CTO route
at CTO entry
at CTO route
One point is assigned if bending> 45 degrees is detected within the CTO segment. Any tortuosity separated from the CTO segment is excluded from this assessment.
Bending >45°
☐ Absence (0)
☐ Presence (1)
point
Occlusion length
collateral
CTO segment
true occlusion length
Using good collateral images, try to measure "true" distance of occulusion, which tends to be shorter than the first im ression.
Occl. Length
☐ <20mm (0)
☐ ≥20mm (1)
point
Re-try lesion
Is this Re-try (2nd attempt) lesion ? (previously attempted but failed)
Re-try lesion
☐ No (0)
☐ Yes (1)
point
Category of difficulty (total point)
☐ easy (0)
☐ Intermediate (1)
☐ difficult (2)
☐ very difficult (≥3)
Total
points

Fig. 28.2 Components of the J-CTO score. A higher score indicates a lower ability to cross the chronic total occlusion within 30 min. Adapted from Morino et al. [25]

Planning a Revascularization Strategy

- Identification of the proximal and distal cap is important, and determining the course of the vessel and its side branches, the presence of calcification and extent of (usable) collateral circulation can all help in planning the strategy that is most likely to be successful (Table 28.1).
- Dual injection coronary angiography (retrograde and antegrade is considered manadatory to demonstrate collateral filling patterns, the length and course of the CTO and the character of the distal cap.
- Some suggest a clearer understanding of the proximal and vessel course can be obtained from CT scanning. It is not suggested that this be done routinely but as an adjunct investigation perhaps after baseline (often single-injection) angiography when the vessel course appears to be particularly tortuous, or after a first attempt failure, if it is felt the chances of success could be improved by a better understanding of the vessel course (Fig. 28.3).

Table 28.1   Lesion-specific and patient-level predictors of procedural success [27]

	Simple	Complex
Vessel diameter (mm)	≥3.0	<3.0
Occlusion length (mm)	≤20	>20
Calcium occluded segment	None to moderate	Severe
Tortuosity occluded segment	Minimal to moderate	Severe
Occlusion stump	Tapered	Blunt or absent
Distal vessel opacification	Good to excellent	Poor
Distal vessel disease	Absent or moderate	Severe
Tandem/multiple occlusions	No	Yes
Tortuosity proximal to occlusion	Minimal to moderate	Severe
Disease of the proximal segment	Absent to moderate	Severe
Expected guiding catheter support	Good	Poor
Ostial location	No	Yes
Previous attempts	No	Yes[a]
Renal insufficiency	Yes	No
Expected patient tolerance[b]	Good	Poor

[a]Previous attempts are not an absolute contraindication but an adequate interval to allow sealing of dissections is desirable
[b]Cardiac or respiratory failure, musculoskeletal pain or psychiatric disorders limiting the patient's ability to lie flat for prolonged periods

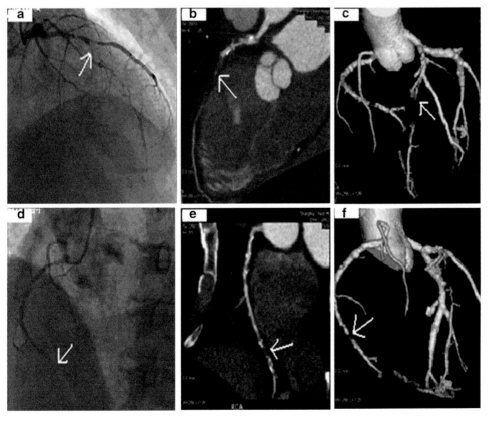

Fig. 28.3   Use of computed tomography to guide chronic total occlusion (CTO) intervention. Reconstructed images of CTO lesions from the left anterior descending artery (plates **a**, **b**, and **c**) and the right coronary artery (plates **d**, **e**, and **f**). From left to right: coronary angiography; multi-planar reconstruction images on CT coronary angiogram and three-dimensional volume rendering. The latter allows for optimal visualization of the tract of the occluded segment (arrows). Reproduced with permission from Qu X, Fang W, Gong K, et al. PLoS One 2014;9(6):e98242

- Key questions to consider when planning a strategy are as follows (Fig. 28.4) [28]:
  - Is the lesion short and are there good antegrade or retrograde collaterals?
  - Does the occluded segment lie in a less tortuous portion of the artery? If so then an antegrade approach with wire escalation (and then de-escalation after crossing) should be the primary approach.
  - Will I need to consider changing to a retrograde approach, and if so should a more experienced operator be involved in the initial attempt? Thus the quality and utility of retrograde collaterals (assessed in a straight RAO view) should be considered at this stage.
  - Will I need access to and be ready to use more specialist devices such as the CrossBoss™ (Boston Scientific, Massachusetts, USA) and Stingray™ (Boston Scientific, Massachusetts, USA) catheters for antegrade dissection and reentry (for example a long lesion with clear landing zone beyond the CTO)?

Procedure Preparation and Equipment

- It is important to ensure that all the necessary equipment is available prior to a planned CTO PCI procedure. Easy access to all CTO equipment stored in the cath lab is mandatory—having to hunt for wires or other kit disrupts the flow of the case. A CTO specific trolley is recommended.

Access

- The selection of access route is largely dependent on patient characteristics as well as operator preference.
- However there is a general move away from use of large (8F) long femoral sheaths since arterial complications may be profound. 6 and 7F radial sheaths are preferred, even for retrograde cases.
- Dual arterial access for contralateral injections should be considered as mandated in most cases—the exceptions being where there are good antegrade collaterals and no retro-

grade collaterals [29], or where the retrograde collateral supply is from the same arterial system (LAD from circumflex, for example).

- A 4–6F sheath can be used for contralateral injections and be up-sized for retrograde approach if needed. However if there is thought that there may be a need to go retrogradely this probably should be set up from the beginning) For most cases combined radial (perhaps for the retrograde injection) and femoral for the procedure may be recommended but each case must be considered individually.

Guide Catheter

- Optimal guide catheter support is crucial for successful crossing of a CTO lesion. Most operators use 7–8F guide catheters as it allows better support along with the insertion of covered stent grafts (in case of perforation).
- It also allows for the use of simultaneous dual Over the Wire (OTW) catheters, use of balloons for trapping or the use of intravascular ultrasound (IVUS) beside along with an OTW balloon.
- The choice of guide catheter is operator dependent but most operators start with Judkins Right (JR) or an Internal Mammary Artery (IMA) catheter for right coronary artery (RCA) lesions so minimizing ostial damage and allowing for deep intubation for extra support, perhaps with a guide catheter extension. Other catheters frequently used are an Amplatz Left (AL) 1.0 or 0.75.
- For left coronary artery (LCA) lesions Extra Back Up (EBU) 3.5 and 4.0 are the most commonly used catheters.

Guide Catheter Extensions

- This technique can be used to further enhance the support provided by the original guide catheter.
- The options include a GuideLiner® (Vascular Solutions Inc., Minnesota, USA), Guidezilla™ (Boston Scientific), and Heartrail® "mother and child" catheter system (Terumo, Shibuya, Japan) (Fig. 28.5).

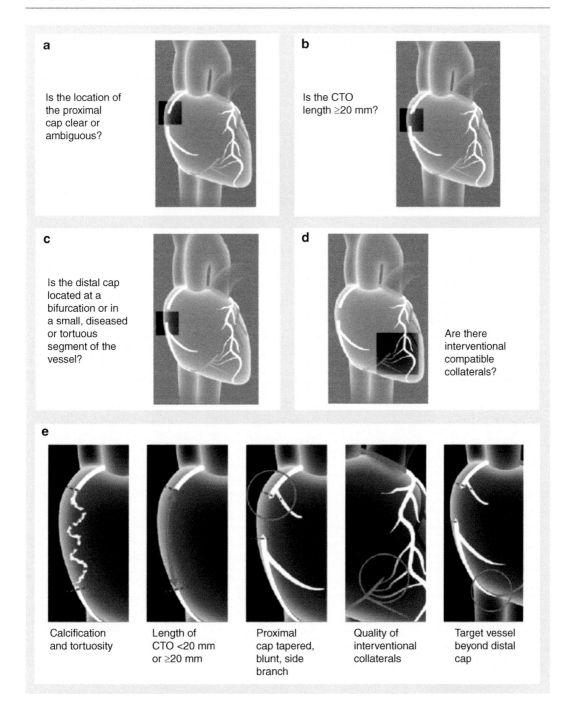

Fig. 28.4 Lesion characteristics of chronic total occlusions to consider when planning revascularization. Key elements of planning CTO intervention are the: (**a**) proximal cap; (**b**) length of the occluded segment; (**c**) distal cap; (**d**) presence or absence of viable interventional collaterals; and (**e**) areas of calcification or tortuosity

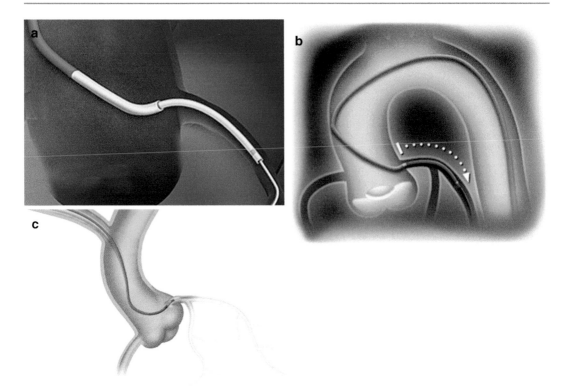

Fig. 28.5 Guide catheter extension systems. Guide catheter extensions are designed to maximize backup force/support and can improve access to discrete regions of the coronary vasculature. Plate **a** = GuideLiner (Vascular Solutions Inc.); plate **b** = Guidezilla (Boston Scientific) and plate **c** = Heartrail (Terumo)

Guide Wires

- Guide wire selection is a very important part of CTO PCI. Having a selection, or more importantly becoming extremely familiar with a few wires that cover all lesion crossing options, is part of learning CTO PCI practice.
- Some of the key features to consider in selecting a guide wire are tip load, tip stiffness, flexibility, trackability, ability to shape, shaping memory, shaft support, torque transmission and resistance to trapping of the wire within the occlusion.
- They can be broadly subdivided into hydrophilic (polymer-coated) and non-hydrophilic (uncoated). Both these groups can be further divided into tapered tip and non-tapered tip (Table 28.2).
- Understanding what is required for any particular scenario (e.g., antegrade wire

Table 28.2 Properties of CTO guide wires

Guide wire property	Uses
Hydrophilic, tapered, low gram force wire	Probing and knuckle wire technique
Hydrophilic, non-tapered, low gram force wire	Retrograde collateral workhorse wire, initial probing
Polymer-jacketed, high gram force, non-tapered wire	Complex lesion crossing, dissection/reentry
Non-jacketed tip, high gram force, tapered wire	Penetration technique, cap puncture, lumen reentry

escalation—Fielder XTA—Gaia 2nd—Confianza Pro—lesion cross—de-escalate to workhorse wire) or variations on these is fundamental, and being expert with a small selection of wires with which the operator is experienced is always the best approach, leading to the best chance of success (Table 28.3).

Table 28.3 Commonly used guide wires for CTO procedures [30]

Name	Tip style	Tip stiffness	Manufacturer	Uses
Polymer covered wires				
Fielder XT	Tapered	1.2 g	Asahi Intecc	Frontline for antegrade crossing, retrograde crossing and to make a knuckle wire
Fielder FC	Straight, non-tapered, low tip stiffness	1.6 g	Asahi Intecc	Crossing collateral vessels during retrograde approach
Whisper LS, MS, ES		0.8, 1.0, 1.2 g	Abbott Vascular	
Pilot 50		1.5 g	Abbott Vascular	
Choice PT Floppy		2.1 g	Boston Scientific	
Pilot 150/200	Straight, non-tapered, high tip stiffness	2.7, 4.1 g	Abbott Vascular	Antegrade crossing (ambiguous vessel course), knuckle wire formation, reentry into true lumen during LAST technique
Crosswire NT		7.7 g	Terumo	
PT Graphix Intermediate		1.7 g	Boston Scientific	
PT2 Moderate Support		2.9 g	Boston Scientific	
Shinobi		7.0 g	Cordis	
Shinobi Plus		6.8 g	Cordis	
Open coil (no polymer jacket)				
SION (hydrophilic)	Straight, low tip stiffness	0.8 g	Asahi Intecc	Antegrade crossing when vessel course is known
Cross-it 100XT	Tapered, low tip stiffness	1.7 g	Abbott vascular	Antegrade crossing when vessel course is known
Runthrough NS tapered		1.0 g	Terumo	
Confianza Pro 9, 12	Tapered, high tip stiffness, hydrophilic coating	9.3, 12.4 g	Asahi Intecc	Antegrade crossing when vessel course is known
Progress 140T, 200T		12.5, 13.3 g	Abbott Vascular	
Persuader 9		9.1 g	Medtronic	
ProVia 9, 12		11.8, 13.5 g	Medtronic	
MiracleBros 3, 4.5, 6	Straight tip, high tip stiffness	3.9, 4.4, 8.8 g	Asahi Intecc	Antegrade crossing when vessel course is known
MiracleBros 12		13.0 g	Asahi Intecc	
PROGRESS 40, 80, 120		5.5, 9.7, 13.9 g	Abbott Vascular	
Persuader 3, 6 (hydrophilic and hydrophobic)		5.1, 8.0 g	Medtronic	
ProVia 3, 6 (hydrophilic and hydrophobic)		8.3, 9.1 g	Medtronic	
Confianza 9 (hydrophobic)	Tapered, high tip stiffness, hydrophobic coating	8.6 g	Asahi Intecc	Antegrade crossing when vessel course is known
Persuader 9 (hydrophobic)		9.1 g	Medtronic	
ProVia 9, 12 (hydrophobic)		11.8, 13.5 g	Medtronic	

| Fielder FC | Fielder | SION | SION blue | Fielder XT | Fielder XT-R | ULTIMATEbros3 |

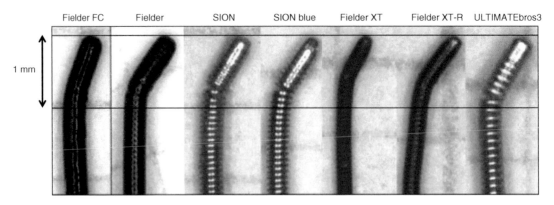

1 mm

Fig. 28.6 Guide wire tips of frequently used guide wires in CTO procedures. This image also shows the types of bend that may be required to cross a proximal CTO cap during antegrade procedures. All wires manufactured by Asahi Intecc (Aichi, Japan)

- It is important to note that knowing which wires are available, while important, is no substitute for mentored learning.

Wire Tip Shaping

- Ideally a shallow bend (30–45°) should be made no more than 1–1.5 mm from tip (primary curve) (Fig. 28.6).
- Occasionally a secondary bend may be required to orientate the tip in the vessel.
- A more acute bend may be required 2–3 mm from the tip in a high gram force wire to aid in lumen reentry.

Gaia Wire Family

- This family of guide wires is gaining popularity in CTO PCI. It has a long hydrophilic coating which allows it to be manipulated smoothly.
- The double coil structure and the round core design at the distal end allow torque transfer and prevent whip motion.
- The micro-cone tip of Gaia wires (Asahi Intecc, Aichi, Japan) is hollow and provides better penetration and allows the wire to penetrate more easily in hard lesions while keeping a flexible tip.

Over the Wire (OTW) Microcatheters

- Finecross® (Terumo) or Quick-Cross™ (Spectranetics, Colorado, USA), Turnpike® (Teleflex Inc, Morrisville, USA) family
- These are now considered mandatory when considering PCI CTO lesion. They allow stiff wires to be delivered to the lesion safely by using a workhorse wire to deliver the microcatheter to the lesion and then swapping the workhorse wire out for a more specialized wire (e.g., Gaia 2, Progress 80, or Confianza Pro 9 or 12 for cap penetration).
- Whenever any wire is removed from the microcatheter, saline via a syringe should replace it as it is being extracted (Fig. 28.7).
- The use of OTW microcatheters and balloons allows better transmission of torque to the tip during a crossing attempt and improved feedback as well as backup support for penetration.
- It also allows for the exchange of wires at any time during the procedure (de-escalation, for example, after stiff wire crossing and to facilitate reshaping of the wire during the crossing attempt).
- Tip injections through the microcatheter may be performed to confirm wire position as being in the true lumen in the absence of obvious collaterals, by carefully injecting 1–2 mL

of contrast to visualize the distal vessel. However any dissection can be easily worsened by such injections and this technique must be considered carefully.

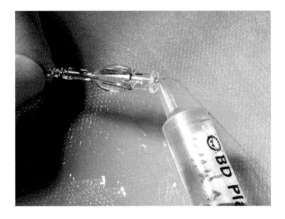

Fig. 28.7 Technique for wire exchange through a microcatheter. The wire is exchanged through the microcatheter at the hub, using a saline-filled syringe to ensure the hub is flushed prior to wire insertion to prevent air entry via the microcatheter. After removal of the wire and perhaps while reshaping the tip or while waiting for another wire, the saline-filled syringe should be placed on the end of the catheter

- The OTW microcatheters can then be safely removed (for example to now dilate the lesion with a balloon) using wire extension, the Nanto technique (attaching an indeflator maintained at 20 atmosphere pressure to maintain wire position) or best of all by balloon trapping, where a balloon is passed adjacent to the wire into the distal guide catheter (but not into the coronary artery). The microcatheter is then withdrawn proximal to the balloon and the balloon is inflated in the guide catheter to trap the wire as the microcatheter is removed. Angiographic screening of the wire tip is critical to ensure it doesn't move (Fig. 28.8).

Corsair Microcatheter

- This is a 2.7 French microcatheter with a lubricious outer coating, bidirectional wire braiding, and tapered soft tip.
- It has excellent ability to cross through collateral channels and obviates the need for col-

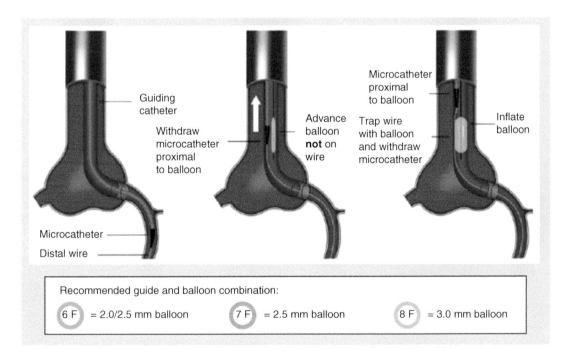

Fig. 28.8 The trapping balloon technique for removing a microcatheter

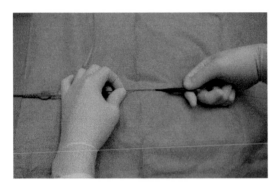

Fig. 28.9 Corsair microcatheter. Here the Corsair (Asahi Intecc) microcatheter is over a guide wire. As the Corsair is advanced with the left hand, the operator performs a clockwise rotation of the hub of the corsair using the right hand

lateral channel dilatation, thus causing less channel injury.

- It provides excellent support for antegrade wire manipulation and has good cross-ability through the lesion. It is advanced by rotation of the catheter (Fig. 28.9).
- However care should be taken not to over-rotate as it can cause the catheter to kink. It can also be used for contrast injection for distal vessel visualization; however, it should be flushed adequately afterward to prevent wire stickiness and trapping.

Tornus

- The Tornus (Asahi-Intecc) is particularly useful when trying to cross a calcified lesion. It is a braided microcatheter with a left-handed thread.
- It is advanced by turning anticlockwise, which allows rotational energy to be transmitted to the tip to create a pathway. It is useful in resistant lesions.
- It can only be used for an antegrade approach and is not useful for contrast injection.
- It is used much less nowadays since accessing the distal artery with the crossing wire usually means that a RotaWire (Boston Scientific) can

be placed distally and then rotablation de-bulking can be deployed.

CrossBoss™ Coronary CTO Crossing Catheter

- The CrossBoss™ (Boston Scientific) is a metal OTW microcatheter with a blunt tip to prevent vessel exit and ensure safe subintimal passage.
- As it is advanced it can be used to either find a path through the occlusion within the true lumen or can be used to track through the subintimal space once a stiff wire has accessed this plane, to create a dissection plane in a controlled manner (a bit like blunt finger dissection during surgery) (Fig. 28.10).
- It is advanced using a rapid spin motion. It can be advanced without the guide wire lead once it is in the subintimal space always ensuring by angiography that it is within the vessel architecture.

Stingray™ Coronary Reentry System

- Stingray™ (Boston Scientific) is a reentry system that utilizes a specific flat balloon, which hugs the vessel architecture (Fig. 28.11).
- Allows the operator to accurately target and reenter the true lumen from a subintimal position.
- There are two wire exit ports on opposite sides of the balloon so that one faces the true lumen and one faces the adventitia when the balloon is inflated.
- Using fluoroscopy a Stingray guide wire (0.014 in., high gram force wire with distal tapered end) can be used to reenter the true lumen.
- This can be then be withdrawn and a more trackable softer wire delivered down the Stingray™ catheter and out of the port and into the distal lumen.

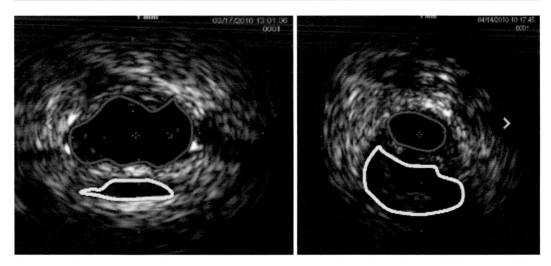

Fig. 28.10 Knuckle wire technique versus CrossBoss™. Intravascular ultrasound images demonstrating the difference in subintimal space formed by a knuckle wire (left) compared to the CrossBoss™ (right) system. There is a more controlled formation of subintimal space with the CrossBoss™ (red circle = true lumen; yellow circle = subintimal space). When there is a CTO lesion with a clear distal segment of normal vessel beyond it and with no bifurcation at the point of reentry, then antegrade dissection reentry can be considered either at first or subsequent PCI CTO attempt.

Antegrade dissection reentry can be achieved by using a routine stiff wire to gain entry into the subintimal space and then knuckle wire progression (e.g., Fielder XT, Pilot 50) can be used to ensure safe tracking through the subintimal space. Attempted reentry into the true lumen with a stiff wire is the final step in the process. This can be less well controlled than is desirable and the subintimal space created can large making control of the wire for reentry difficult. It is for this reason that controlled antegrade subintimal tracking using specialized equipment such as the Crossboss™ is preferred

Fig. 28.11 STINGRAY LP Coronary CTO Re-Entry System. Reproduced with permission from Boston Scientific

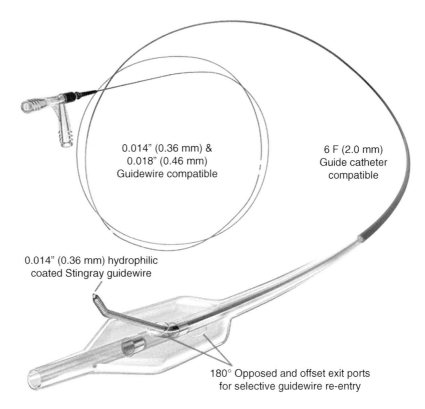

0.014" (0.36 mm) & 0.018" (0.46 mm) Guidewire compatible

6 F (2.0 mm) Guide catheter compatible

0.014" (0.36 mm) hydrophilic coated Stingray guidewire

180° Opposed and offset exit ports for selective guidewire re-entry

Procedural Strategy and Techniques

- Given the potential complexity and hetero-geneity of CTO lesions it is difficult to always have a single strategy. The basic approach to CTO PCI consists of three strategies:
    - Antegrade Wire escalation
    - Retrograde
    - Antergrade Dissection reentry
- All should be considered even at the same sitting although this will depend on a number of factors such as operator and patient fatigue, dye load, and radiation exposure duration.
- The trick is moving rapidly from one to another and not getting caught in the spiral of persisting with a single strategy until it fails [31].
- The contemporary CTO model is thus of a hybrid approach (Fig. 28.12) where all three

techniques can complement each other and can be combined if necessary. The main aim of this approach is not only to improve proce-dural success but also to improve procedural efficiency by reducing procedure time, radia-tion dose, and contrast load.

- As previously discussed, lesion, collaterals, and vessel characteristics will help shape the appropriate strategy.
- Prior to any approach it is essential there are adequate setup shots. If there are retrograde collaterals (Table 28.4) it is critical that bidi-rectional injections are performed starting with the retrograde injection first and the antegrade vessel injected at the point when there is no more filling of the retrograde vessel.
- In this way the maximal apparent length of the occlusion can be estimated as well as giving an idea of initial direction of approach needed for the antegrade wire.

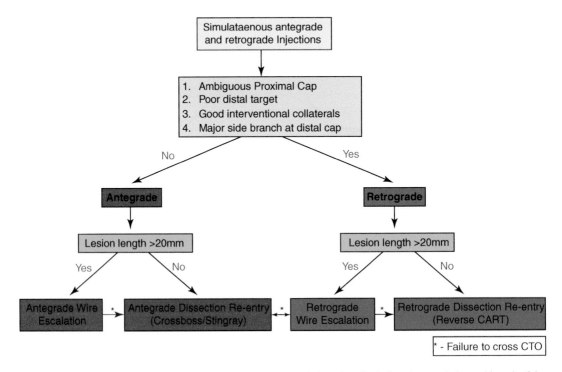

Fig. 28.12 The "Hybrid" CTO Algorithm. The planned strategy is based on the lesion characteristics and length of the CTO, with the option of switching if there is failure to cross with the primary strategy. Adapted from Brilakis et al. [30]

Table 28.4 The Rentrop and Werner classification of coronary collaterals

Rentrop classification	
Grade 0	No filling of collateral vessels
Grade 1	Filling of collateral vessel without any epicardial filling of target artery
Grade 2	Partial epicardial filling of target vessels by collateral vessel
Grade 3	Complete epicardial filling of target artery
Werner collateral connection (CC) grade	
CC0	No continuous connection
CC1	Threadlike continuous connection
CC2	Side branch-like connection (>0.4 mm)
CC3	>1 mm diameter of direct connection

Activated Clotting Time (ACT)

- It is mandatory that following initial heparin administration (70 U/kg) that an ACT is undertaken every 30 min.
- The ACT needs to be maintained at 250–300 s, using appropriate doses of heparin administered after the result becomes available (a guide might be that at 30 min if the ACT is, for example, 190 s, then another 3000 units may be given depending on the weight of the patient and that the ACT is re-checked at 30 min or early if there is concern).
- Thrombus cannot be allowed to form (particularly in the feeder vessel) since having the original occlusion and clot in the feeder artery can be fatal.

Antegrade Approach

- This has been the historic approach to CTO PCI with success rates between 60 and 70%. It is widely applied as a first strategy by many operators.
- Newer wires such as the Gaia series with their penetration success have re-affirmed the role of the antegrade approach.

Single Wire Technique

- This is the most widely used technique. This has two variants:
  - Wire escalation (stiff, stiffer, stiffest)
  - Step up and down (stiff, stiffer, soft)
- The wire is advanced usually over a microcatheter and once at the lesion is progressed through the antegrade cap using forward and backward motion with one (left) hand and clockwise/anticlockwise rotational movement with the other (right) hand, using the attached torquer.
- The torque is placed slightly further away from the Y connector than usual—about 3–4 in. The left hand only pushes using forefinger and thumb when the right hand has turned the wire in the direction considered best for making progress through the cap.
- Care is taken not to over-rotate the wire as this can cause enlargement of any subintimal space entered. The microcatheter can be used to provide support—*however pushing the microcatheter against the proximal cap should be avoided as this can lead to subintimal passage and perforation*. Indeed the microcatheter can impede rotation of the wire if it is too close to the cap.
- Depending on the tactile feedback and vessel tortuosity, wires can be exchanged from tapered soft wires to stiffer wires and similarly the end curve on the wire changed.

Parallel Wire Technique (less used nowadays)

- Can be used when a single wire technique is unsuccessful because of subintimal passage of the wire.
- The wire in the subintimal space is left where it is and a second wire (usually a stiffer wire) with a different bend can be used to cross the lesion using the first wire as a marker.
- If the second wire also tracks into a different subintimal space, then the first wire can be

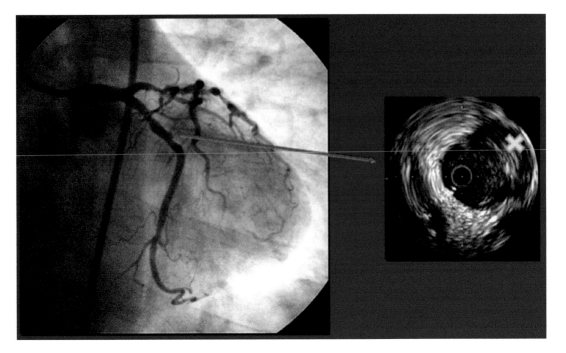

Fig. 28.13 Use of IVUS to identify entry point of a CTO. The IVUS catheter is used to identify the origin of an occluded obtuse marginal branch (cross), that has a blunt stump and thus not immediately identifiable on angiography

withdrawn and used to advance in the true lumen. This is known as the see-saw technique. It has gone out of fashion somewhat.

IVUS-Guided Technique

- IVUS can be used especially if there is a blunt stump next to a side branch to identify more easily the origin of the occlusion site as well as monitoring wire progress.
- The IVUS is placed in the side branch that is at the blunt stump of the main vessel—the images of the ostium of the occlusion are classic (Fig. 28.13).
- The IVUS can be left in situ to enable an understanding of the point and direction of penetration into the occlusion.
- IVUS during a case may really aid an understanding of where the wire (antegrade or retrograde) is positioned—true lumen, intima, sub-intima. As such it can aid connection of spaces to allow completion of the procedure.

Dissection Reentry Technique

- This technique is often used when there is a long section of occlusion or vessel ambiguity within the occlusion and is best considered when there is no significant tortuosity and there is a pre-bifurcation landing zone.
- The principle is to advance a wire within the subintimal space across the lesion and then to reenter the true lumen distal to the occluded segment.
- There has to be no bifurcation in the vicinity of the reentry point since the technique involves making a channel in the subintimal space and then reentering to do so beyond a bifurcation will result in jeopardy of normal flow down the non-reentered limb of the bifurcation.

Subintimal Tracking and Re-Entry (STAR) Technique and Modifications

- This technique is rarely used now since if too long a subintimal track is created it will result in loss of side branch blood supply.

- A looped polymer-coated (knuckle) wire is gently advanced within the subintimal space to traverse the lesion.
- The advantage of a knuckle wire is that it tends to stay within the adventitia. However it can create long subintimal tracks and can cause occlusion of any side branches.
- Furthermore the reentry relies on meeting resistance at the distal end and is uncontrolled.
- A modified or "contrast-guided" STAR technique uses contrast injection via an OTW microcatheter in the subintimal space to create/visualize a dissection plane, which can subsequently be wired with a softer wire. Again it is rarely used now.
- A mini-STAR technique uses the principle of trying to reenter the true lumen as proximally as possible using a softer polymer wire, thus creating a smaller subintimal track.
- Here two curves are placed on the wire, a small curve at the distal end (1–2 mm proximal to the tip of the wire) and a second curve a further 3–5 mm proximal to the tip.
- The wire forms a J-loop once the occluded segment has been crossed through the subintimal space, followed by efforts to reenter the true lumen.

Limited Antegrade Subintimal Tracking (LAST) Technique

- Similar to mini-STAR, in that efforts are made to reenter the true lumen as proximally as possible.
- Here a Confianza Pro 12 (Asahi Intecc) or Pilot 200 (Abbott Vascular, Illinois, USA) with an acute distal bend is often used.

Device-Based Method

- Uses the Stingray™ balloon and guide wire in conjunction with the Crossboss™ microcatheter (see above).

- Best method for controlled antegrade dissection reentry and is recommended as part of any CTO operators acquired skill set.

Retrograde Approach

- Retrograde PCI was first described in 1990 using the saphenous venous graft as access to treat a CTO in the left anterior descending (LAD) artery [32]. Use of collateral vessels to access the distal cap and so cross occluded segments has further revolutionized this field [33, 34]. Since then this technique has become one of the mainstays in CTO angioplasty practice albeit used still in only 30–40% of cases.
- The occluded segment is approached via retrograde, septal collaterals, collaterals from the same system (LAD to LCx, for example—so-called ping-pong technique), or less often (because of the risk of perforation and tamponade) epicardial collaterals.
- The rationale of the retrograde technique is that the lesion is often softer and tapered at the distal end, hence making wiring relatively easier to cross.

Collaterals

- Identifying collaterals is key in success of a retrograde CTO procedure.
- These should be studied in detail in multiple views prior to planning a procedure but best if originating from the LAD to RCA in a RAO 5° cranial view with **no panning**.
- The collaterals can be graded according to the Rentrop classification [35] and/or Werner classification (Table 28.4) [36].
- The Rentrop classification grades the extent of filling of the artery by collaterals rather than the collaterals themselves. The Werner classification grades the collateral channels and is widely accepted.
- The retrograde approach can be considered in CTO cases where the proximal cap cannot be crossed in an antegrade wire escalation

strategy, or where despite an antegrade dissection reentry technique it is still impossible to enter the true lumen distally.

- The presence of an ambiguous proximal cap may also lead to a consideration that an upfront antegrade strategy is likely to fail and favor a primary retrograde approach.
- To successfully perform a retrograde procedure, the following are required:
  - A retrograde donor artery capable of accommodating a guide wire and Corsair microcatheter
  - Suitable interventional collaterals
- Generally the retrograde approach can be divided into two strategies, dependent mostly on the nature of the occlusion:

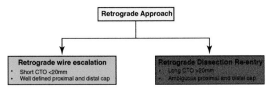

- In some cases, a primary retrograde wire escalation may result in the retrograde wire entering the subintimal space, in which case the strategy is converted to a retrograde dissection reentry with the intention of reentering the true lumen.

Collateral Selection for Retrograde Procedures

- Careful analysis of the diagnostic angiogram is important in determining how the retrograde approach will be achieved (Fig. 28.14). In general, the collateral system can be divided into the following:
  - Septal collaterals
  - Epicardial collaterals
- In general, septal collaterals are preferred to epicardial collaterals, due to a lesser degree of tortuosity and reduced risk of significant cardiac tamponade in the event of wire perforation of the collateral vessel.
- However, epicardial collaterals can be more safely used (but don't exclude tamponade) in

patients who have previously undergone CABG, as the lack of pericardial space makes cardiac tamponade less likely in these patients.

- Use of epicardial collaterals may result in ischemia, particularly where there is little or no septal collateral to the distal CTO.
- Epicardial collaterals can be longer than septal collaterals, a consideration for choosing suitably long enough equipment (Corsair 150 cm, for example) when undertaking retrograde procedures using these collaterals.
- A third potential option is the use of preexisting surgical grafts as "collateral" conduits to open native vessels retrogradely. In such cases (for example, use of a preexisting LIMA graft to LAD) caution must be employed not to dissect the graft as this may result in compromise to the supplied territory.
- Prior to undertaking a retrograde approach, assessment of collateral vessels is crucial to the success of the procedure; in a retrospective analysis of 157 patients who underwent retrograde CTO procedures significant predictors of procedural failure were non-visibility of the recipient vessel angle, a "corkscrew" tortuosity of the collateral channel, and collaterals with Werner CC1 classification [37].

Accessing and Crossing Collaterals

- Dual access with large enough Guide catheters, is mandatory for retrograde procedures, either as a single radial/single femoral or bifemoral procedure.
- As wire externalization can result in deep engagement of the retrograde guide catheter, caution must be employed with use of the catheter shape in the donor artery.
- Use of short 90 cm guide catheters can be useful as this will reduce the distance required for wire externalization, especially if epicardial collaterals are being considered.
- If these catheters are not available, a standard 100 cm guide catheter can be shortened by cutting and removing a segment of the guide catheter shaft and joining the ends

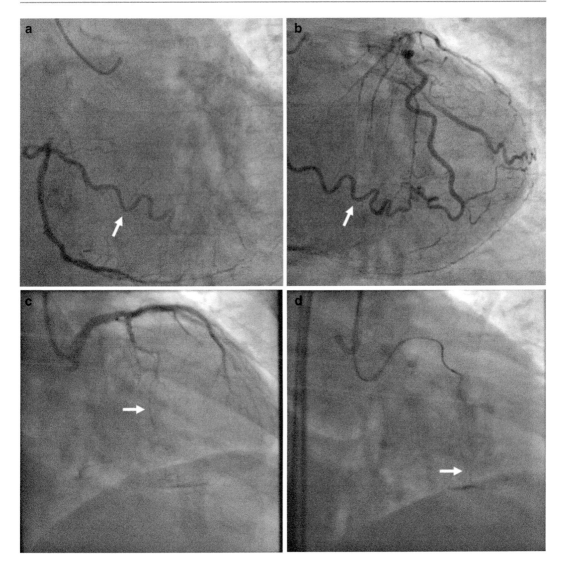

Fig. 28.14 Assessment of the collateral circulation for retrograde CTO intervention. Angiographic images demonstrating epicardial (**a**, **b**) and septal (**c**, **d**) collaterals. Plates A and B show a large epicardial collateral from the LAD supplying the distal RCA (white arrows). Plate C shows a septal collateral from the LAD supplying the dis-tal RCA (white arrow). Plate **d** shows the result of a tip injection from a Corsair microcatheter within the same septal collateral as Plate **c** demonstrating the course of the collateral and connection with an occluded RCA (distal collateral shown with white arrow). Key: *LAD* left anterior descending artery, *RCA* right coronary artery

(at the proximal end of the guide) with an introducer sheath 1 French size smaller than the guide catheter.

- Following engagement of the retrograde guide catheter, the vessel is wired with a standard workhorse wire to the selected collateral. This can require a large "double bend" to ensure the guide wire can then enter the septal collateral of choice. This is done on a micro-catheter that will enter the septal collateral; the most commonly used are the Corsair (Asahi Intecc) or Turnpike spiral that can also act as a channel dilator.

- Once the selected collateral has been entered, the workhorse wire is exchanged for a hydrophilic wire, such as Sion or polymer-

jacketed wires with a low tip load (Fielder FC or Pilot 50).
- Two strategies can be employed in traversing the septal collaterals (Fig. 28.15):
  - Septal surfing or
  - Contrast-guided crossing.
- Most septal collaterals can be entered in the right anterior oblique (RAO) cranial view to identify the entry and course of the collateral, while the exit of the collateral into the distal true lumen of the vessel with the CTO can be sometimes seen by changing the view to an RAO caudal.
- These views are applicable for a classical LAD septal supplying the distal RCA; for other retrograde approaches (such as using grafts or ipsilateral collaterals within an LAD) a different set of views will be required to identify the entry-point and exit of the collateral supply to the distal vessel.
- Common guide wires that can be used for crossing collateral vessels are shown in Table 28.5.

- The Quebec experience with septal surfing has shown this to be a safe and efficient method of traversing septal collaterals, independent of the Werner classification of the collaterals.
- The more recent use of hydrophilic low tip load wires such as the Sion wires with regards to lower risk of perforation [39]. In essence septal surfing requires the wire to be rapidly moved up and down the collateral till it makes progress.
- The Corsair microcatheter can be used to dilate the septal channels while the selected wire (Sion, Fielder FC or Pilot 50) is advanced. A tip injection of contrast through the Corsair can help track the path of the septal network (see Fig. 28.14), this is particularly important when performing contrast-guided crossing to ensure the guide wire is advanced within the septal network to the distal vessel (small volumes: 2–3 mL of neat dye are injected). Suction on the microcatheter to ensure there is no air in the system is mandatory.

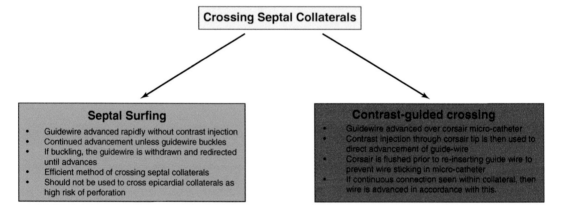

Fig. 28.15 Methods for crossing septal collaterals. Adapted from Brilakis E "The retrograde approach" from "Manual of Coronary Chronic Total Occlusion Interventions", Academic Press, 2014

Table 28.5 Guide wires used to cross collateral vessels. Adapted from Joyal et al. JACC Interv 2012;5:1–11 [38]

Guide wire	Manufacturer	Tip load (g)	Wire properties	Hydrophilicity
Sion	Asahi Intecc Corp	0.7	0.014″ wire with 28 cm spring coil at tip	Hydrophilic tip, hydrophobic shaft
Pilot 50	Abbott Vascular	1.5	0.014″ diameter, core-to-tip stainless steel guide wire with polymer coating	Hydrophilic tip, hydrophobic shaft
Fielder FC	Asahi Intecc Corp	0.8	0.014″ wire, core-to-tip wire with polymer coating	Hydrophilic tip, hydrophobic shaft

Retrograde Wire Escalation (RWE)

- Crossing the CTO retrograde from "true lumen to true lumen" can be successful in only about 30% of cases. The wire escalation should be performed through sequential advancement of the Corsair/Turnpike microcatheter.
- RWE requires initial puncture of the distal cap with a low tip load hydrophilic tip wire such as the Fielder XT, Fielder FC, or Pilot 50. A Gaia 2nd or 3rd might also be considered.
- A low tip load can be tried first given the generally lower strength and tapered nature of the distal cap compared to the tougher proximal cap.
- Crossing the CTO can then be achieved by using either a low tip load hydrophilic wire (Fielder XT) or exchanging to a higher tip load with a hydrophilic tip and hydrophobic shaft (Pilot 200).
- Such wires may be able to track within microchannels within the body of the CTO, however could also be used to form a "knuckle" within the sub-intimal space.
- The proximal cap of the CTO is generally harder than the distal cap, and hence this may require exchange again to a high tip load wire such as a Confianza Pro 9 or 12 wire to puncture the proximal cap and enter the sub-intimal space proximally.
- In contrast to the Fielder/Pilot family of wires, the Confianza Pro wires have a hydrophobic tip with hydrophilic shaft, allowing the operator greater tactile feedback when puncturing the proximal cap (Table 28.6).

- In some cases, where there is a firm CTO plaque with a clear trajectory, the Confianza Pro wire could be used to cross the CTO as well as puncturing through the proximal cap. Equally, the proximal cap may be punctured with the same wire to traverse the CTO plaque. Care must be taken with these stiff wires and crossing sub-intimally retrogradely may be hazardous.
- Following entry into the true lumen, de-escalation should be performed through the microcatheter to avoid dissection or wire perforation of the proximal vessel prior to wire externalization (Fig. 28.16).

Retrograde Dissection Reentry

- In cases where there is a long CTO with an ambiguous course, or if retrograde wire escalation through the "true lumen" is unsuccessful, a dissection reentry strategy can be employed to cross the occlusion.
- Retrograde dissection reentry (RDR) involves entering the subintimal space within the CTO using a polymer-jacketed hydrophilic wire (such as a Fielder XT or Pilot 200) and forming a safe "knuckle" on the wire (Fig. 28.17).
- The knuckle wire is then advanced within the subintimal space by pushing the wire, although rotating the wire at this stage can result in knotting the knuckle wire within the subintimal space making it difficult to then complete the procedure and reenter the true lumen beyond the proximal cap.
- Advancement of the knuckle wire is also aided by progressive advancement of the

Table 28.6 Commonly used guide wires to cross a CTO via the retrograde approach. Adapted from Joyal et al. JACC Interv 2012;5(1):1–11 [38]

Guide wire	Manufacturer	Tip load (g)	Wire properties	Hydrophilicity
Fielder XT	Asahi Intecc Corp	0.8	Polymer-jacket, tapered tip	Hydrophilic tip, hydrophobic shaft
Pilot 200	Abbott Vascular	6	Polymer-jacket, tapered tip	Hydrophilic tip, hydrophilic shaft
Confianza Pro 12	Asahi Intecc Corp	12	Core-to-tip design, tapered spring coil with hydrophobic coating	Hydrophobic tip, hydrophilic shaft

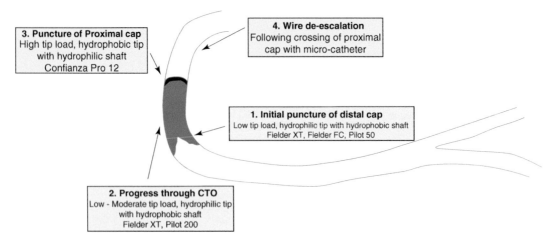

3. Puncture of Proximal cap
High tip load, hydrophobic tip
with hydrophilic shaft
Confianza Pro 12

4. Wire de-escalation
Following crossing of proximal
cap with micro-catheter

1. Initial puncture of distal cap
Low tip load, hydrophilic tip with hydrophobic shaft
Fielder XT, Fielder FC, Pilot 50

2. Progress through CTO
Low - Moderate tip load, hydrophilic tip
with hydrophobic shaft
Fielder XT, Pilot 200

Fig. 28.16 Retrograde wire escalation

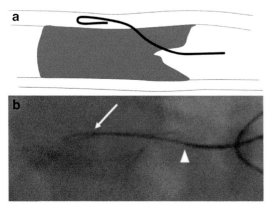

Fig. 28.17 Knuckle wire into subintimal space. Schematic diagram (top) of guide wire entering subintimal space with a knuckle at the tip of the guide wire. Angiographic image (bottom) of a Fielder XT knuckle wire (white arrow) within the subintimal space of a CTO, delivered with a Corsair microcatheter (white triangle)

microcatheter over the wire followed by advancing the knuckle wire further along the subintimal plane.

- The aim of the RDR technique is to join the proximal and distal true lumen across the subintimal space of the CTO. In order to achieve this, a second antegrade wire is taken to either cross the proximal cap of the CTO or be positioned within the subintimal space.
- Reentry from the subintimal space into the true lumen proximal to the CTO can be achieved using the CART (Controlled Antegrade and Retrograde Subintimal Tracking) technique and its variants.

CART and Reverse CART Technique

- First described by Surmeley, Tsuchikane, and Katoh in 2006 [34]. The principle is to create a shared space within the subintimal plane of the CTO to allow connection of the true lumen proximal and true lumen distal to the CTO segment. This is achieved with balloon inflation within the subintimal space of the CTO.
- The traditional CART technique involved balloon inflation on the retrograde wire within the subintimal space, followed by directing the antegrade wire into this subintimal space while the balloon was being deflated. The antegrade wire is then progressed through the same track as the retrograde wire into the distal true lumen (Fig. 28.18).
- Once the antegrade guide wire has been advanced into the distal true lumen, the retrograde wire and balloon can be removed and PCI to the CTO can proceed with delivery of balloons and stent on the antegrade wire.
- A variant of this is the "reverse CART" technique and is the one more commonly used nowadays. While the principle is the same, the difference is that the balloon is delivered and inflated using the antegrade wire, with the retrograde wire directed into the subintimal space following balloon inflation and advanced past the proximal cap into the proximal true lumen (Fig. 28.19).

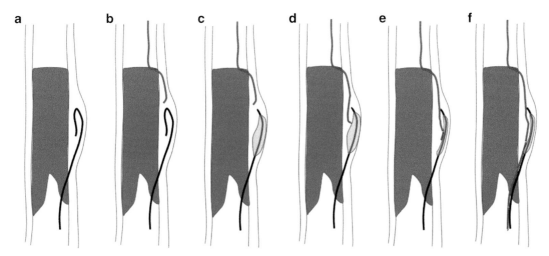

Fig. 28.18 The Controlled Antegrade and Retrograde Subintimal Tracking (CART) Technique. (**a**) Initial subintimal tracking using a knuckled retrograde wire (black line). (**b**) Antegrade wire (red line) into the subintimal plane. (**c**) Inflation of a balloon delivered on the retrograde wire within the subintimal plane to enlarge a subintimal space formed by the track of the retrograde wire. (**d**) Advancement of the antegrade wire to the inflated balloon. (**e**) Deflation of the retrograde balloon with advancement of the antegrade wire into the subintimal space formed by the balloon inflation. (**f**) Advancement of the antegrade wire through the track formed by the retrograde wire across the subintimal space and into the distal true lumen beyond the CTO

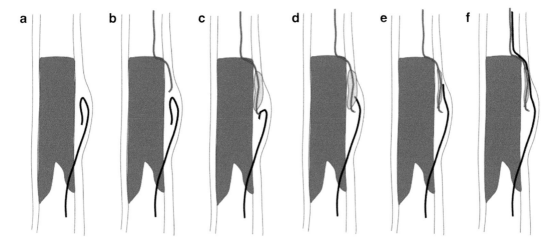

Fig. 28.19 Reverse CART technique. (**a**) Initial subintimal tracking using a knuckled retrograde wire (black line). (**b**) Antegrade wire (red line) into the subintimal plane. (**c**) Inflation of a balloon delivered on the antegrade wire within the subintimal plane to enlarge a subintimal space formed by the track of the antegrade wire. (**d**) Advancement of the retrograde wire to the inflated balloon. (**e**) Deflation of the antegrade balloon with advancement of the retrograde wire into the subintimal space formed by the balloon inflation. (**f**) Advancement of the retrograde wire through the track formed by the antegrade wire across the subintimal space and into the proximal true lumen of the CTO

- The advantage of using the reverse CART technique is that the balloon does not need to pass through the retrograde collaterals. This technique is also aided by use of the microcatheter on the retrograde wire, allowing control of the retrograde wire in advancing this across the subintimal space formed by the antegrade balloon inflation (Fig. 28.20).
- In some cases, a balloon cannot be passed across the proximal cap into the subintimal space

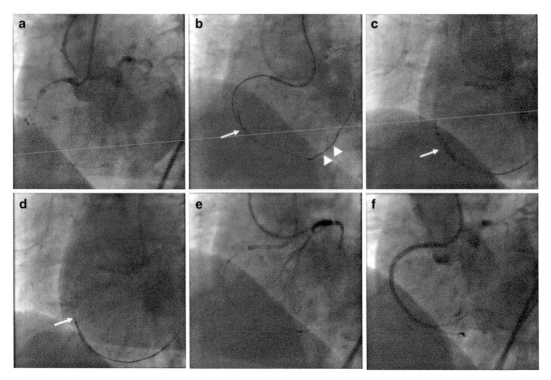

Fig. 28.20 A reverse CART procedure on angiography. (**a**) Simultaneous injection demonstrating a CTO of the RCA with retrograde filling of distal PDA via septal collaterals from the LAD. (**b**) Septal collateral crossed with Corsair microcatheter (white triangles) with knuckled retrograde wire in subintimal space of RCA CTO, overlapping antegrade wire in the shared subintimal space (white arrow). (**c**) Balloon inflation on antegrade wire to enlarge subintimal space. (**d**) Retrograde wire advanced following balloon inflation into CTO proximal true lumen (white arrow shows tip of retrograde wire advanced into a GuideLiner within the true lumen of the RCA proximal to the CTO). (**e**) Following exchange of retrograde wire with RG3 long wire externalized via the RCA guide catheter, stent positioned across the CTO. (**f**) Final angiographic result

parallel to the retrograde wire/micro-catheter. In this case, a Tornus microcatheter can be used on the antegrade wire to enlarge the subintimal track and allow subsequent delivery of the antegrade balloons to complete the reverse CART.

- A key aspect of CART and reverse CART is that both antegrade and retrograde wires are within the subintimal plane, with balloon inflation used to enlarge the space on one of these wires, to facilitate entry of the other wire into this space and exit to the true lumen. IVUS can ensure that the wire(s) position within the vessel is more clearly understood.
- However, in some cases:
  1. The antegrade wire may progress within the "true lumen" of the CTO while the retrograde wire is within the subintimal space. In this situation, balloon inflation on the antegrade wire will expand the track within

the antegrade "true lumen" of the CTO, and the retrograde wire can be exchanged over the micro-catheter for a stiff wire such as a Confianza Pro 12 to reenter from the subintimal retrograde space into the antegrade true lumen.

  2. The antegrade wire may enter the subintimal space; however, the retrograde wire progresses through the "true lumen" of the CTO. In this case, advancement of a knuckle on the retrograde wire should encourage it to advance into the subintimal plane and hence allow the reverse CART to be performed as above. Once the retrograde wire has been advanced past the CTO into the proximal true lumen, the Corsair microcatheter is advanced into the true lumen proximal to the CTO allowing for wire exchange across the CTO.

Table 28.7 Externalization wires for retrograde CTO procedures. Adapted from Joyal et al. JACC Interv 2012;5(1): 1–12 [38]

Guide wire	Manufacturer	Tip load (g)	Wire properties	Hydrophilicity
RG3	Asahi Intecc Corp	3.0	330 cm length, 0.010″ diameter, spring coil tip	Hydrophilic tip, hydrophobic shaft
ViperWire advance	Cardiovascular system	–	330 cm length, 0.014″ wire, strongest shaft for externalization	
R350	CHS interventional specialties	–	350 cm nitinol wire, 0.012″ tapering to 0.006″ at distal coil, 5 cm distal platinum coil for radiopacity	No hydrophilic coating

Wire Externalization

- Whether the CTO has been crossed with retrograde wire escalation or retrograde dissection reentry, both techniques will result in the retrograde wire within the proximal true lumen. In both cases, the next step is to pass the retrograde wire into the antegrade guide catheter.
- The aim is to externalize the retrograde guide wire, such that this can be used as a system to deliver balloons and stents antegradely across the CTO. Specially available long wires are used for this process (Table 28.7).
- A floppy Rota-wire (Boston Scientific) can potentially be used for externalization; however, it is more prone to kinking, and caution must be employed if this is externalized using a snare (see below). The Pilot 200 wire also is available as a 300 cm wire for externalization.

Externalizing the Retrograde Wire: Wiring the Antegrade Guide Catheter

- This requires the antegrade guide catheter to be positioned co-axially with the CTO. Once the antegrade guide wire has been passed into the antegrade guide catheter, it is trapped using an appropriately sized balloon within the guide catheter (2.0 mm for 6 Fr, 2.5 mm for 7 Fr and 8Fr guide catheters).
- Trapping the retrograde wire within the antegrade guide catheter can allow delivery of the Corsair/Turnpike microcatheter across the CTO and proximal vessel lumen into the antegrade guide catheter. Once the Corsair/Turnpike is within the antegrade guide catheter, the retrograde wire is removed and a long wire (RG3 or Viper 200) can be delivered

through the Corsair/Turnpike and externalized through the antegrade guide catheter and Y connector.
- Passing a guide catheter extension (GuideLiner or Guidezilla) through the antegrade guide catheter into the proximal vessel may facilitate this process, by passing the retrograde wire into the guide catheter extension, followed by advancement of the Corsair through extension and thus into the guide catheter. It extends the antegrade Guide Catheter and so there is less distance for the retrograde wire to traverse.
- The potential advantage of this is to prevent the risk of the retrograde wire tracking subintimally in the true lumen proximal to the CTO, with potential resulting compressive hematoma (Fig. 28.21).

Externalizing the Retrograde Wire: Snaring Technique

- In some cases, a wire cannot be passed directly into the antegrade guide catheter or guide catheter extension.
- This can be the case with aorto-ostial CTO or where co-axial engagement of the antegrade guide catheter is not possible.
- In such circumstances, once the retrograde microcatheter has been advanced across the CTO lesion, the retrograde wire is exchanged for a long wire to be externalized (RG3 or Viper).
- This wire is then advanced with the Corsair through the proximal vessel and into the aorta. A snare is then advanced through the antegrade guide catheter and opened in the aorta to capture the externalization wire. Once achieved, the snare is closed and retracted into

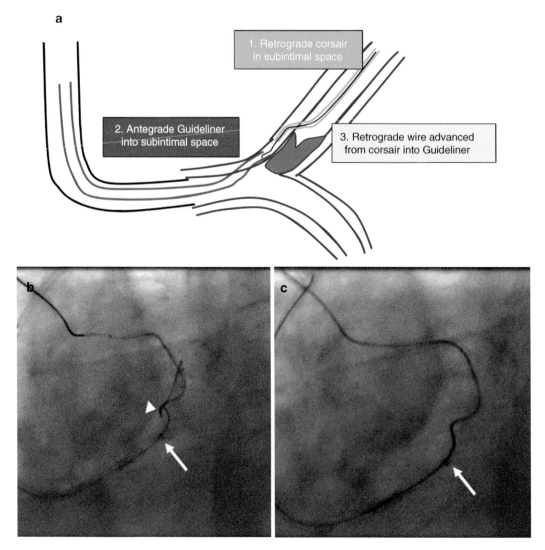

Fig. 28.21 GuideLiner-assisted completion of a reverse CART procedure. This technique can be used to capture the retrograde wire without the need to advance the wire directly into the antegrade guide catheter. (**a**) Following balloon inflation in the subintimal space, the GuideLiner is advanced over the antegrade wire into the shared subintimal space. The retrograde wire is then advanced into the GuideLiner, allowing advancement of the Corsair into the antegrade GuideLiner. This can then facilitate exchange of the retrograde wire with a long externalization wire. (**b**) White arrow shows the GuideLiner within the subintimal space, with the Corsair shown by the white triangle. (**c**) Following advancement of the retrograde wire into the GuideLiner, the Corsair has also been advanced into the antegrade GuideLiner (white arrow)—following this the retrograde wire is exchanged for a long RG3 wire from the retrograde guide catheter and externalized via the antegrade guide catheter

the antegrade guide catheter, hence externalizing the long wire.

- The above is dependent on being able to advance the Corsair/Turnpike into the aorta across the CTO. If this is not possible, then the original retrograde wire is advanced into the aorta and captured using the snare. In this situation, caution must be employed when snaring the retrograde wire:
  - The distal flexible portion of the wire should not be snared as this can result in wire fracture
  - The snared wire may unravel if snared distally

 – At all times being aware of being able to release the snare
- The optimal position to snare a standard retrograde wire is immediately proximal to the radiopaque part of the wire. In comparison, the RG3 or Viper externalization wires are less likely to fracture or unravel with snaring. However, in all cases snaring and capture of the retrograde wire should be performed under direct fluoroscopic guidance [38].
- Regardless of the method by which the retrograde wire is externalized, once in the antegrade guide catheter, the long externalization wire is advanced by pushing within the antegrade catheter. Care must be taken at all times to ensure the retrograde guide catheter is not being dragged into the ostium of the feeder artery as this will risk dissection of the feeder artery and indeed the retrograde catheter should be kept disengaged at all times of long wire manipulation.
- The Y-connector is then removed from the antegrade guide catheter and a finger placed on the end until the tip of the externalization wire is felt. The introducer needle is placed through the Y-connector, and the tip of the externalized wire is then threaded through the introducer needle/Y-connector. The Y-connector is then re-connected to the hub of the antegrade guide catheter over the introducer needle and externalized wire, without flushing to prevent hydraulic dissection.
- The retrograde externalized wire is then advanced until 20 cm is outside the antegrade guide catheter. If the externalized end of the wire is damaged, this can be cut to allow safe mounting, antegradely of rapid exchange balloons and stents.

Opening the CTO Following Wire Externalization

- The externalized wire can be used for delivery of rapid exchange balloons antegradely across the CTO and subsequently stenting of the CTO.
- Prior to this, the retrograde Corsair/Turnpike must be withdrawn to the distal true lumen of the CTO, and it is important to ensure that the antegrade balloons/stents do not interlock with the Corsair/Turnpike or it may not be possible to disentangle them.
- However, the Corsair/Turnpike should not be brought back too far and must be kept within the distal true lumen to cover the collaterals, which could be subject to shear stresses from the externalized wire as equipment is passed on the externalized wire.
- Once the CTO has been opened, the stent can either be delivered on the same system, or an antegrade wire can be delivered across the opened CTO and the retrograde equipment removed prior to delivering the stent on the antegrade wire.

Removal of Retrograde Equipment at the End of the Procedure

- Once the CTO has been treated, the microcatheter is advanced over the externalized guide wire to the mid part of the stented segment.
- Following this, the retrograde guide catheter is disengaged into the aorta, to ensure that this is not pulled into the donor artery to cause dissection during withdrawal of the retrograde wire. The externalized retrograde wire is then withdrawn through the retrograde guide catheter, with fluoroscopy monitoring the retrograde guide catheter for over-engagement of the donor coronary artery.
- The Corsair/Turnpike microcatheter is then withdrawn using clockwise torque.
- At the end of the procedure, a contrast injection should be performed of the donor coronary artery to ensure that there is no evidence of dissection, collateral perforation or collateral thrombosis.

Complications of Retrograde Procedures

- There are important complications that can occur when using the retrograde approach, not only related to the occluded artery itself but

Table 28.8 Potential complications that can occur during a retrograde approach CTO intervention. Compiled from Brilakis E "The retrograde approach" from "Manual of Chronic Coronary Total Occlusions", Academic Press, 2014

Potential complication	Description
Advancing retrograde guide wire into the collateral vessel	
Dissection of donor artery	• Injury to the donor artery can be catastrophic as this can affect both the donor vessel and CTO vessel territory, leading to severe ischemia and rapid hemodynamic compromise • This can be avoided by use of a standard workhorse guide wire over the Corsair microcatheter • Management is stenting of the dissection
Crossing septal collateral with retrograde guide wire	
Collateral dissection	• This can result in loss of collateral • Further attempts at retrograde PCI will require use of a different collateral vessel
Collateral perforation	• This is usually benign and results in intra-myocardial staining. Rarely there may be septal hematoma or perforation into the pericardium • Management is conservative observation, unless evidence of tamponade requiring pericardiocentesis
Guide wire entrapment	• This can be avoided by avoiding large and acute bends on the retrograde wire during advancement of the wire across the septal collaterals • The bend on the wire can be changed following advancement of the microcatheter if required
Crossing epicardial collaterals with retrograde guide wire	
Collateral dissection	• This may compromise retrograde filling to the CTO territory resulting in ischemia • Further attempts at retrograde CTO PCI will require use of a septal collateral
Collateral perforation	• When occurring in an epicardial collateral, this can result in cardiac tamponade necessitating pericardiocentesis and coiling of the epicardial artery
Guide wire entrapment	• This can occur if a loop forms at the end of the retrograde wire within the epicardial artery • Careful advancement of the retrograde wire over the Corsair microcatheter can prevent this from occurring
Crossing the collateral with the microcatheter	
Ischemia	• This is most likely to occur if the collateral used is the only one supplying the CTO territory • Most likely to occur with epicardial collateral use • Analgesia may be required for mild chest discomfort
Dissection of the donor vessel	• This occurs due to inadvertent "back and forth" motion of the retrograde guide catheter during advancement of the microcatheter • Careful attention is required to the ostium of the donor circulation during this step, occasionally with disengagement of the guide catheter or backward tension
Donor vessel thrombosis	• This can be avoided with careful monitoring of the activated clotting time and additional heparin boluses when required
Retrograde wire escalation/retrograde dissection reentry	
Loss of side-branches over dissection area	• This may result in ischemia in the supplied territory
Perforation	• Most likely to occur if an oversized balloon is used within the subintimal space, or if a stiff high tip load wire is used within the proximal vessel following completion of the CART procedure • This can be avoided by using a suitable balloon size and de-escalating wires following crossing the CTO within the proximal true lumen
Wire externalization	
Fracture of retrograde wire during snaring	• This occurs if retrograde wire is snared in the distal flexible portion • Avoidance of snaring at this point, or exchanging to the externalization wire prior to snaring if possible
Unraveling of the snared retrograde wire	• Important to retract the snared retrograde wire under continuous fluoroscopic guidance

Table 28.8 (continued)

Potential complication	Description
PCI of the CTO	
Collateral dissection	• This can occur due to shear caused by the long retrograde wire • To prevent this, the retrograde wire should always be covered either with the Corsair microcatheter or an OTW balloon over the length of the collateral while the balloons/stents are delivered antegradely over the externalized wire
Dissection of target vessel ostia	• This can occur from forward movement of the antegrade guide catheter during wire externalization; this is prevented by pushing the long wire rather than pulling it • During mounting of rapid exchange balloons on the externalized wire, it is important not to hold the externalized wire as this may cause the antegrade guide catheter to move forward and dissect the target vessel
Equipment entrapment	• The antegrade balloons/stents must not meet the retrograde microcatheter, this can result in "interlocking" of the equipment, which may require surgery to remove • To prevent this, it is important that the Corsair is withdrawn following wire externalization to a point distal to the CTO in the true lumen but beyond the collateral circulation

also the donor artery through which the retrograde wires and microcatheter are deployed (Tables 28.8 and 28.9).

- The CTO trolley should have a supply of equipment that can be used emergently to deal with such complications, in particular **coils** (specifically those that the operator is familiar with using) and also **covered stents** for perforations.
- A pericardiocentesis kit should be available always, and access to portable echocardiography mandatory.
- Additional complications related to CTO procedures include:
  - Vascular injury at site of sheath insertion (with consequent hematoma, pseudoaneurysm or retroperitoneal hematoma)—CTO procedures may require larger (7 Fr/8 Fr) sheaths with consequent risk of vascular injury and retroperitoneal haematoma.
  - Contrast-induced nephropathy—the use of dual-injections for CTO procedures can result in a large amount of contrast use during procedures. In spite of this, limited contrast injections, especially when traversing the CTO thorough subintimal planes and IV fluid pre-hydration are important to mitigate this risk.
  - Radiation injury—This can be limited by occasionally altering the views and frame rates for the radiographic projections.

Procedural Success Rates with PCI for Chronic Total Occlusions

- Earlier reports of procedural success with CTO PCI suggested this was approximately 60–70% [42]; however, this review covered procedures between 1980 and 1999 using antegrade techniques with earlier technologies.
- Advancement in techniques and guide wire/microcatheter technology in the intervening time, together with more careful evaluation of CTOs including the use of collaterals for retrograde procedures, has increased the procedural success rates. One center employing contemporary retrograde techniques has reported success rates of 90% [43].
- Similarly, procedural success rate was seen to improve over a 4-year course from 60 to 94%, associated with a reduction in number of guide wires used per case and reduction in procedural times [44].
- Within the UK, an analysis of the CCAD database for CTO procedures between 2005 and 2009 demonstrated a success rate of 70.6% [9]. These reflect the procedural success rates of retrograde CTO procedures seen from the ERCTO registry [42].
- Development of new techniques and technologies, together with careful evaluation of the

Table 28.9 Summary of reported complication rates from CTO procedures [40–42]

Study	Death	MI (Q-wave and non-Q-wave)	CVA	Emergency CABG	Vascular complication	Coronary perforation/ tamponade	Contrast-induced nephropathy	Radiation skin injury
Galassi et al. EuroIntervention 2011;7(4):472–479 Antegrade and retrograde from ERCTO registry: 1914 patients and 1983 CTO lesions.	0.3%	1.3%	0.05%	0.1%	0.7%	3.1%	0.9%	–
Patel VG et al. JACC Interv 2013;6(2):128–136 Weighted meta-analysis of 18,061 patients from 65 studies	0.2%	2.7%	<0.01%	0.1%	0.6%	2.9%	3.8%	<0.01%
Galassi AR et al. JACC 2015;65(22):2388–2400 Analysis of retrograde procedures from ERCTO registry: 1395 patients with 1582 CTO lesions	0.2%	0.4%	0%	0.1%	1.0%	3.6%	–	–

angiograms for CTO patients to determine best strategy for performing CTO PCI within experienced centers should lead to improved outcomes for CTO PCI.

Conclusions

- CTOs remain common and an under-treated subset of coronary lesions. This can result in patients languishing for years on medical therapy but with persistent symptoms.
- Initial procedural success rates have improved over time due to use of new strategies, technology and identification of lesion characteristics that can guide interventionists to decide which upfront strategy would be best to deploy.
- Advances in cardiac imaging not only can indicate which lesions should be treated based on ischemia and viability, but can also track the course of CTOs and provide further information to the operator for successful PCI to these lesions.
- Management of CTO lesions requires dedicated operators with skills and expertise in the use of the CTO equipment.
- Recent data from retrospective registries suggest that the benefit of CTO PCI may extend to more than symptom relief, with reduced long-term mortality especially in multivessel disease where complete revascularization with the CTO is performed.

References

1. Sianos G, Werner GS, Galassi AR, et al. Recanalisation of chronic total coronary occlusions: 2012 consensus document from the EuroCTO club. EuroIntervention. 2012;8(1):139–45.
2. Christofferson RD, Lehmann KG, Martin GV, Every N, Caldwell JH, Kapadia SR. Effect of chronic total coronary occlusion on treatment strategy. Am J Cardiol. 2005;95(9):1088–91.
3. Kahn JK. Angiographic suitability for catheter revascularization of total coronary occlusions in patients from a community hospital setting. Am Heart J. 1993;126(3 Pt 1):561–4.
4. Anderson HV, Shaw RE, Brindis RG, et al. A contemporary overview of percutaneous coronary interventions. The American College of Cardiology-National Cardiovascular Data Registry (ACC-NCDR). J Am Coll Cardiol. 2002;39(7):1096–103.
5. Williams DO, Holubkov R, Yeh W, et al. Percutaneous coronary intervention in the current era compared with 1985-1986: the National Heart, Lung, and Blood Institute Registries. Circulation. 2000;102(24):2945–51.
6. Silber S, Albertsson P, Aviles FF, et al. Guidelines for percutaneous coronary interventions. The Task Force for Percutaneous Coronary Interventions of the European Society of Cardiology. Eur Heart J. 2005;26(8):804–47.
7. Smith SC Jr, Feldman TE, Hirshfeld JW Jr, et al. ACC/AHA/SCAI 2005 guideline update for percutaneous coronary intervention—summary article: a report of the American College of Cardiology/American Heart Association Task Force on Practice Guidelines (ACC/AHA/SCAI writing committee to update the 2001 guidelines for percutaneous coronary intervention). Circulation. 2006;113(1):156–75.
8. Grantham JA, Jones PG, Cannon L, Spertus JA. Quantifying the early health status benefits of successful chronic total occlusion recanalization: results from the FlowCardia's Approach to Chronic Total Occlusion Recanalization (FACTOR) Trial. Circ Cardiovasc Qual Outcomes. 2010;3(3):284–90.
9. George S, Cockburn J, Clayton T, Ludman P, Cotton J, Spratt J, Redwood S, de Belder M, de Belder A, Hill J, Hoye A, Palmer N, Rathore S, Gershlick AH, Di Mario C, Hildick-Smith D. Long-term follow-up of elective chronic total coronary occlusion angioplasty. Analysis from the UK Central Cardiac Audit Database. J Am Coll Cardiol. 2014;64:235–43.
10. Melchior JP, Doriot PA, Chatelain P, et al. Improvement of left ventricular contraction and relaxation synchronism after recanalization of chronic total coronary occlusion by angioplasty. J Am Coll Cardiol. 1987;9(4):763–8.
11. Sirnes PA, Myreng Y, Molstad P, Bonarjee V, Golf S. Improvement in left ventricular ejection fraction and wall motion after successful recanalization of chronic coronary occlusions. Eur Heart J. 1998;19(2):273–81.
12. Werner GS, Surber R, Kuethe F, et al. Collaterals and the recovery of left ventricular function after recanalization of a chronic coronary occlusion. Am Heart J. 2005;149(1):129–37.
13. Dzavik V, Carere RG, Mancini GB, et al. Predictors of improvement in left ventricular function after percutaneous revascularization of occluded coronary arteries: a report from the Total Occlusion Study of Canada (TOSCA). Am Heart J. 2001;142(2):301–8.
14. Valenti R, Migliorini A, Signorini U, et al. Impact of complete revascularization with percutaneous coronary intervention on survival in patients with at least one chronic total occlusion. Eur Heart J. 2008;29(19):2336–42.
15. Elhendy A, Cornel JH, Roelandt JR, et al. Impact of severity of coronary artery stenosis and the collateral

circulation on the functional outcome of dyssynergic myocardium after revascularization in patients with healed myocardial infarction and chronic left ventricular dysfunction. Am J Cardiol. 1997;79(7):883–8.

16. Kirschbaum SW, Baks T, van den Ent M, et al. Evaluation of left ventricular function three years after percutaneous recanalization of chronic total coronary occlusions. Am J Cardiol. 2008;101(2):179–85.

17. Warren RJ, Black AJ, Valentine PA, Manolas EG, Hunt D. Coronary angioplasty for chronic total occlusion reduces the need for subsequent coronary bypass surgery. Am Heart J. 1990;120(2):270–4.

18. Hoye A, van Domburg RT, Sonnenschein K, Serruys PW. Percutaneous coronary intervention for chronic total occlusions: the Thoraxcenter experience 1992–2002. Eur Heart J. 2005;26(24):2630–6.

19. Olivari Z, Rubartelli P, Piscione F, et al. Immediate results and one-year clinical outcome after percutaneous coronary interventions in chronic total occlusions: data from a multicenter, prospective, observational study (TOAST-GISE). J Am Coll Cardiol. 2003;41(10):1672–8.

20. Suero JA, Marso SP, Jones PG, et al. Procedural outcomes and long-term survival among patients undergoing percutaneous coronary intervention of a chronic total occlusion in native coronary arteries: a 20-year experience. J Am Coll Cardiol. 2001;38(2):409–14.

21. Hannan EL, Racz M, Holmes DR, et al. Impact of completeness of percutaneous coronary intervention revascularization on long-term outcomes in the stent era. Circulation. 2006;113(20):2406–12.

22. van der Schaaf RJ, Vis MM, Sjauw KD, et al. Impact of multivessel coronary disease on long-term mortality in patients with ST-elevation myocardial infarction is due to the presence of a chronic total occlusion. Am J Cardiol. 2006;98(9):1165–9.

23. Moreno R, Conde C, Perez-Vizcayno MJ, et al. Prognostic impact of a chronic occlusion in a non-infarct vessel in patients with acute myocardial infarction and multivessel disease undergoing primary percutaneous coronary intervention. J Invasive Cardiol. 2006;18(1):16–9.

24. Shaw LJ, Berman DS, Maron DJ, et al. Optimal medical therapy with or without percutaneous coronary intervention to reduce ischemic burden: results from the Clinical Outcomes Utilizing Revascularization and Aggressive Drug Evaluation (COURAGE) trial nuclear substudy. Circulation. 2008;117(10):1283–91.

25. Morino Y, Abe M, Morimoto T, et al. Predicting successful guidewire crossing through chronic total occlusion of native coronary lesions within 30 minutes: the J-CTO (Multicenter CTO Registry in Japan) score as a difficulty grading and time assessment tool. JACC Cardiovasc Interv. 2011;4(2):213–21.

26. Christopoulos G, Wyman RM, Alaswad K, et al. Clinical utility of the Japan-chronic total occlusion score in coronary chronic total occlusion interventions: results from a multicenter registry. Circ Cardiovasc Interv. 2015;8(7):e002171.

27. Di Mario C, Werner GS, Sianos G, et al. European perspective in the recanalisation of Chronic Total Occlusions (CTO): consensus document from the EuroCTO Club. EuroIntervention. 2007;3(1):30–43.

28. McEntegart M, Spratt JC. Procedure planning for chronic total occlusion percutaneous coronary intervention. Interv Cardiol. 2013;5(5):549–57.

29. Singh M, Bell MR, Berger PB, Holmes DR Jr. Utility of bilateral coronary injections during complex coronary angioplasty. J Invasive Cardiol. 1999;11(2):70–4.

30. Brilakis ES, Grantham JA, Rinfret S, et al. A percutaneous treatment algorithm for crossing coronary chronic total occlusions. JACC Cardiovasc Interv. 2012;5(4):367–79.

31. Sianos G, Konstantinidis NV, Di MC, Karvounis H. Theory and practical based approach to chronic total occlusions. BMC Cardiovasc Disord. 2016;16:33.

32. Kahn JK, Hartzler GO. Retrograde coronary angioplasty of isolated arterial segments through saphenous vein bypass grafts. Catheter Cardiovasc Diagn. 1990;20(2):88–93.

33. Surmely JF, Katoh O, Tsuchikane E, Nasu K, Suzuki T. Coronary septal collaterals as an access for the retrograde approach in the percutaneous treatment of coronary chronic total occlusions. Catheter Cardiovasc Interv. 2007;69(6):826–32.

34. Surmely JF, Tsuchikane E, Katoh O, et al. New concept for CTO recanalization using controlled antegrade and retrograde subintimal tracking: the CART technique. J Invasive Cardiol. 2006;18(7):334–8.

35. Rentrop KP, Cohen M, Blanke H, Phillips RA. Changes in collateral channel filling immediately after controlled coronary artery occlusion by an angioplasty balloon in human subjects. J Am Coll Cardiol. 1985;5(3):587–92.

36. Werner GS, Ferrari M, Heinke S, et al. Angiographic assessment of collateral connections in comparison with invasively determined collateral function in chronic coronary occlusions. Circulation. 2003;107(15):1972–7.

37. Rathore S, Katoh O, Matsuo H, Terashima M, Tanaka N, Kinoshita Y, Kimura M, Tsuchikane E, Nasu K, Ehara M, Asakura K, Asakura Y, Suzuki T. Retrograde percutaneous recanalization of chronic Total occlusion of coronary arteries: procedural outcomes and predictors of success in contemporary practice. Circ Cardiovasc Interv. 2009;2:124–32.

38. Joyal D, Thompson CA, Grantham JA, Buller CEH, Rinfert S. The retrograde tecnhique for recanalization of chronic total occlusions: a step-by-step approach. JACC Cardiovasc Interv. 2012;5(1):1–12.

39. Dautov R, Urena M, Nguyen CM, Gibrat C, Rinfert S. Safety and effectiveness of the surfing technique to cross septal collateral channels during retrograde chronic total occlusion percutaneous coronary intervention. Eurointervention. 2016;Jaa-015-2016. https://doi.org/10.4244/EIJ-D-6-00650.

40. Galassi AF, Tomasello SD, Reifart N, et al. In-hospital outcomes of percutaoneous coronary intervention

in patients with chronic total occlusions: insights from the ERCTO (European Registry of Chronic Total Occlusion) registry. EuroIntervention. 2011;7(4):472–9.

41. Patel VG, Bryaton KM, Tamayo A, MOgabgab O, MIchael TT, Lo N, Alomar M, Shorrock D, Cipher D, Abdullah S, Banerjee S, Brilakis ES. Angiographic success and procedural complications in patients undergoing percutaneous coronary chronic Total occlusion interventions: a weighted meta-analysis of 18,061 patients from 65 studies. JACC Cardiovasc Interv. 2013;6(2):128–36.

42. Galassi AF, Sianos G, Werner GS, et al. Retrograde recanalization of chronic total occlusions in Europe: procedural, in-hospital and long term outcomes from the multi-Centre ERCTO Registry. J Am Coll Cardiol. 2015;65(22):2388–400.

43. Rathore S, Katoh O, Tuschikane E, Oida A, Suzuki T, Takase S. A novel modification of the retrograde approach for the recanalization of chronic total occlusion of the coronary arteries intravascular ultrasound-guided reverse controlled antegrade and retrograde tracking. JACC Cardiovasc Interv. 2010;3(2):155–64.

44. Wang K, Chen C, Chen Y, Tsai J, Lin W, Cheng H, Yeh H, Hou CJ. Improving success rates of percutaneous coronary intervention for chronic total occlusion at a rural Hospital in East Taiwan. Int J Gerontol. 2014;8(3):157–61.

Multivessel Coronary Artery Disease

29

Mina Owlia and Sripal Bangalore

About Us

New York University Langone medical center is one of the USA's premier academic medical centers. It is ranked No. 3 medical school for research (U.S. news 2019), No. 10 in the nation on U.S. News & World Report's "Best Hospitals 2016–2017" Honor Roll. The cardiac catheterization laboratory is among the top in the nation with expertise in coronary intervention including complex coronary intervention, peripheral intervention, and structural heart disease.

Management of Multivessel Coronary Artery Disease in Stable Ischemic Heart Disease

Clinical Vignette: 65 y/o man with hypertension, diabetes mellitus, and obesity presents with stable angina after 3 flights of stairs. The patient undergoes nuclear stress testing which shows reversible ischemia in the anterior and inferior territories with preserved left ventricular ejection fraction. He undergoes a left heart catheterization which shows an 80% mid left anterior descending artery stenosis and a 70% mid right coronary artery stenosis.

Introduction

- Among patients with stable ischemic heart disease (SIHD), multivessel disease (MVD) is not uncommon. Moreover, a greater number of vessel stenosis or occlusions sequentially portends a worse prognosis [1].
- The optimal treatment for SIHD is a topic of ongoing debate, and a number of important clinical characteristics must be considered prior to deciding on a management strategy. The treatment options for MVD in patients with SIHD are shown below in Fig. 29.1.
- The treatment goals in patients with MVD are to: (1) improve survival and/or (2) relieve symptom burden.

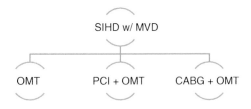

Fig. 29.1 Management options for patients with SIHD and MVD. Key: *SIHD* stable ischemic heart disease, *MVD* multivessel disease, *OMT* optimal medical therapy, *PCI* percutaneous coronary intervention, *CABG* coronary artery bypass grafting

M. Owlia · S. Bangalore (✉)
The Leon H. Charney Division of Cardiology, New York University School of Medicine,
New York, NY, USA

© Springer International Publishing AG, part of Springer Nature 2018
A. Myat et al. (eds.), *The Interventional Cardiology Training Manual*,
https://doi.org/10.1007/978-3-319-71635-0_29

What Are the Management Strategies?

Optimal Medical Therapy (OMT)

- Risk factor modification through a combination of lifestyle interventions and medical therapy is the cornerstone of management of SIHD. Atherosclerosis is a systemic condition and lifestyle and medical therapy can therefore address not only significant coronary plaques but also less significant ones (which are more prone to rupture and result in acute coronary syndromes).
- OMT is also important in patients undergoing revascularization and post hoc analysis has shown lower mortality with OMT in revascularized patients (with either percutaneous coronary intervention—PCI, or coronary artery bypass graft surgery—CABG) when compared with patients without OMT [2].
- In addition to pharmacologic therapy, OMT is aimed at dietary modification, smoking cessation, promoting daily physical activity, weight management, and risk factor control.
- OMT is defined by guidelines as the following [3]:
  - Antianginal medication: beta-blocker or calcium channel blocker as first line
  - Antiplatelet agents: aspirin (or clopidogrel)
  - Lipid lowering therapy: statins (or ezetimibe in statin intolerant patients)
- While the importance of OMT for all patients with SIHD is undisputed, beyond these recommended classes of medication, there is considerable debate on the titration of medical therapy to specific goals, such as systolic blood pressure targets.
- Randomized trials with an OMT arm have widely variable rates of OMT, reflecting challenges with adherence, even in the setting of highly selected populations, such as those participating in clinical trials.
- Moreover, there is no clear consensus as to what constitutes OMT beyond antiplatelet therapy, lipid lowering, and blood pressure reduction, especially as it relates to reduction of hard outcomes such as death or myocardial infarction (MI).

Percutaneous Coronary Intervention

- There has been significant progress in PCI from the early era of plain old balloon angioplasty (POBA) to bare metal stents (BMS) to first and second generation drug-eluting stents (DES).
- In addition to progress in stent technology (see Chap. 11), there has been considerable progress in tools used, antiplatelet and anticoagulant strategies, making the procedure less invasive and more safer.
- Accordingly, the volume of PCI performed for MVD has increased tremendously over the past decade, while CABG surgeries have substantially declined [4].
- PCI in patients with SIHD and MVD targets lesions that are angiographically and/or functionally significant and can potentially relieve areas of ischemia, resulting in faster relief of angina.
- However, PCI alone (without OMT) is a spot treatment of atherosclerosis for a rather systemic problem and is therefore suboptimal.

Coronary Artery Bypass Graft Surgery

- CABG remains the treatment of choice for patients with complex coronary artery disease, including those with left main coronary artery disease and those with three-vessel disease, although this paradigm has been challenged more recently by landmark trials such as NOBLE and EXCEL (see Chap. 27).
- CABG treats not only the severe culprit lesion but also the non-culprit less severe stenosis in the bypass segment.
- Similar to PCI, there has been significant progress in CABG with the advent of less invasive options, off-pump bypass (e.g., CORONARY Trial, N Engl J Med 2016; 375:2359–2368) and multi arterial revascularization.

What Is the Evidence for Each Treatment Strategy in Patients with SIHD and MVD?

Medical Therapy vs. Revascularization

- Whether revascularization reduces cardiovascular events in patients with SIHD is controversial, however overall evidence suggests a greater/more rapid reduction in angina compared to OMT.

- There has been considerable evolution in pharmacological and technological therapies and as such earlier trials (before 2000) comparing medical therapy to revascularization are no longer reflective of contemporary practice.
- Key trials from the current era of OMT and revascularization techniques evaluating are summarized below:

1. **Clinical Outcomes Utilizing Revascularization and Aggressive Drug Evaluation (COURAGE) [5, 6]:**
   - **Study Objective**: Comparison of PCI (mainly BMS) in addition to OMT versus OMT alone in 2287 patients with SIHD for the primary endpoint of death or MI.
   - Two-thirds of patients had MVD (30% of patients had 2-vessel coronary artery disease—CAD, while 39% had 3-vessel CAD).
   - There was no statistically significant difference in the primary outcome (19% PCI vs. 18.5% OMT, $p = 0.62$). The results were similar in patients with MVD (HR = 1.04, 95% CI 0.84–1.30).
   - A greater proportion of patients in the PCI group were angina free but this was no longer statistically significant at 36 months when compared with OMT alone.
   - Study limitations include usage of BMS and high percentage of crossovers from OMT to PCI (33% at 5 years).

2. **Bypass Angioplasty Revascularization Investigation 2 Diabetes (BARI 2D) [7, 8]:**
   - **Study Objective**: Comparison of prompt revascularization with CABG or PCI in addition to OMT versus OMT alone in 2368 diabetic patients with SIHD for the primary endpoint of all-cause mortality.
   - 67% of the randomized patients had 2- or 3-vessel CAD.
   - No difference in the 5-year survival rate among patients in the revascularization arm versus OMT arm.

- Revascularization with PCI did not reduce the risk of death or MACE (death, MI, or stroke), however CABG did lead to a reduction in nonfatal MI in patients with MVD compared to OMT [9].
- Revascularization strategy at 3 years had a lower rate of worsening angina (8% vs. 13%; $P < 0.001$), new angina (37% vs. 51%; $P < 0.001$), and subsequent coronary revascularizations (18% vs. 33%; $P < 0.001$) and a higher rate of angina-free status (66% vs. 58%; $P < 0.003$) when compared with OMT alone, with greater benefit in the subgroup with 3-vessel CAD [8].
- Study limitations include low usage of DES (35%) (all first generation) and high percentage of crossovers from OMT to revascularization (42% at 5 years).

3. **Fractional Flow Reserve Versus Angioplasty for Multivessel Evaluation (FAME 2) [10]:**
   - **Study Objective**: Comparison of outcomes between fractional flow reserve (FFR)-guided PCI with 2nd generation DES + OMT vs. OMT alone.
   - Approximately 24% of the patents had 2 or more angiographically significant lesions.
   - The trial was stopped prematurely after FFR-guided PCI demonstrated a markedly reduced incidence in the primary endpoint of death, MI, or urgent revascularization (4.3% vs. 12.7%, $p = 0.001$), a difference largely driven by a decrease in urgent revascularization (1.6% vs. 11.1%, $p < 0.001$), with no difference in death or MI.

4. **Surgical Treatment for Ischemic Heart Failure (STICH) trial [11]:**
   - **Study Objective**: Comparison of 1212 patients with an ejection fraction of 35% or less and coronary artery disease amenable to CABG randomized to OMT alone versus CABG + OMT.
   - There was no significant difference in the primary endpoint of all-cause mortality between CABG + OMT and OMT

alone (HR = 0.86; 95% CI 0.72–1.04; P = 0.12) at a median of 56 months of follow-up. However, death from cardiovascular causes (HR = 0.81; 95% CI 0.66–1.00; P = 0.05) and death from any cause or hospitalization for cardiovascular causes (HR = 0.74; 95% CI 0.64–0.85; P < 0.001) occurred less frequently in the CABG group.

- Moreover, in the longer term follow-up study (STICHES), at 10 years, CABG was associated with a significant reduction in all of the above endpoints when compared with OMT alone [12].

5. **Meta-Analyses**:
- A number of meta-analyses have evaluated the role of revascularization (especially PCI) when compared with medical therapy alone in patients with SIHD.

- The studies have shown no difference in death or MI with revascularization when compared with medical therapy except for reduction in angina pectoris (Fig. 29.2).

- Other meta-analyses have shown a reduction in spontaneous MI but increase in procedural MI with PCI when compared with OMT (Fig. 29.3). This was also seen in the FAME 2 trial where after 7 days, the rate of death or MI was significantly lower with PCI when compared with OMT alone.

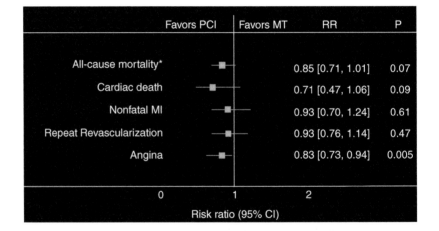

Fig. 29.2 PCI vs. medical therapy (MT) in SIHD. Results from a meta-analysis of 12 randomized trials that enrolled 7182 patients [13]

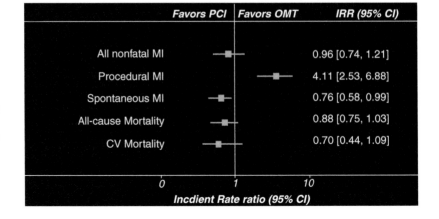

Fig. 29.3 PCI vs. optimal medical therapy (OMT) in SIHD for the outcome of spontaneous MI. Results from a meta-analysis of 12 randomized trials with 37,548 patient-years of follow-up [14]

PCI vs. CABG in MVD

- It is essential to note that several important trials comparing CABG to PCI for patients with MVD compared CABG to PCI using older generation technology (POBA, BMS, or 1st generation DES) [15]. Newer generation DES have thinner struts and more biocompatible polymers and studies have shown a reduction in not only restenosis but also death, MI, and stent thrombosis when compared with first generation DES or BMS. The evolution in technology with newer generation stents has stimulated a shift toward a decreasing "mortality gap" between PCI and CABG, as shown in Fig. 29.4 [16].

1. **Future Revascularization Evaluation in Patients with Diabetes Mellitus (FREEDOM) trial** [17]:
   - **Study Objective**: Comparison of outcomes with CABG vs. PCI using 1st generation DES in 1900 patients with MVD (without left main stenosis) and DM for the reduction of the primary outcome, a composite of all-cause death, nonfatal MI, and stroke
   - Primary outcome was significantly lower in the CABG arm compared to PCI, irrespective of SYNTAX score, with divergence at approximately 2 years, largely driven by reduction of all-cause mortality and significantly lower rates of MI in favor

of CABG. Similar to multiple other studies, the rates of stroke were significantly higher in the CABG arm.
   - Importantly, both PCI and CABG lead to significant improvements in quality of life, but notably more rapid improvement in health status in the PCI group.
   - Limitations include the use of 1st generation DES (especially paclitaxel-eluting stents) that have been shown to be inferior to 2nd generation DES [18].

2. **Synergy between PCI with Taxus and Cardiac Surgery Trial (SYNTAX)** [19]:
   - **Study Objective**: Comparison of CABG versus PCI with Taxus Express (paclitaxel-eluting) first generation DES in 1800 patients with triple vessel or left main disease, designed to show non-inferiority trial of PCI for the rates of major cardiovascular and cerebrovascular events.
   - At 1 year, rates of major adverse cardiovascular and cerebrovascular event (MACCE) rates were significantly lower in the CABG group compared to PCI (12.4% vs. 17.8%, $p = 0.002$), (demonstrating inferiority of PCI compared to CABG), as well as secondary higher rates of repeat revascularization in the PCI group, but higher rates of stroke in the CABG arm.
   - Patients with high SYNTAX scores (≥33), and therefore more complex disease who

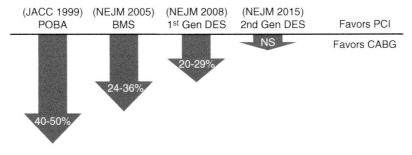

Fig. 29.4 Diminishing mortality gap between PCI and CABG for multivessel disease in a New York Registry. Reproduced from Bangalore S [16]. Outcomes with percutaneous coronary intervention (PCI) versus coronary artery bypass graft (CABG) for multivessel disease from the New York State registries published in the last two decades indicated a diminishing mortality gap between PCI and CABG. There was 40–50% lower mortality with CABG compared with plain old balloon angioplasty (POBA), which has progressively diminished to statistically nonsignificant when CABG is compared with PCI using newer generation drug-eluting stents (DES). Key: *BMS* bare-metal stent, *Gen* generation, *JACC Journal of the American College of Cardiology, NEJM New England Journal of Medicine, NS* not significant

underwent PCI had higher rates of MACCE and the composite of death, stroke and MI compared to those who underwent CABG (11.9% vs. 7.6%, $p = 0.08$). For patients with low (0 to 22) or intermediate SYTAX scores (23 to 32), the 12 month event rates were similar with either revascularization strategy.

- It is important to note that approximately one-fourth of the clinical events occurring in the PCI group were due to stent thrombosis, an outcome that has largely been attributed to the use of 1st generation DES.
- Limitations include the use of 1st generation DES (especially paclitaxel-eluting stents) which have been shown to be inferior to 2nd generation DES [18], and being underpowered for the outcome of death or MI.

3. **The Randomized Comparison of Coronary Artery Bypass Surgery and Everolimus-Eluting Stent Implantation in the Treatment of Patients with Multivessel Coronary Artery Disease (BEST) trial** [20]:
   - **Study Objective**: Comparison of PCI with everolimus-eluting stents (EES) versus CABG on a background of OMT in 880 patients with MVD to show the non-inferiority of PCI for the primary endpoint, a composite of death, MI, or target-vessel revascularization.
   - The study was terminated early secondary to poor enrollment. The primary endpoint occurred in 11% of patients in PCI group versus 7.9% in CABG group at 2 years ($P = 0.32$ for non-inferiority). At longer term follow-up, PCI was associated with a significant increase in the incidence of the primary endpoint, as compared with CABG, a difference largely attributable to target-vessel revascularization. There was no significant difference in the composite safety endpoint of death, MI, or stroke, though rates of new-lesion revascularization and spontaneous MI were higher after PCI compared to CABG.
   - Limitations include premature termination of the trial and hence being grossly underpowered even for the primary composite

outcome and also for the hard endpoint of death or MI.

4. **Observational Studies and Meta-analyses**: To date well-powered randomized trials comparing CABG versus PCI using newer generation DES are lacking. Reliance on prior trials such as SYNTAX and FREEDOM for decision-making is problematic as the stents used in those trials are no longer in clinical practice. If the mortality benefit of CABG as shown in SYNTAX and FREEDOM persists when compared with newer generation DES, CABG should be preferentially used in the majority of patients with MVD. Observational studies therefore provide some insights and are hypothesis generating.

a. In patients with diabetes mellitus, evidence from indirect comparison of 68 randomized trials that enrolled 24,015 diabetic patients with a total of 71,595 patient-years of follow-up showed similar mortality between CABG and PCI using 2nd generation DES (especially cobalt–chromium EES) (Fig. 29.5). CABG was associated with numerically excess stroke and PCI with cobalt–chromium EES with numerically increased repeat revascularization [21].

b. In an analysis from the New York State angioplasty registry, the risk of death associated with PCI with newer generation DES (EES) was similar to that associated with CABG. PCI was associated with a higher risk of MI (among patients with incomplete revascularization) and repeat revascularization but a lower risk of stroke (Fig. 29.6) [22]. Thus PCI with EES is a reasonable option especially if complete revascularization is achieved.

c. Even in patients with diabetes, and contrary to the findings from the FREEDOM trial, analysis from the New York State angioplasty registry showed that PCI with EES was associated with lower up-front risk of death and stroke when compared with CABG surgery (Fig. 29.7). However, in the long-term, EES was associated with a similar risk of death, a higher risk of MI (in those with incomplete revascularization), and repeat revascularization but a lower risk of stroke [23].

Outcome: Mortality

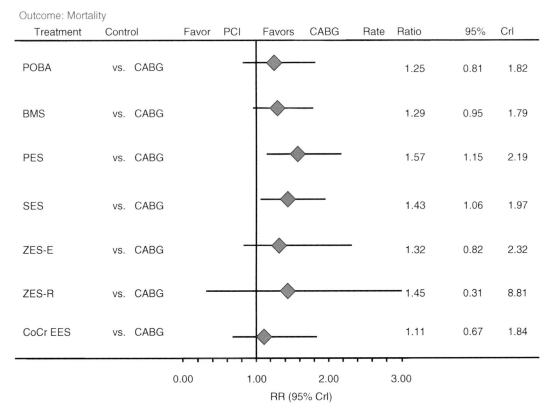

Fig. 29.5 Bridging of the mortality gap between PCI and CABG with newer generation DES. Data from a network analysis of randomized trials. Reproduced from Bangalore et al. [21]. Key: *POBA* plain old balloon angioplasty, *BMS* bare metal stent, *PES* paclitaxel-eluting stent, *SES* sirolimus-eluting stents, *ZES-E* zotarolimus-eluting stent endeavour, *ZES-R* zotarolimus-eluting stent resolute, *CoCr EES* cobalt-chromium everolimus-eluting stent

d. In patients with MVD and left ventricular systolic dysfunction, where CABG has been historically preferred, analysis from the New York State angioplasty registry showed that PCI with EES had comparable long-term survival in comparison with CABG. PCI was associated with a higher risk of MI (in those with incomplete revascularization) and repeat revascularization, and CABG was associated with a higher risk of stroke (Fig. 29.8) [21].

e. The results from these studies suggest that the decision to choose between PCI and CABG should be made after weighing the short-term risk of death or stroke with CABG against the longer-term risk of repeat revascularization with PCI. We should also take into consideration the ability to achieve complete revascularization with PCI and patient preference. The outcomes of CABG when compared with

2nd generation DES should be tested in a well-powered randomized trial.

Focus on Decision-Making

- The decision for a particular elective treatment strategy for the patient with SIHD and MVD, whether with revascularization by either modality or with OMT without revascularization involves an integrated evaluation of the patient's comorbidities, clinical disease burden and anatomic characteristics as well as careful attention to the patient's informed preferences.

- For many patients, decision-making may be based on a balance of the up-front versus long-term risks and benefits with a particular treatment modality.

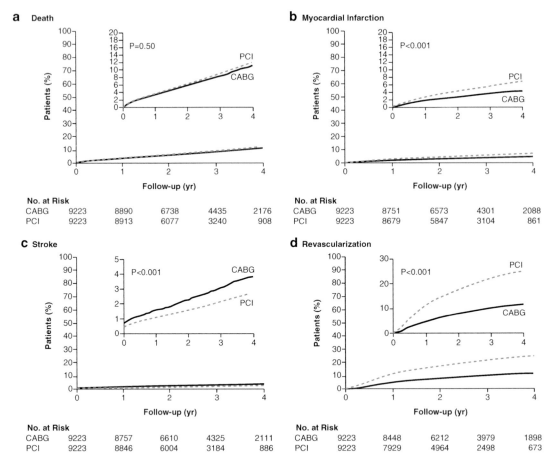

Fig. 29.6 Outcomes with PCI with everolimus-eluting stent (EES) vs. CABG in patients with multivessel disease. Reproduced from Bangalore et al. [22]

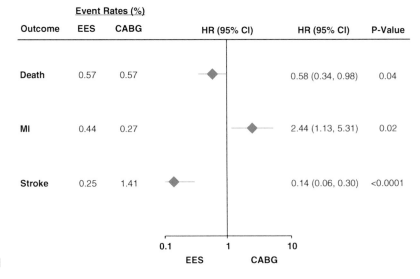

Fig. 29.7 Short-term (within 30 days) outcomes with PCI using everolimus-eluting stents (EES) vs. CABG in patients with diabetes mellitus and multivessel disease. Reproduced from Bangalore et al. [23]

Fig. 29.8 Long-term death with PCI using everolimus-eluting stents (EES) vs. CABG in patients with left ventricular systolic dysfunction and multivessel disease. Reproduced from Bangalore et al. [24]

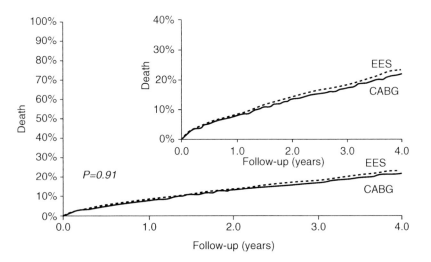

- The physician must exercise caution to avoid bias when presenting options to the patient.
- The cornerstone of the decision-making process should be the discussion of the patient with a multidisciplinary Heart Team, which involves a collaboration of interventional cardiologists, cardiac surgeons and clinical cardiologists [25].
- A Heart Team approach is an evidence-based, class I recommendation for patients with complex CAD that should utilize several of the validated tools for risk stratification listed below prior to selecting a treatment approach [9, 26, 27].
- Key Components of the Heart Team Approach:
  - Risk of periprocedural morbidity and mortality:
    Society of Thoracic Surgeon's (STS) score: Risk calculator for CABG (and valvular surgery) to predict perioperative and 30-day mortality [28]
    EuroSCORE II: Updated model to predict surgical perioperative mortality [29]
    National Cardiovascular Database Registry (NCDR CathPCI) risk score: Can predict risk in PCI patients [30]
  - Coronary anatomy:
    SYNTAX score: A weighted anatomical assessment of lesion complexity in patients with left main or MVD [9, 19].
    SYNTAX II score: Offers a more individualized approach to revascularization

decision-making by incorporating clinical variables in addition to coronary anatomy.
Go to: www.syntaxscore.com
  - Age
    ACEF model: Age, creatinine, and ejection fraction (EF): A simple model that has been shown to predict mortality with PCI [31]
  - Additional comorbidities which may impact the patient's life expectancy
  - Patient preferences
  - Consideration of the patient's symptoms, functional status, and quality of life
  - Institutional protocols and operator experience

Future Directions

- The International Study of Comparative Health Effectiveness with Medical and Invasive Approaches (ISCHEMIA) is an ongoing study which aims to provide outcomes on patients with SIHD including multivessel CAD with at least moderate ischemia on stress testing randomized to a conservative strategy of OMT versus optimal revascularization with PCI or CABG.
- Go to: https://www.ischemiatrial.org/
- Go to: https://clinicaltrials.gov/ct2/show/NCT01471522

Controversies and Considerations in the Management of Multivessel Coronary Artery Disease in Patients Presenting with ST-Segment Elevation Myocardial Infarction

Clinical Vignette: *56 y/o man presents with acute onset typical chest pain for 2 h. EKG shows 3 mm anterior ST-segment elevation. Emergent coronary angiography shows 100% proximal LAD thrombus and an 80% mid RCA lesion. How should this patient be managed?*

Introduction

- Approximately 50% of patients suffering an ST-elevation myocardial infarction (STEMI) have significant MVD, or non-culprit lesions.
- These patients have worse outcomes due to higher mortality and increased risk of recurrent MI when compared with patients with single-vessel disease [32–34].
- The recommendations for culprit-only PCI versus complete or staged revascularization in the setting of STEMI are dynamic, and have been an ongoing area of controversy, in large

part secondary to the lack of adequately powered trials to assess important clinical endpoints.

- Based on the current literature and guidelines, in the case of STEMI with evidence of concomitant severe non-culprit lesions, there are multiple approaches (Fig. 29.9).

Outcomes in Patients with MVD and STEMI

- The clinical significance of MVD in patients presenting with STEMI has been explored previously and has shown a substantial increase in the risk of cardiovascular morbidity and mortality compared to patients with single-vessel disease [35].
- When compared with patients with STEMI and 1-vessel CAD, patients with STEMI and MVD have increase in the incidence of [35–37]:
  - Recurrent acute coronary syndromes
  - Repeat revascularization, particularly of non-culprit lesions
  - CABG surgery
  - MACCE
  - Mortality

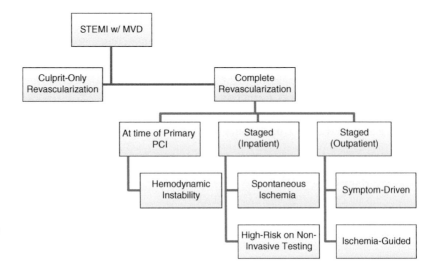

Fig. 29.9 Management options for patients with STEMI and MVD (see also Chap. 16)

Pathophysiology of Increased Risk with MVD in STEMI

- The mechanisms driving increased adverse outcomes in patients with STEMI and MVD are not well elucidated as it is unknown if the presence of a greater burden of disease or inadequately treated and potentially unstable lesions are implicated.
- In the TAMI study, patients with MVD had lower ejection fraction despite having the same extent of infarction as patients with single-vessel disease. This lower ejection fraction was attributed to a significant difference in the function of the non-infarct zone, which was hyperkinetic in the group with minimal or single-vessel disease but was hypocontractile or dyskinetic in those with MVD [38].
- Data from the TAMI trial indicate that enhanced function of the non-infarct zone was associated with preservation of the acute ejection fraction, and the most powerful clinical factor associated with this enhanced function was the absence of MVD [38].
- Inhospital mortality was closely related to function in the non-infarct zone, ejection fraction, and the number of diseased vessels but was not related to infarct zone function. Therefore, it can be hypothesized that a combination of infarcted or stunned myocardium (resulting from culprit artery occlusion) and dysfunctional and hibernating myocardium (from non-culprit artery stenosis) may not be conducive for maintenance of adequate pump function and would lead to adverse clinical outcomes [38].
- Moreover, it has been demonstrated that in patients with acute MI, flow in non-culprit vessels can be slowed, likely due to an enhanced systemic inflammatory response and vasospasm [39]. The presence of severe stenosis in the non-culprit artery in this setting would lead to further hemodynamic compromise to the non-infarct myocardium zone leading to a decrease in left ventricular function and an increase in the risk of cardiovascular events.

- Increase in atherosclerotic burden and ischemia in MVD.
- Decrease in myocardial reserve which may lead to less tolerance to hemodynamic imbalances and for arrhythmias.
- These findings underscore the systemic nature of plaque instability and suggest that patients with MVD may benefit from aggressive clinical strategies aimed at improving/preserving the function of non-infarct-related, but potentially jeopardized, myocardium, as well as by reducing subsequent myocardial ischemia

Culprit-Only Revascularization vs. Complete Revascularization

Two schools of thought exist regarding revascularization strategy for MVD during STEMI.

Opponents of Multivessel Revascularization

- This largely stems from concerns about safety of the second procedure:
  - Concern for increased radiation dose
  - Increased contrast utilization
  - Increased procedural complications
  - Increase in the risk of stent thrombosis given a prothrombotic, proinflammatory state
  - Increase in inhospital adverse outcomes
  - Increased length of hospital stay

Proponents of Multivessel Revascularization

- This is based on the premise that recent advancements in endovascular technology and adjunctive pharmacotherapy have led multivessel PCI to be feasible and safe and hence multivessel revascularization:
  - Avoids staged procedures, with subsequent savings in cost and procedural risks from a second procedure.
  - Would afford protection against plaque rupture of bystander lesions and prevention

of recurrent MI, refractory ischemia, and death (given the systemic nature of the atherosclerotic process, multiple unstable plaques are frequently seen).

- Potentially leads to faster improvement in left ventricular function [40].

Randomized Clinical Trials

Seven randomized clinical trials to date have been performed to evaluate the optimal revascularization strategy at the time of primary PCI (Table 29.1) [41]. The individual results for major outcomes from four of the large contemporary trials are shown in Fig. 29.10.

- These seven trials (2004 patients in total) demonstrate the following for efficacy and safety outcomes:
  - **Death or MI**: reduction of the composite of death or MI with complete vs. culprit-

only revascularization (OR, 0.71; 95% CI, 0.52–0.96; $P = 0.03$). However, more robust analyses taking into consideration the required sample size showed that there was lack of firm evidence for a 25% reduction in death/recurrent MI with multivessel PCI compared with culprit-only revascularization (Fig. 29.11) [49].

- **All-cause mortality and cardiovascular mortality**: insufficient evidence (inadequate power of trials) [41].
- **Non-fatal MI**: insufficient evidence (inadequate power of trials) [41].
- **Repeat revascularization**: reduction with complete vs. culprit-only revascularization (9.6% vs. 20.2%) [41].
- **Contrast-induced nephropathy**: no statistical difference with complete revascularization vs. culprit only, however significantly increased contrast volume and procedure time with complete revascularization [41].

Table 29.1 Summary of randomized controlled trials evaluating culprit vs. multivessel PCI in patients with STEMI

Trial	Year	Sample size	Follow-up (months)	Staged PCI for CR (%)
CvLPRIT [42]	2014	296	12	27
Dambrink et al. [43]	2010	121	6	100
HELP AMI [44]	2004	69	12	0
Politi L et al. [45]	2010	214	30	50
PRAMI [46]	2013	465	23	0
DANAMI-3-PRIMULTI [47]	2015	627	27	100
PRAGUE 13 [48]	2015	214	38	100

Key: *CR* complete revascularization, *CvLPRIT* (complete versus culprit-lesion only primary PCI), *HELP-AMI* (hepacoat for culprit or multivessel stenting for acute myocardial infarction)

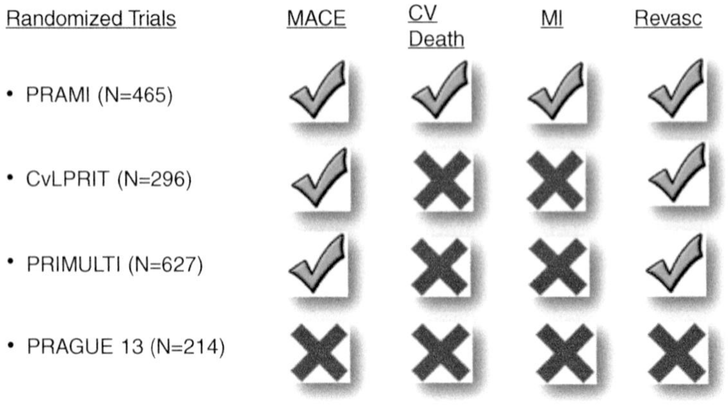

Fig. 29.10 Culprit-only versus complete revascularization for patients with STEMI and MVD from four contemporary trials. A green tick indicates benefit of complete revascularization whilst a red cross indicates no difference when compared with culprit-only revascularization

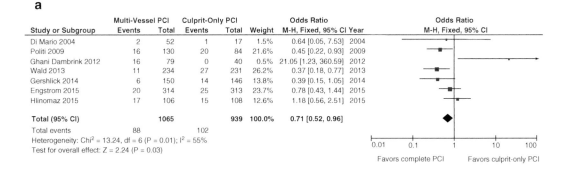

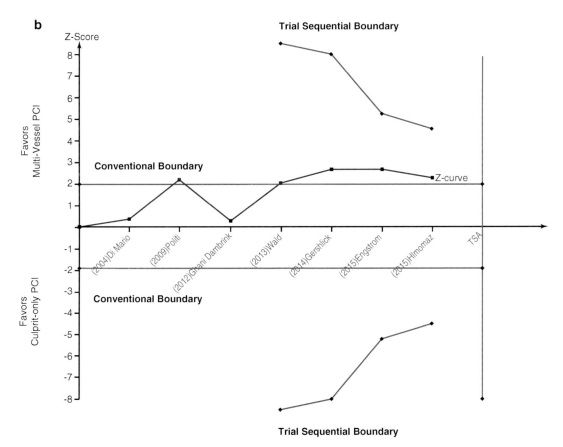

Fig. 29.11 Culprit-only versus complete revascularization for patients with STEMI and MVD for the outcome of death or MI (**a**). Trial sequential analysis shows that the cumulative z-curve crosses the conventional boundary but not the trial sequential monitoring boundary indicating lack of firm evidence for benefit of complete revascularization over culprit revascularization (**b**). Reproduced from Bainey et al. [49]

Guideline Recommendations
(Table 29.2)

- Previously, the ACC/AHA guidelines stated that PCI in a non-culprit artery in patients with STEMI should not be performed at the time of primary PCI, classified as Class IIIB (harm) [50, 51].

- These recommendations were based largely on observational data which suggested an increase in mortality when non-culprit artery revascularization was attempted at the time of primary PCI [51, 52].

- As discussed above, data from randomized trials seem to suggest improved outcomes with

Table 29.2 Summary of current guideline recommendations for revascularization at the time of primary angioplasty

Guideline	Recommendation	Level of recommendation
2015 ACC/AHA/SCAI Focused Update on PPCI for Patients With ST-Elevation Myocardial Infarction [53]	**At time of PPCI (or planned staged)**: PCI of non-IRA may be considered in selected patients with STEMI and MVD who are hemodynamically stable	**Class IIb LOE B-R**[a]
	Before Hospital Discharge: PCI in non-IRA in patients with spontaneous symptoms of myocardial ischemia	**Class I LOE C**
	Before Hospital Discharge: PCI in non-IRA in patients with intermediate or high risk findings on noninvasive testing	**Class IIa LOE B**
2014 ESC/EACTS Guidelines on Myocardial Revascularization [26]	**At the time of PPCI**: PPCI should be limited to IRA with exception of cardiogenic shock and persistent ischemia after PCI of IRA	**Class IIa LOE B**
	At time of PPCI: Immediate revascularization of significant non-IRA may be considered in selected patients	**Class IIb LOE C**
	Staged PCI: Revascularization of non-IRA may be considered in case of symptoms or ischemia within days to weeks after PPCI	**Class IIa LOE B**

[a]Moderate quality evidence from ≥1 RCTs and/or meta-analyses of moderate quality RCTs
Key: *PPCI* primary percutaneous coronary intervention, *IRA* infarct-related artery, *LOE* level of evidence, *STEMI* ST-segment elevation myocardial infarction, *MVD* multivessel disease

regard to MACE and repeat revascularization with complete revascularization and these trials have led to a paradigm shift in the understanding of the safety and efficacy of complete revascularization at the time of primary PCI [53].

Timing of Revascularization: Decision-Making for a Staged Approach to Multivessel Disease

- As reflected in the above guidelines, revascularization can be considered at multiple time frames, either in the inpatient or outpatient setting.
- The optimal timing for revascularization of MVD following a STEMI is not well defined. Overall, data from largely observational studies suggests that staged revascularization leads to superior outcomes with decreased risk of mortality, MACCE, and stent thrombosis with both short- and long-term outcomes compared to revascularization performed during the index PCI [54, 55].
- There are multiple considerations based on patient-related characteristics when deciding on

timing strategy, and both anatomical and functional assessments that should be incorporated.

Anatomic Considerations in STEMI and MVD

- Lesion severity may be overestimated at the time of STEMI secondary to catecholamine-mediated vasoconstriction and endothelial dysfunction.
- Extent of myocardial territories at risk.
- Appearance of multiple plaque ruptures present.
- Lesions more suitable for coronary artery bypass grafting (chronic total occlusions, extensive calcification, or tortuosity).

Functional Assessment

- Ischemia-guided revascularization
- Symptom-guided revascularization
- FFR-guided revascularization

Patient Factors

- Hemodynamic status at the time of index PCI.
- Risk of contrast nephropathy (baseline renal function, age, volume of contrast load administered).
- Risk of congestive heart failure (volume of contrast load, ejection fraction, respiratory status).
- Hospital duration and related costs.

Use of Fractional Flow Reserve in Patients Presenting with STEMI and Non-culprit MVD

- The adjunctive use of Fractional Flow Reserve (FFR) to guide PCI has been well validated in the SIHD population to improve ischemic outcomes and reduce costs when compared to PCI based on angiography alone [56].

- The use of FFR to guide revascularization of non-culprit artery lesions is supported by the DANAMI-3-PRIMULTI trial, which demonstrated a reduction in a composite endpoint of all-cause mortality, nonfatal MI, and ischemia-driven revascularization of non-culprit arteries when performed within 48 h of index PCI [47].

Future Directions

- The ongoing, multicenter randomized Complete vs. Culprit-only Revascularization to Treat Multi-vessel Disease After Primary PCI for STEMI (COMPLETE – NCT01740479) trial aims to determine whether a strategy of complete revascularization with staged PCI of all severe non-culprit arteries is superior to a culprit-only strategy for reducing cardiovascular death or MI in patients with STEMI.

- While there is growing evidence that complete revascularization during the index admission may reduce future events, the optimal timing and value of functional assessment remains unknown.

References

1. Emond M, Mock MB, Davis KB, et al. Long-term survival of medically treated patients in the Coronary Artery Surgery Study (CASS) Registry. Circulation. 1994;90(6):2645–57.
2. Iqbal J, Zhang YJ, Holmes DR, et al. Optimal medical therapy improves clinical outcomes in patients undergoing revascularization with percutaneous coronary intervention or coronary artery bypass grafting: insights from the Synergy Between Percutaneous Coronary Intervention with TAXUS and Cardiac Surgery (SYNTAX) trial at the 5-year follow-up. Circulation. 2015;131(14):1269–77.
3. Task Force M, Montalescot G, Sechtem U, et al. 2013 ESC guidelines on the management of stable coronary artery disease: the Task Force on the management of stable coronary artery disease of the European Society of Cardiology. Eur Heart J. 2013;34(38):2949–3003.
4. Riley RF, Don CW, Powell W, Maynard C, Dean LS. Trends in coronary revascularization in the United States from 2001 to 2009: recent declines in percutaneous coronary intervention volumes. Circ Cardiovasc Qual Outcomes. 2011;4(2):193–7.
5. Boden WE, O'Rourke RA, Teo KK, et al. Optimal medical therapy with or without PCI for stable coronary disease. N Engl J Med. 2007;356(15):1503–16.
6. Weintraub WS, Spertus JA, Kolm P, et al. Effect of PCI on quality of life in patients with stable coronary disease. N Engl J Med. 2008;359(7):677–87.
7. Group BDS, Frye RL, August P, et al. A randomized trial of therapies for type 2 diabetes and coronary artery disease. N Engl J Med. 2009;360(24):2503–515.
8. Dagenais GR, Lu J, Faxon DP, et al. Effects of optimal medical treatment with or without coronary revascularization on angina and subsequent revascularizations in patients with type 2 diabetes mellitus and stable ischemic heart disease. Circulation. 2011;123(14):1492–500.
9. Fihn SD, Gardin JM, Abrams J, et al. ACCF/AHA/ACP/AATS/PCNA/SCAI/STS Guideline for the diagnosis and management of patients with stable ischemic heart disease: a report of the American College of Cardiology Foundation/American Heart Association Task Force on Practice Guidelines, and the American College of Physicians, American Association for Thoracic Surgery, Preventive Cardiovascular Nurses Association, Society for Cardiovascular Angiography and Interventions, and Society of Thoracic Surgeons. J Am Coll Cardiol. 2012;60(24):e44–e164.
10. De Bruyne B, Pijls NH, Kalesan B, et al. Fractional flow reserve-guided PCI versus medical therapy in stable coronary disease. N Engl J Med. 2012;367(11):991–1001.
11. Velazquez EJ, Lee KL, Deja MA, et al. Coronary-artery bypass surgery in patients with left ventricular dysfunction. N Engl J Med. 2011;364(17):1607–16.
12. Velazquez EJ, Lee KL, Jones RH, et al. Coronary-artery bypass surgery in patients with ischemic cardiomyopathy. N Engl J Med. 2016;374(16):1511–20.
13. Pursnani S, Korley F, Gopaul R, et al. Percutaneous coronary intervention versus optimal medical therapy in stable coronary artery disease: a systematic review and meta-analysis of randomized clinical trials. Circ Cardiovasc Interv. 2012;5(4):476–90.
14. Bangalore S, Pursnani S, Kumar S, Bagos PG. Percutaneous coronary intervention versus optimal medical therapy for prevention of spontaneous myocardial infarction in subjects with stable ischemic heart disease. Circulation. 2013;127(7):769–81.
15. Daemen J, Boersma E, Flather M, et al. Long-term safety and efficacy of percutaneous coronary intervention with stenting and coronary artery bypass surgery for multivessel coronary artery disease: a meta-analysis with 5-year patient-level data from

the ARTS, ERACI-II, MASS-II, and SoS trials. Circulation. 2008;118(11):1146–54.

16. Bangalore S. Applicability of the COURAGE, BARI 2D, and FREEDOM trials to contemporary practice. J Am Coll Cardiol. 2016;68(10):996–8.

17. Farkouh ME, Domanski M, Sleeper LA, et al. Strategies for multivessel revascularization in patients with diabetes. N Engl J Med. 2012;367(25):2375–84.

18. Kaul U, Bangalore S, Seth A, et al. Paclitaxel-eluting versus Everolimus-eluting coronary stents in diabetes. N Engl J Med. 2015;373(18):1709–19.

19. Serruys PW, Morice MC, Kappetein AP, et al. Percutaneous coronary intervention versus coronary-artery bypass grafting for severe coronary artery disease. N Engl J Med. 2009;360(10):961–72.

20. Park SJ, Ahn JM, Kim YH, et al. Trial of Everolimus-eluting stents or bypass surgery for coronary disease. N Engl J Med. 2015;372(13):1204–12.

21. Bangalore S, Toklu B, Feit F. Outcomes with coronary artery bypass graft surgery versus percutaneous coronary intervention for patients with diabetes mellitus: can newer generation drug-eluting stents bridge the gap? Circ Cardiovasc Interv. 2014;7(4):518–25.

22. Bangalore S, Guo Y, Samadashvili Z, Blecker S, Xu J, Hannan EL. Everolimus-eluting stents or bypass surgery for multivessel coronary disease. N Engl J Med. 2015;372(13):1213–22.

23. Bangalore S, Guo Y, Samadashvili Z, Blecker S, Xu J, Hannan EL. Everolimus eluting stents versus coronary artery bypass graft surgery for patients with diabetes mellitus and multivessel disease. Circ Cardiovasc Interv. 2015;8(7):e002626.

24. Bangalore S, Guo Y, Samadashvili Z, Blecker S, Hannan EL. Revascularization in patients with multivessel coronary artery disease and severe left ventricular systolic dysfunction: everolimus-eluting stents versus coronary artery bypass graft surgery. Circulation. 2016;133(22):2132–40.

25. Head SJ, Kaul S, Mack MJ, et al. The rationale for Heart Team decision-making for patients with stable, complex coronary artery disease. Eur Heart J. 2013;34(32):2510–8.

26. Kolh P, Windecker S, Alfonso F, et al. ESC/EACTS Guidelines on myocardial revascularization: the Task Force on Myocardial Revascularization of the European Society of Cardiology (ESC) and the European Association for Cardio-Thoracic Surgery (EACTS). Developed with the special contribution of the European Association of Percutaneous Cardiovascular Interventions (EAPCI). Eur J Cardiothorac Surg. 2014;46(4):517–92.

27. Feit F, Brooks MM, Sopko G, et al. Long-term clinical outcome in the Bypass Angioplasty Revascularization Investigation Registry: comparison with the randomized trial. BARI Investigators. Circulation. 2000;101(24):2795–802.

28. Shahian DM, O'Brien SM, Filardo G, et al. The Society of Thoracic Surgeons 2008 cardiac surgery risk models: part 3—valve plus coronary artery bypass grafting surgery. Ann Thorac Surg. 2009;88(1 Suppl):S43–62.

29. Nashef SA, Sharples LD, Roques F, Lockowandt U. EuroSCORE II and the art and science of risk modelling. Eur J Cardiothorac Surg. 2013;43(4):695–6.

30. Peterson ED, Dai D, DeLong ER, et al. Contemporary mortality risk prediction for percutaneous coronary intervention: results from 588,398 procedures in the National Cardiovascular Data Registry. J Am Coll Cardiol. 2010;55(18):1923–32.

31. Wykrzykowska JJ, Garg S, Onuma Y, et al. Value of age, creatinine, and ejection fraction (ACEF score) in assessing risk in patients undergoing percutaneous coronary interventions in the 'All-Comers' LEADERS trial. Circ Cardiovasc Interv. 2011;4(1):47–56.

32. Park DW, Clare RM, Schulte PJ, Pieper KS, Shaw LK, Califf RM, Ohman EM, Van de Werf F, Hirji S, Harrington RA, Armstrong PW, Granger CB, Jeong MH, Patel MR. Extent, location, and clinical significance of non-infarct-related coronary artery disease among patients with ST-elevation myocardial infarction. JAMA. 2014;312:2019–27.

33. van der Schaaf RJ, Timmer JR, Ottervanger JP, Hoorntje JC, de Boer MJ, Suryapranata H, Zijlstra F, Dambrink JH. Long-term impact of multivessel disease on cause-specific mortality after ST elevation myocardial infarction treated with reperfusion therapy. Heart. 2006;92:1760–3.

34. Sorajja P, Gersh BJ, Cox DA, McLaughlin MG, Zimetbaum P, Costantini C, Stuckey T, Tcheng JE, Mehran R, Lansky AJ, Grines CL, Stone GW. Impact of multivessel disease on reperfusion success and clinical outcomes in patients undergoing primary percutaneous coronary intervention for acute myocardial infarction. Eur Heart J. 2007;28:1709–16.

35. Bangalore S, Faxon D. Coronary intervention in patients with acute coronary syndrome: does every culprit lesion require revascularization? Curr Cardiol Rep. 2010;12:330–7.

36. Goldstein JA, Demetriou D, Grines CL, Pica M, Shoukfeh M, O'Neill WW. Multiple complex coronary plaques in patients with acute myocardial infarction. N Engl J Med. 2000;343:915–22.

37. Corpus RA, House JA, Marso SP, Grantham JA, Huber KC Jr, Laster SB, Johnson WL, Daniels WC, Barth CW, Giorgi LV, Rutherford BD. Multivessel percutaneous coronary intervention in patients with multivessel disease and acute myocardial infarction. Am Heart J. 2004;148:493–500.

38. Muller DW, Topol EJ, Ellis SG, Sigmon KN, Lee K, Califf RM. Multivessel coronary artery disease: a key predictor of short-term prognosis after reperfusion therapy for acute myocardial infarction. Thrombolysis and Angioplasty in Myocardial Infarction (TAMI) Study Group. Am Heart J. 1991;121:1042–9.

39. Gibson CM, Ryan KA, Murphy SA, Mesley R, Marble SJ, Giugliano RP, Cannon CP, Antman EM, Braunwald E. Impaired coronary blood flow in non-culprit arteries in the setting of acute myocardial infarction. The TIMI Study Group Thrombolysis in myocardial infarction. J Am Coll Cardiol. 1999;34:974–82.

40. Ochala A, Smolka GA, Wojakowski W, Dudek D, Dziewierz A, Krolikowski Z, Gasior Z, Tendera M. The function of the left ventricle after complete multivessel one-stage percutaneous coronary intervention in patients with acute myocardial infarction. J Invasive Cardiol. 2004;16:699–702.

41. Bangalore S, Toklu B, Wetterslev J. Complete versus culprit-only revascularization for ST-segment-elevation myocardial infarction and multivessel disease: a meta-analysis and trial sequential analysis of randomized trials. Circ Cardiovasc Interv. 2015;8:e002142.

42. Gershlick AH, Khan JN, Kelly DJ, Greenwood JP, Sasikaran T, Curzen N, Blackman DJ, Dalby M, Fairbrother KL, Banya W, Wang D, Flather M, Hetherington SL, Kelion AD, Talwar S, Gunning M, Hall R, Swanton H, McCann GP. Randomized trial of complete versus lesion-only revascularization in patients undergoing primary percutaneous coronary intervention for STEMI and multivessel disease: the CvLPRIT trial. J Am Coll Cardiol. 2015;65:963–72.

43. Dambrink JH, Debrauwere JP, van 't Hof AW, Ottervanger JP, Gosselink AT, Hoorntje JC, de Boer MJ, Suryapranata H. Non-culprit lesions detected during primary PCI: treat invasively or follow the guidelines? EuroIntervention. 2010;5:968–75.

44. Di Mario C, Mara S, Flavio A, Imad S, Antonio M, Anna P, Emanuela P, Stefano DS, Angelo R, Stefania C, Anna F, Carmelo C, Antonio C, Monzini N, Bonardi MA. Single vs multivessel treatment during primary angioplasty: results of the multicentre randomised HEpacoat for cuLPrit or multivessel stenting for Acute Myocardial Infarction (HELP AMI) Study. Int J Cardiovasc Interv. 2004;6:128–33.

45. Politi L, Sgura F, Rossi R, Monopoli D, Guerri E, Leuzzi C, Bursi F, Sangiorgi GM, Modena MG. A randomised trial of target-vessel versus multi-vessel revascularisation in ST-elevation myocardial infarction: major adverse cardiac events during long-term follow-up. Heart. 2010;96:662–7.

46. Wald DS, Morris JK, Wald NJ, Chase AJ, Edwards RJ, Hughes LO, Berry C, Oldroyd KG, Investigators P. Randomized trial of preventive angioplasty in myocardial infarction. N Engl J Med. 2013;369:1115–23.

47. Engstrom T, Kelbaek H, Helqvist S, Hofsten DE, Klovgaard L, Holmvang L, Jorgensen E, Pedersen F, Saunamaki K, Clemmensen P, De Backer O, Ravkilde J, Tilsted HH, Villadsen AB, Aaroe J, Jensen SE, Raungaard B, Kober L, Investigators D-P. Complete revascularisation versus treatment of the culprit lesion only in patients with ST-segment elevation myocardial infarction and multivessel disease (DANAMI-3-PRIMULTI): an open-label, randomised controlled trial. Lancet. 2015;386:665–71.

48. Hlinomaz O. Multivessel coronary disease diagnosed at the time of primary PCI for STEMI: complete revascularization versus conservative strategy: the PRAGUE 13 trial. EuroPCR, May 19, 2015; Paris, France.

49. Bainey KR, Welsh RC, Toklu B, Bangalore S. Complete vs culprit-only percutaneous coronary intervention in STEMI with multivessel disease: a meta-analysis and trial sequential analysis of randomized trials. Can J Cardiol. 2016;32:1542–51.

50. O'Gara PT, Kushner FG, Ascheim DD, Casey DE Jr, Chung MK, De Lemos JA, Ettinger SM, Fang JC, Fesmire FM, Franklin BA, Granger CB, Krumholz HM, Linderbaum JA, Morrow DA, Newby LK, Ornato JP, Ou N, Radford MJ, Tamis-Holland JE, Tommaso CL, Tracy CM, Woo YJ, Zhao DX, Anderson JL, Jacobs AK, Halperin JL, Albert NM, Brindis RG, Creager MA, DeMets D, Guyton RA, Hochman JS, Kovacs RJ, Kushner FG, Ohman EM, Stevenson WG, Yancy CW, American College of Emergency Physicians, Society for Cardiovascular Angiography and Interventions. ACCF/AHA guideline for the management of ST-elevation myocardial infarction: a report of the American College of Cardiology Foundation/American Heart Association Task Force on Practice Guidelines. J Am Coll Cardiol. 2013;61:e78–140.

51. Toma M, Buller CE, Westerhout CM, Fu Y, O'Neill WW, Holmes DR Jr, Hamm CW, Granger CB, Armstrong PW, APEX AMI Investigators. Non-culprit coronary artery percutaneous coronary intervention during acute ST-segment elevation myocardial infarction: insights from the APEX-AMI trial. Eur Heart J. 2010;31:1701–7.

52. Hannan EL, Samadashvili Z, Walford G, Holmes DR Jr, Jacobs AK, Stamato NJ, Venditti FJ, Sharma S, King SB 3rd. Culprit vessel percutaneous coronary intervention versus multivessel and staged percutaneous coronary intervention for ST-segment elevation myocardial infarction patients with multivessel disease. JACC Cardiovasc Interv. 2010;3:22–31.

53. Levine GN, Bates ER, Blankenship JC, Bailey SR, Bittl JA, Cercek B, Chambers CE, Ellis SG, Guyton RA, Hollenberg SM, Khot UN, Lange RA, Mauri L, Mehran R, Moussa ID, Mukherjee D, Ting HH, O'Gara PT, Kushner FG, Ascheim DD, Brindis RG, Casey DE Jr, Chung MK, de Lemos JA, Diercks DB, Fang JC, Franklin BA, Granger CB, Krumholz HM, Linderbaum JA, Morrow DA, Newby LK, Ornato JP, Ou N, Radford MJ, Tamis-Holland JE, Tommaso CL, Tracy CM, Woo YJ, Zhao DX. 2015 ACC/AHA/SCAI focused update on primary percutaneous coronary intervention for patients with ST-elevation myocardial infarction: an update of the 2011 ACCF/AHA/SCAI guideline for percutaneous coronary intervention and the 2013 ACCF/AHA guideline for the management of ST-elevation myocardial infarction. J Am Coll Cardiol. 2016;67:1235–50.

54. Kornowski R, Mehran R, Dangas G, Nikolsky E, Assali A, Claessen BE, Gersh BJ, Wong SC, Witzenbichler B, Guagliumi G, Dudek D, Fahy M, Lansky AJ, Stone GW, Investigators H-AT. Prognostic impact of staged versus "one-time" multivessel percutaneous intervention in acute myocardial infarction: analysis from the HORIZONS-AMI (harmonizing outcomes

with revascularization and stents in acute myocardial infarction) trial. J Am Coll Cardiol. 2011;58:704–11.

55. Vlaar PJ, Mahmoud KD, Holmes DR Jr, van Valkenhoef G, Hillege HL, van der Horst IC, Zijlstra F, de Smet BJ. Culprit vessel only versus multivessel and staged percutaneous coronary intervention for multivessel disease in patients presenting with ST-segment elevation myocardial infarction: a pairwise and network meta-analysis. J Am Coll Cardiol. 2011;58:692–703.

56. Tonino PA, De Bruyne B, Pijls NH, Siebert U, Ikeno F, van' t Veer M, Klauss V, Manoharan G, Engstrom T, Oldroyd KG, Ver Lee PN, MacCarthy PA, Fearon WF, Investigators FS. Fractional flow reserve versus angiography for guiding percutaneous coronary intervention. N Engl J Med. 2009;360:213–24.

Secondary Percutaneous Revascularization After Coronary Artery Bypass Graft Surgery

Jean Paul Vilchez-Tschischke, Hernán David Mejía-Rentería, Nieves Gonzalo, Philip Francis Dingli, Pablo Salinas, and Javier Escaned

About Us

The Interventional Cardiology Unit of Hospital Clinico San Carlos (Madrid, Spain) has an extensive track record in clinical, research and educational aspects of interventional cardiology. Most of the clinical work is performed in 6 catheterization laboratories: 3 located inside HCSC and dedicated to both coronary procedures and structural heart interventions, and 3 additional cath labs for coronary procedures are located out of the main hospital building. The cath labs are fully equipped for functional coronary assessment (integrated pressure wire [FFR and iFR], Doppler velocity and thermodilution [CFR and IMR]) and intracoronary imaging (IVUS and OCT), and are open 24 hours 7 days a week for primary PCI.

The unit runs a very active international research fellowship program (more than 200 fellows from 25 countries since 1995) and a 2-year Masters degree in Interventional Cardiology with the Complutense University of Madrid. Since 1995 the Interventional Cardiology Unit has generated over 900 publications listed in PubMed (more than 60 publications in PubMed per year over the last 4 years). Fellows are encouraged to get involved in clinical research activities. Methodology skills are facilitated by on-site full-time personnel, including a physicist with programming skills and an MD dedicated to research data management. Fellows are invited to get involved in clinical trials (a program supported by 8 full-time study coordinators) and to develop research protocols that will be submitted for Ethics Review Board approval. In addition to major clinical trials our center participates in numerous EU and internationally funded projects. Major areas of research include complex PCI and new devices, physiology of coronary epicardial vessels and the microcirculation, intracoronary imaging, secondary revascularization, primary PCI in STEMI, structural heart interventions, and cell therapy.

From an educational perspective the unit is involved in multiple international courses as a live case center (including EuroPCR and TCT). Over the year multiple workshops with on-site live case transmissions are held, including EuroPCR seminars, dedicated courses on CTO revascularization and complex PCI, and workshops on novel diagnostic and therapeutic techniques.

J. P. Vilchez-Tschischke · H. D. Mejía-Rentería
N. Gonzalo · P. F. Dingli · P. Salinas · J. Escaned (✉)
Interventional Cardiology Unit, Department
of Cardiology, Hospital Universitario Clínico San
Carlos IDISSC and Universidad Complutense de
Madrid, Madrid, Spain
e-mail: escaned@secardiologia.es

© Springer International Publishing AG, part of Springer Nature 2018
A. Myat et al. (eds.), *The Interventional Cardiology Training Manual*,
https://doi.org/10.1007/978-3-319-71635-0_30

Introduction

- Secondary revascularization procedures encompass all interventions following an index coronary revascularization procedure, be it percutaneous or surgical, regardless of whether they relate to the original stenosis or other arterial territory.
- The focus of this chapter is on secondary revascularization procedures in the setting of prior CABG. Secondary revascularization procedures are complex procedures associated with higher procedure-related complications and mortality, as well as higher rates of target vessel failure and need of revascularization.
- Secondary revascularization procedures are associated with the presence of multiple cardiovascular risk factors that trigger aggressive atherosclerosis, resulting in diffuse stenosis and chronic total occlusions which are often calcified and progress rapidly, limiting surgical and percutaneous revascularization options [1–3].
- Furthermore, patients presenting for secondary revascularization are usually older and with a high-risk profile, frequently including left ventricular systolic dysfunction, diabetes mellitus, hypertension, and acute coronary syndromes [2].
- The need for secondary revascularization increases dramatically in the second decade after CABG [1, 2, 4–6]. Between 29 and 68% of SVGs are occluded after 10 years post surgery [7–10].
- Adaptation of vein grafts to their new arterial environment is characterized by structural vessel wall remodelling and intimal thickening [11]. Factors that contribute to long-term failure of SVG are constrictive remodelling, intimal hyperplasia, thrombosis, and unstable atherosclerotic lesions [10]. The systemic arterial pressure stressing the thin wall of the veins contribute to the atherosclerotic degeneration process.
- Over the last three decades secondary revascularization procedures have increased substantially in part due to increased longevity paired with the risk of target vessel failure with time [1]. Another important factor is that accessi-bility to coronary revascularization has increased over the last 20 years, as new laboratories are created, and preexisting ones increase their activity.
- Data on secondary coronary revascularization rates is limited. The 2001–2002 European Heart Survey on coronary revascularization collected the complete data of 5619 consecutive patients undergoing invasive coronary angiography, showing that 11% had a previous CABG surgery, and of those patients, 57.9% required a secondary revascularization procedure, either percutaneous (88.2%) or surgical (11.8%) [12].
- Prior CABG patients represented 17.5% of the total PCI volume (300,902 of 1,721,046) in the National Cardiovascular Data Registry. In the latter the PCI target was a native coronary artery in 62.5% of the cases and a bypass graft in 37.5% (SVG, 34.9%; arterial graft, 2.5%; both SVG and arterial graft, 0.2%) [13].
- The Veterans Affairs Clinical Assessment, Reporting, and Tracking Program reported that patients with prior CABG represented 18.5% of all patients undergoing PCI (11,118 of 60,171), bypass grafts were the target vessel in 26.6% (SVG, 25.0%; arterial graft, 1.5%) [14].
- When considering patients only with STEMI, data from the British Cardiovascular Intervention Society showed that those who had prior CABG represent 3.4% (2658 of 76,637), of whom 44% underwent primary PCI to native vessels and 56% to bypass grafts [15].
- From these observational studies, it is apparent that repeat revascularization procedures in CABG patients makes up a considerable part of the average cath-lab workload.

Decision-Making on Secondary Revascularization After CABG Surgery

- The decision to perform repeat myocardial revascularization in patients with previous coronary surgery should be based on symptoms, response to antiangina medications, extent of ischemia in noninvasive tests, and the presence and location of significant coronary stenosis [16].

- According to the latest European guidelines for myocardial revascularization, routine stress testing may be considered in asymptomatic patients with more than 5 years after CABG [8].
- In certain circumstances, particularly in cases of suboptimal or incomplete revascularization, diabetic or multivessel disease patients with residual intermediate lesions, or where there is a suspicion of silent ischemia, early imaging testing should be considered even when the patient is asymptomatic [17].
- Patients with ischemia at low-workload in stress testing, with multiple zones of high-grade wall motion abnormalities affecting more than 10% of the left ventricle wall or reverse perfusion defect are considered at intermediate to high risk and coronary angiography is recommended.
- Otherwise, in patients with low-risk findings at stress testing, medical therapy optimization and lifestyle changes are recommended [8].
- Due to the complexity of these patients it is important that decisions are taken within the Heart Team, involving interventional and clinical cardiologists, as well as cardiac surgeons.
- The modality of repeat revascularization has shifted over the last 30 years. In the 80s re-do coronary surgery was the preferred treatment [7, 18], followed by a period of conservative

management [2]. Currently only 3–4% of CABG patients undergo re-do CABG [19].

- Even though clinical practice guidelines recommendations have been limited on this issue historically, new guidelines include dedicated sections on secondary revascularization. The 2009 Appropriateness Criteria for Coronary Revascularization document endorsed by several American scientific societies [20], updated in 2012 [16], has a specific section regarding patients with prior bypass surgery.
- The ESC guidelines on myocardial revascularization also provide new recommendations on secondary revascularization [8, 21]. In general, the level of evidence in many of the recommendations is C, meaning that evidence supporting expert opinions is limited (Table 30.1). There are several contributory factors to this lack of evidence, most importantly being that patients with prior CABG have been systematically excluded from RCTs.
- The 2014 ESC clinical guidelines recommend that the decision on re-do CABG or PCI should be made by ad hoc consultation in the Heart Team, based on the feasibility of revascularization, area at risk, comorbidities, and clinical status (class I, level of evidence C), considering PCI as the first choice if technically feasible rather than re-do surgery (class IIa, level of evidence C), if PCI is performed, revascularization of the native vessels or ITA grafts rather than SVGs should be considered (class IIa, level of evidence C) [8].

Table 30.1 2014 ESC Guideline recommendations for disease progression and late graft failure [8]

Recommendations	Class	LoE
Repeat revascularization is indicated in patients with severe symptoms or extensive ischemia despite medical therapy if technically feasible	I	B
PCI should be considered as a first choice if technically feasible, rather than re-do CABG	IIa	C
PCI of the bypassed native vessels should be the preferred approach, if technically feasible	IIa	C
ITA, if available, is the conduit of choice for redo-CABG	I	B
Re-do CABG should be considered for patients without a patent ITA graft to the LAD	IIa	B
Re-do CABG may be considered in patients with lesions and anatomy not suitable for revascularization by PCI	IIb	C
PCI may be considered in patients with patent ITA graft if technically feasible	IIb	C
DES are recommended for PCI of SVGs	I	A
Distal protection devices are recommended for PCI of SVG lesions if technically feasible	I	B

LoE level of evidence, *ITA* internal thoracic artery, *PCI* percutaneous coronary intervention, *CABG* coronary artery bypass graft surgery, *LAD* left anterior descending artery, *DES* drug-eluting stents, *SVG* saphenous vein graft

- Retrospective studies have demonstrated that both secondary PCI and re-do CABG have a significantly higher risk than de novo revascularization procedures. Five-year mortality has been found to be twice as high in patients undergoing secondary revascularization, either percutaneous (25% vs. 16%) or surgical (21% vs. 14%) compared with de novo procedures [22–24].

- Bypass graft PCI is associated with 30% higher mortality, 61% higher risk for MI, and 60% higher risk for repeat revascularization during long-term follow-up [13, 14, 25, 26]. Surgical series also consistently identified re-do CABG as a predictor of risk [1, 5], with higher inhospital mortality, myocardial infarction (MI), and prolonged ventilation [19].

- Such outcomes are associated with the increased complexity and risk derived from sternum reentry, pericardial adhesions, patent internal mammary artery, and patent but diseased SVGs [27]. Advances in perioperative management, such as minimally invasive incisions, new modalities of myocardial protection, and off-pump interventions, have contributed to a modest reduction in the risk of re-do CABG [22].

- It remains to be seen whether other novel surgical techniques developed to improve the long-term patency of SVG reduce the need of re-do CABG [28, 29].

- Decision-making on the modality of secondary revascularization is influenced by a number of anatomical and clinical features. Surgical re-intervention is preferred in patients at higher risk, with fewer functional grafts, more chronic total occlusions (CTOs), and lower systolic function, as well as the presence of valvular disease likely to require future surgery.

- On the other hand, PCI is the technique of choice in patients with a patent LIMA and favorable coronary anatomy [8]. However, the benefits of choosing one modality over another appear to be limited as prognosis is mostly affected by age and left ventricular ejection fraction.

- Moreover, it seems that patients with patent LIMA to left anterior descending artery (LAD) presenting with ischemia in non-LAD myocardial territories, re-intervention with CABG or PCI of such territories may relieve symptoms but do not provide survival benefits [30].

- In the registry group of the AWESOME trial (Angina With Extremely Serious Operative Mortality Evaluation) [31], a RCT dedicated to secondary revascularization after CABG, both physicians and patients preferred PCI over re-CABG and survival was uniformly higher with PCI, although statistically significant only for the patient-choice registry.

- In this study, patients with previous CABG presenting with refractory ischemic symptoms that underwent re-do CABG had higher inhospital mortality than those that underwent PCI. However, long-term survival (3-year follow-up) was similar between both groups.

- Results regarding long-term outcomes have been confirmed in another observational study (median follow-up of 3.9 years) in which clinical outcomes were similar in both re-PCI and re-do CABG in patients with graft failure, in the composite of all-cause death, MI, or TVR, even though repeat revascularization occurred more frequently after PCI [32]. These results have indicated PCI to be the preferred strategy of re-intervention in patients with patent LIMA and favorable anatomy [8].

- PCI of the bypassed native artery should be the preferred approach provided the native vessel is not chronically occluded. PCI for CTO may be indicated in symptomatic patients with evidence of significant ischemia and viable myocardium. If PCI of the native vessel fails, PCI of the diseased SVG can be an option [8].

- As discussed previously, CABG is preferred for patients with extensively diseased or occluded bypass grafts, reduced systolic LV function, several total occlusions of native arteries, and absence of patent arterial grafts.

- Regarding re-do CABG, LIMA grafts show the best clinical outcomes in patients who did not receive a LIMA during their first CABG [33]. Clinical guidelines recommend LIMA as the conduit of choice for re-do CABG if available, with a class I, level of evidence B [8].

- In patients with a prior LIMA graft, the radial artery seems to have better outcomes at long-term in re-do CABG compared with SVG [34].
- New modalities of percutaneous interventions have been described for the anatomically challenging vascular circuits created by surgical grafting of the coronary arteries [35]; for example, magnetic navigation has been used in complex PCI of patients with prior CABG and other scenarios [36–41]. How these novel techniques will influence outcomes is still uncertain.

Treatment of Native Coronary Arteries in Patients with Prior CABG

- Percutaneous treatment of stenosis located in native vessels constitutes the first alternative to re-do CABG. Long-term failure of SVG more frequently affects the right or circumflex coronary arteries with concomitant patency of a LIMA graft to the LAD. Due to observed better short- and long-term outcomes, PCI of the bypassed native vessel should be the preferred approach whenever feasible [8].
- Typically, however, native coronary vessels in these patients have unfavorable characteristics for PCI, such as diffuse vessel calcification, left main disease, or CTOs.
- The main objectives of native vessel treatment are: (1) restoring vessel patency without affecting functional grafts and (2) optimizing the procedure in order to ensure long-term success.
- Special techniques, such as rotational atherectomy or cutting balloons, may be required to ensure stent crossing and facilitate adequate stent expansion.
- Multi-slice CT imaging may be helpful to map the location of coronary calcifications and determine the characteristics of total occlusions (see Chap. 28). In patients with high atherosclerotic burden, intracoronary imaging is strongly recommended to guide the procedure and to optimize luminal dimensions.

- Drug-eluting stents should be considered to minimize the risk of restenosis. Collateral filling from a functional graft can be useful to guide crossing the wire through a CTO; in some cases, experienced operators use surgical conduits as an alternative to collateral channels to perform retrograde recanalization of CTOs, with high technical success rates, but this may carry an increased risk for complications [42, 43].
- Competitive flow plays a crucial role in arterial graft functionality and this must be taken in consideration when revascularizing a patient; IMAs are the best arterial conduits to withstand competitive flow, thanks to their endothelial function; radial and right gastroepiploic arteries support much less competitive flow due to their different anatomy, histology, and endothelial function, that leads to spasm and occlusion.
- SVGs are not significantly affected by competitive flow, mainly because of its non-resistivity and reimplantation in the aorta. Special consideration must be taken with sequential arterial anastomoses as they are very sensitive to competitive flow [44].

Percutaneous Revascularization of Saphenous Vein Grafts

- Percutaneous intervention of SVG poses a unique set of challenges:
  - The thinner venous wall with coexistent calcified (Fig. 30.1) and soft plaque areas may favor SVG rupture during dilatation, an important consideration in the management of under-expanded stents (Fig. 30.2) [45–47].
  - Furthermore, pericardial tamponade may occur after a vessel or graft perforation even in patients with prior pericardiectomy [48].
- It is important to stress that patients with failing SVG undergoing PCI are at high risk of cardiac events. A very large recent observational study found high rates of adverse clinical outcomes at 3 years follow-up in older patients (median age of 75 years) subjected to

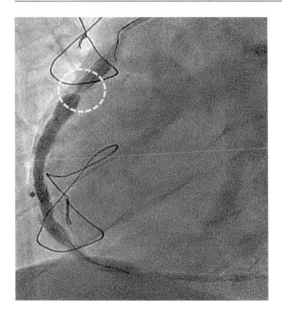

Fig. 30.1 Calcified severe focal stenosis in a degenerated saphenous vein graft (yellow circle) during contrast injection to locate best landing zone for stent deployment; red asterisk shows radiopaque distal filter loop location

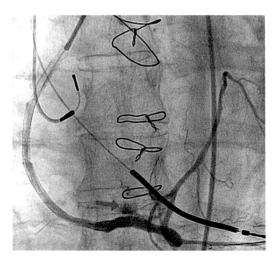

Fig. 30.2 Saphenous vein graft perforation after implantation of a drug-eluting stent, the red arrow points to contrast leakage during control angiography, the bleeding was controlled with 10 min of balloon occlusion and heparin reversion with protamine

SVG PCI: death in 24.5%; MI in 14.6%; urgent revascularization in 29.5% [49].

- Atheroembolism is a frequent cause of complications in SVG PCI. As vein graft degeneration is caused by an accelerated form of atherosclerosis [50], lesions are more concentric, diffuse, and friable and prone to be dislodged by intracoronary devices [11, 51].

- Major CK-MB elevation occurs in 15% of otherwise successful SVG interventions, which is associated with increased mortality at 1-year follow-up [52]. Given this high risk, embolic protection is an important component of SVG PCI.

- The pivotal trial regarding embolic protection was the SAFER trial (Saphenous vein graft Angioplasty Free of Emboli Randomized), an 801-patient, US multicenter study, in which patients undergoing SVG intervention were randomized to undergo either stenting with a conventional guidewire, or with the GuardWire (Medtronic Vascular, Santa Rosa, CA, USA), a distal protection device that enables temporary occlusion of the distal artery and also contains an aspiration system. There was a 42% relative risk reduction (6.9% absolute reduction) in 30-day MI, with greater rates of TIMI 3 flow and a reduction of no-reflow events [53].

- Several RCTs have demonstrated non-inferiority of new devices, compared against the GuardWire or other protection devices, being approved by the FDA, but none against non-protection as it is considered nonethical to perform SVG PCI without the use of EPDs [54–56].

- The guidelines of the American College of Cardiology granted a class I, level of evidence B, recommendation for EPD use in PCI of failed SVG [57]; in 2014 the ESC guidelines on myocardial revascularization made the same recommendation [8].

- Recent data has confirmed EPD use to be a strong predictor of improved postprocedural TIMI flow with lower TVR and a trend towards lower mortality at 1 year. But these associations were not confirmed after 2-year follow-up [58].

- On the other hand, an analysis of the Medicare-linked National Cardiovascular Data Registry CathPCI Registry (49.325 senior patients), between 2005 and 2009, failed to demonstrate any short- or long-term benefits of EPDs.

However, this study has major limitations that preclude definitive conclusions [59].

- It is important to highlight that the use of EPD in real life is only around 21% [59–61]. This limited use of EPD in SVG PCI cannot be justified by technical difficulties such as small vessel diameter or aorto-ostial location, since current technology makes possible both proximal and distal SVG protection [9].

- Embolic protection devices can be categorized according to their mechanism of operation [53, 62–64]:

  - Distal occlusion devices (e.g., GuardWire, PercuSurge, TriActiv system): a balloon is inflated in the SVG several centimeters beyond the target lesion so that the possible liberated plaque remains suspended in the resulting stagnant column of blood. The column of blood and debris generated are aspirated before releasing the occlusion (Fig. 30.3).

  - Distal filters (e.g., FilterWire—Figs. 30.3 and 30.4): they trap particulate debris, especially those of more than 100 μm, allowing distal perfusion, maintaining the possibility of contrast imaging during operation. As the device has to cross the lesion, there is a potential risk of dislodgement before the device can be deployed.

  - Proximal occlusion devices (e.g., Proxis system): they occlude the inflow proximal to a target lesion to suspend antegrade flow during PCI (Fig. 30.3). As with distal occlusion devices, stagnant blood containing suspended debris particles must be evacuated before restoring flow. Potential benefits include complete recovery of particles of all sizes, including humoral substances, the establishment of protection before any device is passed across the target lesion, the ability to protect vessels with multiple side branches or distal lesions prohibitive for distal protection devices, and compatibility with conventional guidewires. To use these devices the patient should have adequate collaterals that ensure distal perfusion during occlusion.

- Local plaque trapping has been considered another option to prevent distal embolism. Several randomized clinical trials have compared covered stents with BMS in the treatment of SVG stenosis.

- The JoMed polytetrafluoroethylene (PTFE) covered stainless steel stent (JoMed, Abbott Vascular, Santa Clara, CA, USA) was tested in 3 trials (RECOVERS [Randomized Evaluation of polytetrafluoroethylene COVERed Stent in SVG], STING [STents IN Grafts trial], and BARRICADE [Barrier Approach to Restenosis: Restrict Intima to Curtail ADverse Events]) enrolling a total of 755 patients in SVG [65–67].

- In the RECOVERS trial the incidence of 30-day MACE was higher in the PTFE group (10.9% vs. 4.1%), mainly attributed to MI (10.3% vs. 3.4%). The restenosis rate at 6-month follow-up was similar between the 2 groups. The 6-month non-Q-wave MI rate was higher in the PTFE group (12.8% vs. 4.1%) [65].

- In the STING trial restenosis rate was not significantly different between the Flex (20%) and the Stentgraft (29%) groups, although there was a nonsignificant trend towards a higher late occlusion rate in the Stentgraft group (7% vs. 16%) at follow-up. After 14 months of follow-up, cumulative event rates were comparable in the two groups (31% vs. 31%) [66].

- In the BARRICADE study, that included 243 patients, restenosis occurred in 31.8% of lesions treated with the Jostent versus 28.4% of lesions treated with BMS ($p = 0.63$). At 9 months, the major secondary endpoint of target vessel failure occurred in 32.2% of patients treated with the Jostent versus 22.1% of patients treated with BMS ($p = 0.08$). During long-term follow-up, significantly more events occurred in the Jostent arm, such that by 5 years target vessel failure had occurred in 68.3% of Jostent patients versus 51.8% of BMS patients ($p = 0.007$), despite high pressure implantation and prolonged dual antiplatelet therapy [67].

- The PTFE-covered stent Symbiot™ (Boston Scientific, Natick, MA, USA) was tested in

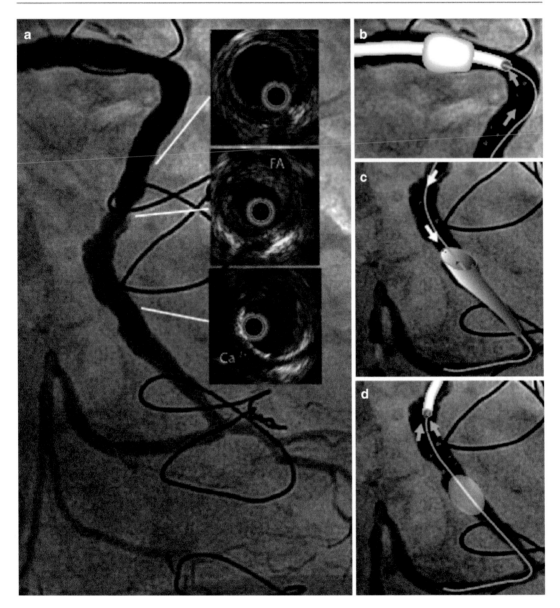

Fig. 30.3 Embolic protection devices (EPD) used in percutaneous revascularization of saphenous vein grafts. EPD increase safety of percutaneous revascularization by decreasing the risk of embolism of dislodged atheroma during intervention. Panel **a** shows angiographic and intravascular ultrasound (IVUS) images obtained during PCI in a degenerated SVG anastomosed to an obtuse marginal branch. IVUS images reveal the heterogeneity of atheromatous graft involvement, with abundant soft fibroatheroma (FA) at the location of the target stenosis and calcification (Ca^{2+}) in a more distal segment. Right panels (**b–d**) illustrate schematically the mechanism of action of the three different EPD devices. Proximal EPD (**b**) use an atraumatic compliant balloon occluder to block antegrade flow during PCI, with manual aspiration (yellow arrows) of dislodged atheromatous particles before restoring antegrade flow. The balloon and/or stent are not shown in the picture. Filter EPD (**c**) are made of porous synthetic material that allow antegrade blood flow (white arrows) during the intervention but impede distal embolization of debris. Distal occlusive EPD (**d**) are compatible with PCI equipment and used similarly to conventional PCI guidewires. An atraumatic distal balloon occluder is inflated before and during the SVG intervention. Following coronary intervention, an aspiration catheter (shown in panel **d**) is advanced and manual aspiration (yellow arrows) of the accumulated debris is performed with a dedicated intracoronary catheter (shown in the picture) before the balloon is deflated (First published: Escaned, J. Secondary revascularization after CABG surgery. Nat. Rev. Cardiol. 9, 540–9; 2012) [42]

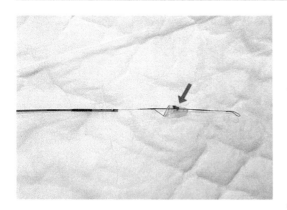

Fig. 30.4 Atherothrombotic particle (red arrow) captured in the filtration system of the FilterWire EZ™ during PCI of an SVG

the randomized SYMBIOT III trial [68]. This study included 400 patients undergoing SVG PCI, showing no benefit over BMS, but a trend towards higher TVR in the Symbiot arm at 8 months follow-up. Moreover, the Symbiot stent failed to show advantages regarding clinical outcomes at long-term (mean 7 years) compared with BMS [69].

- The MGuard™ stent (InspireMD, Boston, MA, USA), a balloon-expandable close-cell design bare metal stent with a polyethylene terephthalate microfiber sleeve attached to its outer surface, has been tested in two clinical trials with an excellent rate of procedural success [70], but a high rate of MACE (23%) in 20-months follow-up [71], or 20% need of ischemia-driven repeat target vessel revascularization at 12 months [72].

- The AneuGraft® (ITGI Medical, Or Akiva, Israel) is a pericardium-covered stent, composed of an equine pericardium cylinder covering a stainless steel stent, pre-mounted on a delivery catheter, evaluated in the SLEEVE II registry, that included 47 patients and showed a technical success of 89.1%, with a cumulative MACE incidence at 30 days of 10.6% [73]. Neither of these covered stent designs have been tested in randomized clinical trials in SVG PCI.

- The use of mesh-covered stents in SVG is not reflected in the 2014 Guidelines focused update based on the very limited experience with these devices [8]. Due to the lack of evidence on the safety of these stent designs to prevent distal embolization [74], *their use should not be considered as an alternative to EPDs in SVG PCI.*

- The most sensible recommendation at the present time is to use them in combination or under occasional circumstances, which might preclude the use of available EPDs. Covered stents, particularly of the membrane-covered type, are extremely useful in treating SVG perforations during PCI [75, 76].

- Other techniques have been tested or proposed to prevent atheroembolism during SVG treatment, but none have adequately proved clinical benefits in RCTs. For example, excimer laser coronary angioplasty (ELCA), because of its ability to debulk and vaporize thrombus, has been tested as an alternative method to prevent atheroembolism.

- A case-control study of 71 consecutive patients with non-ST elevation acute coronary syndrome, undergoing PCI of degenerated SVG, was performed, comparing ELCA with EPD. ELCA was associated with a trend for better myocardial reperfusion and a less incidence of periprocedural necrosis. Controlled randomized trials are warranted to confirm these early observations [77].

- The recently published Japanese registry ULTRAMAN (Utility of Laser for Transcatheter Atherectomy-Multicenter Analysis around Naniwa) evaluated ELCA efficacy and safety in different clinical scenarios, demonstrating that it is a safe and effective treatment for different types of lesions, but only 1.8% of the patients included were treated for an SVG [78].

- Stenting constitutes the standard treatment of SVG stenosis (Fig. 30.5). In 1997, the first trial demonstrating that coronary stents resulted in superior procedural outcomes, larger gain in luminal diameter, and a reduction in major cardiac events was the SAVED (Saphenous Vein De Novo Trial Investigators) trial, which compared, in a randomized fashion, the use of the Palmaz-Schatz stent versus standard balloon angioplasty in 220 patients with SVG stenosis.

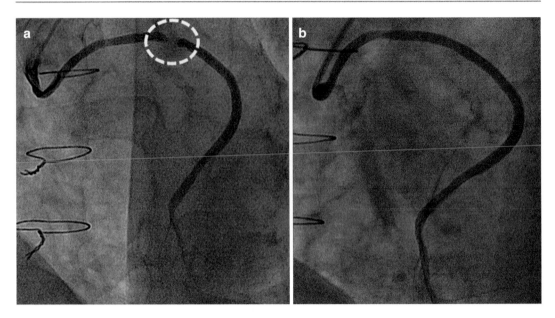

Fig. 30.5 A severe focal stenosis (panel **a**, yellow circle) in a saphenous vein graft to an occluded left anterior descending artery treated with a drug-eluting stent achieving an excellent acute angiographic result (panel **b**). See Fig. 30.6 for long-term follow-up

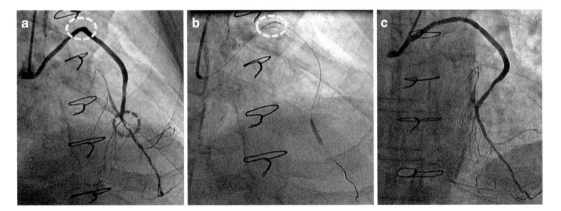

Fig. 30.6 Three-year follow-up of the patient shown in Fig. 30.5. The patient presented this time with non-ST segment elevation myocardial infarction. Coronary angiography showed a severe stenosis in the left anterior descending artery, distal to the anastomosis of the saphenous vein graft (panel **a**, red circle), and a good long-term result of the drug-eluting stent implanted in the graft previously (panels **a** and **b**, yellow circle). The stenosis was treated with a drug-eluting stent (panel **b**) implanted through the graft with an excellent angiographic result (panel **c**)

- However, the restenosis rate of stents implanted in SVGs was substantially higher than in native coronary vessels, with a 37% angiographic restenosis rate 6 months after BMS treatment, which was not significantly lower than in the balloon angioplasty group, where the stenosis rate was of 47%. Major cardiac events occurred less frequently in the stent group [79].

- Drug-eluting stents have offered a solution to this problem. Currently, evidence supports the superiority of DES over BMS in SVG PCI to reduce the rates of mortality, TLR, and TVR without increasing the risk of MI and stent thrombosis (Fig. 30.6) [32, 49, 80–92].
- A recent meta-analysis of 4 RCTs that included 812 patients demonstrated that DES can minimize the risk of short-term MACEs,

TLR, TVF, and TVR when compared with BMS but without difference in the incidence of long-term MACE, MI, mortality, cardiac death, and stent thrombosis [93].

- Another meta-analysis of 4 RCTs, with 1077 patients, compared second-generation with first-generation DES in SVG disease. Second-generation DES-treated patients had significantly lower MACE rates at 12 months, with similar levels of safety. No differences in the two groups were seen in all-cause mortality, MI, TVR, stent thrombosis, and TLR [94].

- *The European Guidelines on Myocardial Revascularization recommend DES for PCI of SVGs with a class I, level of evidence A recommendation [8].*

- Pathological characteristics of SVG attrition must be taken into consideration when analyzing safety and efficacy of stent use in this context. Atheromas in SVGs frequently present extensive areas of necrotic core that may interfere with endothelialization and neointimal coverage of stent struts.

- The long-term benefit of stenting may be limited due to progression of attrition or thrombus formation in non-stented segments of the SVG, which occurs as part of the natural history of SVG degeneration.

- As rapid progression of intermediate nonobstructive lesions has been observed in SVG, a randomized controlled trial was conducted to assess the efficacy of sealing intermediate nonobstructive coronary SVG lesions with drug-eluting stents (paclitaxel- or everolimus-eluting stents) for reducing MACE, compared with medical treatment, concluding that this strategy was safe but not associated with a significant reduction of cardiac events at 3-year follow-up [95].

- The use of undersized drug-eluting stents, defined as a ratio of the stent diameter to the average IVUS reference lumen diameter of less than 0.9, to treat patients with SVG lesions has been associated with a reduction in the frequency of post-PCI creatine kinase-MB elevation, without significant differences in the incidence of 1-year TLR or TVR [96].

- When feasible, direct stenting should be the preferred approach when treating SVG stenosis, as it is associated with less CK-MB release, less non-Q-wave MI, and significantly lower TLR-MACE in the DS group at 1 year [97].

- Intensive antithrombotic treatment with abciximab, an inhibitor of the glycoprotein IIb/IIIa, in an attempt to prevent thromboembolic events, has not improved clinical outcomes in terms of death, MI, or revascularization at 30 days or 6 months, but increases the risk of major bleeding. This lack of efficacy was consistent in different trials [98, 99].

- Finally, the treatment of stent restenosis in SVG is safer than treatment of de novo stenosis, due to the different pathological substrate, which in the case of restenosis, does not have the feared athero-embolic characteristics of SVG atheroma.

Percutaneous Revascularization of Arterial Grafts

- The pathophysiology of luminal narrowing in the internal mammary artery (IMA) graft is completely different from saphenous vein attrition. In most cases, lumen loss is the result of neointimal hyperplasia, secondary to vascular trauma during the surgery.

- Therefore, percutaneous treatment of IMA grafts does not carry the risk of atheroembolism present with SVG PCI.

- On many occasions, IMA stenosis responds favorably to balloon dilatation [100–102].

- In around 60% of cases, stenosis develops at the anastomotic site [103]. The overall success of balloon angioplasty in this setting, according to a review of more than 1000 published cases is around 90% [104].

- Stents may be needed in case of dissection or suboptimal results of balloon angioplasty, with similar results using BMS and DES [105, 106].

- Currently, there is little evidence regarding the best percutaneous interventional approach for treating late IMA graft failure. A recent multicenter observational study of 268 patients with IMA failure treated with different drug-eluting stents showed a very high immediate success of implantation; after 41 months follow-up, the all-cause mortality was 16.5%

(9% cardiac, 7.5% non-cardiac) and 11.9% required repeat revascularization [107].

- Evidence regarding the treatment of stenoses in radial artery grafts is lacking, the most frequent mode of angiographic failure is a complete occlusion, and less often a string-like appearance.
- Focal stenosis of radial artery grafts are a rare angiographic finding, and its meaning is uncertain as radial artery grafts are particularly prone to spasm [108].
- It has been recommended to perform balloon angioplasty alone in the early postoperative period during which spasm is difficult to exclude, while stenting is preferred in all the other settings, on the grounds of excellent and durable results [109].

Percutaneous Coronary Intervention for Early Postoperative CABG Failure

- Ischemia in the early postoperative setting is mostly due to surgical problems such as incomplete revascularization or vascular injury [6]. Perioperative MI is associated with highly increased perioperative morbidity and mortality as well as poor long-term outcomes [110].

- Early graft failure after CABG may occur in 7–30% of cases [111, 112]. Systematic perioperative angiography showed that 12% of all grafts had some form of angiographic defect, with major defects in 8% of SVGs and in 7% of LIMA grafts [113].
- In up to 75% of symptomatic patients after CABG, the main cause of chest pain was ischemia due to early graft failure, while other causes included pericarditis or coronary spasm [17].
- When the diagnosis of early graft failure is suspected and the hemodynamic condition of the patient allows it, an urgent coronary angiogram should be performed.
- Possible findings include:
  – Occluded graft(s) due to thrombosis,
  – Poor distal runoff in the grafted coronary artery,
  – Graft stenosis,
  – Suboptimal or failed anastomoses,
  – Competitive flow with native vessels including left mammary artery subclavian artery steal,
  – Bypass kinking,
  – Conduit mechanical issues (tension or overstretching) or spasm (Fig. 30.7), or
  – Grafting of the wrong coronary artery [114].

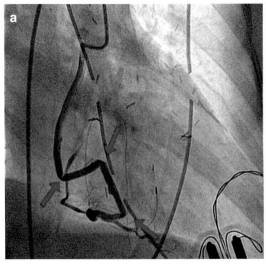 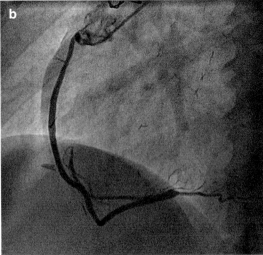

Fig. 30.7 Panel **a**: Saphenous vein graft kinking observed in an early postoperative angiography (red arrows), as the distal coronary flow was preserved no intervention was deemed necessary. Panel **b**: 3 months later repeat angiography demonstrates that the graft is functional without kinking

- In cases where angiography does not show any graft failure or new artery occlusion, ischemia may have been caused by air or plaque embolization, microcirculatory damage, or inappropriate myocardial protection (non-graft-related injuries), precluding the need for additional revascularization.

- Between 3 and 5% of all CABG patients undergo coronary angiography during the postoperative inhospital stay, with an important increase over the past 10 years, partially as a result of existing 24 h primary angioplasty programs in many hospitals [115, 116].

- Up to 30% of these patients present elevated myocardial damage markers, and a similar proportion of patients develop electrocardiographic changes following revascularization procedures [117].

- Cardiac biomarkers for myocardial damage do not distinguish between graft-related and non-graft-related perioperative MI until 12 h after CABG, reaching an accurate discrimination capability only at 24 h, with levels of troponin I significantly increased in patients with graft failure compared with patients with non-graft-related perioperative myocardial infarction, suggesting that the size of the infarction when a graft is involved is of greater size [110].

- PCI plays a very important role as a rescue procedure for CABG [118–128]. Patients presenting with cardiac arrest immediately after CABG do better with early re-intervention either by re-do CABG or PCI rather than a non-interventional approach.

- Emergency revascularization leads to a reduction in: hemodynamic stabilization time; duration of hospitalization, and less use of mechanical support.

- During a mean follow-up period of 37 ± 25 months, long-term mortality and event-free survival rates significantly favored the revascularization group [128]. Few studies have directly compared conservative treatment with re-do CABG and bailout PCI in perioperative MI.

- A report on 118 patients who underwent coronary angiography within the first 24 h after CABG found nonsignificant differences between acute PCI, emergency reoperation, or conservative treatment groups regarding 30-day mortality (12%, 20%, and 14.8% respectively) and 1-year follow-up (20%, 27%, and 18.5%) [126].

- A retrospective chart review on 46 patients with recurrent ischemia within 3 months post-CABG showed that 40% of the grafts were occluded or stenotic with successful PCI possible in 54% of them.

- PCI was performed upon native vessels and occluded grafts with equal frequency. At 1-year follow-up there was a 14% restenosis rate of the target vessel in the PCI group, while nearly 48% of the non-PCI group (including surgical and conservative treatments) were readmitted with recurrent ischemia [125].

- Another study in patients with early graft failure showed a trend towards reduction in the extent of myocardial damage with early re-intervention (PCI or CABG) compared with a conservative approach [129].

- Only one small study has reported on the use of DES for immediate post-CABG complications, showing that angiographic results were improved but with an increase in major bleeding complications [127]. Our group has reported a mortality rate of 21% (15% inhospital and 6% during follow-up period) associated with bailout PCI after CABG [115].

- In this emergency context it is difficult to extrapolate any conclusions from the available evidence on whether PCI offers benefits over re-do CABG. In many cases a complex native coronary anatomy was the reason to choose CABG in the first instance.

- On the other hand, organizing an operating room in emergency circumstances may require more time, which means more extensive necrosis and a bigger risk of hemodynamic instability; while the accessibility of the catheterization laboratory can save precious time leading to increased myocardial salvage.

- Likewise, it is not possible to infer whether the use of DES in bailout PCI provides additional benefits. It is clear that early diagnosis of perioperative ischemic complications and fast decision-making are of extreme importance

Table 30.2 2014 ESC Guideline recommendations for early postoperative ischemia and graft failure [8]

Recommendations	Class	LoE
Coronary angiography is recommended for patients with: • Symptoms of ischemia and/or abnormal biomarkers suggestive of perioperative myocardial infarction • Ischemic ECG changes indicating large area of risk • New significant wall motion abnormalities • Hemodynamic instability	I	C
It is recommended to make the decision on re-do CABG or PCI by ad hoc consultation in the Heart Team and based on feasibility of revascularization, area at risk, comorbidities, and clinical status	I	C
PCI should be considered over reoperation in patients with early ischemia after CABG if technically feasible	IIa	C
If PCI is performed, revascularization of the native vessels or ITA grafts rather than occluded or heavily diseased SVGs should be considered	IIa	C

LoE level of evidence, *PCI* percutaneous coronary intervention, *CABG* coronary artery bypass graft surgery, *ECG* electrocardiogram, *ITA* internal thoracic artery, *SVG* saphenous vein graft

since they influence short- and long-term prognosis [126].

- Significant predictors of inhospital mortality in patients with perioperative myocardial ischemia are hemodynamic deterioration, pre-angiography creatine kinase-MB isoenzyme rise >2 times the cutoff value and a delay of more than 30 h between primary CABG and coronary angiography [116].

- To identify such complications may be challenging, as ECG changes and myocardial markers rises are common after CABG; signs of perioperative myocardial ischemia such as new ST-segment abnormalities or new Q waves, new regional wall motion abnormalities on echocardiography, the presence of refractory ventricular arrhythmias, troponin elevation and persistent cardiogenic shock should lead to suspect early graft failure and prompt an urgent coronary angiography.

- Care should be taken, as working with new implanted grafts seems to be associated with a higher risk of graft rupture or anastomotic dehiscence than in the chronically implanted setting.

- Finally, since hemodynamic instability is frequently present or may occur during PCI, a low threshold for using the intra-aortic balloon pump during PCI is appropriate [130].

- The ESC guidelines recommendations for early postoperative ischemia and graft failure are summarized in Table 30.2.

Conclusions

- Secondary revascularization in patients with previous CABG usually takes place in complex clinical and anatomical contexts.

- Decisions regarding repeat revascularization should be made within Heart Team meetings, taking into account symptoms, personal characteristics of the patient, comorbidities, and previous procedures.

- When percutaneous revascularization is deemed to be required, the first option to treat should be native coronary vessels, followed by addressing surgical grafts.

- When treating SVGs, special care must be held to prevent distal embolism using dedicated devices, and drug-eluting stents should be used.

- Even though great advances have been achieved in this increasingly important subset of patients, many gaps in knowledge remain and more evidence is needed.

References

1. Sabik JF, Blackstone EH, Gillinov AM, Smedira NG, Lytle BW. Occurrence and risk factors for reintervention after coronary artery bypass grafting. Circulation. 2006;114:I454–60.
2. Brener SJ, et al. Predictors of revascularization method and long-term outcome of percutaneous coronary intervention or repeat coronary bypass surgery in patients with multivessel coronary disease and previous coronary bypass surgery. Eur Heart J. 2006;27:413–8.

3. Sprecher DL, Pearce GL. How deadly is the 'deadly quartet'? A post-CABG evaluation. J Am Coll Cardiol. 2000;36:1159–65.
4. Eagle KA, et al. ACC/AHA 2004 guideline update for coronary artery bypass graft surgery: a report of the American College of Cardiology/American Heart Association Task Force on Practice Guidelines (Committee to Update the 1999 Guidelines for Coronary Artery Bypass Graft S). Circulation. 2004;110:e340–437.
5. Sergeant P, Blackstone E, Meyns B, Stockman B, Jashari R. First cardiological or cardiosurgical reintervention for ischemic heart disease after primary coronary artery bypass grafting. Eur J Cardio-Thoracic Surg. 1998;14:480–7.
6. Noyez L. The evolution of repeat coronary artery surgery. EuroIntervention. 2009;5(Suppl D):D30–3.
7. Tatoulis J, Buxton BF, Fuller JA. Patencies of 2127 arterial to coronary conduits over 15 years. Ann Thorac Surg. 2004;77:93–101.
8. Windecker S, et al. 2014 ESC/EACTS guidelines on myocardial revascularization: The Task Force on Myocardial Revascularization of the European Society of Cardiology (ESC) and the European Association for Cardio-Thoracic Surgery (EACTS). Developed with the special contribution of the European Association of Percutaneous Cardiovascular Interventions (EAPCI). Eur Heart J. 2014;35:2541–619.
9. Morís C, Lozano I, Martín M, Rondán J, Avanzas P. Embolic protection devices in saphenous percutaneous intervention. EuroIntervention. 2009;5(Suppl D):D45–50.
10. Tatoulis J. Total arterial coronary revascularization-patient selection, stenoses, conduits, targets. Ann Cardiothorac Surg. 2013;2:499–506.
11. de Vries MR, Simons KH, Jukema JW, Braun J, Quax PHA. Vein graft failure: from pathophysiology to clinical outcomes. Nat Rev Cardiol. 2016;13:451–70.
12. Lenzen MJ, et al. Management and outcome of patients with established coronary artery disease: the Euro Heart Survey on coronary revascularization. Eur Heart J. 2005;26:1169–79.
13. Brilakis ES, et al. Percutaneous coronary intervention in native arteries versus bypass grafts in prior coronary artery bypass grafting patients: a report from the National Cardiovascular Data Registry. JACC Cardiovasc Interv. 2011;4:844–50.
14. Brilakis ES, et al. Percutaneous coronary intervention in native coronary arteries versus bypass grafts in patients with prior coronary artery bypass graft surgery: insights from the veterans affairs clinical assessment, reporting, and tracking program. JACC Cardiovasc Interv. 2016;9:884–93.
15. Iqbal J, et al. Outcomes following primary percutaneous coronary intervention in patients with previous coronary artery bypass surgery. Circ Cardiovasc Interv. 2016;9:e003151.
16. Patel MR, Dehmer GJ, Hirshfeld JW, Smith PK, Spertus JA. ACCF/SCAI/STS/AATS/AHA/ASNC/HFSA/SCCT 2012 appropriate use criteria for coronary revascularization focused update: a report of the American College of Cardiology Foundation Appropriate Use Criteria Task Force, Society for Cardiovascular Angiography and Interventions. J Am Coll Cardiol. 2012;59:857–81.
17. Scarsini R, Zivelonghi C, Pesarini G, Vassanelli C, Ribichini FL. Repeat revascularization: percutaneous coronary intervention after coronary artery bypass graft surgery. Cardiovasc Revasc Med. 2016;17:272–8.
18. Tatoulis J, Buxton BF, Fuller JA, Royse AG. Total arterial coronary revascularization: techniques and results in 3,220 patients. Ann Thorac Surg. 1999;68:2093–9.
19. Yap C-H, et al. Contemporary results show repeat coronary artery bypass grafting remains a risk factor for operative mortality. Ann Thorac Surg. 2009;87:1386–91.
20. Patel MR, et al. ACCF/SCAI/STS/AATS/AHA/ASNC 2009 appropriateness criteria for coronary revascularization: a report by the American College of Cardiology Foundation Appropriateness Criteria Task Force, Society for Cardiovascular Angiography and Interventions, Society of T. J Am Coll Cardiol. 2009;53:530–53.
21. Task Force on Myocardial Revascularization of the European Society of Cardiology (ESC) and the European Association for Cardio-Thoracic Surgery (EACTS), et al. Guidelines on myocardial revascularization. Eur Heart J. 2010;31:2501–55.
22. Sabik JF, Blackstone EH, Houghtaling PL, Walts PA, Lytle BW. Is reoperation still a risk factor in coronary artery bypass surgery? Ann Thorac Surg. 2005;80:1719–27.
23. Brener SJ, et al. Propensity analysis of long-term survival after surgical or percutaneous revascularization in patients with multivessel coronary artery disease and high-risk features. Circulation. 2004;109:2290–5.
24. Kohl LP, et al. Outcomes of primary percutaneous coronary intervention in ST-segment elevation myocardial infarction patients with previous coronary bypass surgery. JACC Cardiovasc Interv. 2014;7:981–7.
25. Varghese I, Samuel J, Banerjee S, Brilakis ES. Comparison of percutaneous coronary intervention in native coronary arteries vs. bypass grafts in patients with prior coronary artery bypass graft surgery. Cardiovasc Revasc Med. 2009;10:103–9.
26. Liu W, et al. Long-term outcome of native artery versus bypass graft intervention in prior coronary artery bypass graft patients with ST-segment elevation myocardial infarction. Chin Med J (Engl). 2013;126:2281–5.
27. Maroto LC, Silva JA, Rodríguez JE. Assessment of patients with previous CABG. EuroIntervention. 2009;5(Suppl D):D25–9.

28. Taggart DP, et al. A randomized trial of external stenting for saphenous vein grafts in coronary artery bypass grafting. Ann Thorac Surg. 2015;99:2039–45.

29. Meirson T, et al. Flow patterns in externally stented saphenous vein grafts and development of intimal hyperplasia. J Thorac Cardiovasc Surg. 2015;150:871–8.

30. Subramanian S, et al. Decision-making for patients with patent left internal thoracic artery grafts to left anterior descending. Ann Thorac Surg. 2009;87:1392–1398; discussion 1400.

31. Morrison DA, et al. Percutaneous coronary intervention versus repeat bypass surgery for patients with medically refractory myocardial ischemia: AWESOME randomized trial and registry experience with post-CABG patients. J Am Coll Cardiol. 2002;40:1951–4.

32. Harskamp RE, et al. Clinical outcome after surgical or percutaneous revascularization in coronary bypass graft failure. J Cardiovasc Med (Hagerstown). 2013;14:438–45.

33. Sabik JF, Raza S, Blackstone EH, Houghtaling PL, Lytle BW. Value of internal thoracic artery grafting to the left anterior descending coronary artery at coronary reoperation. J Am Coll Cardiol. 2013;61:302–10.

34. Zacharias A, et al. Late outcomes after radial artery versus saphenous vein grafting during reoperative coronary artery bypass surgery. J Thorac Cardiovasc Surg. 2010;139:1511–1518.e4.

35. Herrera-Nogueira RS, et al. How should I treat a DES restenosis in a graft anastomosis with challenging access and multiple previous coronary interventions? EuroIntervention. 2016;11:1565–8.

36. Ramcharitar S, van Geuns R-J. Magnetic navigation in patients with coronary artery bypass grafting. EuroIntervention. 2009;5(Suppl D):D58–63.

37. Patterson M. 3D reconstruction from contrast coronary angiography in magnetic percutaneous coronary intervention. Catheter Cardiovasc Interv. 2010;76:532–5.

38. Weisz G, et al. Magnetic positioning system in coronary angiography and percutaneous intervention: a feasibility and safety study. Catheter Cardiovasc Interv. 2013;82:1084–90.

39. Sandhu GS, et al. Magnetic navigation facilitates percutaneous coronary intervention for complex lesions. Catheter Cardiovasc Interv. 2014;84:660–7.

40. Safian RD. Magnetic navigation: what's the attraction? Catheter Cardiovasc Interv. 2014;84:668–9.

41. Roth C, et al. Comparison of magnetic wire navigation with the conventional wire technique for percutaneous coronary intervention of chronic total occlusions: a randomised, controlled study. Heart Vessel. 2015;31:1266.

42. Escaned J. Secondary revascularization after CABG surgery. Nat Rev Cardiol. 2012;9(9):540.

43. Nguyen-Trong P-KJ, et al. Use of saphenous vein bypass grafts for retrograde recanalization of coronary chronic Total occlusions: insights from a multicenter registry. J Invasive Cardiol. 2016;28:218–24.

44. Glineur D, Hanet C. Competitive flow in coronary bypass surgery. Curr Opin Cardiol. 2012;27:620–8.

45. Lorusso R, et al. Emergency surgery after saphenous vein graft perforation complicated by catheter balloon entrapment and hemorrhagic shock. Ann Thorac Surg. 2008;86:1002–4.

46. Shammas NW, Thondapu VR, Winniford MD, Kalil DA. Perforation of saphenous vein graft during coronary stenting: a case report. Catheter Cardiovasc Diagn. 1996;38:274–6.

47. Lozano I, Rondan J, Avanzas P. Vessel diameter should be taken into account in saphenous stenting. EuroIntervention. 2010;5:991–3.

48. Lowe R, Hammond C, Perry RA. Prior CABG does not prevent pericardial tamponade following saphenous vein graft perforation associated with angioplasty. Heart. 2005;91:1052.

49. Brennan JM, et al. Safety and clinical effectiveness of drug-eluting stents for saphenous vein graft intervention in older individuals: results from the medicare-linked National Cardiovascular Data Registry(®) CathPCI registry(®) (2005–2009). Catheter Cardiovasc Interv. 2015;87:43.

50. Abdel-Karim A-RR, et al. Prevalence and outcomes of intermediate saphenous vein graft lesions: findings from the stenting of saphenous vein grafts randomized-controlled trial. Int J Cardiol. 2013;168:2468–73.

51. Yahagi K, et al. Pathophysiology of native coronary, vein graft, and in-stent atherosclerosis. Nat Rev Cardiol. 2015;13:79–98.

52. Hong MK, et al. Creatine kinase-MB enzyme elevation following successful saphenous vein graft intervention is associated with late mortality. Circulation. 1999;100:2400–5.

53. Baim DS, et al. Randomized trial of a distal embolic protection device during percutaneous intervention of saphenous vein Aorto-coronary bypass grafts. Circulation. 2002;105:1285–90.

54. Stone GW, et al. Randomized comparison of distal protection with a filter-based catheter and a balloon occlusion and aspiration system during percutaneous intervention of diseased saphenous vein Aorto-coronary bypass grafts. Circulation. 2003;108:548.

55. Coolong A, et al. Saphenous vein graft stenting and major adverse cardiac events. Circulation. 2008;117, 790–7.

56. Mauri L, et al. The PROXIMAL trial: proximal protection during saphenous vein graft intervention using the proxis embolic protection system: a randomized, prospective, multicenter clinical trial. J Am Coll Cardiol. 2007;50:1442–9.

57. Levine GN, et al. ACCF/AHA/SCAI guideline for percutaneous coronary intervention: executive summary. Catheter Cardiovasc Interv. 2011;79(2012):453–95.

58. Iqbal MB, et al. Embolic protection device use and its association with procedural safety and long-term

outcomes following saphenous vein graft intervention: an analysis from the British Columbia Cardiac registry. Catheter Cardiovasc Interv. 2016;88:73–83.

59. Brennan JM, et al. Three-year outcomes associated with embolic protection in saphenous vein graft intervention: results in 49 325 senior patients in the Medicare-Linked National Cardiovascular Data Registry CathPCI Registry. Circ Cardiovasc Interv. 2015;8:e001403.

60. Mehta SK, et al. Utilization of distal embolic protection in saphenous vein graft interventions (an analysis of 19,546 patients in the American College of Cardiology-National Cardiovascular Data Registry). Am J Cardiol. 2007;100:1114–8.

61. Lim MJ, Young JJ, Senter SR, Klein LW, Interventional Committee for The Society for Cardiovascular Angiography and Interventions. Determinants of embolic protection device use: case study in the acceptance of a new medical technology. Catheter Cardiovasc Interv. 2005;65:597–9.

62. Mauri L, Rogers C, Baim DS. Devices for distal protection during percutaneous coronary revascularization. Circulation. 2006;113:2651.

63. Naidu SS, et al. Contemporary incidence and predictors of major adverse cardiac events after saphenous vein graft intervention with embolic protection (an AMEthyst trial substudy). Am J Cardiol. 2010;105:1060–4.

64. Carrozza JP, et al. Randomized evaluation of the TriActiv balloon-protection flush and extraction system for the treatment of saphenous vein graft disease. J Am Coll Cardiol. 2005;46:1677–83.

65. Stankovic G, et al. Randomized evaluation of polytetrafluoroethylene-covered stent in saphenous vein grafts: the Randomized Evaluation of polytetrafluoroethylene COVERed stent in Saphenous vein grafts (RECOVERS) Trial. Circulation. 2003;108:37–42.

66. Schächinger V, et al. A randomized trial of polytetrafluoroethylene-membrane-covered stents compared with conventional stents in aortocoronary saphenous vein grafts. J Am Coll Cardiol. 2003;42:1360–9.

67. Stone GW, et al. 5-year follow-up of polytetrafluoroethylene-covered stents compared with bare-metal stents in aortocoronary saphenous vein grafts the randomized BARRICADE (barrier approach to restenosis: restrict intima to curtail adverse events) trial. JACC Cardiovasc Interv. 2011;4:300–9.

68. Turco MA, et al. Pivotal, randomized U.S. study of the Symbiottrade mark covered stent system in patients with saphenous vein graft disease: eight-month angiographic and clinical results from the Symbiot III trial. Catheter Cardiovasc Interv. 2006;68:379–88.

69. Bennett J, et al. Long-term follow-up after percutaneous coronary intervention with polytetrafluoroethylene-covered Symbiot stents compared to bare metal stents, with and without FilterWire embolic protection, in diseased saphenous vein grafts. Acta Cardiol. 2013;68:1–9.

70. Maia F, et al. Preliminary results of the INSPIRE trial with the novel MGuard™ stent system containing a protection net to prevent distal embolization. Catheter Cardiovasc Interv. 2010;76:86–92.

71. Grube E, Hauptmann KE, Müller R, Uriel N, Kaluski E. Coronary stenting with MGuard: extended follow-up of first human trial. Cardiovasc Revasc Med. 2011;12:138–46.

72. Costa JR, et al. One-year results of the INSPIRE trial with the novel MGuard stent: serial analysis with QCA and IVUS. Catheter Cardiovasc Interv. 2011;78:1095–100.

73. Colombo A, Almagor Y, Gaspar J, Vonderwalde C. The pericardium covered stent (PCS). EuroIntervention. 2009;5:394–9.

74. Yassin I, Thuesen L. Distal embolization after net protective stent (MGUARD) implantation in a degenerated saphenous vein graft lesion. Catheter Cardiovasc Interv. 2010;75:639–41.

75. Latsios G, Tsioufis K, Tousoulis D, Kallikazaros I, Stefanadis C. Perforation of a saphenous vein graft during percutaneous angioplasty: demonstration by means of intravascular ultrasound and consequent treatment with a polytetrafluoroethylene-covered stent. Int J Cardiol. 2009;134:e15–6.

76. Romaguera R, Gomez-Hospital JA, Cequier A. Novel use of the Mguard mesh-covered stent to treat coronary arterial perforations. Catheter Cardiovasc Interv. 2012;80:75–8.

77. Niccoli G, et al. Case-control registry of excimer laser coronary angioplasty versus distal protection devices in patients with acute coronary syndromes due to saphenous vein graft disease. Am J Cardiol. 2013;112:1586–91.

78. Nishino M, et al. Indications and outcomes of excimer laser coronary atherectomy: efficacy and safety for thrombotic lesions—the ULTRAMAN registry. J Cardiol. 2016;69:314. https://doi.org/10.1016/j.jjcc.2016.05.018.

79. Savage MP, et al. Stent placement compared with balloon angioplasty for obstructed coronary bypass grafts. Saphenous Vein De Novo Trial Investigators. N Engl J Med. 1997;337:740–7.

80. Wiisanen ME, Abdel-Latif A, Mukherjee D, Ziada KM. Drug-eluting stents versus bare-metal stents in saphenous vein graft interventions: a systematic review and meta-analysis. JACC Cardiovasc Interv. 2010;3:1262–73.

81. Alam M, et al. Clinical outcomes of percutaneous interventions in saphenous vein grafts using drug-eluting stents compared to bare-metal stents: a comprehensive meta-analysisof all randomized clinical trials. Clin Cardiol. 2012;35:291–6.

82. Aggarwal V, et al. Safety and effectiveness of drug-eluting versus bare-metal stents in saphenous vein bypass graft percutaneous coronary interventions: insights from the Veterans Affairs CART program. J Am Coll Cardiol. 2014;64:1825–36.

83. Tolerico PH, et al. In-hospital and 1-year outcomes with drug-eluting versus bare metal stents

in saphenous vein graft intervention: a report from the EVENT registry. Catheter Cardiovasc Interv. 2012;80:1127–36.

84. Sanchez-Recalde A, et al. Safety and efficacy of drug-eluting stents versus bare-metal stents in saphenous vein grafts lesions: a meta-analysis. EuroIntervention. 2010;6:149–60.

85. Brodie BR, et al. Outcomes with drug-eluting versus bare-metal stents in saphenous vein graft intervention results from the STENT (strategic transcatheter evaluation of new therapies) group. JACC Cardiovasc Interv. 2009;2:1105–12.

86. Fröbert O, Scherstén F, James SK, Carlsson J, Lagerqvist B. Long-term safety and efficacy of drug-eluting and bare metal stents in saphenous vein grafts. Am Heart J. 2012;164:87–93.

87. Brilakis ES, et al. Continued benefit from paclitaxel-eluting compared with bare-metal stent implantation in saphenous vein graft lesions during long-term follow-up of the SOS (Stenting of Saphenous Vein Grafts) trial. JACC Cardiovasc Interv. 2011;4:176–82.

88. Hakeem A, et al. Safety and efficacy of drug eluting stents compared with bare metal stents for saphenous vein graft interventions: a comprehensive meta-analysis of randomized trials and observational studies comprising 7,994 patients. Catheter Cardiovasc Interv. 2011;77:343–55.

89. Mamas MA, et al. A comparison of drug-eluting stents versus bare metal stents in saphenous vein graft PCI outcomes: a meta-analysis. J Interv Cardiol. 2011;24:172–80.

90. Mehilli J, et al. Drug-eluting versus bare-metal stents in saphenous vein graft lesions (ISAR-CABG): a randomised controlled superiority trial. Lancet (London, England). 2011;378:1071–8.

91. Brilakis ES, et al. A randomized controlled trial of a paclitaxel-eluting stent versus a similar bare-metal stent in saphenous vein graft lesions the SOS (Stenting of Saphenous Vein Grafts) trial. J Am Coll Cardiol. 2009;53:919–28.

92. Jeger RV, et al. Drug-eluting stents compared with bare metal stents improve late outcome after saphenous vein graft but not after large native vessel interventions. Cardiology. 2009;112:49–55.

93. Gao J, Ren M, Liu Y, Gao M, Sun B. Drug-eluting versus bare metal stent in treatment of patients with saphenous vein graft disease: a meta-analysis of randomized controlled trials. Int J Cardiol. 2016;222:95–100.

94. Shi H, et al. Second-generation versus first-generation drug-eluting stents in saphenous vein graftdisease: a meta-analysis of randomized controlled trials. Int J Cardiol. 2016;214:393–7.

95. Rodés-Cabau J, et al. Sealing intermediate non-obstructive coronary saphenous vein graft lesions with drug-eluting stents as a new approach to reducing cardiac events. Circ Cardiovasc Interv. 2016;9:e004336.

96. Hong YJ, et al. Outcome of undersized drug-eluting stents for percutaneous coronary intervention of saphenous vein graft lesions. Am J Cardiol. 2010;105:179–85.

97. Leborgne L, et al. Effect of direct stenting on clinical outcome in patients treated with percutaneous coronary intervention on saphenous vein graft. Am Heart J. 2003;146:501–6.

98. Roffi M, et al. Lack of benefit from intravenous platelet glycoprotein IIb/IIIa receptor inhibition as adjunctive treatment for percutaneous interventions of aortocoronary bypass grafts: a pooled analysis of five randomized clinical trials. Circulation. 2002;106:3063–7.

99. Harskamp RE, et al. Procedural and clinical outcomes after use of the glycoprotein IIb/IIIa inhibitor abciximab for saphenous vein graft interventions. Cardiovasc Revasc Med. 2015;17:19.

100. Sketch MH, et al. Angiographic follow-up after internal mammary artery graft angioplasty. Am J Cardiol. 1992;70:401–3.

101. Kereiakes DJ, George B, Stertzer SH, Myler RK. Percutaneous transluminal angioplasty of left internal mammary artery grafts. Am J Cardiol. 1985;55:1215–6.

102. Bell MR, Holmes DR, Vlietstra RE, Bresnahan DR. Percutaneous transluminal angioplasty of left internal mammary artery grafts: two years' experience with a femoral approach. Br Heart J. 1989;61:417–20.

103. Shimshak TM, et al. Application of percutaneous transluminal coronary angioplasty to the internal mammary artery graft. J Am Coll Cardiol. 1988;12:1205–14.

104. Douglas JS. In: Topol E, editor. Textbook of interventional cardiology. Philadelphia: Saunders/Elsevier; 2008. p. 443–74.

105. Buch AN, et al. Comparison of outcomes between bare metal stents and drug-eluting stents for percutaneous revascularization of internal mammary grafts. Am J Cardiol. 2006;98:722–4.

106. Zavalloni D, et al. Drug-eluting stents for the percutaneous treatment of the anastomosis of the left internal mammary graft to left anterior descending artery. Coron Artery Dis. 2007;18:495–500.

107. Lozano I, et al. Immediate and long-term results of drug-eluting stents in mammary artery grafts. Am J Cardiol. 2015;116:1695–9.

108. Kulkarni NM, Thomas MR. Severe spasm of a radial artery coronary bypass graft during coronary intervention. Catheter Cardiovasc Interv. 1999;47:331–5.

109. Goube P, et al. Radial artery graft stenosis treated by percutaneous intervention. Eur J Cardio-Thorac Surg. 2010;37:697–703.

110. Thielmann M, et al. Diagnostic discrimination between graft-related and non-graft-related perioperative myocardial infarction with cardiac troponin I after coronary artery bypass surgery. Eur Heart J. 2005;26:2440.

111. PREVENT IV Investigators, Alexander JH, et al. Efficacy and safety of edifoligide, an E2F transcription factor decoy, for prevention of vein graft failure following coronary artery bypass graft surgery. JAMA. 2005;294:2446.
112. Balacumaraswami L, et al. Intraoperative imaging techniques to assess coronary artery bypass graft patency. Ann Thorac Surg. 2007;83:2251–7.
113. Zhao DX, et al. Routine intraoperative completion angiography after coronary artery bypass grafting and 1-stop hybrid revascularization results from a fully integrated hybrid catheterization laboratory/operating room. J Am Coll Cardiol. 2009;53:232–41.
114. Rasmussen C, et al. Significance and management of early graft failure after coronary artery bypass grafting: feasibility and results of acute angiography and re-re-vascularization. Eur J Cardiothorac Surg. 1997;12:847–52.
115. Babiker A, et al. Rescue percutaneous intervention for acute complications of coronary artery surgery. EuroIntervention. 2009;5(Suppl D):D64–9.
116. Davierwala PM, et al. Impact of expeditious management of perioperative myocardial ischemia in patients undergoing isolated coronary artery bypass surgery. Circulation. 2013;128:S226–34.
117. Califf RM, et al. Myonecrosis after revascularization procedures. J Am Coll Cardiol. 1998;31:241–51.
118. Hanratty CG, Koyama Y, Ward MR. Angioplasty and stenting of the distal coronary anastomosis for graft failure immediately after coronary artery bypass grafting. Am J Cardiol. 2002;90:1009–11.
119. Khurana S, O'Neill WW, Sakwa M, Safian RD. Acute occlusion of a left internal mammary artery graft immediately after redo coronary artery bypass surgery: successful rescue PTCA. Catheter Cardiovasc Diagn. 1997;41:166–9.
120. Dorogy ME, Highfill WT, Davis RC. Use of angioplasty in the management of complicated perioperative infarction following bypass surgery. Catheter Cardiovasc Diagn. 1993;29:279–82.
121. Piana RN, et al. Rescue percutaneous coronary intervention immediately following coronary artery bypass grafting. Chest. 2001;120:1417–20.
122. Reifart N, Störger H, Schwarz F, Besser R, Iversen S. [From surgical to interventional standby?]. Z Kardiol. 1998:87(Suppl 3):8–11; discussion 14–5.
123. Gobel FL, et al. Safety of coronary arteriography in clinically stable patients following coronary bypass surgery. Post CABG Clinical Trial Investigators. Cathet Cardiovasc Diagn. 1998;45:376–81.
124. Adams MR, et al. Rescue percutaneous coronary intervention following coronary artery bypass graft—a descriptive analysis of the changing interface between interventional cardiologist and cardiac surgeon. Clin Cardiol. 2002;25:280–6.
125. Abdulmalik A, Arabi A, Alroaini A, Rosman H, Lalonde T. Feasibility of percutaneous coronary interventions in early postcoronary artery bypass graft occlusion or stenosis. J Interv Cardiol. 2007;20:204–8.
126. Thielmann M, et al. Emergency re-revascularization with percutaneous coronary intervention, reoperation, or conservative treatment in patients with acute perioperative graft failure following coronary artery bypass surgery. Eur J Cardio-Thorac Surg. 2006;30:117–25.
127. Price MJ, Housman L, Teirstein PS. Rescue percutaneous coronary intervention early after coronary artery bypass grafting in the drug-eluting stent era. Am J Cardiol. 2006;97:789–91.
128. Guney MR, et al. Results of treatment methods in cardiac arrest following coronary artery bypass grafting. J Card Surg. 2009;24:227–33.
129. Laflamme M, et al. Management of early postoperative coronary artery bypass graft failure. Interact Cardiovasc Thorac Surg. 2012;14:452–6.
130. Rubino AS, et al. Early intra-aortic balloon pumping following perioperative myocardial injury improves hospital and mid-term prognosis. Interact Cardiovasc Thorac Surg. 2009;8:310–5.

In-Stent Restenosis

31

Roisin Colleran and Robert A. Byrne

About Us

The Deutsches Herzzentrum München (German Heart Center Munich) was founded in 1972/73 as the first heart center in Europe—offering state-of-the-art medical treatment of cardiovascular diseases in one centralized location. It is now one of the leading centers for cardiac care in Germany and Europe. The department of cardiovascular diseases serves the greater Munich area (population ca. 3 million) and is also a referral center for the state of Bavaria (population ca. 12.5 million). The number of therapeutic coronary and structural interventions continues to increase each year, with ca. 2000 PCI procedures, >600 transcatheter aortic valve implantations, and >100 percutaneous mitral valve interventions being performed per year. There is a 24-h chest pain

unit and primary PCI service. Scientifically, the German Heart Center is one of the most successful in Germany. Key research interests are the investigation of novel coronary stent and balloon devices, antithrombotic treatment of stable coronary disease and acute coronary syndromes, as well as basic research on molecular and genetic causes of atherosclerosis and myocardial infarction. The ISAResearch Centre of the German Heart Centre also has a full-time imaging core laboratory specializing in quantitative coronary angiography and optical coherence tomography analysis.

Introduction

- Restenosis is an arterial wall healing response to mechanical injury at the site of a previously treated coronary segment.
- In-stent restenosis (ISR) is an angiographic diagnosis, defined as recurrent diameter stenosis >50% within a stent or at its edges (5 mm segments proximal and distal to the stent).
- It is the most common cause of stent failure and the most common reason for target lesion revascularization (TLR). Moreover, its treatment is challenging owing to a relatively high rate of recurrence at follow-up.

R. Colleran
Deutsches Herzzentrum München, Technische Universität München, Munich, Germany

R. A. Byrne (✉)
Deutsches Herzzentrum München, Technische Universität München, Munich, Germany

DZHK (German Centre for Cardiovascular Research), partner site Munich Heart Alliance, Munich, Germany
e-mail: byrne@dhm.mhn.de

© Springer International Publishing AG, part of Springer Nature 2018
A. Myat et al. (eds.), *The Interventional Cardiology Training Manual*,
https://doi.org/10.1007/978-3-319-71635-0_31

Classification of ISR

- Classification of ISR based on angiographic lesion morphology has been shown to aid in the prediction of TLR.
- The Mehran system classifies lesions from I to IV based on length, location, and presence or absence of vessel occlusion, with increasing class correlating with increasing rates of TLR at follow-up:
  I. Focal
  II. Diffuse (confined within stent)
  III. Proliferative (diffuse within and beyond stent)
  IV. Occlusive [1]
- Although the correlation with clinical outcomes was originally demonstrated in bare metal stent (BMS)-ISR, it was subsequently shown to also apply to drug-eluting stent (DES)-ISR [2].
- The American College of Cardiology/ American Heart Association classification of coronary stenosis has also been validated in ISR, with B2-C lesions being associated with higher ISR rates and poorer long-term outcomes [3].

Clinical Presentation

- With current generation DES, the rate of ISR in patients undergoing planned surveillance angiography in routine practice is ca. 10% and the rate of TLR in randomized trials is typically <5% at 12 months [4, 5].
- ISR may be symptomatic or asymptomatic. In a study of 10,004 patients with routine surveillance angiography 6–8 months post-BMS or DES implantation, 52% of patients with ISR were asymptomatic, 43% had stable angina, and 5% presented with acute coronary syndrome [6]. In one study of symptomatic patients with BMS-ISR, 64% of patients presented with stable angina, and the remaining 36% with acute coronary syndrome [7].

Pathophysiology: BMS-ISR Versus DES-ISR

- ISR is a multifactorial process. The key contributing factors are shown in Table 31.1. The pathophysiology of ISR differs from that of restenosis after balloon angioplasty, the latter being caused by a combination of tissue prolapse, elastic recoil, negative vascular remodeling, and neointimal hyperplasia (NIH).
- Although stenting addresses the first three of these issues, neointimal hyperplasia is, in fact, enhanced in response to the increased vessel wall injury induced by stent implantation. By inhibiting neointimal hyperplasia through the release of locally acting cytotoxic or immunosuppressive drugs, DES succeeded in reducing ISR rates considerably compared with BMS.
- Despite this, when DES-ISR does occur, treatment tends to be more challenging and outcomes are generally less favorable than with BMS-ISR [8].
- The difference in outcomes after intervention for BMS-ISR and DES-ISR may be explained by differences in the pathophysiology. Histopathologically, BMS-ISR is typically composed of intimal hyperplasia and smooth muscle cell proliferation; DES-ISR usually

Table 31.1 Factors contributing to BMS-ISR and DES-ISR

Mechanical factors
• Stent under-expansion (malapposition)
• Strut fracture
• Stent gap
• Geographic miss (where the stent does not fully cover the lesion; may result in edge restenosis giving a "candy-wrapper" angiographic appearance)
• Edge dissection
• Uneven/undelivered drug (DES-ISR: Stent damage; non-uniform strut distribution)
Biological factors (DES-ISR only)
• Drug resistance (often implicated in NIH)
• Hypersensitivity reaction (often in response to polymer coating)

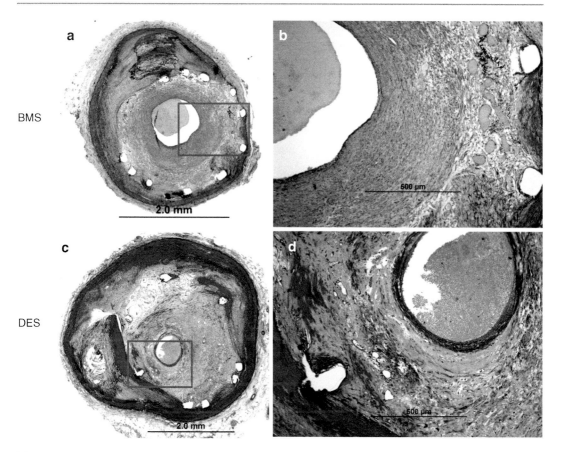

Fig. 31.1 (**a**) Low power magnification of a bare metal stent with severe in-stent restenosis. (**b**) High power magnification shows typical neointimal hyperplasia with predominance of smooth muscle cells. (**c**) Low power magnification of a drug-eluting stent showing severe in-stent restenosis with almost complete occlusion. (**d**) High power magnification section shows a stent strut with surrounding proteoglycan-rich neointimal tissue and presence of foam cells, typical of neoatherosclerotic change, as well as neovascularization

has a hypocellular composition, and more often shows fibrin deposition and neoatherosclerosis or high atherosclerotic plaque content (Fig. 31.1).

- Neoatherosclerosis develops over months to years following stenting and usually has a more accelerated time course compared with *de novo* atherosclerosis. For reasons that are poorly understood, it tends to occur more rapidly and twice as frequently in DES compared with BMS [9].

- Differences between BMS-ISR and DES-ISR are also apparent on angiography and intracoronary imaging (Table 31.2). Angiographically, BMS-ISR tends to be more diffuse and DES-ISR more focal, a phenomenon explained by the overall more effective suppression of neointimal hyperplasia with DES, which means that focal mechanical issues—such as local under-expansion or stent fracture—play a relatively more important role.

Table 31.2 Comparison of principle features of bare metal and drug-eluting stent restenosis

Characteristic	Bare metal stent restenosis	Drug-eluting stent restenosis
Histopathological features		
Smooth muscle cellularity	Rich	Hypocellular
Proteoglycan content	Moderate	High
Peri-strut fibrin and inflammation	Occasional	Frequent
Complete endothelialization	3–6 months	Up to 48 months
Presence of thrombus	Occasional	Occasional
Neoatherosclerosis	Relatively infrequent, late after stenting	Relatively frequent, accelerated course
Imaging features		
Angiographic appearance	Diffuse pattern more common	Focal pattern more common
Time course of late luminal loss	Late loss maximal by 6–8 months	Ongoing late loss out to 5 years
Optical coherence tomography tissue properties	Homogenous, high-signal band typical	Layered structure or heterogeneous typical

Role of Intravascular Imaging

- Intracoronary imaging is important for the evaluation of patients with ISR. It may be used to:
  - Assess the underlying mechanism of ISR (i.e., mechanical versus biological)
  - To characterize the restenotic tissue type (i.e., NIH versus neoatherosclerosis)
- This information can be important to guide therapy, though clinical trial evidence showing an advantage with systematic use of imaging in ISR is lacking. Current European guidelines give a IIa recommendation, level of evidence C for use of IVUS or OCT for detection of stent-related mechanical problems in this setting.
- The two most frequently used intravascular imaging modalities for assessment of ISR are intravascular ultrasound (IVUS) and optical coherence tomography (OCT). The relative merits of each modality are discussed below.

Intravascular Ultrasound (IVUS)

Advantages
- Deeper tissue penetration compared with OCT, allowing visualization of the external elastic lamina behind stent struts, thereby facilitating more accurate vessel sizing.

- Ability to detect stent under-expansion and edge problems.
- No need for a blood-free imaging field (obviating the need for contrast).

Disadvantage
- Lower spatial resolution compared with OCT (~150 μm).

Optical Coherence Tomography (OCT)

Advantages
- High spatial resolution (12–15 μm) allowing more detailed visualization of the lumen-neointima interface, unrivaled in vivo tissue characterization and better strut visualization compared with IVUS
- Allows visualization of unstable features such as plaque rupture or nonocclusive intracoronary thrombus, which may influence clinical decision-making

Disadvantages
- The need for a blood-free imaging field necessitates the use of contrast
- Reduced ability to detect external elastic lamina in diseased or stented segments and potential for less accurate vessel sizing compared with IVUS

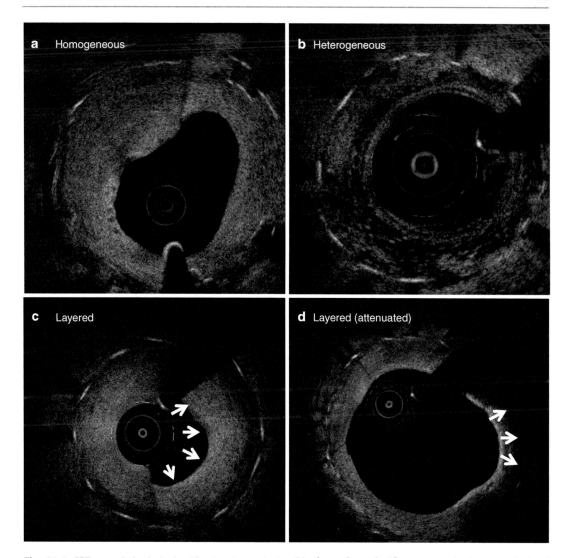

Fig. 31.2 ISR morphological classification by optical coherence tomography (OCT); (**a**): Homogeneous tissue typical of neointimal hyperplasia; (**b**) heterogeneous, (**c**) layered, and (**d**) attenuated tissue typical of neoatherosclerosis

Representative examples of OCT tissue morphologies are displayed in Fig. 31.2. Findings may be broadly classified into two categories:

1. Homogeneous—high-signal intensity tissue with low backscatter characteristic of smooth muscle cell-rich NIH and typical of BMS-ISR.
2. Heterogeneous, attenuated, or layered tissue—areas of both high and low signal intensity representing a spectrum of tissue types ranging from granulation tissue to hypocellular neointima with a high proteoglycan or fibrin content to in-stent fibroatheroma typical of neoatherosclerosis and more commonly observed in DES-ISR.

Treatment

- European guidelines recommend repeat PCI as the strategy of choice for treatment of restenosis if technically feasible (Class I recommendation, level of evidence C) [10].
- Many percutaneous therapies have been investigated, including balloon angioplasty, ather-

Fig. 31.3 Treatment algorithm for in-stent restenosis. Key: *BMS* bare metal stent, *DES* drug-eluting stent, *G2* second generation, *IVUS* intravascular ultrasound, *OCT* optical coherence tomography. *Randomized trial data relates specifically to durable polymer everolimus-eluting stent. §Randomized trial data relates specifically to iopromide excipient paclitaxel-coated balloon and BTHC excipient paclitaxel-coated balloon

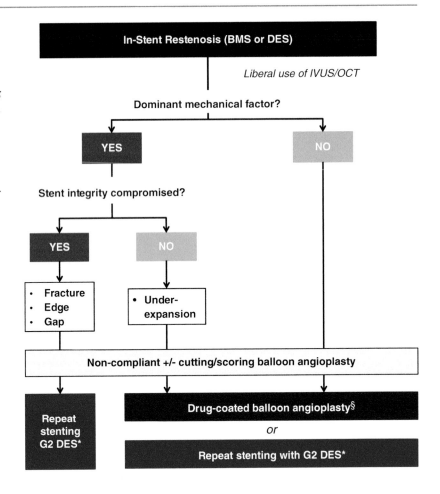

- ectomy, brachytherapy, repeat stenting with BMS, repeat stenting with DES, and drug-coated balloon (DCB) angioplasty [11].
- Ultimately, only the latter two therapies—repeat stenting with DES and DCB angioplasty—have proven successful and are recommended for routine clinical use (both Class I recommendations, level of evidence A) in current European guidelines [10, 12].
- Figure 31.3 depicts a proposed treatment algorithm for ISR.

Repeat Stenting with DES

- Repeat stenting with DES is established as the standard of care in many centers. Repeat stenting with BMS implantation is not recommended for treatment of ISR.

- In fact, the early randomized RIBS trial (*n* = 450) of repeat stenting with BMS failed to show clear benefit over simple balloon angioplasty in BMS-ISR [13].
- The advent of DES was an important development in the treatment of patients with ISR. Two initial randomized trials (discussed below) provided evidence of clear benefit of DES over balloon angioplasty.
- In terms of the choice of DES, it is intuitive that use of a DES eluting an alternative class of anti-restenotic agent ("hetero-DES") might result in lower risk of repeat restenosis because of the potential contribution of drug-hyporesponsiveness to the index ISR [14]. However, in view of the almost exclusive use of limus-based DES in conventional clinical practice, this issue is now of limited relevance.

ISAR-DESIRE (sirolimus-eluting stent versus paclitaxel-eluting stent versus balloon angioplasty)

- The ISAR-DESIRE trial enrolled patients with BMS-ISR ($n = 300$) and showed that both sirolimus-eluting stents (SES; $n = 100$) and paclitaxel-eluting stents (PES; $n = 100$) were superior to balloon angioplasty ($n = 100$) at preventing recurrent restenosis at 6 months, with SES demonstrating a greater risk reduction than PES [15].

RIBS II (SES versus balloon angioplasty)

- This trial enrolled patients with BMS-ISR ($n = 150$) and showed superior 9-month angiographic, IVUS, and 1-year clinical outcomes with SES compared with balloon angioplasty for the treatment of BMS-ISR. The primary endpoint of binary angiographic restenosis occurred in 11% versus 39%, respectively, $p < 0.001$ [16].

Angioplasty with Drug-Coated Balloons

- Angioplasty with drug-coated balloons (DCB) has emerged as a valuable alternative therapy to repeat stenting with DES.
- A DCB is a balloon angioplasty catheter coated with a mixture of an anti-restenotic drug (paclitaxel is the only anti-restenotic agent used on current commercially available devices) and a spacer or excipient (such as iopromide, shellac, or BTHC) that facilitates uptake of the drug into the vessel wall [17].
- The ability to deliver antiproliferative drug to the arterial wall without the need for a permanent metallic implant is particularly attractive in the setting of ISR where the mechanical integrity of the underlying stent is intact.
- Indeed, a number of randomized trials (discussed below) have also shown a benefit with DCB over balloon angioplasty. It is important to realize that the DCB is merely a vehicle for drug delivery; underlying mechanical factors must be first corrected, typically with angioplasty with noncompliant balloons. In

addition, where stent integrity is lacking—e.g., in cases of fracture or gap—repeat stenting should be preferred.

PACCOCATH-ISR (DCB versus balloon angioplasty)

- For the treatment of BMS-ISR, Paccocath-ISR I ($n = 52$) and II ($n = 56$) compared the efficacy of the Paccocath DCB versus balloon angioplasty. The primary endpoint of in-segment late lumen loss at 6 months was lower after treatment with DCB compared with balloon angioplasty (0.81 vs. 0.11, $p < 0.001$). Clinical event rates were also significantly lower with DCB at 12 months, an effect that persisted at 5-year follow-up [18, 19].

PEPCAD-DES (DCB versus balloon angioplasty)

- For treatment of DES-ISR, PEPCAD-DES ($n = 110$) showed superiority of DCB angioplasty over plain balloon angioplasty in terms of the angiographic primary endpoint (late lumen loss 0.43 mm versus 1.03 mm, respectively, $p < 0.001$) and 1-year clinical outcomes [20], an effect which was maintained out to 3 years [21].

Habara et al. (DCB versus balloon angioplasty)

- Two randomized trials ($n = 50$; $n = 207$) were conducted in Japan comparing these two therapies for the treatment of DES-ISR, both showing better angiographic and clinical outcomes with DCB [22, 23]. One of these trials included both patients with DES-ISR and BMS-ISR and showed a worse prognosis for patients with DES-ISR as compared with BMS-ISR after DCB therapy.

Head-to-Head Trials of DCB Versus DES for the Treatment of ISR

- Multiple randomized trials have compared DCB and repeat stenting with DES for the treatment of ISR. In general, broadly comparable results were observed with both therapies, though a marginal advantage is seen for repeat stenting in terms of angiographic endpoints [12].

- In addition, a slight advantage in terms of TLR in some studies must be interpreted in light of the open-label design of trials and possible bias because operators may have been more reluctant to perform repeat stenting in a segment that already had two stent layers compared with one treated with stent implantation followed by DCB angioplasty.

PEPCAD II ISR (DCB Versus PES)

- In patients with BMS-ISR, PEPCAD II ISR (n = 131) showed broadly comparable results between DCB and PES in terms of angiographic efficacy. Although superiority for DCB was seen in terms of the primary endpoint of late lumen loss at 6 months (0.17 vs. 0.38, p = 0.03) [24], late loss is not a suitable endpoint when comparing stents with balloons—because of the higher acute gain achieved with stenting tends to be associated, per se, with more late loss (the "the more you gain, the more you lose" law).
- Nevertheless the broadly comparable findings mean that ISR could be successfully treated by DCB without the need for an additional stent layer. Subsequent clinical event rates between 12 months and 3 years were low and comparable in both groups [25].

RIBS V (DCB Versus EES)

- RIBS V (n = 189) compared DCB with second-generation EES for treatment for BMS-ISR and found EES to be superior in terms of the primary endpoint of MLD at 6–9 months. Clinical outcomes were comparable at 12 months [26], though at 3-year follow-up TLR was lower for EES (2% vs. 8%, p = 0.04) [27].

ISAR DESIRE 3 (DCB Versus PES Versus Balloon Angioplasty)

- ISAR-DESIRE 3 showed that in patients with DES-ISR (n = 402), both DCB and repeat stenting with PES were superior to balloon angioplasty for treatment of DES-ISR, in terms of the primary endpoint of % diameter stenosis at 6–8 months; in addition, DCB was non-inferior to PES in terms of the primary endpoint and clinical outcomes were broadly comparable between these two approaches (Fig. 31.4) [28].
- Subsequent long-term follow-up to 3 years showed that TLR was not significantly different between DCB and PES (although it was numerically higher with DCB). There was a trend however toward lower death or myocardial infarction with DCB vs. PES (HR: 0.55,

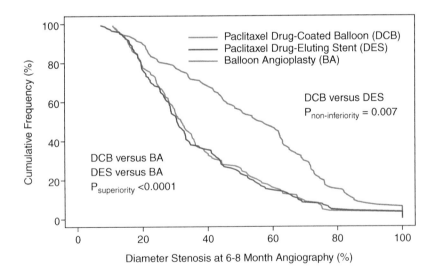

Fig. 31.4 Primary endpoint of the ISAR DESIRE 3 Trial

95% CI: 0.28 to 1.07; $p = 0.08$), supporting some concerns about the long-term effects of DES-in-DES [29].

RIBS IV (DCB Versus EES)

- In patients with DES-ISR enrolled in the RIBS IV trial ($n = 309$), second-generation EES was found superior to DCB in terms of the primary endpoint of minimal lumen diameter (MLD) at 6–9 months and the composite clinical outcome at 1 year, driven by reduced TLR.

Network Meta-Analyses

- A number of network meta-analyses comparing the merits of multiple percutaneous treatment strategies for BMS- and DES-ISR have been published [12, 30, 31].
- The largest included 27 randomized trials and 5923 patients and reported that EES and DCB were the first and second most effective therapies, respectively, in terms of percent diameter stenosis, angiographic restenosis, and TLR.
- The authors concluded that both of these therapies should be considered for the treatment of patients with ISR, given the superiority of EES over alternative therapies (with a slight efficacy advantage over DCB), and the favorable results seen with DCB without the need for an additional stent layer [12].

Lesion Preparation Prior to Drug-Eluting Therapy

- It is important to thoroughly prepare restenotic lesions prior to definitive treatment with local drug delivery devices—either DES or DCB.
- High-pressure noncompliant balloon angioplasty is generally recommended. Balloon angioplasty results in tissue extrusion and additional stent expansion in the case of under-expansion.
- Care must be taken, however, to avoid edge-related complications or slippage of the balloon outside of the stent ("watermelon seeding"), which may result in geographic miss, with potential suboptimal acute and long-term results.
- Cutting or scoring balloon lesion preparation offers less potential for balloon slippage and more effective compression or extrusion of restenotic tissue. A cutting balloon is a balloon catheter with mounted lateral metallic blades that incise the restenotic tissue when the balloon is inflated.
- The blades help to anchor the balloon in the lesion to prevent slippage and the deep incisions may improve subsequent delivery of anti-restenotic drug from DCB or DES deep into the restenotic tissue. There is one commercially available cutting balloon in Europe and the USA at this time (Fig. 31.5). As of yet, there is no randomized data to date that shows an advantage of cutting balloon angioplasty over balloon angioplasty for lesion preparation in ISR.
- Scoring balloons work along a similar principle as cutting balloons but instead of blades have low profile wires in a spiral arrangement on the surface of the balloon catheter. This allows greater flexibility and deliverability of the device, with the trade-off of less plaque incision compared with a cutting balloon. There are three commercially available devices in widespread clinical use at this time (Fig. 31.5). In the recent ISAR DESIRE 4 randomized trial, lesion preparation with scoring balloons increased the efficacy of DCB therapy in terms of the primary endpoint of percentage diameter stenosis at 6–8 month surveillance angiography [32].
- Rotablation is occasionally required for lesion preparation and can be safely performed within a restenosed stent.

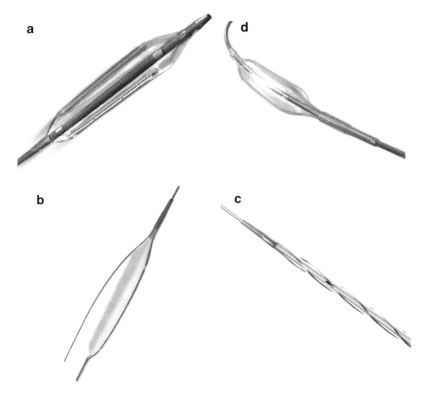

Fig. 31.5 Cutting and scoring balloons. (**a**) Flextome cutting balloon catheter (Boston Scientific); (**b**) Scoreflex scoring balloon catheter (Orbus Neich); (**c**) Angiosculpt scoring balloon catheter (Biotronik); (**d**): NSE Alpha scoring balloon catheter (B Braun)

Alternative Therapies for ISR

Bioresorbable Scaffolds

- Some observational studies suggest acceptable results using fully bioresorbable scaffolds (BRS) to treat patients with BMS-ISR and DES-ISR [33]. However, comparative efficacy data in this setting is lacking.
- Moreover, data from randomized trials in patients with *de novo* disease demonstrated an increase in adverse events with BRS compared with conventional DES [34], and at present this approach cannot be recommended for the treatment of ISR.

Brachytherapy

- Brachytherapy refers to a form of intracoronary radiotherapy delivered at the time of balloon angioplasty, using radioactive seeds or liquid. Beta and gamma radiation have both been shown to successfully treat ISR.
- Superiority of brachytherapy over balloon angioplasty in terms of angiographic and clinical endpoints was demonstrated in a randomized trial. However, the need for specialized laboratory equipment and concerns regarding subsequent systemic impaired arterial healing made brachytherapy unattractive for routine use. Although once a promising therapy, it

was ultimately superseded by DES. Indeed, two randomized trials comparing first-generation DES with brachytherapy for the treatment of BMS-ISR both showed superiority of DES [35, 36].

Coronary Artery Bypass Grafting Surgery

- As ISR often presents as focal pattern disease, it tends to be amenable to PCI. However, bypass surgery may be considered as first-line therapy in selected patients, such as those with recurrent episodes of diffuse ISR or associated significant disease in other vessels, especially if complex.

Conclusion

- Considerable progress has been made in terms of the refinement of percutaneous coronary intervention over the four decades since its introduction into clinical practice.
- Nowadays, rates of clinically significant restenosis in randomized trials with DES, including patients broadly representative of those treated in routine practice, are around 5% or less at one year.
- When DES-ISR does occur, however, pathological findings can be quite different from BMS-ISR and treatment can be more challenging.
- Intravascular imaging plays an important role in the evaluation and treatment of all forms of ISR and should be liberally used.
- Although bypass surgery is occasionally indicated, repeat PCI with DES or DCB is the mainstay of treatment.
- Both repeat stenting with new generation DES and DCB should be considered options for the treatment of patients with ISR:
  - Repeat stenting with DES due its superiority over alternative therapies in ran-

domized trials (including a marginal efficacy advantage over DCB).
  - Angioplasty with DCB due to the favorable results seen without the need for an additional stent layer.

References

1. Mehran R, Dangas G, Abizaid AS, et al. Angiographic patterns of in-stent restenosis: classification and implications for long-term outcome. Circulation. 1999;100:1872–8.
2. Solinas E, Dangas G, Kirtane AJ, et al. Angiographic patterns of drug-eluting stent restenosis and one-year outcomes after treatment with repeated percutaneous coronary intervention. Am J Cardiol. 2008;102:311–5.
3. Alfonso F, Cequier A, Angel J, et al. Value of the American College of Cardiology/American Heart Association angiographic classification of coronary lesion morphology in patients with in-stent restenosis. Insights from the Restenosis Intra-stent Balloon angioplasty versus elective Stenting (RIBS) randomized trial. Am Heart J. 2006;151:681.e1–9.
4. Cassese S, Byrne RA, Tada T, et al. Incidence and predictors of restenosis after coronary stenting in 10004 patients with surveillance angiography. Heart. 2014;100:153–9.
5. Byrne RA, Serruys PW, Baumbach A, et al. Report of a European Society of Cardiology-European Association of Percutaneous Cardiovascular Interventions task force on the evaluation of coronary stents in Europe: executive summary. Eur Heart J. 2015;36:2608–20.
6. Cassese S, Byrne RA, Schulz S, et al. Prognostic role of restenosis in 10 004 patients undergoing routine control angiography after coronary stenting. Eur Heart J. 2015;36:94–9.
7. Chen MS, John JM, Chew DP, Lee DS, Ellis SG, Bhatt DL. Bare metal stent restenosis is not a benign clinical entity. Am Heart J. 2006;151:1260–4.
8. Byrne RA, Cassese S, Windisch T, et al. Differential relative efficacy between drug-eluting stents in patients with bare metal and drug-eluting stent restenosis; evidence in support of drug resistance: insights from the ISAR-DESIRE and ISAR-DESIRE 2 trials. EuroIntervention. 2013;9:797–802.
9. Otsuka F, Byrne RA, Yahagi K, et al. Neoatherosclerosis: overview of histopathologic findings and implications for intravascular imaging assessment. Eur Heart J. 2015;36:2147–59.
10. Windecker S, Kolh P, Alfonso F, et al. 2014 ESC/EACTS Guidelines on myocardial revascularization: The Task Force on Myocardial Revascularization of

the European Society of Cardiology (ESC) and the European Association for Cardio-Thoracic Surgery (EACTS) Developed with the special contribution of the European Association of Percutaneous Cardiovascular Interventions (EAPCI). Eur Heart J. 2014;35:2541–619.

11. Alfonso F, Byrne RA, Rivero F, Kastrati A. Current treatment of in-stent restenosis. J Am Coll Cardiol. 2014;63:2659–73.

12. Siontis GC, Stefanini GG, Mavridis D, et al. Percutaneous coronary interventional strategies for treatment of in-stent restenosis: a network meta-analysis. Lancet. 2015;386:655–64.

13. Alfonso F, Zueco J, Cequier A, et al. A randomized comparison of repeat stenting with balloon angioplasty in patients with in-stent restenosis. J Am Coll Cardiol. 2003;42:796–805.

14. Mehilli J, Byrne RA, Tiroch K, et al. Randomized trial of paclitaxel- versus sirolimus-eluting stents for treatment of coronary restenosis in sirolimus-eluting stents: the ISAR-DESIRE 2 (Intracoronary Stenting and Angiographic Results: Drug Eluting Stents for In-Stent Restenosis 2) study. J Am Coll Cardiol. 2010;55:2710–6.

15. Kastrati A, Mehilli J, von Beckerath N, et al. Sirolimus-eluting stent or paclitaxel-eluting stent vs balloon angioplasty for prevention of recurrences in patients with coronary in-stent restenosis: a randomized controlled trial. JAMA. 2005;293:165–71.

16. Alfonso F, Perez-Vizcayno MJ, Hernandez R, et al. A randomized comparison of sirolimus-eluting stent with balloon angioplasty in patients with in-stent restenosis: results of the Restenosis Intrastent: Balloon Angioplasty Versus Elective Sirolimus-Eluting Stenting (RIBS-II) trial. J Am Coll Cardiol. 2006;47:2152–60.

17. Byrne RA, Joner M, Alfonso F, Kastrati A. Drug-coated balloon therapy in coronary and peripheral artery disease. Nat Rev Cardiol. 2014;11:13–23.

18. Scheller B, Clever YP, Kelsch B, et al. Long-term follow-up after treatment of coronary in-stent restenosis with a paclitaxel-coated balloon catheter. JACC Cardiovasc Interv. 2012;5:323–30.

19. Scheller B, Hehrlein C, Bocksch W, et al. Two year follow-up after treatment of coronary in-stent restenosis with a paclitaxel-coated balloon catheter. Clin Res Cardiol. 2008;97:773–81.

20. Rittger H, Brachmann J, Sinha AM, et al. A randomized, multicenter, single-blinded trial comparing paclitaxel-coated balloon angioplasty with plain balloon angioplasty in drug-eluting stent restenosis: the PEPCAD-DES study. J Am Coll Cardiol. 2012;59:1377–82.

21. Rittger H, Waliszewski M, Brachmann J, et al. Long-term outcomes after treatment with a paclitaxel-coated balloon versus balloon angioplasty: insights from the PEPCAD-DES study (treatment of drug-eluting stent [DES] in-stent restenosis with SeQuent please paclitaxel-coated percutaneous transluminal coro-

nary angioplasty [PTCA] catheter). JACC Cardiovasc Interv. 2015;8:1695–700.

22. Habara S, Mitsudo K, Kadota K, et al. Effectiveness of paclitaxel-eluting balloon catheter in patients with sirolimus-eluting stent restenosis. JACC Cardiovasc Interv. 2011;4:149–54.

23. Habara S, Iwabuchi M, Inoue N, et al. A multicenter randomized comparison of paclitaxel-coated balloon catheter with conventional balloon angioplasty in patients with bare-metal stent restenosis and drug-eluting stent restenosis. Am Heart J. 2013;166:527–533 e2.

24. Unverdorben M, Vallbracht C, Cremers B, et al. Paclitaxel-coated balloon catheter versus paclitaxel-coated stent for the treatment of coronary in-stent restenosis. Circulation. 2009;119:2986–94.

25. Unverdorben M, Vallbracht C, Cremers B, et al. Paclitaxel-coated balloon catheter versus paclitaxel-coated stent for the treatment of coronary in-stent restenosis: the three-year results of the PEPCAD II ISR study. EuroIntervention. 2015;11:926–34.

26. Alfonso F, Perez-Vizcayno MJ, Cardenas A, et al. A randomized comparison of drug-eluting balloon versus everolimus-eluting stent in patients with bare-metal stent-in-stent restenosis: the RIBS V Clinical Trial (Restenosis Intra-stent of Bare Metal Stents: paclitaxel-eluting balloon vs. everolimus-eluting stent). J Am Coll Cardiol. 2014;63:1378–86.

27. Alfonso F, Perez-Vizcayno MJ, Garcia Del Blanco B, et al. Long-term results of everolimus-eluting stents versus drug-eluting balloons in patients with bare-metal in-stent restenosis: 3-year follow-up of the RIBS V clinical trial. JACC Cardiovasc Interv. 2016;9:1246–55.

28. Byrne RA, Neumann FJ, Mehilli J, et al. Paclitaxel-eluting balloons, paclitaxel-eluting stents, and balloon angioplasty in patients with restenosis after implantation of a drug-eluting stent (ISAR-DESIRE 3): a randomised, open-label trial. Lancet. 2013;381:461–7.

29. Kufner S, Cassese S, Valeskini M, et al. Long-term efficacy and safety of paclitaxel-eluting balloon for the treatment of drug-eluting stent restenosis: 3-year results of a randomized controlled trial. JACC Cardiovasc Interv. 2015;8:877–84.

30. Giacoppo D, Gargiulo G, Aruta P, Capranzano P, Tamburino C, Capodanno D. Treatment strategies for coronary in-stent restenosis: systematic review and hierarchical Bayesian network meta-analysis of 24 randomised trials and 4880 patients. BMJ. 2015;351:h5392.

31. Lee JM, Park J, Kang J, et al. Comparison among drug-eluting balloon, drug-eluting stent, and plain balloon angioplasty for the treatment of in-stent restenosis: a network meta-analysis of 11 randomized, controlled trials. JACC Cardiovasc Interv. 2015;8:382–94.

32. Kufner S, Joner M, Schneider S, et al. Neointimal modification with scoring balloon and efficacy of drug-coated balloon therapy in patients with

restenosis in drug-eluting coronary stents: a randomized controlled trial. JACC Cardiovasc Interv. 2017;10:1332–40.

33. Moscarella E, Ielasi A, Granata F, et al. Long-term clinical outcomes after bioresorbable vascular scaffold implantation for the treatment of coronary in-stent restenosis: a multicenter Italian experience. Circ Cardiovasc Interv. 2016;9:e003148.

34. Cassese S, Byrne RA, Ndrepepa G, et al. Everolimus-eluting bioresorbable vascular scaffolds versus everolimus-eluting metallic stents: a meta-analysis of randomised controlled trials. Lancet. 2016;387:537–44.

35. Stone GW, Ellis SG, O'Shaughnessy CD, et al. Paclitaxel-eluting stents vs vascular brachytherapy for in-stent restenosis within bare-metal stents: the TAXUS V ISR randomized trial. JAMA. 2006;295:1253–63.

36. Holmes DR Jr, Teirstein P, Satler L, et al. Sirolimus-eluting stents vs vascular brachytherapy for in-stent restenosis within bare-metal stents: the SISR randomized trial. JAMA. 2006;295:1264–73.

Percutaneous Coronary Intervention: Management of Complications

Robert T. Gerber, Athanasios Kosovitsas, and Carlo Di Mario

About Us

The Cardiology Department at East Sussex Healthcare Trust (ESHT) is situated in a beautiful coastal corner of England on two sites in large district general hospitals (>500 beds) close to Hastings and Eastbourne. The catchment area is 500,000 and comprises predominantly an elderly population and so recruitment to the RINCAL trial looking at revascularization in the Elderly (>80 years) vs. medical treatment is ongoing. Over 800 PCI are performed annually and there is a 24/7 PPCI rota with sizeable device implantation and electrophysiology programs. The department has contributed to multicenter randomized trials in acute coronary syndromes (TAO, ATLANTIC, PEGASUS), hemodynamic assessment of inter-

mediate coronary lesions (ORBITA and FLAIR), and PCSK9 inhibition (ODYSSEY Outcomes). The department has been involved in investigating the role of renal denervation (RDN) in the treatment of resistant hypertension and heart failure (REACH) and is currently enrolling patients in PARADISE HTN. Finally, ESHT was the top UK site for the recently completed multicenter MASCOT Registry.

Royal Brompton Hospital is located in central London in Chelsea and has a long distinguished history of being a tertiary referral center for cardiovascular and respiratory disease. Along with Harefield Hospital near Uxbridge, it forms the Royal Brompton and Harefield NHS Foundation Trust, which is the largest specialist heart and lung center in the UK. There are 2800 angiograms and 2300 angioplasties taking place in the Trust annually. The department has expertise in intravascular imaging using IVUS, OCT, and more recently NIRS IVUS. There are well-established CTO and structural, TAVI and Mitraclip programs. It has the largest experience of Mitraclip implants in the UK with more than 150 cases and it achieved a world first by implanting a Tendyne transcatheter mitral valve system to treat mitral regurgitation. The department is involved in several trials such as DEFINE-FLAIR, the Lipid Rich Plaque Study, the ABSORB Registry, the Shockwave study, the BLADE study, and the UK TAVI trial.

The University Hospital of Florence Careggi is a large tertiary referral center serving a popula-

R. T. Gerber
Department of Cardiology, Conquest Hospital
Hastings and Eastbourne DGH, East Sussex
Healthcare NHS Trust, East Sussex, UK

NIHR Cardiovascular Biomedical Research Unit,
Royal Brompton Hospital, London, UK
e-mail: r.gerber@nhs.net; rtgerber@doctors.org.uk

A. Kosovitsas
NIHR Cardiovascular Biomedical Research Unit,
Royal Brompton Hospital, London, UK

C. Di Mario (✉)
NIHR Cardiovascular Biomedical Research Unit,
Royal Brompton Hospital, London, UK

Careggi University Hospital, Florence, Italy
e-mail: C.DiMario@rbht.nhs.uk

© Springer International Publishing AG, part of Springer Nature 2018
A. Myat et al. (eds.), *The Interventional Cardiology Training Manual*,
https://doi.org/10.1007/978-3-319-71635-0_32

tion of 1.9 million inhabitants in the heart of Tuscany. It started one of the first and most efficient primary angioplasty services back in the 1990s and has been running for almost 10 years an interventional stroke unit with dedicated CT and immediate transfer direct from the ambulance service. It performed seminal studies on the arachidonic acid pathway and the role of aspirin, with an active basic science cardiovascular unit dedicated to platelet and coagulation as well as genetic identification of cardiomyopathies.

Background

- In 1980 Gruentzig said, *"If I had an enemy I would teach him angioplasty"* [1], which no doubt refers to the trials and tribulations that a busy Interventional Cardiologist faces in day-to-day practice. The reality is that any coronary invasive procedure (PCI) carries risks which can range from 1 to 20% mortality depending on patient and lesion subgroups alongside acute presentation (acute coronary syndromes—ACS), chronic kidney disease (CKD), diabetes, sex, and advanced age, all having an impact on occurrence of complications [2].
- In the previous chapters of this manual, patient selection and choice of revascularization mode have been discussed in detail but we must emphasize that once the decision to perform PCI is made by the operator (and/or heart multidisciplinary team) a successful outcome depends on several crucial factors:
  - The cath lab team must be appropriately trained to face unexpected complications, regularly rehearsing and simulating events. The emergency pericardiocentesis kit, temporary wires, and covered stents must be kept in a visible well-identified location and everybody must be familiar on how to use dedicated bailout devices. Part of the cath lab meetings should be dedicated to "complication troubleshooting," thereby ensuring protocols are regularly updated, cases discussed, and devices reviewed.
  - Operator skill and expertise is also important in determining a favorable outcome

and regular morbidity and mortality audit meetings should be an essential part of managing PCI complications. Interventionalists should attend the PCI complication forums at congresses and familiarize themselves with newer devices and the complications that can arise with their use (see device capture section). Nobody should be allowed to work as independent operator unless he learns to deploy embolization coils, covered stents with the use of buddy wire or guideliner devices and microcatheters. The emergency bypass rate from PCI has now decreased to much less than 0.1% (Fig. 32.1) [3] which is an attestation to the improvements in Heart Team-delivered percutaneous revascularization.

- PCI complications can be broadly grouped into:
  - Coronary ischemia:
    Dissection
    No-reflow, air or thrombotic embolism
  - Device-related factors:
    Coronary perforation
    Stent, wire, or catheter misadventures
  - Patient-related factors:
    Contrast-induced nephropathy (CIN)
    Contrast allergy/anaphylaxis
- We describe a systematic process with which to recognize and manage the aforementioned complications associated with PCI and adopt a pragmatic "tips and tricks" approach on how to deal with these acutely.
- We also provide, where possible, evidence and case report experience from the literature to help the interventionalist when faced with the daunting task of tackling a life-threatening complication.

Coronary Ischemia

- The short-term consequences of acute vessel closure will result in myocardial infarction (MI), ischemic arrhythmias, and if survived ischemic left ventricular dysfunction.
- Rapid restoration of TIMI 3 flow is one of the most important predictors of long-term

Fig. 32.1 BCIS National Audit 1991–2015. Emergency bypass rate following PCI and mortality from emergency CABG. Key: *em CABG* emergency coronary artery bypass grafting, *BCIS* British Cardiovascular Intervention Society

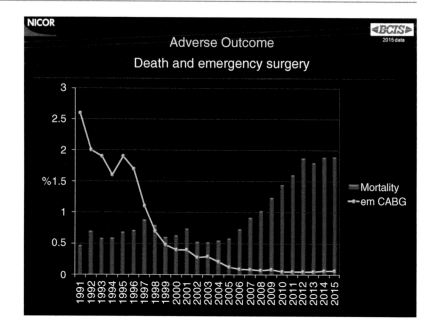

event-free survival following vessel closure [4], and so every effort should be made to restore flow.

Dissection

- Dissection of the coronary artery is a consequence of separation of the different layers of the arterial wall causing luminal obstruction. This usually involves separation of the intima from the media (Figs. 32.2 and 32.3).
- Unlike periprocedural dissections with dissection planes through the intima or between intima and media, in spontaneous dissections separation of the media from the adventitia can also occur.
- Flow impairment, presence of dissection flaps and thrombus have characteristic angiographic appearances which have been categorized into a morphological classification (Types A–F—Table 32.1) [5].
- Primary dissections are spontaneous and have very different management [6] compared to secondary dissections which develop as a consequence of vessel injury from PCI, CABG or aortic root or chest trauma (Figs. 32.4, 32.5, 32.6, 32.7, 32.8, and 32.9).

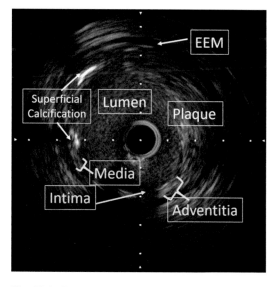

Fig. 32.2 Intravascular ultrasound (IVUS) image demonstrating the structures of intima, media, and adventitia within the vessel wall surrounded by the external elastic membrane (EEM)

- Major dissections with poor outcome are generally regarded as Types C-F with additional features such as luminal staining in two projections and defects greater than 20 mm.
- Persistent complications from Types C-F dissections have become much less frequent in the stent era but still develop in 12–17% of

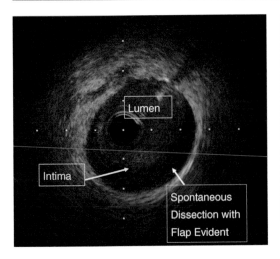

Fig. 32.3 IVUS image of a spontaneous coronary artery dissection (SCAD) in a young woman presenting with an acute coronary syndrome

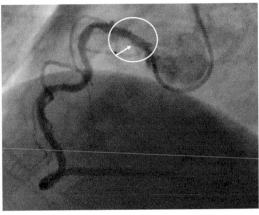

Fig. 32.4 Type A dissection. Radiolucent areas within the coronary lumen during contrast injection that do not persist after dye clearance with normal coronary flow (white circle and arrow). Note the Amplatz-shaped catheter

Table 32.1 National Heart, Lung, and Blood Institute (NHLBI) Angiographic Dissection Classification [5]

Dissection type	Angiographic description of dissection
Type A	Radiolucent areas within the coronary lumen during contrast injection that do not persist after dye clearance with normal coronary flow
Type B	Parallel tracks or double lumen evident on contrast injection with minimal or no persistence of dye after injection
Type C	Dissection evident after dye injection in extraluminal space with persistence of dye
Type D	Spiral dissection—As with type C but with spiral luminal dissections with extensive contrast staining of the vessel
Type E	Dissections appear as new persistent filling defects with impaired coronary flow
Type F	Result in impaired flow and total occlusion of the coronary artery with no anterograde flow

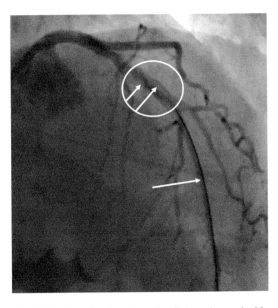

Fig. 32.5 Type B dissection. Parallel tracks or double lumen evident on contrast injection with minimal or no persistence of dye after injection (white circle and arrows). Note the coronary wire (arrow)

cases and include abrupt vessel closure, emergency CABG, and MI.

- Iatrogenic dissection from the guide catheter is observed more frequently when intubation is performed with coexisting disease at the coronary ostia. Use of Amplatz guides, deep intubation, vigorous contrast injection, and stiffer angioplasty wires are also associated with this potentially life-threatening complication.
- The usual treatment option for dissections is coronary stenting although some success can occur from conservative management if, in particular, the dissection is not extensive, TIMI flow is preserved, and the vessel is not extensively diseased.
- *Intravascular ultrasound (IVUS) can help in guiding treatment strategies. If there is associated intramural hematoma, then stenting is usually the preferred option.*

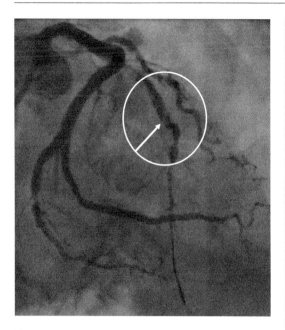

Fig. 32.6 Type C dissection. Dissection evident after dye injection in extraluminal space with persistence of dye (white circle and arrow)

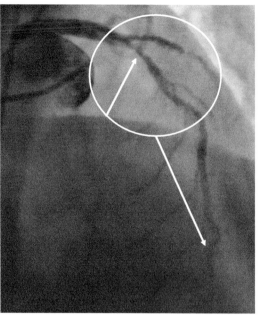

Fig. 32.8 Type E dissection. Dissections appear as new persistent filling defects with impaired coronary flow (white circle and arrows)

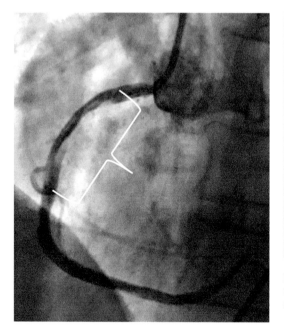

Fig. 32.7 Type D dissection. Spiral dissection—as with Type C (Fig. 32.6) but with spiral luminal dissections with extensive contrast staining of the vessel (large parenthesis)

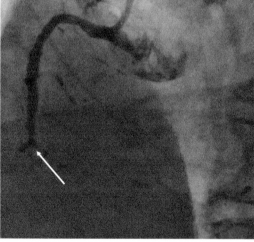

Fig. 32.9 Type F dissection. Dissection causes impaired flow and total occlusion of the coronary artery with no anterograde flow (white arrow)

No-Reflow

- The description of no-reflow relates to impaired or absent coronary flow without any evidence of vessel obstruction or high-grade stenosis. If dissection is excluded as described above, then the cause of no-reflow needs to be established as this has implications on treatment strategies.
- The most common cause is embolism of debris from a plaque rupture, which is usually friable material released at the time of PCI for ACS.
- IVUS studies have suggested that plaques with higher amounts of thin-cap fibroatheromas (TCFAs) and large necrotic cores are more prone to result in no-reflow [7].
- Meticulous PCI "housekeeping" is also important to avoid thrombus or air embolism related to the guide catheters, multiple wires, aspiration catheters, and microcatheters by ensuring adequate ACT monitoring (every 30–45 min; ACT ≥250) and diligent preparation of equipment to stop air entry into Y-connectors or injected directly from contrast syringes.
- The pathophysiology relates to a combination of distal embolization and microvascular obstruction due to spasm and inflammation. The inflammatory mediators implicated are thromboxane A2, serotonin, free radicals, and plasmin activator inhibitor-1 (PAI-1).
- Another rarer phenomenon describes no-reflow from reflex sympathetic microvascular obstruction after aggressive post-dilatation [8].
- Restoration of TIMI 3 flow is paramount as persistent no-reflow is associated with inhospital events (e.g., malignant ventricular arrhythmias and MI) and long-term LV impairment and death [9].
- It is more common in men than women and in one study around 20% of patients that did not receive timely pharmacotherapy developed a clinical composite of heart failure, cardiogenic shock, and death. This reduced to less than half (9%) if flow restoration was achieved after pharmacotherapy [10].

- It must be emphasized that while working on the restoration of flow with vasopressors, regular ACT monitoring should be made and aim for values around 300 to prevent thrombus formation in segments with stagnant blood.
- Normal blood pressure must be maintained using hemodynamic support with intravenous fluids or IABP with correction of any electrophysiological instability by using temporary pacing wires, amiodarone, or atropine.
- In general proven treatment strategies involve intracoronary administration of arteriolar vasodilators such as nitroprusside, verapamil, or adenosine. It is also worth mentioning that nitrates, nicardipine, papaverine, diltiazem, and ephedrine have also been used in this scenario. Nitrates are in fact predominantly venodilators but do have an action on arterial endothelium-independent relaxation through the secondary messenger cGMP.
- Nitroprusside is a direct nitric oxide (NO) donor, which needs to be prepared in a syringe covered in foil to prevent light degradation, and is less manageable causing severe hypotension in the doses needed (50–200 mcg) to restore flow, so an intracoronary infusion through a microcatheter is required.
- Nitrates are usually the first-line agent due to familiarity and they do increase the minimum lumen diameter of the epicardial vessel [11], however it is not effective on the coronary microvasculature with little impact in the treatment of no-reflow demonstrated in several studies [12, 13].
- This is not the case for nitroprusside, which has been shown to be very effective. This agent is best utilized if given through either a microcatheter or multipurpose catheter placed distally in the coronary bed with incremental dose escalation (100–200 mcg boluses, up to a maximum of five applications).
- This is therefore not a practical solution for most cath labs and nitroprusside use is not favored over the calcium channel blockers.
- Intracoronary verapamil has been shown to improve microvascular perfusion, reduce

platelet aggregation, and increase the ischemic tolerance of the myocardium. It is a better alternative to nitroprusside and nitrate,
especially in SVG intervention [14].

- These mechanisms go beyond calcium
channel-mediated actions and involve its role
in reduction of catecholamine responses. It
should be used with caution however since it
can cause transient heart block and hypotension as it has a negative inotropic action.

- Verapamil is simply prepared by diluting 1 mg
in a 10 mL syringe (100 mcg/mL). Most laboratories use verapamil as part of the radial
artery cocktail. The primary operator can then
bolus a dose of 2 mL intracoronary verapamil
to a maximum of five applications.

- Adenosine, which is familiar to most operators due to its use in pressure wire studies, has
a short half-life (10–15 s) and works by opening K$^+$ channels in vascular smooth muscle
cells. This is mediated by A2A and A2B
receptors and in several studies has successfully reversed no-reflow with a synergistic
effect if used with nitroprusside in combination [15].

- Our experience is to use 50–100 mcg boluses
with up to 10–15 applications. Rarely, transient atrioventricular block may occur but this
tends to resolve spontaneously.

- If air embolus is identified as the etiology,
then immediate aspiration should be
attempted. Energetic flushing with saline
(avoid contrast!) can dislodge the microbub-
bles (Fig. 32.10).

- If no-reflow persists despite the use of vasodilators described above, then sitting the patient
upright has been proposed as this is thought to
siphon through the air particles from the
microvasculature.

- Thromboembolic material is commonly associated with SVG intervention, rotablator use,
and incomplete thrombo-aspiration in the context of ACS.

- If SVG intervention is performed evidence
from at least one randomized trial suggests the
use of filter wires and pretreatment of vessels

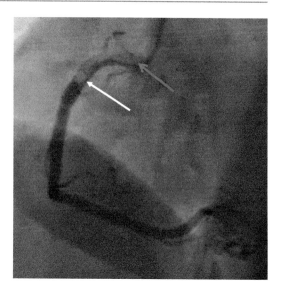

Fig. 32.10 Angiogram demonstrating air embolus.
Iatrogenic air embolus evident (white arrow) after contrast
injection from the guide catheter, which also has residual
air within it proximally (blue arrow)

with verapamil to prevent no-reflow (see
Chap. 30). The older the SVG (>7 years), the
more likely no-reflow is observed.

- No-reflow as a consequence of thromboembo-
lism is more likely to respond to glycoprotein
IIb/IIa inhibitors and these agents should be
used if the etiology is thrombus.

- However, if no-reflow is due to microvascular
causes as outlined above, then IIb/IIIa infusion is contraindicated and can indeed be detrimental due to promoting microvascular
hemorrhage at sites of poor perfusion [16].

Device-Related Factors

Coronary Perforation

- Sir William Osler wrote, *'Medicine is a science of uncertainty and an art of probability,'*
which encapsulates the unpredictable nature
of the most feared cath lab complication.

- We have all embarked on straightforward
cases with the intention and expectation of
achieving an optimal result only to be faced

Table 32.2 Ellis classification of coronary perforations

Perforation type	Ellis classification of coronary perforations
Type I	Extraluminal crater without extravasation
Type II	Pericardial or myocardial blush without contrast jet Extravasation
Type III	Extravasation through frank (>1 mm) perforation
Cavity spilling	Perforation into an anatomic cavity chamber, coronary sinus, etc.

with a perforation. The incidence is 0.1–1.3% of PCIs.

- Perforation is more common in elderly patients, previous CABG subjects and females more prone to perforation. The use of higher inflation pressures in compliant balloons with higher balloon-to-artery ratios, hydrophilic stiff wires, and athero-ablative devices all promote perforation [17].
- The Ellis classification for describing coronary perforations can be seen in Table 32.2. This is similar to the NHLBI dissection classification in terms of grade equating to severity but has a more practical and widespread understanding within the interventional community [18].
- Ellis Type I perforations are essentially the same as localized dissections and are angiographically indistinguishable from dissections. They tend to be benign and careful monitoring or stenting of the vessel is usually all that is required.
- Rotablation with or without the use of scoring or cutting devices often result in Ellis I angiographic images, which are often regarded as a sign of adequate vessel preparation prior to stenting.
- Ellis Type II and Type III perforations carry the worse prognosis with up to 40% MACE and 16% mortality reported in one single center contemporary experience [19].
- Mechanistically the increment in vessel size is a combination of epicardial vessel stretch and lumen increase from plaque modification/displacement. Overstretching of the epicardial vessel will result in rupture and so it stands to

reason that post-dilatation to high pressure of calcific vessels will cause rupture as the vessel dilates away from the non-modifiable calcific plaque.

- Other scenarios to be mindful of are balloon ruptures and the associated high pressure jet causing rupture and over dilation of negatively remodeled vessels with the risk of stent strut protruding through the vessel wall.
- Clinically the patient feels an acute pain due to disruption of epicardial sensory nerves and not from myocardial ischemia. Experienced operators are aware of this forewarning and leave the balloon in the guide catheter while taking a quick fluoro-acquisition. The management of Ellis III perforations is nicely described in the flowchart from Al-Lamee et al. (Fig. 32.11) [19].
- Pericardiocentesis is usually required but can be delayed if timely sealing of the perforation can occur, as described below, and is performed in approximately one-third of cases.

Case-Based Scenarios with "Tips and Tricks" to Dealing with ELLIS III Perforations

Case 1

- A 65-year-old female presented with worsening angina and after a positive stress test was listed for angiography. There was a tight lesion in the mid RCA (Fig. 32.12) and pre-dilatation resulted in a Type D spiral dissection extending proximal and distal to the lesion (Fig. 32.7).
- The vessel was eventually stented. There was some difficulty passing the stent, so buddy wires were used but the dissection was sealed adequately. The vessel was then post-dilated with a 4.0 mm noncompliant balloon to 18 atmospheres, as there was some concern about under-expansion of the proximal stent.
- This resulted in an Ellis III perforation (Fig. 32.13), which was initially managed by prolonged balloon inflation (Fig. 32.14) using a balloon-to-artery ratio of 1:1. Prolonged balloon inflation is an effective technique and can be effective alone if the vessel is small and if

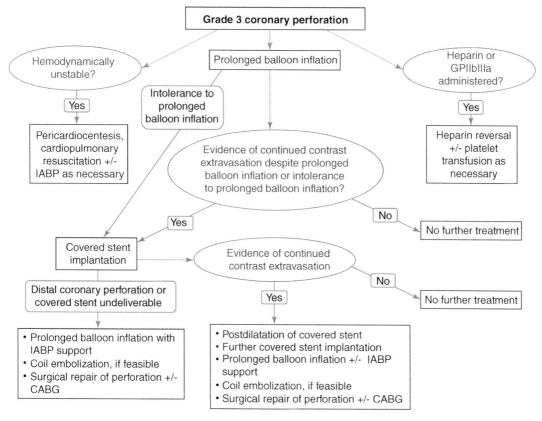

Fig. 32.11 Algorithm for the management of Ellis Grade (Type) III coronary perforations. Key: *CABG* coronary artery bypass grafting, *GPIIb/IIIa* glycoprotein IIbIIIa inhibitors, *IABP* intra-aortic balloon pumps. Reproduced with permission from Al-Lamee et al. [19]

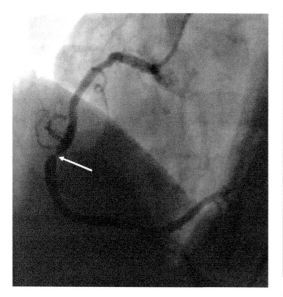

Fig. 32.12 Tight concentric lesion in the mid portion of a large dominant right coronary artery (white arrow)

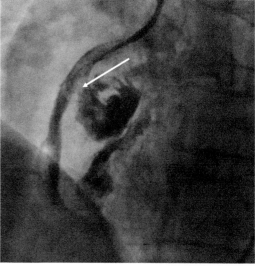

Fig. 32.13 An Ellis type/grade III perforation (white arrow) following stent deployment and post-dilatation with a noncompliant balloon resulting in extravasation of blood into the pericardial space. Also refer to Fig. 32.7

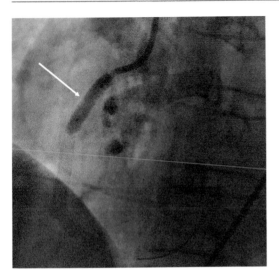

Fig. 32.14 The Ellis III perforation was managed initially by prolonged balloon inflation using a balloon-to-artery ratio of 1:1 (white arrow)

the amount of the myocardium supplied by the vessel is not too extensive, thereby limiting the degree of MI.

- The comprehensive flow chart (Fig. 32.11) provides a useful "road map" to operators when faced with alarming and unexpected angiographic Ellis III perforations. In this case the stent struts protruded through the dissection planes and resulted in perforation of the vessel with most likely a longitudinal tear of the vessel within the stented area.
- The operator thought prior to the perforation that post-dilatation was necessary due to stent under-expansion angiographically but this was most likely an area where the stent was passing sub-intimally and the vessel layers at the mid-point of the stent were outside the device giving the appearance of under-expansion.
- In fact, the stent was placed in an abluminal position in its midcourse and so traversing from true lumen proximally to false lumen (intra-stent) and then into true lumen distally.
- The diagnosis and cause of the Ellis III is important and the operator in this scenario

became aware of this issue and so prolonged balloon inflation alone was unlikely to be successful and so a covered stent was implanted.

- The different types of covered stent are discussed below but it is important to emphasize in this scenario that heparin was not reversed with protamine and no pericardiocentesis was performed.
- It must be highlighted that it is now NOT usual practice to reverse heparin immediately and perform emergency pericardiocentesis with IABP insertion +/− emergency CABG.
- These measures are utilized if prolonged balloon inflation, covered stent implantation, or embolization prove ineffective. Efforts must be made to arrest the perforation and determining the etiology and site of perforation are crucial in this regard.
- Reversal of heparin can in fact be deleterious in this circumstance when further stenting or distal embolization is necessary as this could result in stent thrombosis or catheter-related thrombosis which is a scenario best avoided, i.e., hemorrhage and thrombosis in the same patient.
- There are several types of covered stent available but predominantly the two most effective types are a polytetrafluoroethylene-covered stent (PTFE) which is a bare metal stent with PTFA overlay and a further bare metal stent on the outside producing a "stent sandwich" with PTFE as the filler. The other device is an equine pericardium-covered stent and has the advantage of being more deliverable.
- Prior to the introduction of covered stents in the late 1990s the emergency CABG rate was around 50% [17].
- The PTFE device is very bulky and difficult to deliver and it may require use of a larger guide for support and sizing needs to be accurate as overexpansion is difficult and apposition to the vessel wall is essential.
- Use of "ping pong" guiding catheters are helpful if the operator anticipates difficulty with fast exchange of devices.

Case 2

- A 72-year-old presented to her primary care physician with chest pain and the ECG demonstrated transient anterior ST elevation. She was brought to the cath lab for primary angioplasty and preloaded with dual antiplatelet therapy in the ambulance.

- Angiography demonstrated TIMI 3 flow on arrival and a high-grade lesion in the mid left anterior descending (LAD) artery. Significant angulation and some calcification meant the lesion required preparation and the use of buddy wires for stent implantation (Fig. 32.15).

- After stenting, distal blush at the very distal portion of the LAD was noted at the point where the terminal portion of the stiff buddy wire had been (Fig. 32.16). An appearance like this should always cause concern as often wire exit perforations have consequences which are often delayed and result in tamponade and

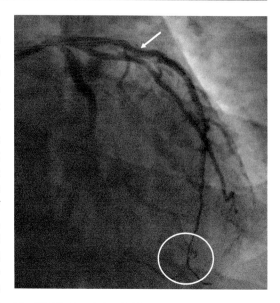

Fig. 32.15 Angulation (white arrow) and some calcification within the LAD artery meant the lesion required the use of buddy wires (white circle) for stent implantation

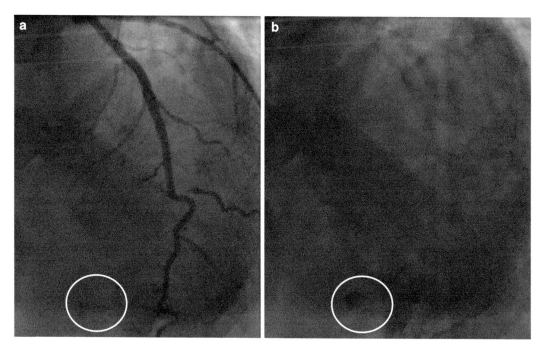

Fig. 32.16 Myocardial blush evident at the very distal portion of the LAD artery post stenting (white circles). This was at the location of the terminal part of the stiff part of the buddy wire (Plate **a**). Contrast staining was noted to be more pronounced after contrast injection, suggesting late extravasation of dye/blood (Plate **b**)

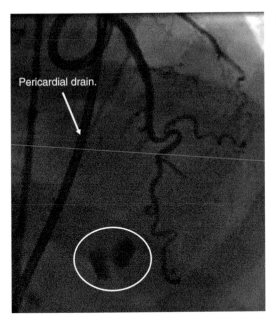

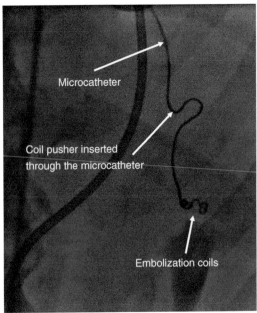

Fig. 32.17 Wire exit perforation with brisk outflow into the pericardium (white circle)

Fig. 32.18 Through the microcatheter embolization coils, fat or glue can be administered. The use of either a stylet or coil pusher through the microcatheter provides more control for delivery of devices

hemodynamic instability hours later (3–5 h) rather than acutely and have surprisingly a worse the prognosis.

- In this instance the patient developed tamponade on the coronary care unit 1 h later which required emergency pericardiocentesis.
- Hemodynamic instability ensued so a decision was made to return to the cath lab. On angiography, a wire exit perforation with brisk outflow into the pericardium was found (Fig. 32.17).
- Here the preferred method is to place a microcatheter into the vessel and perform an intracoronary angiogram to identify the leakage. Through the microcatheter embolization coils, fat or glue can be administered. The use of either a stylet or coil pusher through the microcatheter provides more control for delivery of devices (Fig. 32.18).
- In this case more than two coils were required to halt leakage and we recommend spending time with your local coil manufacturer representative or interventional radiologist who can

explain the differing coil types, delivery methods, and sizes which can be used safely in coronary arteries (Fig. 32.19).

- It should be emphasized that in the case of chronic total occlusion (CTO) intervention, wire exit perforations can occur from both the antegrade and retrograde distal vessels and so coil implantation to stem flow may be required from both antegrade and retrograde CTO wire exits.

Case 3

- An 82-year-old gentleman presented with lateral ST-elevation MI and underwent primary PCI. This demonstrated an occluded diagonal (Fig. 32.20). The vessel was recanalized after wiring and thrombus aspiration and a stent inserted to cover the sequential lesion (Fig. 32.21).
- An Ellis III perforation became evident after stenting (Fig. 32.22) with brisk extravasation

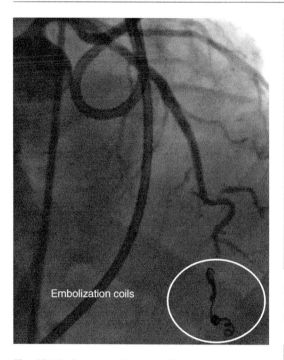

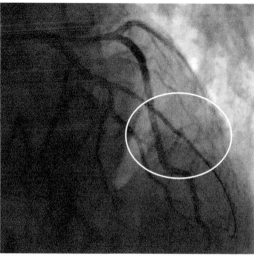

Fig. 32.21 The diagonal was recanalized after wiring and thrombus aspiration and a stent inserted to open the occlusion (white circle)

Fig. 32.19 Two embolization coils were necessary to arrest the flow and extravasation of blood into the pericardium. Check angiography either through the microcatheter or the guide confirms this. If at any stage ongoing leakage is suspected, then further coils can be subsequently placed

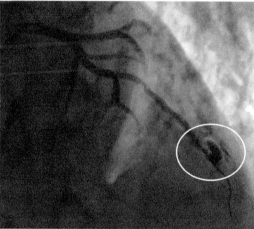

Fig. 32.22 An Ellis III perforation became evident after stent implantation with brisk extravasation of contrast (white circle)

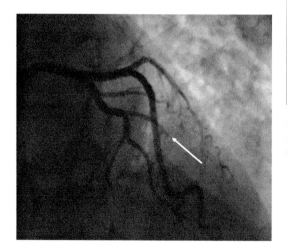

Fig. 32.20 A patient who presented with a lateral ST-elevation myocardial infarction with angiography demonstrating an occluded diagonal branch vessel (arrow)

of contrast and so balloon tamponade with the stent balloon was performed immediately (Fig. 32.23). This gave the cath lab team and operator time to think about the appropriate strategy to deal with this and also prevented hemodynamic instability and obviated the need for pericardiocentesis.

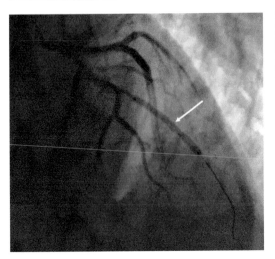

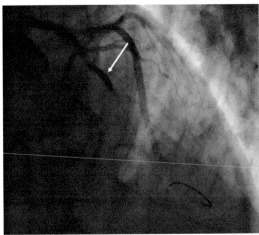

Fig. 32.23 Balloon tamponade with the stent balloon (white arrow) proximal to the point of perforation was performed, immediately arresting extravasation of blood from the distal vessel

Fig. 32.25 The LAD artery was wired and a pericardium-covered stent was inserted to cover the ostium of the diagonal (white arrow) with removal of the diagonal balloon and wire

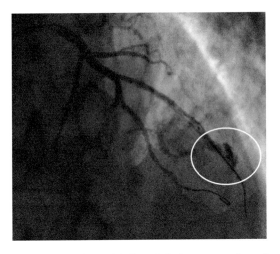

Fig. 32.24 Prolonged balloon inflation was performed for 10–15 min but proved ineffective as extravasation was still evident after brief deflation of the balloon (white circle)

- Prolonged balloon inflation was performed for 10–15 min but was ineffective at sealing the perforation (Fig. 32.24). Further interrogation of the coronary angiogram suggested two causes for the perforation: namely a wire exit perforation and a simultaneous vessel rupture caused by the stent.
- It was felt that in this scenario the safest option was to sacrifice the diagonal vessel

rather than attempt to insert a covered stent in the diagonal artery, which would be ineffective in dealing with the wire exit perforation. Additionally, it could potentially promote further extravasation by extending the rupture and facilitating flow into the disrupted vasculature distally.

- The LAD was wired and a pericardium-covered stent was inserted to cover the ostium of the diagonal with removal of the diagonal balloon and wire (Fig. 32.25).
- Covered stents in general need post-dilating once inserted to arrest flow, as they are not well opposed by their stent delivery balloons. Post-dilation must be performed by noncompliant balloons to ensure safe expansion of the device and the post dilation needs to be for a prolonged time (>30 s) to allow the stent to imbed within the vessel media adequately to arrest flow.
- The covered stent arrested flow in the diagonal in this scenario (Fig. 32.26) and the patient returned to the coronary care unit where he was monitored and eventually made a full recovery albeit having sustained a lateral Q-wave MI. However, he did not require emergency CABG, pericardiocentesis or IABP and the antiplatelets and heparin were never interrupted.

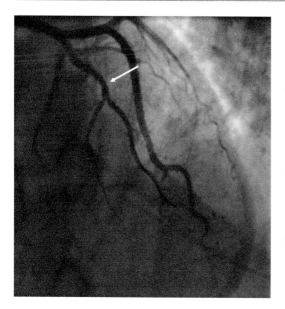

Fig. 32.26 The covered stent arrested flow in the diagonal (white arrow) and pericardiocentesis was not required with minimal pericardial fluid demonstrated on subsequent echocardiography

- These cases highlight the three types of maneuvers necessary to deal with perforation, namely:
    - Sealing a perforation with a covered stent
    - Embolizing a distal leak from a perforation using coils
    - Sacrificing a small vessel by arresting blood flow through to the artery

Device Misadventures

- The inevitable consequence of performing PCI can be loss or incorrect device implantation either due to inability to deploy or unpredictable dislodgment of devices in the coronary tree. We describe here some strategies that help with wire, catheter, and stent misadventures.
- Stent retrieval is always a challenge. If the stent comes away from a stent delivery balloon but remains on the coronary guide wire, then several maneuvers are possible in order of escalation. The simplest method is to pass a smaller CTO type balloon (1.0–1.5 mm) through the stent, inflate the smaller balloon distally, and then remove the stent and distal balloon together.
- If the balloon will not cross the stent, then use of a GuideLiner to envelope the device and then placing a trapping balloon on a parallel wire to trap the stent onto the GuideLiner can also be successful.
- Similar strategies utilizing parallel balloons adjacent to dislodged stents are also effective and can be used for stents that are still mounted on or off their coronary guide wires.
- However, if the stent is lodged in an angulated or calcific part of the vessel, then it is difficult to retrieve even with the use of a snare. It can be useful to pass an IVUS catheter as it will give you some idea about the device and also if it is adherent to the vessel wall.
- Figure 32.27 demonstrates IVUS with Chromaflow of a stent floating in the distal left main stem which was dislodged into an angulated circumflex distally. In this instance the safest outcome was to effectively deploy the stent onto the vessel rather than attempt retrieval as the angulation and anatomical location of the device would preclude a straightforward retrieval procedure.
- Catheters can become twisted or fractured. They can be retrieved by either placing a balloon within the catheter (remembering that you need a 2.5 mm balloon for a 6 French catheter) or with a snare.
- There are several snares but the long gooseneck is the easiest to manipulate and if not successful the Ensnare, which is a device made of three adjacent loops, should be tried.
- GuideLiners can come off the delivery stylet and balloon retrieval is an easy solution to this problem.
- Diagnostic catheters can be untwisted. This is best performed by pushing the catheter to a more proximal larger vessel where it can be unwound or snared (Fig. 32.28). It is easier to unwind the catheter by placing a straight 0.36-in. wire through the lumen or a stiff angioplasty wire.

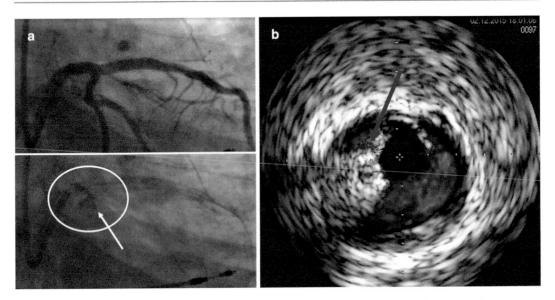

Fig. 32.27 Plate (**a**). Angiography with and without contrast demonstrating a lodged device within the distal left main stem (LMS) extending into the ostial left circumflex vessel. Plate (**b**). IVUS with Chromaflow demonstrating the device seen on angiography is a stent floating in the LMS

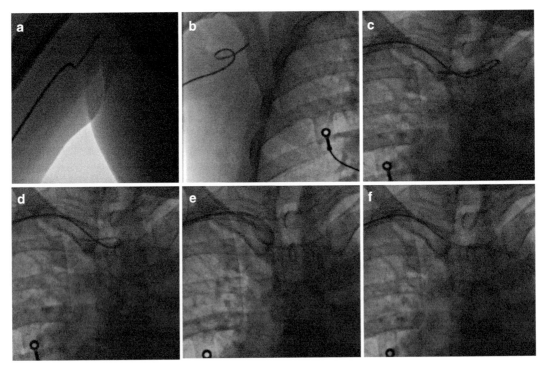

Fig. 32.28 Technique to remove a twisted catheter. (**a**) A diagnostic catheter was over-torqued and became twisted. (**b**) Push the diagnostic catheter into a wider, more proximal position to allow for easier manipulation. (**c**) Exchange the standard J wire for either a straight-tipped 0.36-in. wire or stiff angioplasty wire. (**d**) Manipulate the stiffer wire within the catheter to pass through the kinked section. (**e**) Once the stiffer wire traverses the twisted section, the catheter will start to straighten out. (**f**) Withdraw the catheter while simultaneously advancing the wire

Patient-Related Factors

Contrast-Induced Nephropathy (CIN)

- CIN is the third leading cause of acute kidney injury (AKI), accounting for approximately 14% of hospital-acquired renal failure [20].
- CIN is generally defined as a ≥25% relative increase or ≥44 μmol/L absolute increase in serum creatinine (SCr) within 72 h of contrast exposure in the absence of other identifiable causes.
- Various mechanisms contribute in the development of CIN [21]:
  - Renal medullary hypoxia due to vasoconstriction
  - Oxygen free radical-induced endothelial cell injury and dysfunction
  - Microvessel constriction
  - Increased viscosity from contrast agents producing further reduction in medullary blood flow and glomerular filtration rate
  - Direct cytotoxic effect of the contrast agent on the renal tubular cells
- There are several risk factors described and Mehran et al. have developed a risk scoring system (Fig. 32.29) [22].
- Once contrast-induced AKI develops, the treatment is mainly supportive. AKI prevention is therefore essential and once a patient is identified to be at risk, steps must be taken to minimize contrast volume and avoid repetitive studies in a short period of time.

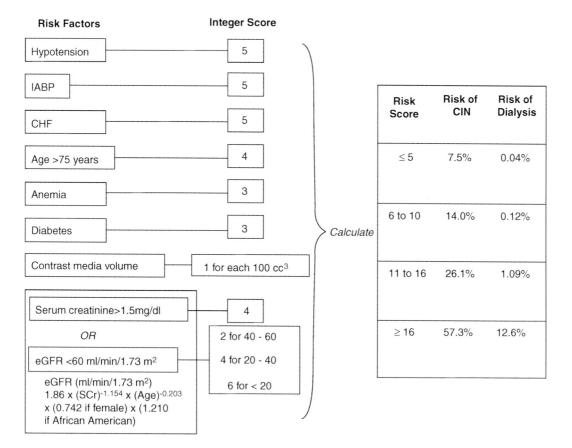

Fig. 32.29 Scheme to calculate a contrast-induced nephropathy (CIN) risk score. Key: *Anaemia* baseline hematocrit value <39% for men and <36% for women; *CHF* congestive heart failure class III/IV by New York Heart Association classification and/or history of pulmonary edema, *eGFR* estimated glomerular filtration rate; hypotension = systolic blood pressure <80 mmHg for at least 1 h requiring inotropic support with medications or intra-aortic balloon pump (IABP) within 24 h periprocedurally

- Nonessential nephrotoxic medications should be stopped for 24 h prior to and 48 h post procedure.
- Metformin should be withheld in patient with an eGFR <60 mL/min/1.73 m^2 and restarted once CIN is excluded due to the risk of lactic acidosis.
- Diagnostic images should be limited with the use of biplane imaging if possible. Ideally one should stage the treatment of complex multivessel disease and use IVUS to optimize stent expansion. The use of automated injector systems can help reduce contrast volume [23].
- There is data suggesting that isosmolar agents are superior to low-osmolar iodinated agents; however, some studies refute this [24, 25].
- Volume expansion is important to prevent CIN but the optimal intravenous hydration regimen is unclear. One simple strategy includes normal saline: 1 mL/kg/h for 12 h pre and post procedure. Moreover, there are trials assessing post procedure induced diuresis and analogous hydration that have demonstrated benefit [26, 27].
- Another strategy that involves less total volume is utilizing sodium bicarbonate (154 mEq/L) 3 mL/kg/h for 1 h before and 1 mL/kg/h for 6 h post procedure [28].
- N-Acetylcysteine (NAC) has been extensively investigated. NAC was widely used in the past as it is well tolerated with low cost but The Acetylcysteine for Contrast-Induced Nephropathy Trial (ACT) failed to show any benefit and so consequently its use now is limited [29].
- The administration of high-dose statins [30] appears to be beneficial which is recommended in the ESC guidelines. Other medications (such as theophylline, calcium channel blockers, dopamine, fenoldopam, L-arginine, atrial natriuretic peptide, ascorbic acid, and alprostadil) have also been studied but their efficacy is still controversial and so consequently their use is not seen in general clinical practice.
- Hemofiltration has shown some benefit [31] but it requires intensive care unit admission, is

expensive, and is associated with significant risks. As a result, this treatment should be reserved for pre-dialysis patients and those with severe kidney disease undergoing complex procedures.

Contrast Allergy/Anaphylaxis

- Contrast reactions are more common to ionic contrast agents compared to nonionic ones and they can be immediate or delayed.
- An immediate reaction will take place within an hour after administration and can be life threatening and a delayed one hours to days. The risk for a severe immediate reaction is 0.01–0.04% [32] while the delayed ones are usually self-limiting and restricted to cutaneous manifestation.
- Risk factors include previous reaction to contrast, asthma and food/drug allergies. However, allergy to seafood is not associated with an increased risk of allergic contrast reactions as often perceived by the cath lab team [33].
- Corticosteroid prophylaxis is only suggested by European guidelines [34] and not recommended by UK guidelines [35]. The discrepancy in recommendation is due to knowledge that despite corticosteroids, severe reactions can still occur.
- However, premedication can reduce the overall risk of a contrast reaction and is generally administered in patients who are at risk. The premedication regime generally used in cath lab protocols is as follows [36]:
  - Prednisone orally 50 mg, 13, 7, and 1 hour(s) before the use of contrast medium. Some operators prefer to use intravenous hydrocortisone 100 mg prior to the procedure but this may not be as effective as steroids require longer administration periods to exert their effects.
  - Diphenhydramine 50 mg, intravenously, intramuscularly, or orally 7 and 1 hour(s) before the procedure.

Conclusions

- Despite meticulous planning, accrued experience, and operator skill, complications associated with PCI can and do occur.
- It is incumbent upon the entire cath lab team to be aware of the potential for adverse periprocedural events and to be in a position where definitive management of complications can be exercised in an efficient, rapid, and methodical manner.
- Awareness of all aspects of cardiovascular monitoring during the procedure is mandatory, not only by the primary and secondary operators but also by nursing, radiography, and cardiac physiology team members.
- A cath lab environment in which all members of the team feel able to speak freely without the fear of recrimination should be actively encouraged.

References

1. Kereiakes D, Kuntz R, Mauri L, MD M, Krucoff M. Surrogates, substudies, and real clinical end points in trials of drug-eluting stents. J Am Coll Cardiol. 2005;45(8):1206.
2. Force m A/T, Windecker S, Kolh P, Alfonso F, Collet JP, Cremer J, et al. 2014 ESC/EACTS guidelines on myocardial revascularization: the task force on myocardial revascularization of the European Society of Cardiology (ESC) and the European Association for Cardio-Thoracic Surgery (EACTS) developed with the special contribution of the European Association of Percutaneous Cardiovascular Interventions (EAPCI). Eur Heart J. 2014;35(37):2541–619.
3. Ludman PF, British Cardiovascular Intervention Society. British cardiovascular intervention society registry for audit and quality assessment of percutaneous coronary interventions in the United Kingdom. Heart. 2011;97(16):1293–7.
4. Resnic FS, Wainstein M, Lee MK, Behrendt D, Wainstein RV, Ohno-Machado L, et al. No-reflow is an independent predictor of death and myocardial infarction after percutaneous coronary intervention. Am Heart J. 2003;145(1):42–6.
5. Huber MS, Mooney JF, Madison J, Mooney MR. Use of a morphologic classification to predict clinical outcome after dissection from coronary angioplasty. Am J Cardiol. 1991;68(5):467–71.
6. Vrints CJ. Spontaneous coronary artery dissection. Heart. 2010;96(10):801–8.
7. Hong YJ, Jeong MH, Choi YH, Ko JS, Lee MG, Kang WY, et al. Impact of plaque components on no-reflow phenomenon after stent deployment in patients with acute coronary syndrome: a virtual histology-intravascular ultrasound analysis. Eur Heart J. 2011;32(16):2059–66.
8. Rezkalla SH, Kloner RA. No-reflow phenomenon. Circulation. 2002;105(5):656–62.
9. Lee CH, Wong HB, Tan HC, Zhang JJ, Teo SG, Ong HY, et al. Impact of reversibility of no reflow phenomenon on 30-day mortality following percutaneous revascularization for acute myocardial infarction-insights from a 1,328 patient registry. J Interv Cardiol. 2005;18(4):261–6.
10. Rezkalla SH, Dharmashankar KC, Abdalrahman IB, Kloner RA. No-reflow phenomenon following percutaneous coronary intervention for acute myocardial infarction: incidence, outcome, and effect of pharmacologic therapy. J Interv Cardiol. 2010;23(5):429–36.
11. Airoldi F, Briguori C, Cianflone D, Cosgrave J, Stankovic G, Godino C, et al. Frequency of slow coronary flow following successful stent implantation and effect of Nitroprusside. Am J Cardiol. 2007;99(7):916–20.
12. Kaul S, Ito H. Microvasculature in acute myocardial ischemia: part I: evolving concepts in pathophysiology, diagnosis, and treatment. Circulation. 2004;109(2):146–9.
13. Kaul S, Ito H. Microvasculature in acute myocardial ischemia: part II: evolving concepts in pathophysiology, diagnosis, and treatment. Circulation. 2004;109(3):310–5.
14. Kaplan BM, Benzuly KH, Kinn JW, Bowers TR, Tilli FV, Grines CL, et al. Treatment of no-reflow in degenerated saphenous vein graft interventions: comparison of intracoronary verapamil and nitroglycerin. Catheter Cardiovasc Diagn. 1996;39(2):113–8.
15. Parikh KH, Chag MC, Shah KJ, Shah UG, Baxi HA, Chandarana AH, et al. Intracoronary boluses of adenosine and sodium nitroprusside in combination reverses slow/no-reflow during angioplasty: a clinical scenario of ischemic preconditioning. Can J Physiol Pharmacol. 2007;85(3–4):476–82.
16. Klein LW, Kern MJ, Berger P, Sanborn T, Block P, Babb J, et al. Society of cardiac angiography and interventions: suggested management of the no-reflow phenomenon in the cardiac catheterization laboratory. Catheter Cardiovasc Interv. 2003;60(2):194–201.
17. Romaguera R, Waksman R. Covered stents for coronary perforations: is there enough evidence? Catheter Cardiovasc Interv. 2011;78(2):246–53.
18. Ellis SG, Ajluni S, Arnold AZ, Popma JJ, Bittl JA, Eigler NL, et al. Increased coronary perforation in the new device era. Incidence, classification, management, and outcome. Circulation. 1994;90(6):2725–30.
19. Al-Lamee R, Ielasi A, Latib A, Godino C, Ferraro M, Mussardo M, et al. Incidence, predictors, management, immediate and long-term outcomes following

grade III coronary perforation. JACC Cardiovasc Interv. 2011;4(1):87–95.

20. Bartholomew BA, Harjai KJ, Dukkipati S, Boura JA, Yerkey MW, Glazier S, et al. Impact of nephropathy after percutaneous coronary intervention and a method for risk stratification. Am J Cardiol. 2004;93(12):1515–9.

21. Persson PB, Hansell P, Liss P. Pathophysiology of contrast medium-induced nephropathy. Kidney Int. 2005;68(1):14–22.

22. Mehran R, Aymong ED, Nikolsky E, Lasic Z, Iakovou I, Fahy M, et al. A simple risk score for prediction of contrast-induced nephropathy after percutaneous coronary intervention: development and initial validation. J Am Coll Cardiol. 2004;44(7):1393–9.

23. Kelly SC, Li S, Stys TP, Thompson PA, Stys AT. Reduction in contrast nephropathy from coronary angiography and percutaneous coronary intervention with ultra-low contrast delivery using an automated contrast injector system. J Invasive Cardiol. 2016;28(11):446–50.

24. McCullough PA, Bertrand ME, Brinker JA, Stacul F. A meta-analysis of the renal safety of isosmolar iodixanol compared with low-osmolar contrast media. J Am Coll Cardiol. 2006;48(4):692–9.

25. Reed M, Meier P, Tamhane UU, Welch KB, Moscucci M, Gurm HS. The relative renal safety of iodixanol compared with low-osmolar contrast media: a meta-analysis of randomized controlled trials. JACC Cardiovasc Interv. 2009;2(7):645–54.

26. Briguori C, Visconti G, Focaccio A, Airoldi F, Valgimigli M, Sangiorgi GM, et al. Renal Insufficiency After Contrast Media Administration Trial II (REMEDIAL II): RenalGuard System in high-risk patients for contrast-induced acute kidney injury. Circulation. 2011;124(11):1260–9.

27. Marenzi G, Ferrari C, Marana I, Assanelli E, De Metrio M, Teruzzi G, et al. Prevention of contrast nephropathy by furosemide with matched hydration: the MYTHOS (induced diuresis with matched hydration compared to standard hydration for contrast induced nephropathy prevention) trial. JACC Cardiovasc Interv. 2012;5(1):90–7.

28. Merten GJ, Burgess WP, Gray LV, Holleman JH, Roush TS, Kowalchuk GJ, et al. Prevention of contrast-induced nephropathy with sodium bicarbonate: a randomized controlled trial. JAMA. 2004;291(19):2328–34.

29. ACT Investigators. Acetylcysteine for prevention of renal outcomes in patients undergoing coronary and peripheral vascular angiography: main results from the randomized Acetylcysteine for Contrast-induced nephropathy Trial (ACT). Circulation. 2011;124(11):1250–9.

30. Leoncini M, Toso A, Maioli M, Tropeano F, Villani S, Bellandi F. Early high-dose rosuvastatin for contrast-induced nephropathy prevention in acute coronary syndrome: results from the PRATO-ACS study (protective effect of Rosuvastatin and antiplatelet therapy on contrast-induced acute kidney injury and myocardial damage in patients with acute coronary syndrome). J Am Coll Cardiol. 2014;63(1):71–9.

31. Marenzi G, Lauri G, Campodonico J, Marana I, Assanelli E, De Metrio M, et al. Comparison of two hemofiltration protocols for prevention of contrast-induced nephropathy in high-risk patients. Am J Med. 2006;119(2):155–62.

32. Namasivayam S, Kalra MK, Torres WE, Small WC. Adverse reactions to intravenous iodinated contrast media: a primer for radiologists. Emerg Radiol. 2006;12(5):210–5.

33. Leder R. How well does a history of seafood allergy predict the likelihood of an adverse reaction to i.v. contrast material? AJR Am J Roentgenol. 1997;169(3):906–7.

34. Thomsen HS. European Society of Urogenital Radiology (ESUR) guidelines on the safe use of iodinated contrast media. Eur J Radiol. 2006;60(3):307–13.

35. Standards for intravascular contrast administration to adult patients. 3rd ed. Royal College of Radiology; 2015.

36. Greenberger PA, Patterson R. The prevention of immediate generalized reactions to radiocontrast media in high-risk patients. J Allergy Clin Immunol. 1991;87(4):867–72.

Bleeding Associated with Angiography and Percutaneous Coronary Intervention

Serdar Farhan, Usman Baber, and Roxana Mehran

About Us

The cardiac catheterization laboratory at Mount Sinai Heart is a premier center delivering a complete range of clinical and research options to patients suffering from cardiovascular diseases. It is a high-volume center with over 5000 coronary, peripheral, and valvular interventions annually. The Center of Interventional Cardiovascular Research and Clinical Trials at The Zena and Michael A. Wiener Cardiovascular Institute serves as the epicenter of innovative ideas in cardiovascular medicine at Mount Sinai. Under the direction of *Prof. Roxana Mehran*, a world-renowned and experienced clinical trialist and outcomes researcher, the center has grown into a full-service academic research organization, encompassing project management, clinical research site expertise, biostatistical analysis, data management and programming services, angiographic and imaging core labs, clinical events committees, and an extensive range of administrative and support services. Prof. Mehran led the Bleeding Academic Research Consortium

(BARC) writing committee, which established a uniform bleeding scale in 2011. Furthermore, Prof. Mehran and her team recently developed the "PARIS risk-scores" for the prediction of coronary thrombotic and bleeding events, respectively. *Dr. Usman Baber* is the director of Clinical Biometrics. *Dr. Serdar Farhan*, a trained cardiologist from Vienna, Austria, is currently working as a research fellow with Prof. Mehran and her team at the Center of Interventional Cardiovascular Research and Clinical Trials.

S. Farhan · U. Baber · R. Mehran (✉)
Interventional Cardiovascular Research and Clinical Trials, Icahn School of Medicine at Mount Sinai, The Zena and Michael A. Wiener Cardiovascular Institute, New York, NY, USA
e-mail: Serdar.farhan@mountsinai.org;
usman.baber@mountsinai.org;
Roxana.mehran@mountsinai.org

Introduction

- A mandatory and necessary component of any coronary intervention is the use of antiplatelet and anticoagulant therapy, which lowers thrombotic risk yet simultaneously exposes patients to potential bleeding harm.
- Over the last several decades numerous antithrombotic drugs have been investigated and received approval based upon lowering thrombotic events, albeit at an excess cost of bleeding.
- Currently bleeding is the most common early complication associated with percutaneous coronary intervention (PCI). Beside the higher healthcare costs, bleeding complications are associated with a higher risk of mortality [1].
- In order to improve quality of care and outcomes, several studies have been conducted to

© Springer International Publishing AG, part of Springer Nature 2018
A. Myat et al. (eds.), *The Interventional Cardiology Training Manual*,
https://doi.org/10.1007/978-3-319-71635-0_33

better stratify bleeding risk, implement uniform bleeding scales, and develop preventive measures. In this chapter we provide a review on definition, risk assessment, prevention, and treatment of bleeding complications associated with interventional procedures.

Definition of Bleeding Complications in Interventional Cardiology

- In 1987 Chesebro et al. developed a bleeding definition for patients with acute myocardial infarction (AMI) treated with fibrinolytic therapy [2]. The *Thrombolysis In Myocardial Infarction* (TIMI) (Table 33.1) bleeding scale is based on laboratory findings (hemoglobin drop) and intracranial bleeding.
- Several years later *The Global Utilization of Streptokinase and Tissue Plasminogen Activator for Occluded Coronary Arteries* (GUSTO) trial investigators established a new bleeding definition (Table 33.1) [3].
- The GUSTO bleeding definition focuses on the clinical context of the bleeding event, thereby categorizing hemorrhagic complications as mild, moderate, and severe. With the development of interventional techniques for treatment of CAD, both TIMI and GUSTO bleeding definitions became increasingly inappropriate as they were designed for medically treated patients receiving thrombolysis.
- This limitation led to the development of several individual bleeding definitions derived from studies and trials conducted in patients with coronary artery disease treated by PCI [4, 5] (Table 33.1).
- The growing number of studies fostered our understanding of the association between bleeding and mortality in this patient population. Nevertheless, heterogeneity in bleeding

Table 33.1 Bleeding definition according to various established criteria

Bleeding criteria	
TIMI Bleeding Definitions [2]	
• Major	Intracranial hemorrhage or a 5 g/dL decrease in the hemoglobin concentration or a 15% absolute decrease in the hematocrit
• Minor	Observed blood loss (including imaging): 3 g/dL decrease in the hemoglobin concentration or 10% decrease in the hematocrit No observed blood loss: 4 g/dL decrease in the hemoglobin concentration or 12% decrease in the hematocrit
• Minimal	Any clinically overt sign of hemorrhage (including imaging) that is associated with a <3 g/dL decrease in the hemoglobin concentration or <9% decrease in the hematocrit
GUSTO Bleeding Definitions [3]	
• Severe or life-threatening	Either intracranial hemorrhage or bleeding that causes hemodynamic compromise and requires intervention
• Moderate	Bleeding that requires blood transfusion but does not result in hemodynamic compromise
• Mild	Bleeding that does not meet the criteria for severe or moderate
ACUITY/HORIZONS Bleeding Definitions [5, 27]	
• Major bleeding	Intracranial hemorrhage, intraocular hemorrhage, bleeding at the access site, with a hematoma that was 5 cm or larger or that required intervention A decrease in the hemoglobin level of 4 g/dL or more without an overt bleeding source A decrease in the hemoglobin level of 3 g/dL or more with an overt bleeding source Reoperation for bleeding Transfusion of any blood products
• Minor bleeding	Any bleeding worthy of clinical mention (e.g., access site hematoma) that does not qualify as life-threatening, disabling or major

Table 33.1 (continued)

Bleeding criteria	
PLATO [4]	
• Major life-threatening bleeding	Fatal bleeding
	Intracranial bleeding
	Intrapericardial bleeding with cardiac tamponade
	Hypovolemic shock or severe hypotension due to bleeding and requiring pressors or surgery
	Decline in the hemoglobin level of 5.0 g/dL or more, or the need for transfusion of at least four units of red cells
• Other major bleeding	Bleeding that led to clinically significant disability (e.g., intraocular bleeding with permanent vision loss)
	Bleeding either associated with a drop in the hemoglobin level of at least 3.0 g/dL but less than 5.0 g/dL or requiring transfusion of 2–3 units of red cells
• Any major	Any bleeding requiring medical intervention but not meeting the criteria for major bleeding
• Minor	Requiring medical intervention to stop or treat bleeding (e.g., epistaxis requiring visit to medical facility for packing)
• Minimal	All others (e.g., bruising, bleeding gums, oozing from injection sites) not requiring intervention or treatment

scales precluded valid comparisons of therapeutic interventions tested across different populations in different time periods.

- Within this context, the Bleeding Academic Research Consortium (BARC) established a uniform bleeding definition in an effort to standardize and accurately quantify the incidence and risk associated with bleeding (Table 33.2) [6].

- In contrast, the *Can Rapid risk stratification of Unstable angina patients Suppress ADverse outcomes with Early implementation of the ACC/AHA guidelines* (CRUSADE) study reported the incidence of major bleeding as 12.0% [9]. The twofold higher rate of bleeding reported by CRUSADE compared with NCDR is attributable to the different bleeding definitions used and the different patient populations investigated.

Incidence of Bleeding Complications

- Notwithstanding the variability in bleeding scales, the incidence and risk associated with bleeding varies according to time (periprocedural versus out of hospital), patient population, study type (randomized vs. observational), the intensity of antithrombotic therapy, and access site (Table 33.3).

- The incidence of bleeding is lowest in elective and highest in primary PCI [5, 7]. Rao et al. published data derived from the US National Cardiovascular Data Registry (NCDR) [8]. Among 60,000 PCI patients the incidence of post-PCI bleeding, defined as bleeding within 72 hours of PCI or before discharge, was 5.8%.

Association of Bleeding with Clinical Outcome

- Numerous studies have consistently shown strong, significant, and durable risks associated with bleeding and both short- and long-term morality [9, 10]. Such patients are also at higher risk for rehospitalization, thus increasing healthcare costs and resource utilization [10].

- It remains unclear whether the increased mortality is attributable to the bleeding itself or to the comorbidities associated with the bleeding event. Indeed, several reports have also shown that mortality risk subsequent to an episode of bleeding is comparable to, or even higher than, that of MI [11, 12].

Table 33.2 Bleeding Academic Research Consortium (BARC) criteria

Bleeding Academic Research Consortium (BARC) criteria [6]	
0	No evidence of bleeding
1	Bleeding that is not actionable and patient does not have unscheduled studies, hospitalization or treatment by a healthcare professional
2	Any clinically overt sign of hemorrhage that is actionable but does not meet criteria for type 3, 4 or 5 bleeding, meeting at least one of the following criteria: 1. requiring medical or percutaneous intervention guided by a healthcare professional, includes (but are not limited to) temporary/permanent cessation or reversal of a medication, coiling, compression, local injection 2. leading to hospitalization or an increased level of care 3. prompting evaluation defined as an unscheduled visit to a healthcare professional resulting in diagnostic testing (laboratory or imaging)
3	Clinical, laboratory and/or imaging evidence of bleeding with specific healthcare provider responses
3a	• Any transfusion with overt bleeding • Overt bleeding plus hemoglobin (Hb) drop ≥ 3 to <5 g/dL* (provided Hb drop is related to bleeding)
3b	• Overt bleeding plus Hb drop ≥ 5 g/dL* (where Hb drop is related to bleed) • Cardiac tamponade • Bleeding requiring surgical intervention for control (excluding dental/nasal/skin/hemorrhoid) • Bleeding requiring intravenous vasoactive drugs
3c	• Intracranial hemorrhage (does not include micro bleeds or hemorrhagic transformation; does include intraspinal). Subcategories: confirmed by autopsy, imaging or lumbar puncture • Intraocular bleed compromising vision
4	CABG-Related Bleeding • Perioperative intracranial bleeding within 48 h • Reoperation following closure of sternotomy for the purpose of controlling bleeding • Transfusion of ≥ 5 units of whole blood or packed red blood cells within a 48 h period • Chest tube output ≥ 2 L within a 24 h period
5	Categorized further as either definite or probable 5a Probable fatal bleeding is bleeding that is clinically suspicious as the cause of death, but the bleeding is not directly observed and there is no autopsy or confirmatory imaging 5b Definite fatal bleeding is bleeding that is directly observed (either by clinical specimen—blood, emesis, stool, etc.—or by imaging) or confirmed on autopsy

Table 33.3 Incidence of bleeding across presentation, type of study and bleeding definition

Study	Study design	Presentation	Primary definition	Bleeding events in %
Amlani et al. [66]	Registry	STEMI	Protocol defined	10.9
Matic et al. [67]	Registry	STEMI	BARC	6.4 BARC ≥ 2
GRACE [68]	Registry	ACS	GRACE	3.9
CRUSADE [20]	Registry	NSTEMI	CRUSADE	11.9
Kinnaird et al. [69]	Registry	Urgent PCI	TIMI	5.4 major 12.7 minor
CathPCI Registry, NCDR [70]	Registry	Urgent PCI	CathPCI Registry bleeding criteria	1.7
ACUITY [27]	RCT	ACS	ACUITY	4.7
HORIZONS-AMI, ACUITY, REPLACE-2 pooled analysis [21]	Pooled RCT	ACS (STEMI, NSTEMI, UA)	TIMI	1.6 major
EVENT [71]	Registry	Elective PCI	TIMI	0.7 major 2.3 minor
REPLACE-2 [28]	RCT	Elective PCI	REPLACE-2 = ISAR-REACT 3	3.2 major
ISAR-REACT 3 [72]	RCT	Elective PCI	ISAR-REACT 3 = REPLACE-2	3.8 major 8.3 minor

STEMI ST-segment elevation myocardial infarction, *ACS* acute coronary syndrome, *NSTEMI* non-ST-segment elevation myocardial infarction, *PCI* percutaneous coronary intervention, *UA* unstable angina, *RCT* randomized clinical trial

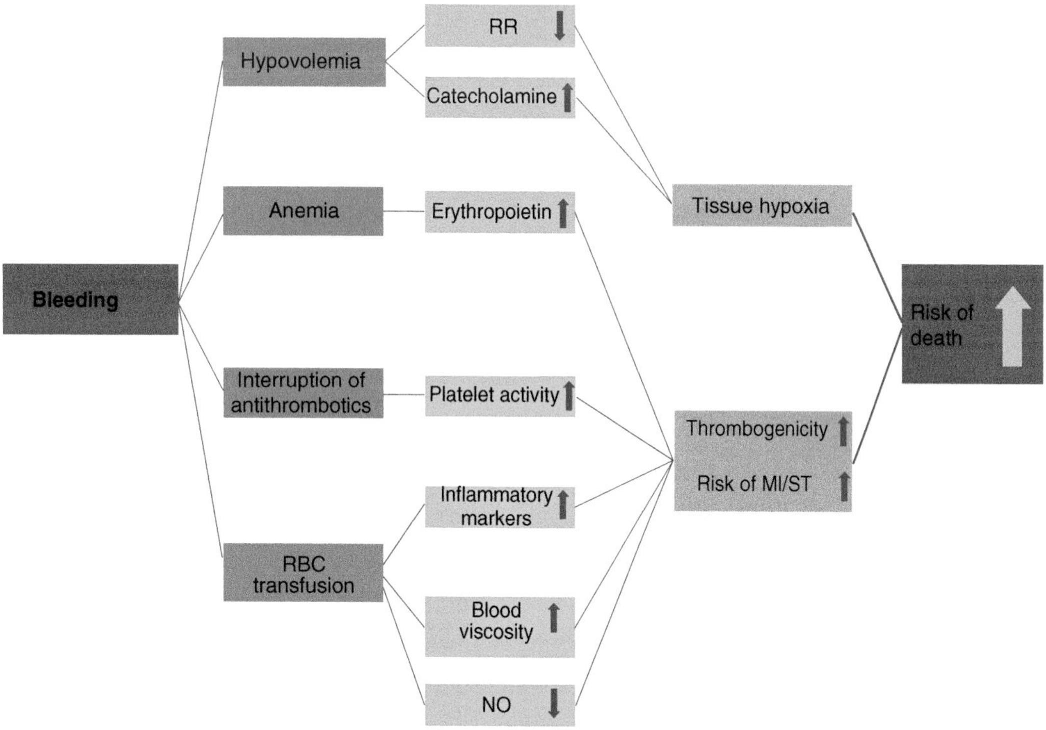

Fig. 33.1 Illustration of consequences of bleeding complications. Key: *RBC* red blood cells, *RR* respiratory rate, *NO* nitric oxide, *MI* myocardial infarction, *ST* stent thrombosis

- Figure 33.1 illustrates several putative pathophysiological mechanisms that may directly lead to excess mortality risk in the setting of a bleeding event. Hypovolemia with subsequent hypotension and anemia leads to reduced tissue oxygenation. Anemia also causes secretion of erythropoietin which may enhance blood thrombogenicity via modulation of prothrombotic factors (e.g., plasminogen activator inhibitor type 1) [13].
- In addition, the occurrence of bleeding might lead to the cessation of antithrombotic agents, which was shown to be associated with a higher risk of ischemic events (e.g., MI or stent thrombosis) [14].
- Finally, bleeding might require the substitution of erythrocytes, which has been linked to higher mortality in patients undergoing PCI [15]. Whether the transfusion of blood cells itself or other factors associated with this clinical scenario are accountable for the increased mortality risk is still under debate.

Table 33.4 European Society of Cardiology and American Heart Association/American College of Cardiology recommendation for blood transfusion for patients with bleeding in the setting of acute coronary syndrome

European Society of Cardiology [39]	
Blood transfusion is only recommended in the case of compromised hemodynamic status or hematocrit <25% or hemoglobin level <7/g/dL	Class I LoE B
American Heart Association/American College of Cardiology [24]	
There is no benefit of routine blood transfusion in hemodynamically stable patients with hemoglobin levels >8 g/dL	Class III LoE B

- There are no robust data to support a liberal (transfusion at hemoglobin level 9–10 g/dL) over a restrictive (transfusion at hemoglobin level 7–8 g/dL) transfusion strategy due to the limited sample size of these investigations [16, 17]. Nevertheless, international guidelines recommend a more restrictive transfusion protocol for hemodynamically stable patients (Table 33.4).

Assessment of Bleeding Risk

- A variety of conditions and factors are consistently associated with higher bleeding risk, and can be subdivided into patient- and procedure-related factors, respectively (Fig. 33.2).
- For example, female sex was found to be associated with increased risk of bleeding [18]. The risk of bleeding associated with femoral access and antithrombotic drug overdose were found to be significantly higher in women compared with men [19]. Despite measures for bleeding avoidance females were still at

higher risk of bleeding [18]. Based on various risk factors reported in Fig. 33.2 several bleeding risk scores were developed.

- Table 33.5 summarizes various bleeding risk scores, which investigated different patient populations and bleeding time points. The CRUSADE Quality Improvement Initiative developed an inhospital bleeding risk score ranging from 1 to 100 points according to risk [20].
- Similarly, Mehran et al. developed a bleeding risk score based on pooled data from the REPLACE 2, ACUTIY, and HORIZONS-AMI trials [21]. Both the CRUSADE and

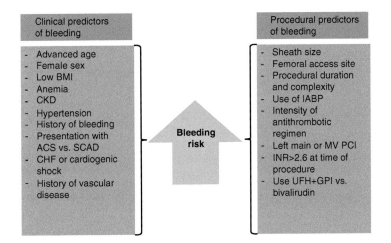

Fig. 33.2 Clinical and procedural predictors of bleeding complications associated with percutaneous coronary intervention. Key: *CKD* chronic kidney disease, *ACS* acute coronary syndrome, *SCAD* stable coronary artery disease, *CHF* congestive heart failure, *IABP* intra-aortic balloon pump, *INR* international normalized ratio, *UFH* unfractioned heparin, *GPI* glycoprotein IIb/IIIa inhibitor, *BMI* boday mass index, *MV PCI* multivessel percutaneous coronary intervention

Table 33.5 Available risk scores for estimation of bleeding hazard in patients undergoing percutaneous coronary intervention

Risk score	Population type	c-statistic	Time of bleeding	Definition of bleeding used	Strongest 3 predictors
CRUSADE [20]	ACS	0.72	Inhospital	Per protocol	– CrCl – HR – Systolic BP
Mehran et al. [73]	SCAD and ACS	0.74	Out of hospital	TIMI	– Age – Serum creatinine – WBC
NCDR [8]	SCAD and ACS	0.78	Inhospital	Per protocol	– PCI urgency Shock – CKD

Key: *CRUSADE* Can Rapid risk stratification of Unstable angina patients Suppress ADverse outcomes with Early implementation of the ACC/AHA guidelines, *ACS* acute coronary syndrome, *CrCl* creatinine clearance, *HR* heart rate, *BP* blood pressure, *SCAD* stable coronary artery disease, *TIMI* Thrombolysis In Myocardial Infarction, *WBC* white blood cell count, *NCDR* National Cardiovascular Data Registry CathPCI Registry, *PCI* percutaneous coronary intervention, *CKD* chronic kidney disease

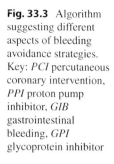

Fig. 33.3 Algorithm suggesting different aspects of bleeding avoidance strategies. Key: *PCI* percutaneous coronary intervention, *PPI* proton pump inhibitor, *GIB* gastrointestinal bleeding, *GPI* glycoprotein inhibitor

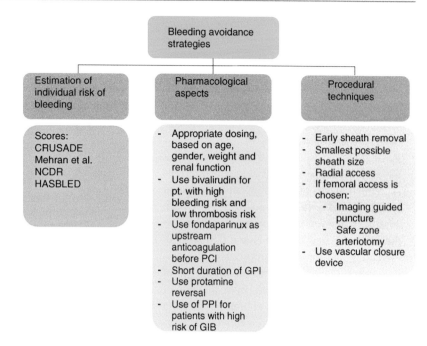

Mehran bleeding scores were developed in patients with ACS. In contrast, the National Cardiovascular Data Registry (NCDR) developed a bleeding score also including patients referred for elective PCI [8].

- Implementing bleeding risk scores to inform clinical decisions surrounding the type and intensity of antithrombotic therapy and/or vascular closure device use may translate to a significant reduction in post-PCI bleeding [18].
- Application of bleeding avoidance strategies in contemporary clinical practice have led to significantly lower bleeding, improved clinical outcomes, and a reduction of healthcare costs in patients after PCI [22]. A proposed algorithm is presented in Fig. 33.3.

Pharmacotherapy

- The benefit of a more potent antithrombotic therapy in reducing ischemic events comes at the cost of increased bleeding risk. Especially, overdosing of antithrombotic therapies has been reported to be associated with excess risk of bleeding and mortality [23]. A reduction of ischemic events while keeping the risk of bleed-

ing at a minimum is the main target of a periprocedural antithrombotic pharmacotherapy.

Anticoagulant Therapy

- *Unfractionated heparin (UFH)* is still the cornerstone of interventional cardiology. Using dosing scales and measuring activated clotting time (ACT) is critical in order to avoid overdosing. An ACT 250–300 s for those treated with heparin monotherapy is considered standard of care, while 200–250 s should be targeted when a glycoprotein IIb/IIIa inhibitor (GPI) is used [24].
- *Enoxaparin* is a low molecular weight heparin. Therapeutic levels of enoxaparin can be achieved using a dosing regimen of 1 mg/kg twice daily via subcutaneous administration. Dose adjustments (0.75 mg/kg twice daily) are required for patients of advanced age (>75 years) and chronic kidney disease (CKD). Enoxaparin has been compared to UFH in several trials, showing inconsistent results [7, 25]. Most recently the *Acute Myocardial Infarction Treated with Primary Angioplasty and Intravenous Enoxaparin or*

Unfractionated Heparin to Lower Ischemic and Bleeding Events at Short- and Long-term Follow-up (ATOLL) trial showed a reduction in the combined ischemic and bleeding endpoint (30 days incidence of death, complication of MI, procedure failure, or major bleeding) with the use of 0.5 mg/kg intravenous enoxaparin vs. UFH [26].

- *Bivalirudin* is a direct thrombin inhibitor which was compared to UFH in several trials. A reduction of bleeding events associated with bivalirudin vs. UFH could be shown [5, 27–29]. However, an association of bivalirudin use compared with UFH and GPI with an increased risk for stent thrombosis (ST) was demonstrated [30]. Patients at high risk of bleeding might still benefit from the use of bivalirudin, while patients at high risk of stent thrombosis should not be treated with an alternate antithrombotic strategy [31].

- *Fondaparinux* is a selective antithrombin. *The Fifth Organization to Assess Strategies in Acute Ischemic Syndrome* (OASIS-5) trial demonstrated a beneficial effect of fondaparinux compared with enoxaparin on the reduction of bleeding events without an increase in ischemic events [32]. However, increased rates of catheter-related thromboses were more frequent among fondaparinux compared to enoxaparin treated patients (0.9% vs. 0.4%) [32].

Antiplatelet Therapy

- *Glycoprotein IIb/IIIa inhibitors (GPI):* Abciximab (monoclonal antibody), eptifibatide (cyclic heptapeptide), and tirofiban (non-peptide tyrosine derivate) are currently in use. GPI are not recommended for routine use in patients pretreated with dual antiplatelet therapy (DAPT). Several trials in the pre-DAPT era showed beneficial effects of GPI use in terms of ischemic events [33]. However, with the advent of DAPT and thereafter the novel and more potent antiplatelet drugs (prasugrel

and ticagrelor) the use GPI has declined from 41 to 28% [5, 27, 34]. Early upstream use of GPI (eptifibatide) increased bleeding risk without a relevant reduction in ischemic events in patients pretreated with DAPT [35]. Currently, the European Society of Cardiology (ESC) recommends the use of GPI only for bailout situations (thrombotic complications or no-reflow) (Class IIa, level of evidence C) [36].

- *Oral P2Y$_{12}$ inhibitors:* Two irreversible (clopidogrel and prasugrel) and one reversible (ticagrelor) inhibitors of the platelet P2Y$_{12}$ receptor are available for treatment of patients undergoing PCI. The *Platelet inhibition and Patient Outcomes* (PLATO) trial compared ticagrelor with clopidogrel in an ACS population [4]. Treatment with ticagrelor was associated with a reduction in ischemic events as well as mortality without increasing the risk of bleeding (per protocol defined bleeding, see Table 33.1). However, considering non-CABG-related bleedings only, ticagrelor was associated with higher rates of bleeding compared to clopidogrel. The *Therapeutic Outcomes by Optimizing Platelet Inhibition with Prasugrel—Thrombolysis in Myocardial Infarction 38* (TRITON TIMI 38) trial compared prasugrel with clopidogrel and found the rate of major bleeding events (TIMI criteria) to be 2.4% for prasugrel and 1.8% for clopidogrel-treated patients, respectively ($p = 0.03$) [37].

- *Intravenous P2Y$_{12}$ inhibitor:* In the *Cangrelor versus Standard Therapy to Achieve Optimal Management of Platelet Inhibition* (CHAMPION PHOENIX) trial, cangrelor, a fast acting reversible P2Y$_{12}$ inhibitor, has been investigated in patients undergoing elective and urgent PCI [38]. Treatment with cangrelor compared to clopidogrel reduced ischemic events with no excess in bleeding complications. Current ESC guidelines recommend the use of cangrelor only in P2Y$_{12}$ inhibitor-naïve patients undergoing PCI (Class IIb, LoE A) [39].

Gastrointestinal Bleeding (GIB)

- GIB accounts for 15% of all bleeding complications associated with interventional procedures [40, 41]. Increased risk of GIB is associated not only with the intensity of antithrombotic therapy but also triggered by several conditions summarized in Fig. 33.4 [41–44].
- Both aspirin and $P2Y_{12}$ inhibitors are associated with an increased risk of GIB. In an observational study of 75,000 subjects, the risk of GIB was lowest for those not taking any antiplatelet agent, followed by patients on aspirin and clopidogrel (1.6% vs. 4.1% vs. 6.1%) [45].
- Novel antiplatelet drugs compared to clopidogrel were reported to be associated with an increased risk of GIB (hazard ratio—HR 1.32 for ticagrelor and 1.46 for prasugrel, respectively) [4, 37].
- GIB is a serious medical condition with high risk of mortality in patients after PCI. Preventive strategies have led to a significant reduction of GIB [46]. In the *Clopidogrel and the Optimization of Gastrointestinal Events Trial* (COGENT) the use of proton pump inhibitors (PPI) was associated with a reduction in gastrointestinal endpoints (composite of overt or occult GI bleeding, symptomatic gastroduodenal ulcers or erosion, obstruction, or perforation) at 6 months [47].
- Currently, international guidelines recommend the use of PPIs in patients treated with DAPT during the initial phase of an ACS (Class I, LoE A) [48]. The management of GIB should include the following considerations:
  - Discontinuing aspirin while keeping patients on $P2Y_{12}$ inhibitors has not been shown to reduce GIB reoccurrence [49].
  - Disruption of DAPT puts the patient at increased risk of ischemic events (e.g., ST) [14].
  - Patients with suspected GIB can be evaluated safely by endoscopy [50, 51].
  - In case of upper GIB prompt administration of PPIs may expedite healing of a potential gastroduodenal ulcer [52].
  - No robust data is available to support a liberal over a restrictive transfusion strategy (Table 33.4).

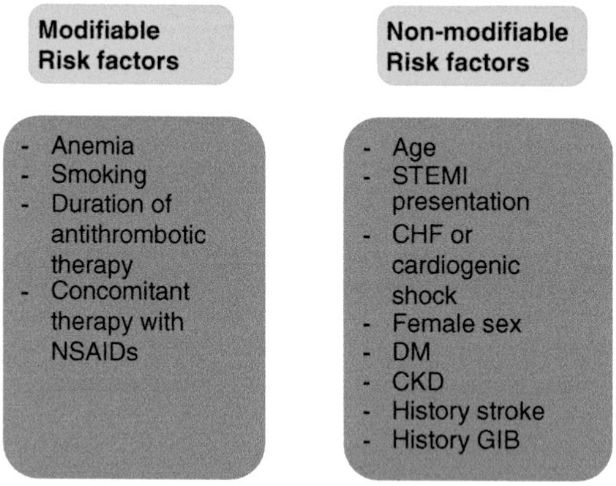

Modifiable Risk factors	Non-modifiable Risk factors
- Anemia - Smoking - Duration of antithrombotic therapy - Concomitant therapy with NSAIDs	- Age - STEMI presentation - CHF or cardiogenic shock - Female sex - DM - CKD - History stroke - History GIB

Fig. 33.4 Modifiable and non-modifiable risk factors for gastrointestinal bleeding complication in patients undergoing coronary intervention. Key: *NSAID* non-steroidal anti-inflammatory drugs, *STEMI* ST-segment elevation myocardial infarction, *CHF* congestive heart failure, *DM* diabetes mellitus, *CKD* chronic kidney disease, *GIB* gastrointestinal bleeding

Acute Coronary Syndromes

- ACS occur on the basis of an acute thrombosis in a coronary vessel. Plaque rupture and subsequent contact of the subendothelial layer with platelets results in activation of the adenosine diphosphate receptors (ADP). ADP in turn upregulates glycoprotein IIb/IIIa receptors, which lead to inter-platelet aggregation and occlusion of the coronary vessel.
- In order to sufficiently antagonize this physiologic cascade, intensive anticoagulant and antiplatelet drugs are needed. However, a potent antithrombotic regimen inevitably leads to an increased bleeding risk.
- Both randomized clinical trials and observational studies provided evidence of an increased risk of bleeding associated with ACS [53]. Table 33.6 presents bleeding events associated with different antiplatelet drugs investigated in patients with ACS.

Table 33.6 Bleeding risk in trials investigating different antiplatelet drugs in patients with acute coronary syndrome undergoing percutaneous coronary intervention

Trial name	Principal aim	Investigated population	Bleeding definition	Major Bleeding in treatment and control arm
CURE [74]	Clopidogrel and aspirin vs. aspirin alone	All ACS	Per protocol	3.7% vs. 2.7%; RR 1.38 P = 0.001
CURRENT OASIS 7 [75]	High- vs. standard-dose of clopidogrel and aspirin	All ACS	Per protocol TIMI	2.5% vs. 2.0%; RR 1.24 P = 0.01 1.7% vs. 1.3%; RR 1.26 P = 0.03
CREDO [76]	Pre-procedural clopidogrel loading dose on top of aspirin compared to aspirin alone	Elective PCI with high percentage of post-ACS patients	TIMI	8.8% vs. 6.7% P = 0.07
TRITON-TIMI-38 [37]	DAPT with prasugrel and aspirin vs. clopidogrel and aspirin	NSTEMI and STEMI	TIMI	2.4% vs. 1.8% RR 1.32 P = 0.03
ACCOAST [77]	Prasugrel (30 mg loading dose) before angiography vs. placebo At time of PCI, additional 30 mg of prasugrel for the pretreatment group vs. loading with 60 mg for the placebo group	NSTEMI	TIMI	2.8% vs. 1.5%; RR 1.97 P = 0.002
PLATO [4]	DAPT with ticagrelor and aspirin vs. clopidogrel and aspirin	All ACS	Per protocol (PLATO)	11.6% vs. 11.2%; RR 1.04; P = 0.43
ATLANTIC [78]	Prehospital administration of ticagrelor	STEMI	PLATO	1.3% vs. 1.3% P = 0.91
EARLY ACS [35]	Early routine vs. delayed, provisional administration of eptifibatide	High-risk ACS	TIMI GUSTO	2.6% vs. 1.8% RR 1.42 P = 0.02 0.8% vs. 0.9% RR 0.99 P = 0.97
FINESSE [79]	Facilitated PCI with a combination of abciximab and reduced-dose reteplase vs. facilitated PCI with abciximab vs. primary PCI	STEMI	TIMI	4.8% vs. 4.1% vs. 2.6%; P < 0.05
CHAMPION-PCI [38]	IV cangrelor vs. clopidogrel	PCI patients (mostly ACS)	TIMI ACUITY	0.4% vs. 0.3% RR 1.36 P = 0.39. 3.6% vs. 2.9% RR 1.26 P = 0.06

ACS acute coronary syndrome, *RR* relative risk, *DAPT* dual antiplatelet therapy, *NSTEMI* non-ST-segment elevation myocardial infarction, *STEMI* ST-segment elevation myocardial infarction, *PCI* percutaneous coronary intervention, *TIMI* thrombolysis in myocardial infarction, *IV* intravenous

Patient with Atrial Fibrillation (AF) Undergoing PCI

- AF is the most common sustained arrhythmia with increasing prevalence in our aging population. Nearly 34% of AF patients suffer from coronary artery disease requiring PCI [54]. Treatment of such patients requires a combination of oral anticoagulation with antiplatelet therapy to avoid athero-embolic and thrombotic events.
- Triple therapy (TT) consisting of oral antico-agulation and DAPT was shown to significantly increase bleeding risk [55]. In order to mitigate the excess bleeding risk related to triple therapy the *What Is the Optimal antiplatelet and anticoagulant therapy in patients with oral anticoagulation and coronary StenTing* (WOEST) trial investigated the withdrawal of aspirin and showed a reduction in bleeding events without an excess in ischemic events comparing TT with dual therapy (DT) [56] (Fig. 33.5).
- A short period (6 weeks) of TT follwed by DT was compared to 6 months of TT in the *Triple Therapy in Patients on Oral Anticoagulation After Drug Eluting Stent Implantation* (ISAR-TRIPLE) trial [57]. The primary composite endpoint of death, MI, definite ST, stroke, or TIMI-major bleeding at 9 months occurred in 9.8% in the 6 weeks group and 8.8% in the 6 months group (HR: 1.14; 95% CI: 0.68 to 1.91; $p = 0.63$) [57].

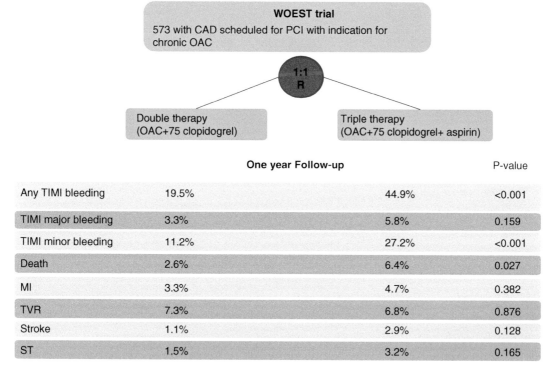

	Double therapy (OAC+75 clopidogrel)	Triple therapy (OAC+75 clopidogrel+ aspirin)	P-value
Any TIMI bleeding	19.5%	44.9%	<0.001
TIMI major bleeding	3.3%	5.8%	0.159
TIMI minor bleeding	11.2%	27.2%	<0.001
Death	2.6%	6.4%	0.027
MI	3.3%	4.7%	0.382
TVR	7.3%	6.8%	0.876
Stroke	1.1%	2.9%	0.128
ST	1.5%	3.2%	0.165

Fig. 33.5 Safety and efficacy of triple therapy compared to dual therapy (WOEST trial) [56]. Key: *CAD* coronary artery disease, *PCI* percutaneous coronary intervention, *OAC* oral anticoagulant, *R* randomization, *MI* myocardial infarction, *TVR* target vessel revascularization, *ST* stent thrombosis

- Most recently, the *Prevention of Bleeding in Patients with Atrial Fibrillation Undergoing PCI* (PIONEER AF-PCI) trial investigated several antithrombotic strategies in PCI patients requiring OAC due to AF [58]. Comparative arms included: rivaroxaban 15 mg daily and antiplatelet monotherapy with a P2Y$_{12}$ inhibitor alone; rivaroxaban 2.5 mg twice daily with conventional DAPT; warfarin with conventional DAPT. Both of the arms that included DAPT were allowed to transition to ASA once the mandatory DAPT duration was completed. The findings showed substantial reductions with the P2Y$_{12}$ inhibitor monotherapy arm compared with either triple therapy strategies (Fig. 33.6).

- Data on combinations including novel P2Y$_{12}$ inhibitors are limited. Observational data showed a significant increase of bleeding associated with prasugrel [59].

- A joint consensus document of the European Society of Cardiology Working Group on Thrombosis, European Heart Rhythm Association (EHRA), European Association of Percutaneous Cardiovascular Interventions (EAPCI) and European Association of Acute Cardiac Care (ACCA) endorsed by the Heart Rhythm Society (HRS) and Asia-Pacific Heart Rhythm Society (APHRS) have proposed an algorithm for treatment of patients with AF and CAD who need PCI (Fig. 33.7).

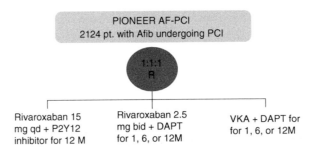

	PIONEER AF-PCI 2124 pt. with Afib undergoing PCI		
	Rivaroxaban 15 mg qd + P2Y12 inhibitor for 12 M	Rivaroxaban 2.5 mg bid + DAPT for 1, 6, or 12M	VKA + DAPT for for 1, 6, or 12M

	Kaplan-Meier event rates			Group 1 vs. 3	Group 2 vs. 3
Primary safety endpoint					
Clinically significant bleeding	16.8	18	26.7	<0.0001	<0.0001
TIMI major bleeding	2.1	1.9	3.3	0.23	0.23
TIMI minor bleeding	1.1	1.1	2.2	0.14	0.14
Bleeding requiring medical attention	14.6	15.8	22.6	<0.0001	<0.0001
Secondary efficacy endpoint					
MACE (CV-death, MI, stroke)	6.5	5.6	6	<0.0001	<0.0001

Fig. 33.6 Safety and efficacy of rivaroxaban and P2Y$_{12}$ inhibitors compared with triple therapy including dual antiplatelet therapy and vitamin K-antagonist (PIONEER AF-PCI) [58]. Key: *Afib* atrial fibrillation, *PCI* percutane-ous coronary intervention, *VKA* vitamin K-antagonist, *DAPT* dual antiplatelet therapy, *TIMI* Thrombolysis in Myocardial Infarction, *MACE* major adverse cardiac events, *CV* cardiovascular, *MI* myocardial infarction

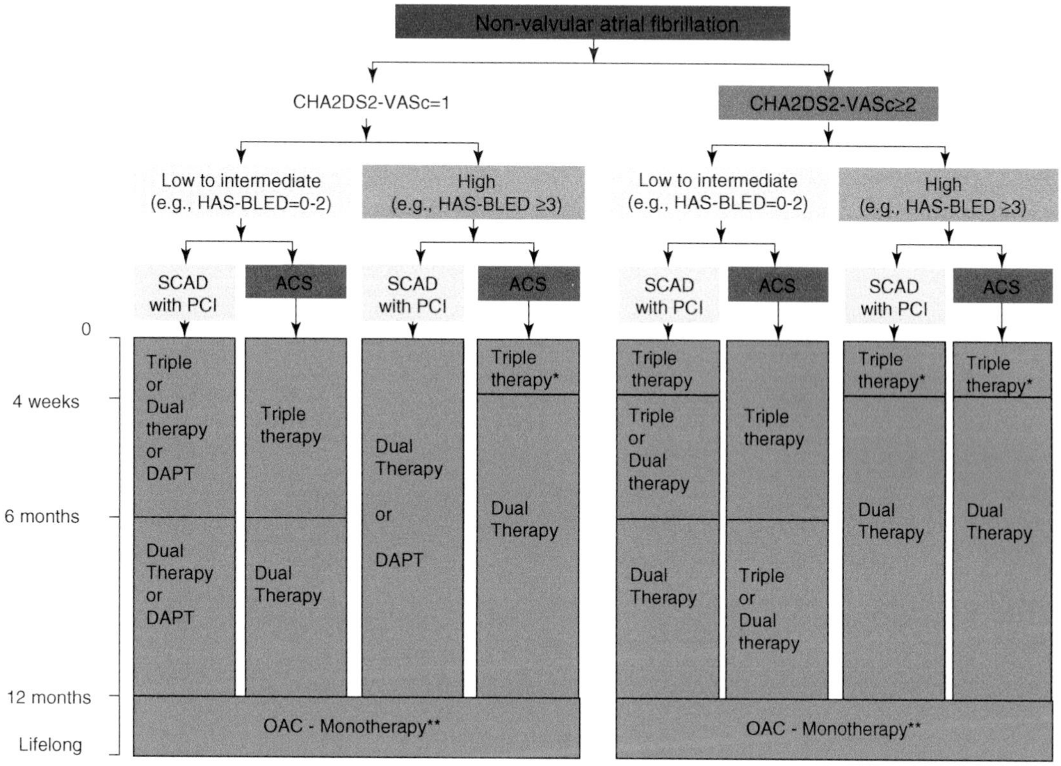

Fig. 33.7 Algorithm for the treatment of AF patients after ACS and/or PCI proposed by the European Society of Cardiology [53]. Key: *SCAD* stable coronary artery dis-ease, *ACS* acute coronary syndrome, *PCI* percutaneous coronary intervention, *DAPT* dual antiplatelet therapy, *OAC* oral anticoagulation

Vascular Access

- Access site bleeding accounts for approximately one-third of all post-PCI bleeding complications [19]. The most important development associated with a reduction in the rate of bleeding was the introduction of angiography and PCI via radial access.
- In contrast to the femoral artery, the radial artery is located more superficially and therefore easier to compress after sheath removal. The advantages of PCI via radial access in patients with ACS have been reported in several studies and meta-analyses [60, 61] (Fig. 33.8).
- The risk of bleeding was reduced by more than half with radial versus femoral access. In patients with STEMI, radial versus femoral PCI was associated with lower rates of major vascular complications, major bleeding, and cardiac mortality [62]. Current guidelines recommend PCI via radial access with a Class IIa LoE A [63]. See also Chap. 5.
- To mitigate potential bleeding complications in patients where femoral access is required, the following should be considered:
  - Proper artery puncture (e.g., ultrasound guided or use middle third of the femoral head as a landmark).
  - Introduction of smallest possible sheath size.
  - Use of vascular closure devices [64, 65] (Fig. 33.9).

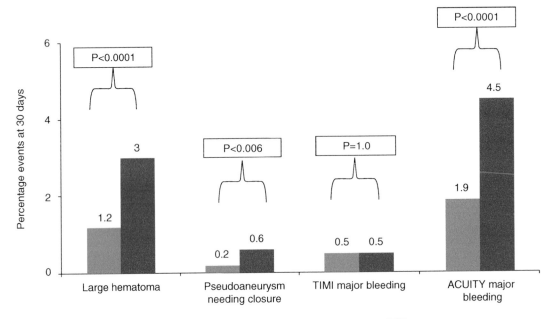

Fig. 33.8 Safety endpoints of the RIVAL trial comparing radial vs. femoral access [60]

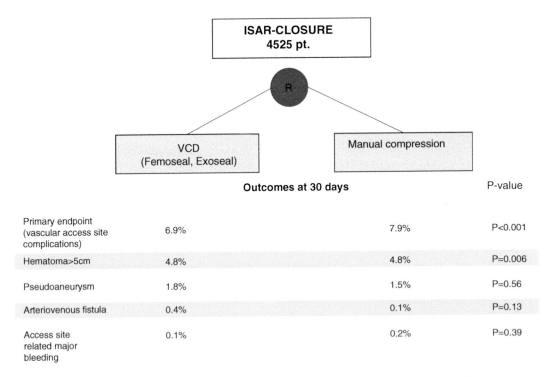

Outcomes at 30 days	VCD (Femoseal, Exoseal)	Manual compression	P-value
Primary endpoint (vascular access site complications)	6.9%	7.9%	P<0.001
Hematoma>5cm	4.8%	4.8%	P=0.006
Pseudoaneurysm	1.8%	1.5%	P=0.56
Arteriovenous fistula	0.4%	0.1%	P=0.13
Access site related major bleeding	0.1%	0.2%	P=0.39

Fig. 33.9 Randomized comparison of vascular closure devices and manual compression after femoral artery puncture (ISAR-CLOSURE) [65]. Key: *VCD* vascular closure device

Conclusion

- Bleeding complications occur in 5–12% of patients undergoing PCI depending on the population investigated. GIB account for 15% of all bleeding complications.
- Bleeding complications after PCI are associated with a higher risk of mortality.
- With the BARC definition, a uniform definition of bleeding complications has been introduced to facilitate a easier comparison between studies and therapy regimes.
- Several risk factors are associated with increased risk and considered in bleeding risk scores (e.g., CRUSADE, Mehran et al. and NCDR scores).
- Dosing of antiplatelet and anticoagulation therapy should be chosen carefully considering specific recommendations for patients with high bleeding risk.
- Radial access is superior over femoral access in terms of bleeding avoidance.
- PPIs should be administered in patients treated with DAPT during the initial phase of an acute coronary syndrome.
- Minor bleeding usually does not require a cessation and/or a reversal of the effect of the anticoagulation.
- Patients experiencing major bleedings should be monitored closely, preferably on an intensive care unit.
- Bleeding avoidance strategies significantly reduce bleeding and improved clinical outcomes, respectively.

References

1. Aggarwal B, Ellis SG, Lincoff AM, Kapadia SR, Cacchione J, Raymond RE, Cho L, Bajzer C, Nair R, Franco I, Simpfendorfer C, Tuzcu EM, Whitlow PL, Shishehbor MH. Cause of death within 30 days of percutaneous coronary intervention in an era of mandatory outcome reporting. J Am Coll Cardiol. 2013;62:409–15.
2. Chesebro JH, Knatterud G, Roberts R, Borer J, Cohen LS, Dalen J, Dodge HT, Francis CK, Hillis D, Ludbrook P, et al. Thrombolysis in myocardial infarction (TIMI) trial, phase I: a comparison between intravenous tissue plasminogen activator and intravenous streptokinase. Clinical findings through hospital discharge. Circulation. 1987;76:142–54.
3. The GUSTO Investigators. An international randomized trial comparing four thrombolytic strategies for acute myocardial infarction. N Engl J Med. 1993;329:673–82.
4. Wallentin L, Becker RC, Budaj A, Cannon CP, Emanuelsson H, Held C, Horrow J, Husted S, James S, Katus H, Mahaffey KW, Scirica BM, Skene A, Steg PG, Storey RF, Harrington RA, Investigators PLATO, Freij A, Thorsen M. Ticagrelor versus clopidogrel in patients with acute coronary syndromes. N Engl J Med. 2009;361:1045–57.
5. Stone GW, Witzenbichler B, Guagliumi G, Peruga JZ, Brodie BR, Dudek D, Kornowski R, Hartmann F, Gersh BJ, Pocock SJ, Dangas G, Wong SC, Kirtane AJ, Parise H, Mehran R, HORIZONS-AMI Trial Investigators. Bivalirudin during primary PCI in acute myocardial infarction. N Engl J Med. 2008;358:2218–30.
6. Mehran R, Rao SV, Bhatt DL, Gibson CM, Caixeta A, Eikelboom J, Kaul S, Wiviott SD, Menon V, Nikolsky E, Serebruany V, Valgimigli M, Vranckx P, Taggart D, Sabik JF, Cutlip DE, Krucoff MW, Ohman EM, Steg PG, White H. Standardized bleeding definitions for cardiovascular clinical trials: a consensus report from the Bleeding Academic Research Consortium. Circulation. 2011;123:2736–47.
7. Montalescot G, White HD, Gallo R, Cohen M, Steg PG, Aylward PE, Bode C, Chiariello M, King SB 3rd, Harrington RA, Desmet WJ, Macaya C, Steinhubl SR, STEEPLE Investigators. Enoxaparin versus unfractionated heparin in elective percutaneous coronary intervention. N Engl J Med. 2006;355:1006–17.
8. Rao SV, McCoy LA, Spertus JA, Krone RJ, Singh M, Fitzgerald S, Peterson ED. An updated bleeding model to predict the risk of post-procedure bleeding among patients undergoing percutaneous coronary intervention: a report using an expanded bleeding definition from the National Cardiovascular Data Registry CathPCI Registry. JACC Cardiovasc interv. 2013;6:897–904.
9. Lopes RD, Subherwal S, Holmes DN, Thomas L, Wang TY, Rao SV, Magnus Ohman E, Roe MT, Peterson ED, Alexander KP. The association of in-hospital major bleeding with short-, intermediate-, and long-term mortality among older patients with non-ST-segment elevation myocardial infarction. Eur Heart J. 2012;33:2044–53.
10. Suh JW, Mehran R, Claessen BE, Xu K, Baber U, Dangas G, Parise H, Lansky AJ, Witzenbichler B, Grines CL, Guagliumi G, Kornowski R, Wohrle J, Dudek D, Weisz G, Stone GW. Impact of in-hospital major bleeding on late clinical outcomes after primary percutaneous coronary intervention in acute myocardial infarction the HORIZONS-AMI (Harmonizing Outcomes With Revascularization and Stents in Acute Myocardial Infarction) trial. J Am Coll Cardiol. 2011;58:1750–6.

11. Ndrepepa G, Berger PB, Mehilli J, Seyfarth M, Neumann FJ, Schomig A, Kastrati A. Periprocedural bleeding and 1-year outcome after percutaneous coronary interventions: appropriateness of including bleeding as a component of a quadruple end point. J Am Coll Cardiol. 2008;51:690–7.

12. Sharma SK, Baber U. The shifting pendulum for DAPT after PCI: balancing long-term risks for bleeding and thrombosis. J Am Coll Cardiol. 2015;66:1046–9.

13. Stasko J, Drouet L, Soria C, Mazoyer E, Caen J, Kubisz P. Erythropoietin and granulocyte colony-stimulating factor increase plasminogen activator inhibitor-1 release in HUVEC culture. Thromb Res. 2002;105:161–4.

14. Mehran R, Baber U, Steg PG, Ariti C, Weisz G, Witzenbichler B, Henry TD, Kini AS, Stuckey T, Cohen DJ, Berger PB, Iakovou I, Dangas G, Waksman R, Antoniucci D, Sartori S, Krucoff MW, Hermiller JB, Shawl F, Gibson CM, Chieffo A, Alu M, Moliterno DJ, Colombo A, Pocock S. Cessation of dual antiplatelet treatment and cardiac events after percutaneous coronary intervention (PARIS): 2 year results from a prospective observational study. Lancet. 2013;382:1714–22.

15. Sherwood MW, Wang Y, Curtis JP, Peterson ED, Rao SV. Patterns and outcomes of red blood cell transfusion in patients undergoing percutaneous coronary intervention. JAMA. 2014;311:836–43.

16. Cooper HA, Rao SV, Greenberg MD, Rumsey MP, McKenzie M, Alcorn KW, Panza JA. Conservative versus liberal red cell transfusion in acute myocardial infarction (the CRIT Randomized Pilot Study). Am J Cardiol. 2011;108:1108–11.

17. Carson JL, Brooks MM, Abbott JD, Chaitman B, Kelsey SF, Triulzi DJ, Srinivas V, Menegus MA, Marroquin OC, Rao SV, Noveck H, Passano E, Hardison RM, Smitherman T, Vagaonescu T, Wimmer NJ, Williams DO. Liberal versus restrictive transfusion thresholds for patients with symptomatic coronary artery disease. Am Heart J. 2013;165:964–71. e961

18. Daugherty SL, Thompson LE, Kim S, Rao SV, Subherwal S, Tsai TT, Messenger JC, Masoudi FA. Patterns of use and comparative effectiveness of bleeding avoidance strategies in men and women following percutaneous coronary interventions: an observational study from the National Cardiovascular Data Registry. J Am Coll Cardiol. 2013;61:2070–8.

19. Ndrepepa G, Kastrati A. Bleeding complications in patients undergoing percutaneous coronary interventions: current status and perspective. Coron Artery Dis. 2014;25:247–57.

20. Subherwal S, Bach RG, Chen AY, Gage BF, Rao SV, Newby LK, Wang TY, Gibler WB, Ohman EM, Roe MT, Pollack CV Jr, Peterson ED, Alexander KP. Baseline risk of major bleeding in non-ST-segment-elevation myocardial infarction: the CRUSADE (can rapid risk stratification of unstable angina patients suppress ADverse outcomes with early implementation of the ACC/AHA guidelines) bleeding score. Circulation. 2009;119:1873–82.

21. Mehran R, Pocock S, Nikolsky E, Dangas GD, Clayton T, Claessen BE, Caixeta A, Feit F, Manoukian SV, White H, Bertrand M, Ohman EM, Parise H, Lansky AJ, Lincoff AM, Stone GW. Impact of bleeding on mortality after percutaneous coronary intervention results from a patient-level pooled analysis of the REPLACE-2 (randomized evaluation of PCI linking angiomax to reduced clinical events), ACUITY (acute catheterization and urgent intervention triage strategy), and HORIZONS-AMI (harmonizing outcomes with revascularization and stents in acute myocardial infarction) trials. JACC Cardiovasc Interv. 2011;4:654–64.

22. Marso SP, Amin AP, House JA, Kennedy KF, Spertus JA, Rao SV, Cohen DJ, Messenger JC, Rumsfeld JS, National Cardiovascular Data R. Association between use of bleeding avoidance strategies and risk of periprocedural bleeding among patients undergoing percutaneous coronary intervention. JAMA. 2010;303:2156–64.

23. Alexander KP, Chen AY, Roe MT, Newby LK, Gibson CM, Allen-LaPointe NM, Pollack C, Gibler WB, Ohman EM, Peterson ED, CRUSADE Investigators. Excess dosing of antiplatelet and antithrombin agents in the treatment of non-ST-segment elevation acute coronary syndromes. JAMA. 2005;294:3108–16.

24. Amsterdam EA, Wenger NK, Brindis RG, Casey DE Jr, Ganiats TG, Holmes DR Jr, Jaffe AS, Jneid H, Kelly RF, Kontos MC, Levine GN, Liebson PR, Mukherjee D, Peterson ED, Sabatine MS, Smalling RW, Zieman SJ, American College of Cardiology, American Heart Association Task Force on Practice Guidelines, Society for Cardiovascular Angiography, Interventions, Society of Thoracic Surgeons, American Association for Clinical C 2014 AHA/ACC Guideline for the Management of Patients with Non-ST-Elevation Acute Coronary Syndromes: a report of the American College of Cardiology/American Heart Association Task Force on Practice Guidelines. J Am Coll Cardiol. 2014;64:e139–228.

25. Ferguson JJ, Califf RM, Antman EM, Cohen M, Grines CL, Goodman S, Kereiakes DJ, Langer A, Mahaffey KW, Nessel CC, Armstrong PW, Avezum A, Aylward P, Becker RC, Biasucci L, Borzak S, Col J, Frey MJ, Fry E, Gulba DC, Guneri S, Gurfinkel E, Harrington R, Hochman JS, Kleiman NS, Leon MB, Lopez-Sendon JL, Pepine CJ, Ruzyllo W, Steinhubl SR, Teirstein PS, Toro-Figueroa L, White H, SYNERGY Trial Investigators. Enoxaparin vs unfractionated heparin in high-risk patients with non-ST-segment elevation acute coronary syndromes managed with an intended early invasive strategy: primary results of the SYNERGY randomized trial. JAMA. 2004;292:45–54.

26. Montalescot G, Zeymer U, Silvain J, Boulanger B, Cohen M, Goldstein P, Ecollan P, Combes X, Huber K, Pollack C, Jr., Benezet JF, Stibbe O, Filippi E,

Teiger E, Cayla G, Elhadad S, Adnet F, Chouihed T, Gallula S, Greffet A, Aout M, Collet JP, Vicaut E, ATOLL Investigators. Intravenous enoxaparin or unfractionated heparin in primary percutaneous coronary intervention for ST-elevation myocardial infarction: the international randomised open-label ATOLL trial. Lancet 2011;378:693-703.

27. Stone GW, McLaurin BT, Cox DA, Bertrand ME, Lincoff AM, Moses JW, White HD, Pocock SJ, Ware JH, Feit F, Colombo A, Aylward PE, Cequier AR, Darius H, Desmet W, Ebrahimi R, Hamon M, Rasmussen LH, Rupprecht HJ, Hoekstra J, Mehran R, Ohman EM, for the ACUITY Investigators. Bivalirudin for patients with acute coronary syndromes. N Engl J Med. 2006;355:2203–16.

28. Lincoff AM, Kleiman NS, Kereiakes DJ, Feit F, Bittl JA, Jackman JD, Sarembock IJ, Cohen DJ, Spriggs D, Ebrahimi R, Keren G, Carr J, Cohen EA, Betriu A, Desmet W, Rutsch W, Wilcox RG, de Feyter PJ, Vahanian A, Topol EJ, REPLACE Investigators. Long-term efficacy of bivalirudin and provisional glycoprotein IIb/IIIa blockade vs heparin and planned glycoprotein IIb/IIIa blockade during percutaneous coronary revascularization: REPLACE-2 randomized trial. JAMA. 2004;292:696–703.

29. Steg PG, van 't Hof A, Hamm CW, Clemmensen P, Lapostolle F, Coste P, Ten Berg J, Van Grunsven P, Eggink GJ, Nibbe L, Zeymer U, Campo dell' Orto M, Nef H, Steinmetz J, Soulat L, Huber K, Deliargyris EN, Bernstein D, Schuette D, Prats J, Clayton T, Pocock S, Hamon M, Goldstein P, EUROMAX Investigators. Bivalirudin started during emergency transport for primary PCI. N Engl J Med. 2013;369:2207–17.

30. Cavender MA, Sabatine MS. Bivalirudin versus heparin in patients planned for percutaneous coronary intervention: a meta-analysis of randomised controlled trials. Lancet. 2014;384:599–606.

31. Singh M. Bleeding avoidance strategies during percutaneous coronary interventions. J Am Coll Cardiol. 2015;65:2225–38.

32. Fifth Organization to Assess Strategies in Acute Ischemic Syndromes Investigators, Yusuf S, Mehta SR, Chrolavicius S, Afzal R, Pogue J, Granger CB, Budaj A, Peters RJ, Bassand JP, Wallentin L, Joyner C, Fox KA. Comparison of fondaparinux and enoxaparin in acute coronary syndromes. N Engl J Med. 2006;354:1464–76.

33. Boersma E, Harrington RA, Moliterno DJ, White H, Theroux P, Van de Werf F, de Torbal A, Armstrong PW, Wallentin LC, Wilcox RG, Simes J, Califf RM, Topol EJ, Simoons ML. Platelet glycoprotein IIb/IIIa inhibitors in acute coronary syndromes: a meta-analysis of all major randomised clinical trials. Lancet. 2002;359:189–98.

34. Subherwal S, Peterson ED, Dai D, Thomas L, Messenger JC, Xian Y, Brindis RG, Feldman DN, Senter S, Klein LW, Marso SP, Roe MT, Rao SV. Temporal trends in and factors associated with bleeding complications among patients undergoing percutaneous coronary intervention: a report from the National Cardiovascular Data CathPCI Registry. J Am Coll Cardiol. 2012;59:1861–9.

35. Giugliano RP, White JA, Bode C, Armstrong PW, Montalescot G, Lewis BS, van 't Hof A, Berdan LG, Lee KL, Strony JT, Hildemann S, Veltri E, Van de Werf F, Braunwald E, Harrington RA, Califf RM, Newby LK, EARLY ACS Investigators. Early versus delayed, provisional eptifibatide in acute coronary syndromes. N Engl J Med. 2009;360:2176–90.

36. Authors/Task Force Members, Windecker S, Kolh P, Alfonso F, Collet JP, Cremer J, Falk V, Filippatos G, Hamm C, Head SJ, Juni P, Kappetein AP, Kastrati A, Knuuti J, Landmesser U, Laufer G, Neumann FJ, Richter DJ, Schauerte P, Sousa Uva M, Stefanini GG, Taggart DP, Torracca L, Valgimigli M, Wijns W, Witkowski A. 2014 ESC/EACTS guidelines on myocardial revascularization: the task force on myocardial revascularization of the European Society of Cardiology (ESC) and the European Association for Cardio-Thoracic Surgery (EACTS) developed with the special contribution of the European Association of Percutaneous Cardiovascular Interventions (EAPCI). Eur Heart J. 2014;35:2541–619.

37. Wiviott SD, Braunwald E, McCabe CH, Montalescot G, Ruzyllo W, Gottlieb S, Neumann FJ, Ardissino D, De Servi S, Murphy SA, Riesmeyer J, Weerakkody G, Gibson CM, Antman EM, TRITON–TIMI 38 Investigators. Prasugrel versus clopidogrel in patients with acute coronary syndromes. N Engl J Med. 2007;357:2001–15.

38. Bhatt DL, Stone GW, Mahaffey KW, Gibson CM, Steg PG, Hamm CW, Price MJ, Leonardi S, Gallup D, Bramucci E, Radke PW, Widimsky P, Tousek F, Tauth J, Spriggs D, McLaurin BT, Angiolillo DJ, Genereux P, Liu T, Prats J, Todd M, Skerjanec S, White HD, Harrington RA, for the CHAMPION PHOENIX Investigators. Effect of platelet inhibition with cangrelor during PCI on ischemic events. N Engl J Med. 2013;368:1303–13.

39. Roffi M, Patrono C, Collet JP, Mueller C, Valgimigli M, Andreotti F, Bax JJ, Borger MA, Brotons C, Chew DP, Gencer B, Hasenfuss G, Kjeldsen K, Lancellotti P, Landmesser U, Mehilli J, Mukherjee D, Storey RF, Windecker S, Baumgartner H, Gaemperli O, Achenbach S, Agewall S, Badimon L, Baigent C, Bueno H, Bugiardini R, Carerj S, Casselman F, Cuisset T, Erol C, Fitzsimons D, Halle M, Hamm C, Hildick-Smith D, Huber K, Iliodromitis E, James S, Lewis BS, Lip GY, Piepoli MF, Richter D, Rosemann T, Sechtem U, Steg PG, Vrints C, Luis Zamorano J. Management of acute coronary syndromes in patients presenting without persistent STSEotESoC. 2015 ESC guidelines for the management of acute coronary syndromes in patients presenting without persistent ST-segment elevation: task force for the management of acute coronary syndromes in patients presenting without persistent ST-segment elevation of the European Society of Cardiology (ESC). Eur Heart J. 2016;37:267–315.

40. Abbas AE, Brodie B, Dixon S, Marsalese D, Brewington S, O'Neill WW, Grines LL, Grines CL. Incidence and prognostic impact of gastrointestinal bleeding after percutaneous coronary intervention for acute myocardial infarction. Am J Cardiol. 2005;96:173–6.

41. Nikolsky E, Stone GW, Kirtane AJ, Dangas GD, Lansky AJ, McLaurin B, Lincoff AM, Feit F, Moses JW, Fahy M, Manoukian SV, White HD, Ohman EM, Bertrand ME, Cox DA, Mehran R. Gastrointestinal bleeding in patients with acute coronary syndromes: incidence, predictors, and clinical implications: analysis from the ACUITY (Acute Catheterization and Urgent Intervention Triage Strategy) trial. J Am Coll Cardiol. 2009;54:1293–302.

42. Gaglia MA Jr, Torguson R, Gonzalez MA, Ben-Dor I, Maluenda G, Collins SD, Syed AI, Delhaye C, Wakabayashi K, Belle L, Mahmoudi M, Hanna N, Xue Z, Kaneshige K, Suddath WO, Kent KM, Satler LF, Pichard AD, Waksman R. Correlates and consequences of gastrointestinal bleeding complicating percutaneous coronary intervention. Am J Cardiol. 2010;106:1069–74.

43. Kelly JP, Kaufman DW, Jurgelon JM, Sheehan J, Koff RS, Shapiro S. Risk of aspirin-associated major upper-gastrointestinal bleeding with enteric-coated or buffered product. Lancet. 1996;348:1413–6.

44. Lanas A, Scheiman J. Low-dose aspirin and upper gastrointestinal damage: epidemiology, prevention and treatment. Curr Med Res Opin. 2007;23:163–73.

45. Grove EL, Wurtz M, Schwarz P, Jorgensen NR, Vestergaard P. Gastrointestinal events with clopidogrel: a nationwide population-based cohort study. J Gen Intern Med. 2013;28:216–22.

46. Koskinas KC, Raber L, Zanchin T, Wenaweser P, Stortecky S, Moschovitis A, Khattab AA, Pilgrim T, Blochlinger S, Moro C, Juni P, Meier B, Heg D, Windecker S. Clinical impact of gastrointestinal bleeding in patients undergoing percutaneous coronary interventions. Circ Cardiovasc Interv. 2015;8:e002053.

47. Bhatt DL, Cryer BL, Contant CF, Cohen M, Lanas A, Schnitzer TJ, Shook TL, Lapuerta P, Goldsmith MA, Laine L, Scirica BM, Murphy SA, Cannon CP, COGENT Investigators. Clopidogrel with or without omeprazole in coronary artery disease. N Engl J Med. 2010;363:1909–17.

48. Agewall S, Cattaneo M, Collet JP, Andreotti F, Lip GY, Verheugt FW, Huber K, Grove EL, Morais J, Husted S, Wassmann S, Rosano G, Atar D, Pathak A, Kjeldsen K, Storey RF. Pharmacology ESCWGoC, Drug Therapy, Thrombosis ESCWGo. Expert position paper on the use of proton pump inhibitors in patients with cardiovascular disease and antithrombotic therapy. Eur Heart J. 2013;34:1708–13, 1713a–1713b

49. Sung JJ, Lau JY, Ching JY, Wu JC, Lee YT, Chiu PW, Leung VK, Wong VW, Chan FK. Continuation of low-dose aspirin therapy in peptic ulcer bleeding: a randomized trial. Ann Intern Med. 2010;152:1–9.

50. Cappell MS. Safety and efficacy of colonoscopy after myocardial infarction: an analysis of 100 study patients and 100 control patients at two tertiary cardiac referral hospitals. Gastrointest Endosc. 2004;60:901–9.

51. Badar A, Scaife J, Yan AT, Robinson SD, Zaman AG, Purcell IF, Ahmed JM, Egred M, Edwards RJ, Spyridopoulos I, Keavney BD, Bagnall AJ. Provision of gastroprotective medication and bleeding risk following acute coronary syndrome. J Invasive Cardiol. 2013;25:397–401.

52. Ng FH, Chan P, Kwanching CP, Loo CK, Cheung TK, Wong SY, Kng C, Ng KM, Lai ST, Wong BC. Management and outcome of peptic ulcers or erosions in patients receiving a combination of aspirin plus clopidogrel. J Gastroenterol. 2008;43:679–86.

53. Steg PG, Huber K, Andreotti F, Arnesen H, Atar D, Badimon L, Bassand JP, De Caterina R, Eikelboom JA, Gulba D, Hamon M, Helft G, Fox KA, Kristensen SD, Rao SV, Verheugt FW, Widimsky P, Zeymer U, Collet JP. Bleeding in acute coronary syndromes and percutaneous coronary interventions: position paper by the Working Group on Thrombosis of the European Society of Cardiology. Eur Heart J. 2011;32:1854–64.

54. Kralev S, Schneider K, Lang S, Suselbeck T, Borggrefe M. Incidence and severity of coronary artery disease in patients with atrial fibrillation undergoing first-time coronary angiography. PLoS One. 2011;6:e24964.

55. Dewilde WJ, Janssen PW, Verheugt FW, Storey RF, Adriaenssens T, Hansen ML, Lamberts M, Ten Berg JM. Triple therapy for atrial fibrillation and percutaneous coronary intervention: a contemporary review. J Am Coll Cardiol. 2014;64:1270–80.

56. Dewilde WJ, Oirbans T, Verheugt FW, Kelder JC, De Smet BJ, Herrman JP, Adriaenssens T, Vrolix M, Heestermans AA, Vis MM, Tijsen JG, van 't Hof AW, ten Berg JM, WOEST Study Investigators. Use of clopidogrel with or without aspirin in patients taking oral anticoagulant therapy and undergoing percutaneous coronary intervention: an open-label, randomised, controlled trial. Lancet. 2013;381:1107–15.

57. Fiedler KA, Maeng M, Mehilli J, Schulz-Schupke S, Byrne RA, Sibbing D, Hoppmann P, Schneider S, Fusaro M, Ott I, Kristensen SD, Ibrahim T, Massberg S, Schunkert H, Laugwitz KL, Kastrati A, Sarafoff N. Duration of triple therapy in patients requiring oral anticoagulation after drug-eluting stent implantation: the ISAR-TRIPLE trial. J Am Coll Cardiol. 2015;65:1619–29.

58. Gibson CM, Mehran R, Bode C, Halperin J, Verheugt FW, Wildgoose P, Birmingham M, Ianus J, Burton P, van Eickels M, Korjian S, Daaboul Y, Lip GY, Cohen M, Husted S, Peterson ED, Fox KA. Prevention of bleeding in patients with atrial fibrillation undergoing PCI. N Engl J Med. 2016;375:2423–34.

59. Sarafoff N, Martischnig A, Wealer J, Mayer K, Mehilli J, Sibbing D, Kastrati A. Triple therapy with aspirin, prasugrel, and vitamin K antagonists in patients with drug-eluting stent implantation and an indication for oral anticoagulation. J Am Coll Cardiol. 2013;61:2060–6.

60. Jolly SS, Yusuf S, Cairns J, Niemela K, Xavier D, Widimsky P, Budaj A, Niemela M, Valentin V, Lewis BS, Avezum A, Steg PG, Rao SV, Gao P, Afzal R, Joyner CD, Chrolavicius S, Mehta SR, RIVAL Trial Group. Radial versus femoral access for coronary angiography and intervention in patients with acute coronary syndromes (RIVAL): a randomised, parallel group, multicentre trial. Lancet. 2011;377:1409–20.

61. Karrowni W, Vyas A, Giacomino B, Schweizer M, Blevins A, Girotra S, Horwitz PA. Radial versus femoral access for primary percutaneous interventions in ST-segment elevation myocardial infarction patients: a meta-analysis of randomized controlled trials. JACC Cardiovasc Interv. 2013;6:814–23.

62. Bernat I, Horak D, Stasek J, Mates M, Pesek J, Ostadal P, Hrabos V, Dusek J, Koza J, Sembera Z, Brtko M, Aschermann O, Smid M, Polansky P, Al Mawiri A, Vojacek J, Bis J, Costerousse O, Bertrand OF, Rokyta R. ST-segment elevation myocardial infarction treated by radial or femoral approach in a multicenter randomized clinical trial: the STEMI-RADIAL trial. J Am Coll Cardiol. 2014;63:964–72.

63. Levine GN, Bates ER, Blankenship JC, Bailey SR, Bittl JA, Cercek B, Chambers CE, Ellis SG, Guyton RA, Hollenberg SM, Khot UN, Lange RA, Mauri L, Mehran R, Moussa ID, Mukherjee D, Nallamothu BK, Ting HH, American College of Cardiology Foundation/American Heart Association Task Force on Practice Guidelines and the Society for Cardiovascular Angiography and Interventions. 2011 ACCF/AHA/SCAI Guideline for Percutaneous Coronary Intervention. A report of the American College of Cardiology Foundation/American Heart Association Task Force on Practice Guidelines and the Society for Cardiovascular Angiography and Interventions. J Am Coll Cardiol. 2011;58:e44–122.

64. Sanborn TA, Ebrahimi R, Manoukian SV, McLaurin BT, Cox DA, Feit F, Hamon M, Mehran R, Stone GW. Impact of femoral vascular closure devices and antithrombotic therapy on access site bleeding in acute coronary syndromes: The Acute Catheterization and Urgent Intervention Triage Strategy (ACUITY) trial. Circ Cardiovasc Interv. 2010;3:57–62.

65. Schulz-Schupke S, Helde S, Gewalt S, Ibrahim T, Linhardt M, Haas K, Hoppe K, Bottiger C, Groha P, Bradaric C, Schmidt R, Bott-Flugel L, Ott I, Goedel J, Byrne RA, Schneider S, Burgdorf C, Morath T, Kufner S, Joner M, Cassese S, Hoppmann P, Hengstenberg C, Pache J, Fusaro M, Massberg S, Mehilli J, Schunkert H, Laugwitz KL, Kastrati A. Instrumental sealing of arterial puncture site CDvMCTI. Comparison of vascular closure devices vs manual compression after femoral artery puncture: the ISAR-CLOSURE randomized clinical trial. JAMA. 2014;312:1981–7.

66. Amlani S, Nadarajah T, Afzal R, Pal-Sayal R, Eikelboom JW, Natarajan MK. Mortality and morbidity following a major bleed in a registry population with acute ST elevation myocardial infarction. J Thromb Thrombolysis. 2010;30(4):434–40.

67. Matic DM, Milasinovic DG, Asanin MR, Mrdovic IB, Marinkovic JM, Kocev NI, Marjanovic MM, Antonijevic NM, Vukcevic VD, Savic LZ, Zivkovic MN, Mehmedbegovic ZH, Dedovic VM, Stankovic GR. Prognostic implications of bleeding measured by Bleeding Academic Research Consortium (BARC) categorisation in patients undergoing primary percutaneous coronary intervention. Heart. 2014;100(2):146–52.

68. Moscucci M, Fox KA, Cannon CP, Klein W, Lopez-Sendon J, Montalescot G, White K, Goldberg RJ. Predictors of major bleeding in acute coronary syndromes: the Global Registry of Acute Coronary Events (GRACE). Eur Heart J. 2003;24(20):1815–23.

69. Kinnaird TD, Stabile E, Mintz GS, Lee CW, Canos DA, Gevorkian N, Pinnow EE, Kent KM, Pichard AD, Satler LF, Weissman NJ, Lindsay J, Fuchs S. Incidence, predictors, and prognostic implications of bleeding and blood transfusion following percutaneous coronary interventions. Am J Cardiol. 2003;92(8):930–5.

70. Chhatriwalla AK, Amin AP, Kennedy KF, House JA, Cohen DJ, Rao SV, Messenger JC, Marso SP, National Cardiovascular Data R. Association between bleeding events and in-hospital mortality after percutaneous coronary intervention. JAMA. 2013;309(10):1022–9.

71. Lindsey JB, Marso SP, Pencina M, Stolker JM, Kennedy KF, Rihal C, Barsness G, Piana RN, Goldberg SL, Cutlip DE, Kleiman NS, Cohen DJ, Investigators ER. Prognostic impact of periprocedural bleeding and myocardial infarction after percutaneous coronary intervention in unselected patients: results from the EVENT (evaluation of drug-eluting stents and ischemic events) registry. JACC Cardiovasc Interv. 2009;2(11):1074–82.

72. Schulz S, Mehilli J, Ndrepepa G, Neumann FJ, Birkmeier KA, Kufner S, Richardt G, Berger PB, Schomig A, Kastrati A. Intracoronary S and antithrombotic regimen: rapid early action for Coronary Treatment 3 Trial I. Bivalirudin vs. unfractionated heparin during percutaneous coronary interventions in patients with stable and unstable angina pectoris: 1-year results of the ISAR-REACT 3 trial. Eur Heart J. 2010;31(5):582–7.

73. Mehran R, Pocock SJ, Nikolsky E, Clayton T, Dangas GD, Kirtane AJ, Parise H, Fahy M, Manoukian SV, Feit F, Ohman ME, Witzenbichler B, Guagliumi G, Lansky AJ, Stone GW. A risk score to predict bleeding in patients with acute coronary syndromes. J Am Coll Cardiol. 2010;55(23):2556–66.

74. Yusuf S, Zhao F, Mehta SR, Chrolavicius S, Tognoni G, Fox KK, the CURE investigators. Effects of clopidogrel in addition to aspirin in patients with acute coronary syndromes without ST-segment elevation. New Engl J Med. 2001;345(7):494–502.

75. CURRENT-OASIS 7 Investigators, Mehta SR, Bassand JP, Chrolavicius S, Diaz R, Eikelboom JW, Fox KA, Granger CB, Jolly S, Joyner CD, Rupprecht HJ, Widimsky P, Afzal R, Pogue J, Yusuf S. Dose comparisons of clopidogrel and aspirin in acute coronary syndromes. New Engl J Med. 2010;363(10):930–42.

76. Steinhubl SR, Berger PB, Mann JT 3rd, Fry ET, DeLago A, Wilmer C, Topol EJ, CREDO Investigators. Clopidogrel for the reduction of events during observation. Early and sustained dual oral antiplatelet therapy following percutaneous coronary intervention: a randomized controlled trial. JAMA. 2002;288(19):2411–20.

77. Montalescot G, Bolognese L, Dudek D, Goldstein P, Hamm C, Tanguay JF, ten Berg JM, Miller DL, Costigan TM, Goedicke J, Silvain J, Angioli P, Legutko J, Niethammer M, Motovska Z, Jakubowski JA, Cayla G, Visconti LO, Vicaut E, Widimsky P, Investigators A. Pretreatment with prasugrel in non-ST-segment elevation acute coronary syndromes. New Engl J Med. 2013;369(11):999–1010.

78. Montalescot G, van't Hof AW, Lapostolle F, Silvain J, Lassen JF, Bolognese L, Cantor WJ, Cequier A, Chettibi M, Goodman SG, Hammett CJ, Huber K, Janzon M, Merkely B, Storey RF, Zeymer U, Stibbe O, Ecollan P, Heutz WM, Swahn E, Collet JP, Willems FF, Baradat C, Licour M, Tsatsaris A, Vicaut E, Hamm CW, Investigators A. Prehospital ticagrelor in ST-segment elevation myocardial infarction. New Engl J Med. 2014;371(11):1016–27.

79. Ellis SG, Tendera M, de Belder MA, van Boven AJ, Widimsky P, Janssens L, Andersen HR, Betriu A, Savonitto S, Adamus J, Peruga JZ, Kosmider M, Katz O, Neunteufl T, Jorgova J, Dorobantu M, Grinfeld L, Armstrong P, Brodie BR, Herrmann HC, Montalescot G, Neumann FJ, Effron MB, Barnathan ES, Topol EJ, Investigators F. Facilitated PCI in patients with ST-elevation myocardial infarction. New Engl J Med. 2008;358(21):2205–17.

Index

Printed by Printforce, the Netherlands